Handbook of
Optical Coherence
Tomography

Handbook of
Optical Coherence Tomography

edited by

Brett E. Bouma
Guillermo J. Tearney

Harvard Medical School and
Wellman Laboratories of Photomedicine
Massachusetts General Hospital
Boston, Massachusetts

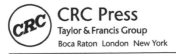

CRC Press
Taylor & Francis Group
Boca Raton London New York

CRC Press is an imprint of the
Taylor & Francis Group, an **informa** business

CRC Press
Taylor & Francis Group
6000 Broken Sound Parkway NW, Suite 300
Boca Raton, FL 33487-2742

First issued in paperback 2019

© 2009 by Taylor & Francis Group, LLC
CRC Press is an imprint of Taylor & Francis Group, an Informa business

No claim to original U.S. Government works

ISBN-13: 978-0-8247-0558-9 (hbk)
ISBN-13: 978-0-367-39678-7 (pbk)

Visit the Taylor & Francis Web site at
http://www.taylorandfrancis.com

and the CRC Press Web site at
http://www.crcpress.com

Preface

Optical coherence tomography (OCT) is a recently developed imaging technology that has stimulated considerable interest in the fields of medicine, biology, and material science. The unique capability of OCT to noninvasively explore microstructure within turbid media using nonionizing radiation has opened the door to applications such as optical biopsy, surgical guidance, studies of developmental biology, and quality control of advanced composites in situ.

The technological innovations that have led to the current success of OCT are manifold and have been published in the scientific literature of optical communications, optical engineering, applied physics, and biomedical engineering. Similarly, the applications of OCT have been separately described in the publications of the relevant fields. The diversity of these publications has led to a need for a comprehensive handbook describing OCT and detailing the advances. The aim of this book, then, is to address this need and to serve as a repository for engineers and scientists involved with the development of OCT technology. Sufficient detail is given to enable newcomers to the field to construct a state-of-the-art OCT imaging system. In addition, the book will serve as a reference for medical clinicians wishing to understand the fundamentals of OCT and its capabilities and limitations.

Chapter 1 presents historical background describing the development of OCT and includes citations to the primary literature. The following five chapters provide a summary of the technology specific to each of the major subcomponents of a typical OCT system, including optical sources, fiber optics, temporal delay scanning, OCT probe design, detection, and system integration. Chapters 7 through 13 are devoted to new imaging concepts spawned from OCT research, such as the reduction of speckle in OCT images, polarization-sensitive OCT, the detection of Doppler-shifted backreflection to determine flow, the combined use of OCT and confocal microscopy, spectral radar, and alternative imaging geometries for OCT.

The applications section (Chapters 14 to 28) begins with a summary of the use of OCT for measuring optical properties and a discussion of nonbiological applications of OCT such as monitoring advanced composites and optical data storage. Biological and medical applications are grouped by topic, beginning with developmental biology and continuing through the major human tissue systems that have been investigated. While the development of OCT has enjoyed widespread interest and has been pursued by many research groups throughout the world, the technology is still young. We hope the readers of this book will be motivated to explore new directions for this promising imaging modality.

Brett E. Bouma
Guillermo J. Tearney

Contents

Contributors

P. Andretzky *University of Erlangen-Nuernberg, Erlangen, Germany*

H. T. Aretz *Harvard Medical School and Wellman Laboratories of Photomedicine, Massachusetts General Hospital, Boston, Massachusetts*

E. Beaurepaire *CNRS, ESPCI, Paris, France*

Reginald Birngruber *Medical Laser Center Lübeck, Lübeck, Germany*

T. J. Brady *Harvard Medical School and Wellman Laboratories of Photomedicine, Massachusetts General Hospital, Boston, Massachusetts*

Stephan Brand *Harvard Medical School and Wellman Laboratories of Photomedicine, Massachusetts General Hospital, Boston, Massachusetts*

Mark E. Brezinski *Harvard Medical School, Massachusetts General Hospital, Boston, Massachusetts*

A. C. Boccara *CNRS, ESPCI, Paris, France*

Stephen A. Boppart *Massachusetts Institute of Technology, Cambridge, Massachusetts*

Brett E. Bouma *Harvard Medical School and Wellman Laboratories of Photomedicine, Massachusetts General Hospital, Boston, Massachusetts*

Zhongping Chen *University of California at Irvine, Irvine, California*

Stephen R. Chinn* *Lincoln Laboratory, Massachusetts Institute of Technology, Lexington, Massachusetts*

Bill W. Colston, Jr. *Lawrence Livermore National Laboratory, Livermore, California*

Current affiliation: Malachite Technologies, Methuen, Massachusetts

Carolyn C. Compton *Harvard Medical School and Wellman Laboratories of Photomedicine, Massachusetts General Hospital, Boston, Massachusetts*

Luiz B. Da Silva *Lawrence Livermore National Laboratory, Livermore, California*

Johannes F. de Boer* *University of California at Irvine, Irvine, California*

Rebekah Drezek *The University of Texas at Austin, Austin, Texas*

A. Dubois *CNRS, ESPCI, Paris, France*

Mathieu G. Ducros *University of Texas at Austin, Austin, Texas*

Joy P. Dunkers *National Institute of Standards and Technology, Gaithersburg, Maryland*

Ralf Engelhardt *Medical Laser Center Lübeck, Lübeck, Germany*

Matthew J. Everett *Lawrence Livermore National Laboratory, Livermore, California*

Felix I. Feldchtein *Institute of Applied Physics, Nizhny Novgorod, Russia*

Adolf F. Fercher *University of Vienna, Vienna, Austria*

James G. Fujimoto *Massachusetts Institute of Technology, Cambridge, Massachusetts*

G. V. Gelikonov *Institute of Applied Physics, Nizhny Novgorod, Russia*

V. M. Gelikonov *Institute of Applied Physics, Nizhny Novgorod, Russia*

N. D. Gladkova *Nizhny Novgorod Medical Academy, Nizhny Novgorod, Russia*

G. Häusler *University of Erlangen-Nuernberg, Erlangen, Germany*

Michael R. Hee *University of California, San Francisco, California*

Christoph K. Hitzenberger *University of Vienna, Vienna, Austria*

Hans Hoerauf *Medical University of Lübeck, Lübeck, Germany*

S. Houser *Harvard Medical School and Wellman Laboratories of Photomedicine, Massachusetts General Hospital, Boston, Massachusetts*

Joseph A. Izatt *Case Western Reserve University, Cleveland, Ohio*

I.-K. Jang *Harvard Medical School and Wellman Laboratories of Photomedicine, Massachusetts General Hospital, Boston, Massachusetts*

D.-H. Kang *Harvard Medical School and Wellman Laboratories of Photomedicine, Massachusetts General Hospital, Boston, Massachusetts*

F. Kiesewetter *University of Erlangen-Nuernberg, Erlangen, Germany*

F. Koenig *Charité Medical School, Humboldt University Berlin, Berlin, Germany*

* *Current affiliation:* Harvard Medical School and Wellman Laboratories of Photomedicine, Massachusetts General Hospital, Boston, Massachusetts

Manish D. Kulkarni *Zeiss Humphrey Systems, Dublin, California*

Eva Lankenau *Medical Laser Center Lübeck, Lübeck, Germany*

M. Lebec *CNRS, CPE, Université Claude Bernard, Villeurbanne, France*

T. Lindmo *Norwegian University of Science and Technology, Trondheim, Norway*

M. W. Lindner *University of Erlangen-Nuernberg, Erlangen, Germany*

Thomas E. Milner *University of Texas at Austin, Austin, Texas*

J. Stuart Nelson *University of California at Irvine, Irvine, California*

Norman S. Nishioka *Harvard Medical School and Wellman Laboratories of Photomedicine, Massachusetts General Hospital, Boston, Massachusetts*

Joachim Noack *Medical Laser Center Lübeck, Lübeck, Germany*

Constantinos Pitris *Massachusetts Institute of Technology, Cambridge, Massachusetts*

Carmen A. Puliafito *University of Miami School of Medicine, Miami, Florida*

Rebecca Richards-Kortum *The University of Texas at Austin, Austin, Texas*

Mark J. Rivellese *Tufts University School of Medicine, Boston, Massachusetts*

Andrew M. Rollins *Case Western Reserve University, Cleveland, Ohio*

H. Saint-Jalmes *Université Claude Bernard-Lyon I, Villeurbanne, France*

Ujwal S. Sathyam *Lawrence Livermore National Laboratory, Livermore, California*

K. Schlendorf *Harvard Medical School and Wellman Laboratories of Photomedicine, Massachusetts General Hospital, Boston, Massachusetts*

J. M. Schmitt *Hong Kong University of Science and Technology, Hong Kong, People's Republic of China*

A. M. Sergeev *Institute of Applied Physics, Nizhny Novgorod, Russia*

A. V. Shakhov *Nizhny Novgorod Medical Academy, Nizhny Novgorod, Russia*

N. M. Shakhova *Nizhny Novgorod Medical Academy, Nizhny Novgorod, Russia*

M. S. Shishkov *Harvard Medical School and Wellman Laboratories of Photomedicine, Massachusetts General Hospital, Boston, Massachusetts*

Shyam M. Srinivas *University of California at Irvine, Irvine, California*

Eric A. Swanson* *Coherent Diagnostic Technology, Concord, Massachusetts*

Guillermo J. Tearney *Harvard Medical School and Wellman Laboratories of Photomedicine, Massachusetts General Hospital, Boston, Massachusetts*

Rujchai Ung-Arunyawee *Case Western Reserve University, Cleveland, Ohio*

---

* *Current affiliation:* Sycamore Networks, Chelmsford, Massachusetts

Hsing-Wen Wang   *Case Western Reserve University, Cleveland, Ohio*

Xiao-jun Wang   *Georgia Southern University, Statesboro, Georgia*

Julia Welzel   *Medical University of Lübeck, Lübeck, Germany*

S. H. Xiang   *Hong Kong University of Science and Technology, Hong Kong, People's Republic of China*

Siavash Yazdanfar   *Case Western Reserve University, Cleveland, Ohio*

K. M. Yung   *Hong Kong University of Science and Technology, Hong Kong, People's Republic of China*

Andrés F. Zuluaga   *The University of Texas at Austin, Austin, Texas*

Handbook of Optical Coherence Tomography

1

Optical Coherence Tomography: Introduction

JAMES G. FUJIMOTO

Massachusetts Institute of Technology, Cambridge, Massachusetts

1.1 INTRODUCTION

Optical coherence tomography (OCT) is a fundamentally new type of optical imaging modality. OCT performs high resolution, cross-sectional tomographic imaging of the internal microstructure in materials and biological systems by measuring backscattered or backreflected light. Image resolutions of $1-15\,\mu$m can be achieved, one to two orders of magnitude higher than with conventional ultrasound. Imaging can be performed in situ and in real time. The unique features of this technology enable a broad range of research and clinical applications. This book, with chapters written by leading research groups in the field, provides a comprehensive description of OCT technology as well as the current and future research and clinical applications of OCT. This introductory chapter provides an overview of OCT technology, background, and applications.

1.2 OPTICAL COHERENCE TOMOGRAPHY VERSUS ULTRASOUND

Optical coherence tomography (OCT) imaging is somewhat analogous to ultrasound B mode imaging except that it uses light instead of sound. In OCT, the first step in constructing a tomographic image is the measurement of axial distance or range information within the material or tissue. There are several different embodiments of OCT, but in essence OCT performs imaging by measuring the echo time delay and intensity of backscattered or backreflected light. An OCT image is a two-dimensional or three-dimensional data set that represents differences in optical backscattering or backreflection in a cross-sectional plane or volume. Because of the analogy between OCT and ultrasound, it is helpful to consider the processes that govern OCT versus ultrasound imaging.

Ultrasound is an established clinical modality for internal body imaging [1–5]. Ultrasound is used in many clinical applications, including imaging of internal organs, transluminal endoscopic imaging, and catheter-based intravascular imaging. In ultrasound, a high frequency sound wave is launched into the material or tissue being imaged by using an ultrasonic probe transducer. The sound wave travels into the tissue and is reflected or backscattered from internal structures that have different acoustic properties. Depending upon the frequency, significant attenuation of the sound wave may occur with propagation. The time behavior or echo structure of the reflected sound waves is detected by the ultrasonic probe, and the ranges and dimensions of the internal structures are determined from the echo delay.

In optical coherence tomography, measurements of distance and microstructure are performed using light that is backreflected and backscattered from microstructural features within the material or tissue [6]. For the purposes of illustration, it is possible to visualize the operation of OCT by thinking of the light beam as being composed of short optical pulses. However, it is important to note that although OCT may be performed using short-pulse light, most OCT systems operate using continuous wave short coherent length light. In addition, other OCT measurement approaches have been demonstrated that measure the spectral properties of low coherence light or use rapidly tunable narrow linewidth light.

The dimensions of structures can be determined by measuring the "echo" time it takes for sound or light to be backreflected or backscattered from the different structures at varying axial (longitudinal) distances. In ultrasound, the axial measurement of distance or range is referred to as A-mode scanning. The principal difference between ultrasound and optical imaging is that the velocity of light is approximately a million times faster than the velocity of sound. Because distances within the material or tissue are determined by measuring the "echo" time delay of backreflected or backscattered light waves, this implies that distance measurement using light requires ultrafast time resolution. Figure 1 compares the characteristic distance and time scales for light and sound propagation. The velocity of sound in water is approximately 1500 m/s, whereas the velocity of light is approximately 3×10^8 m/s. Distance or spatial information may be determined from the time delay of reflected echoes according to the formula $\Delta T = z/v$, where ΔT is the echo delay, z is the distance the echo travels, and v is the velocity of sound or light.

The measurement of distances or dimensions with a resolution on the 100 μm scale, which would be typical for ultrasound, corresponds to a time resolution of approximately 100 ns. One advantage of ultrasound is that echo time delays are on the nanosecond time scale and are well within the limits of electronic detection. Ultrasound technology has dramatically advanced in recent years with the availability of high performance and low cost digital signal processing technology. It is also important to note that because ultrasound imaging depends on sound waves, it requires direct contact with the material or tissue being imaged or immersion in a liquid to transmit the sound waves. In contrast, optical imaging techniques such as OCT can be performed without physical contact or

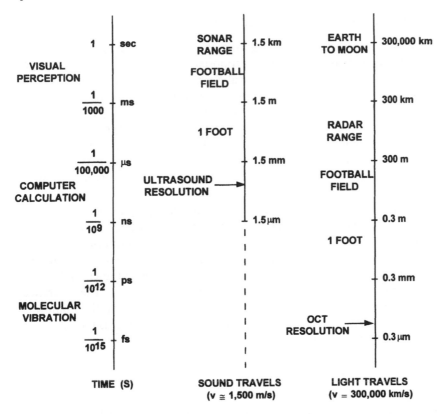

Figure 1 Echo time delay of light and sound. This figure shows the characteristic time and distance scales that govern ultrasound and optical ranging techniques. Optical coherence tomography (OCT) is analogous to ultrasound except that it performs imaging by measuring the echo delay of light rather than that of sound. The velocity of sound in water is ~ 1500 ms/, whereas the velocity of light is $\sim 3 \times 10^8$ m/s. Because of this large difference in velocities, OCT and ultrasound use very different detection technologies.

the need for a special transducing medium. In applications such as ophthalmology, the use of noncontact imaging is important for reducing patient discomfort during examination. In endoscopy or bronchoscopy, imaging without a sound-transducing medium means that contact with or occlusion of the lumen is not required.

The echo time delays associated with light are extremely short. For example, the measurement of a structure with a resolution on the $10 \, \mu$m scale, which is typical in OCT, corresponds to a time resolution of approximately 30 fs. Direct electronic detection is not possible on this time scale. Thus, OCT measurements of echo time delay are based on correlation techniques that compare the backscattered or back-reflected light signal to reference light traveling a known path length. Although OCT imaging is analogous to ultrasound, the core technology upon which it is based is quite different.

1.3 MEASURING ULTRAFAST OPTICAL ECHOES

The concept of using high speed optical gating to perform imaging in scattering systems such as biological tissues was first proposed by M. Duguay 30 years ago [7–9]. Duguay demonstrated an ultrafast optical Kerr shutter to photograph light in flight. The Kerr shutter can achieve picosecond or femtosecond resolution and operates by using an intense ultrashort light pulse to induce birefringence (Kerr effect) in an optical medium placed between crossed polarizers. Duguay recognized that optical scattering limits imaging in biological tissues and that a high speed shutter could be used to gate out unwanted scattered light and detect light echoes from internal structures. This technology could see through tissues and noninvasively image internal biological structures.

The principal disadvantage of the Kerr shutter is that it requires high intensity laser pulses to induce the Kerr effect and operate the shutter. An alternative approach for high speed gating is to use second harmonic generation or parametric conversion. The objective or specimen being imaged is illuminated with short pulses, and the backscattered or backreflected light is upconverted or parametrically converted with a reference pulse in a nonlinear optical crystal [10,11]. The reference pulse is delayed by a variable time τ from the illuminating pulse, and the nonlinear process creates a high speed optical gate. If $I_s(t)$ is the signal and $I_r(t)$ is the reference pulse, the response function $S(\tau)$ is given as

$$S(\tau) \sim \int_{-\infty}^{\infty} I_s(t) I_r(t - \tau)\, dt \tag{1}$$

Nonlinear optical gating measures the time delay and intensity of a high speed optical signal. The time resolution is determined by the pulse duration, and the sensitivity is determined by the conversion efficiency of the nonlinear process. Optical time-of-flight ranging measurements were first demonstrated in biological tissues to measure corneal thickness and the depth of the stratum corneum and epidermis [12]. Dynamic ranges of 10^6 or higher can be achieved. Nonlinear cross correlation does not require pulses of as high intensity as the Kerr shutter but still requires the use of short pulses. It is also important to note that this technique detects the intensity (rather than the field) of the backscattered or backreflected light.

Interferometric detection overcomes many of the limitations of nonlinear gating techniques and can measure the echo time delay or backreflected or backscattered light with high dynamic range and high sensitivity. These techniques are analogous to coherent optical detection in optical communications (in contrast to direct detection). OCT is based on low coherence interferometry or white light interferometry, first described by Sir Isaac Newton. More recently, low coherence interferometry has been used to characterize optical echoes and backscattering in optical fibers and waveguide devices [13–15]. The first biological application of low coherence interferometry was in ophthalmologic biometry for measurement of eye length [16]. Since then, related versions of this technique have been developed for noninvasive high precision and high resolution biometry [17,18]. A dual beam interferometer was used to perform the first in vivo measurements of axial eye length in ophthalmology [19]. High resolution measurements of corneal thickness in vivo were demonstrated by using standard low coherence interferometry [20].

Low coherence interferometry measures the field of the optical beam rather than its intensity. In vacuum, the velocity of light is $c = 3 \times 10^8$ m/s, whereas in water, biological tissues, or materials, the velocity of propagation of light is reduced from its speed in vacuum according to the index of refraction n of the medium, $v = c/n$. The functional form of the electric field in a light wave is

$$E_t(t) = E_i \cos\left(2\pi v t - \frac{2\pi}{\lambda} z\right) \tag{2}$$

When two beams of light are combined, their fields rather than their intensities add and produce interference. Figure 2 shows a schematic diagram of a simple Michelson interferometer. The incident optical wave is directed onto a partially reflecting mirror or beamsplitter that splits the beam into a reference beam and a measurement or signal beam. The reference beam $E_r(t)$ is reflected from a reference mirror whereas the measurement or signal beam $E_s(t)$ is reflected from the biological specimen or tissue that is to be imaged. The beams then recombine and interfere at the beamsplitter. The output of the interferometer is the sum of the electromagnetic fields from the reference beam and the signal beam reflected from the specimen or tissue:

$$E_O(t) \sim E_r(t) + E_s(t) \tag{3}$$

A detector measures the intensity of the output optical beam, which is proportional to the square of the electromagnetic field. If the distance that light travels in the reference path is l_R and the distance in the measurement path, reflected from the

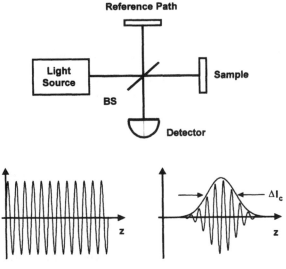

Figure 2 Optical coherence tomography is based on interferometry. OCT performs imaging by measuring the echo time delay and magnitude of backreflected or backscattering light using interferometry. The most common detection method is based upon a Michelson interferometer with a scanning reference delay arm. Backreflected or backscattered light from the object being imaged is correlated with light that travels a known reference path delay.

specimen, is l_S, then the intensity of the interferometer output will oscillate as a function of $\Delta l = l_R - l_S$:

$$I_O(t) \sim \frac{1}{4}|E_R|^2 + \frac{1}{4}|E_S|^2 + \frac{1}{2}E_R E_S \cos\left(2\frac{2\pi}{\lambda}\Delta l\right) \qquad (4)$$

If the position of the reference mirror is varied, then the path length that the optical beam travels in the reference arm changes, and interference will occur. This is shown schematically in Fig. 2. If the light is highly coherent (narrow linewidth) or has a long coherence length, then interference oscillations will be observed for a wide range of relative path lengths of the reference and measurement arms. For applications in optical ranging or optical coherence tomography, it is necessary to measure absolute distance and dimensions of structures within the material or tissue. In this case, low coherence length light (broad bandwidth) is used. Low coherence light may be thought of as a superposition of electromagnetic fields with statistical discontinuities in phase as a function of time. The field is composed of different frequencies or wavelengths rather than a single wavelength. Low coherence light can be characterized by its coherence length (l_c). The coherence length is inversely proportional to the bandwidth. When low coherence light is used in the interferometer, interference is observed only when the path lengths of the reference and measurement arms are matched to within the coherence length. This phenomenon is shown schematically in Fig. 2. The interferometer measures the field autocorrelation of the light. For the purposes of ranging and imaging, the coherence length of the light determines the resolution with which optical range or distance can be measured. The echo time delay and magnitude of reflected light can be determined by scanning the reference mirror position and demodulating the interference signal from the interferometer.

1.4 RESOLUTION LIMITS OF OPTICAL COHERENCE TOMOGRAPHY

The next sections describe mechanisms that govern the performance of optical coherence tomography. Because OCT is based on modern optical communications technology, its performance can be predicted using well-established theories and engineered with high accuracy. Detailed specifications are not given here because specifications are dependent on instrument design and will change as different embodiments of this technology are developed.

In contrast to conventional microscopy, in OCT the mechanisms that govern the axial and transverse image resolution are independent. The axial resolution in OCT imaging is determined by the coherence length of the light source, and high axial resolution can be achieved independently of the beam-focusing conditions. The coherence length is the spatial width of the field autocorrelation produced by the interferometer. The envelope of the field autocorrelation is equivalent to the Fourier transform of the power spectrum. Thus, the width of the autocorrelation function, or the axial resolution, is inversely proportional to the width of the power spectrum. For a source with a Gaussian spectral distribution, the axial resolution Δz is

$$\Delta z = \frac{2\ln 2}{\pi}\left(\frac{\lambda^2}{\Delta\lambda}\right) \qquad (5)$$

where Δz and $\Delta \lambda$ are the full width at half-maximum (FWHM) of the autocorrelation function and power spectrum, respectively, and λ is the source center wavelength. The axial resolution is inversely proportional to the bandwidth of the light source, and thus broad-bandwidth optical sources are required to achieve high axial resolution.

The transverse resolution for optical coherence tomography imaging is the same as for conventional optical microscopy and is determined by the focusing properties of an optical beam. The minimum spot size to which an optical beam can be focused is inversely proportional to the numerical aperture of the angle of focus of the beam. The transverse resolution is

$$\Delta x = \frac{4\lambda}{\pi}\left(\frac{f}{d}\right) \tag{6}$$

where d is the spot size on the objective lens and f is its focal length. High transverse resolution can be obtained by using a large numerical aperture and focusing the beam to a small spot size. In addition, the transverse resolution is also related to the depth of focus or the confocal parameter b, which is $2z_R$, two times the Rayleigh range:

$$2z_R = \pi \, \Delta x^2 / 2\lambda \tag{7}$$

Thus, increasing the transverse resolution produces a decrease in the depth of focus, similar to that produced in conventional microscopy.

Figure 3 shows schematically the relationship between focused spot size and depth of field for low and high numerical aperture focusing. The focusing conditions

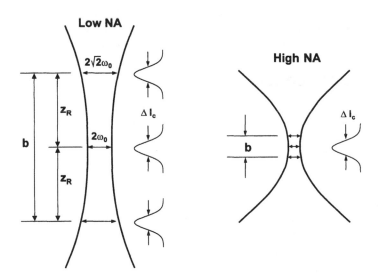

Figure 3 Low and high numerical aperture focusing limits of OCT. Most OCT imaging is performed with low NA focusing, where the confocal parameter is much longer than the coherence length. There is a trade-off between transverse resolution and depth of field. The high NA focusing limit achieves excellent transverse resolution with reduced depth of field. Low coherence detection provides more effective rejection of scattered light than confocal detection.

define two limiting cases for OCT imaging. Typically, OCT imaging is performed with low numerical aperture focusing to have a large depth of field, and low coherence interferometry is used to achieve axial resolution. In this limit the confocal parameter is larger than the coherence length, $b > \Delta z$. The axial image resolution is determined by the coherence length, and the transverse resolution by the spot size. In contrast to conventional microscopy, this mode of operation achieves high axial resolution independently of the available numerical aperture. This feature is particularly powerful for applications such as retinal imaging in ophthalmology or in catheter-endoscope-based imaging where the available numerical aperture may be limited. However, operation in the low numerical aperture limit yields low transverse resolution.

Conversely, it is also possible to focus with high numerical aperture and achieve high transverse resolution at the expense of reduced depth of focus. This operating regime is typical for conventional microscopy or confocal microscopy. Depending upon the coherence length of the light, the depth of field can be shorter than the coherence length, $b < \Delta z$. In this case the depth of field can be used to differentiate backscattered or backreflected signals from different depths. This regime of operation has been referred to as optical coherence microscopy (OCM). This mode of operation can be useful for imaging scattering systems because the coherence gating effect removes the contributions from scattering in front and in back of the focal plane more effectively than confocal gating. A comprehensive discussion of high transverse resolution OCT is provided in Chapter 10.

Although high transverse resolutions can be achieved in OCT, the depth of field will be limited. To perform imaging over a range of depths it is necessary to track the focal depth along with the axial range (reference delay) that is being detected [21]. Alternatively, it is possible to use a technique analogous to ultrasound C-mode scanning and acquire multiple images with different zones of focus and fuse these images together to create a single image with an extended depth of field [22].

1.5 SENSITIVITY LIMITS FOR OPTICAL COHERENCE TOMOGRAPHY

Optical coherence tomography can achieve high detection sensitivity because interferometry measures the field rather than the intensity of light using optical heterodyne detection. This effect can be seen from Eq. (4), which describes the intensity of the interferometer output signal. The oscillating interference term is the result of the backscattered or backreflected electric field from the sample (which can be very weak) multiplied by the electric field of the reference beam. Because the beam from the reference mirror can have a large field amplitude, the weak electric field from the sample beam is multiplied by the large field, thereby increasing the magnitude of the oscillating term that is detected by the detector. The interferometer thus produces heterodyne gain for weak optical signals.

Backreflected or backscattered optical echoes from the specimen are detected by electronically demodulating the signal from the photodetector as the reference mirror is translated. In most OCT embodiments the reference mirror is scanned at a constant velocity v that Doppler shifts the reflected light. This modulates the interference signal at the Doppler beat frequency $f_D = 2v/\lambda$, where v is the reference mirror velocity. By electronically filtering the detected signal at this frequency, the presence of echoes from different reflecting surfaces in the biological specimen may be detected. In addition, it is interesting to note that if the light is backreflected or backscattered from a moving structure, it will also be Doppler shifted and result in a shift of the beat frequency. This principle has been used to perform OCT measurements of Doppler flow.

The signal-to-noise performance can be calculated using well-established methods from optical communication. The signal-to-noise ratio (SNR) is given by the expression

$$SNR = 10 \log(\eta P/2h\nu NEB) \tag{8}$$

where η is the detector quantum efficiency, $h\nu$ is the photon energy, P is the signal power, and NEB is the noise equivalent bandwidth of the electronic filter used to demodulate the signal. This expression implies that the signal-to-noise ratio scales as the detected power divided by the noise equivalent bandwidth of the detection. This means that high image acquisition speeds or higher image resolutions require higher optical powers for a given signal-to-noise ratio. The performance of optical coherence tomography systems varies widely according to their design and data acquisition speed requirements. However, for typical measurement parameters, sensitivities to reflected signals in the range of -90 to -100 dB can be achieved, corresponding to the detection of signals that are 10^{-9} or 10^{-10} of the incident optical power.

1.6 IMAGE GENERATION AND DISPLAY IN OPTICAL COHERENCE TOMOGRAPHY

Optical coherence tomographic cross-sectional imaging is achieved by performing successive axial measurements of backreflected or backscattered light at different transverse positions [6]. Figure 4 shows one example of how optical coherence tomography is performed. A two-dimensional cross-sectional image is acquired by scanning the incident optical beam, performing successive rapid axial measurements of optical backscattering or backreflection profiles at different transverse positions. The result is a two-dimensional data set in which each trace represents the magnitude of reflection or backscattering of the optical beam as a function of depth in the tissue.

A wide range of OCT scan patterns are possible as shown in Fig. 5. The most common method of OCT scanning acquires data with depth priority. However, it is also possible to acquire data with transverse priority, by detecting backreflections or backscattering at a given depth or range while transversely scanning the imaging beam. A cross-sectional image can be generated by detecting the backscattering along successive x scans for different z depths. It is also possible to perform OCT imaging in an *en face* plane [23,24]. In this case the backreflected or backscattered signals are detected at a fixed z depth, scanning along successive x and y directions. This mode of imaging is analogous to that used in confocal microscopy. A comprehensive discussion of OCT imaging using other scanning protocols is presented in Chapter 11.

For purposes of visualization, OCT data are usually acquired by computer and displayed as a two-dimensional gray-scale or false color image. Figure 6 shows an example of a tomographic image of the retina displayed in gray scale. The image displayed consists of 200 pixels (horizontal) by 500 pixels (vertical). The vertical direction corresponds to the direction of the incident optical

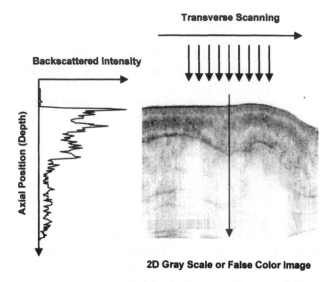

Figure 4   Image generation in OCT. Cross-sectional images are constructed by performing axial measurements of the echo time delay and magnitude of backscattered or backreflected light at different transverse positions. This results in a two-dimensional data set that represents the backscattering in a cross-sectional plane of the material or tissue being imaged.

beam and the axial data sets. The optical beam was scanned in the transverse direction, and 200 axial measurements were performed. The backscattered signal ranges from approximately $-50\,\text{dB}$, the maximum signal, to $-100\,\text{dB}$, the sensitivity limit. Because the signal varies over five orders of magnitude, it is convenient to use the logarithm of the signal to display the image. This expands the dynamic range of the display but results in compression of relative variations in signal. In general the signal fluctuation in an OCT image is relatively high, so OCT has a limited capability for detecting small relative changes in backscattering, and it is difficult to detect relative changes in signal on the percent scale. In contrast, conventional imaging using charge-coupled devices (CCD) detectors can differentiate relative changes in signal of 10^{-4}–10^{-6}.

The intensity of the backscattered optical signal in an OCT image is typically represented on a logarithmic scale. The white level corresponds to the highest reflection or backscatter in the signal, and the black level corresponds to the weakest backreflection. The background noise in the image is typically thresholded and set to black. The gray-scale tomographic image differentiates structure in the retina including intraretinal layers and the retinal nerve fiber layer. The retinal pigment epithelium is highly scattering because it contains melanin. The choroid is highly vascular and is also highly scattering.

The dynamic range of gray-scale images is extremely limited. Most computer monitors provide only 8 bits or 256 gray levels. In addition, the eye has a limited ability to differentiate gray levels, so gray-scale images do not faithfully represent the full dynamic range of information available in OCT images. To enhance the differentiation of different structures within the image, the image may also be displayed in a false color representation as shown in Fig. 7. In this case, the logarithm of the

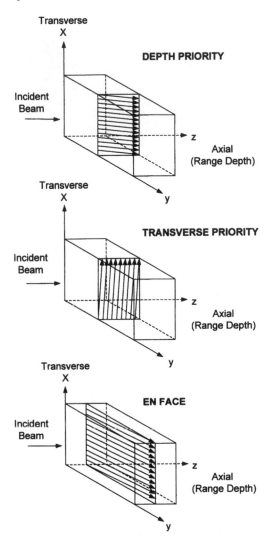

Figure 5 Different scanning protocols for OCT imaging. There are numerous scanning protocols that can be used for OCT imaging depending upon the imaging engine and application. Cross-sectional images may be acquired using either depth- or transverse-priority scanning. In depth-priority scanning, axial scans are acquired at successive transverse positions. In transverse-priority scanning, the beam is scanned rapidly in the transverse direction and light from successive axial depths (or ranges) is detected. Transverse-priority scanning in two transverse dimensions may be used to acquire *en face* images at a given depth.

optical reflection or backscattering is mapped to different colors. In this image, the intensity of the optical signal is mapped to the color scale using the standard "rainbow" order of colors. The highest backreflection or backscattering is represented by red and white and typically corresponds to $-100\,dB$ of the incident signal, whereas the lowest backscattering is represented by blue and black and typically corresponds to $-100dB$ of the incident signal. This image demonstrates that the use of false color can improve the differentiation of different structures. In contrast to gray-level

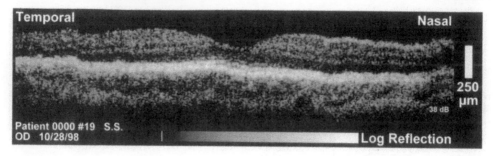

Figure 6   Gray-scale OCT image. Example of an OCT image of the fovea region of retina in a normal human subject. The image shows the differentiation of retinal layers that is possible using gray-scale display. The logarithm of the backscattered or backreflected signal is mapped into the gray scale. Typical ophthalmic images span approximately a 40–50 dB dynamic range. The ability of the eye to differentiate different gray levels is limited, and monitors support only 8-bit gray levels, so the fidelity of the image formation is lost.

monitors, color monitors can have 24-bit color levels, and the human eye can differentiate millions of different colors. The principal disadvantage of using false color display is that it can produce artifacts in the image. If the signal intensity is changed, this produces a color shift of structures in the image. Thus careful normalization of signal levels is required. In addition, different signal levels in the image are mapped to different colors that do not necessarily correspond to different physical structures.

The images of the retina presented in Figs. 6 and 7 (see color plate) are examples of imaging media that have weak reflections. Figure 8 shows a gray-scale OCT image of the human ectocervix in vitro as an example of an image in a highly scattering tissue. In a highly scattering material or tissue, light is rapidly attenuated with propagation depth, resulting in a gradation of signal in the image. Also, there can be significant levels of speckle noise or other noise arising from the microstructural

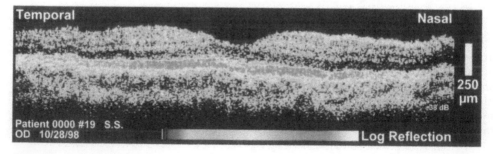

Figure 7   False color OCT image. Example of an OCT image of the fovea region of the retina in a normal human subject. The image shows the differentiation of retinal layers that is possible using false color display (compare to gray-scale display of Fig. 6). The logarithm of the backscattering or backreflected signal is mapped to a false color scale. The retinal pigment epithelium, choroid, and retinal nerve fiber layers are visible as highly backscattered red layers. Typical ophthalmic images span a 40–50 dB dynamic range. Because the eye can differentiate many more colors than gray levels and monitors can support 24-bit colormaps, false color improves the ability to differentiate structures. (See color plate.)

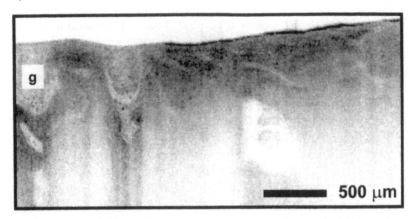

Figure 8 Gray-scale image in scattering tissue. Example of an OCT image of the ectocervix in vitro that illustrates features common to many scattering materials and tissues. These images show strong attenuation of the signal with depth as well as speckle noise. They are more prone to display artifacts than OCT images in weakly scattering tissues. Images in scattering materials or tissues are often displayed using a gray scale. Note the presence of glandular (g) structures that have different backscattering properties.

features of the material or specimen. These image properties can produce display artifacts if the image is displayed using a false color scale. Thus it is more common to use a gray scale to display OCT images in highly scattering materials or tissues.

It is important to note that although the tomographic image represents the true dimensions of the structure (correcting for index of refraction and refraction effects) being measured, the coloring of different structures represents different optical properties and not necessarily different tissue morphology. Thus, OCT images should be interpreted analogously to conventional histopathology. A comprehensive discussion of the theory of OCT imaging is presented in Chapter 2.

1.7 PIXEL DENSITIES AND IMAGE ACQUISITION TIME

The pixel density of an OCT image is determined by the image acquisition conditions and analog-to-digital (A/D) sampling parameters. Assuming that each axial scan covers a depth L_z, then if the axial resolution is Δz the axial scan data should be sampled at a density of two times the resolution or higher. Thus it is desirable to have at least $N_z = 2L_z/\Delta z$ image pixels in the axial direction. The number of pixels in the transverse direction is determined by the number of axial scans, N_x, used to construct the OCT image. For optimum resolution, the number of transverse pixels should be chosen according to the transverse resolution Δx. Thus if an OCT image with a transverse dimension of L_x is required, the optimum resolution image should have $N_x = 2L_x/\Delta x$ pixels. However, in most cases this is a preclusively high number of transverse pixels, and OCT images are undersampled in the transverse direction. With improvements in technology, the pixel dimensions of OCT images have been steadily increasing. Early ophthalmic OCT imaging was performed with 100 transverse pixels and 500 longitudinal pixels or 50k image sizes [25], whereas now ultrahigh resolution OCT images can have more than 1000 transverse pixels and 1500 longitudinal pixels, resulting in megapixel image sizes [22].

The pixel density of an image is closely related to the image acquisition time. Achieving rapid image acquisition time is important for imaging in vivo specimens and for clinical applications. Rapid imaging is necessary to minimize the image distortion produced by motion. In addition, the time available to perform the examination is limited, and it is desirable to maximize the amount of data obtained. The imaging time is directly related to the detection sensitivity, because performing imaging more rapidly (i.e., increasing the noise equivalent bandwidth of the detection) results in reduced signal-to-noise performance in the image. At the same time, in order to distinguish weak reflections from different intraocular structures in ophthalmic imaging or to achieve sufficient image penetration in scattering tissues that are strongly attenuating, it is necessary to image with a sufficient signal-to-noise ratio.

The signal-to-noise ratio may be improved by using higher incident optical power. However, for clinical applications the maximum permissible light exposure is determined by safety standards. For eye and skin exposure the American National Standards Institute (ANSI) has developed criteria for determining the maximum permissible exposure [26]. Unfortunately, no systematic or accepted criteria exist that govern the safe exposure of epithelial surfaces such as those in the gastrointestinal, pulmonary, urinary, or reproductive tracts that are exposed in internal body imaging applications. Thus, the establishment of exposure standards for scanned focused spot illumination of the type performed in OCT imaging (as well as in confocal microscopy) remains an important scientific and regulatory problem.

The image acquisition time is determined by a combination of incident power and signal-to-noise ratio that is required to achieve images of sufficiently high quality for given applications. Image acquisition time increases in proportion to the size of the image and the number of transverse resolution elements or pixels. The image acquisition time is given by the amount of time it takes to perform each axial scan times the number of axial scans in the image, $T = N_x f_s$, where N_x is the number of transverse pixels in each tomograph and f_s is the repetition rate of the axial scanning. This also determines the velocity of the axial scanning, because the distance L_z in the axial direction must be scanned in a time of $1/f_s$ or less. The scan velocity is thus $v_s = L_z/f_s$.

If higher resolution imaging is desired in the transverse direction, i.e., a greater number of transverse pixels are desired, then the image acquisition time increases proportionally. Conversely, if very low resolution imaging is performed—if, for example, only topographic information is required—then the number of transverse pixels may be reduced, resulting in proportionally faster image acquisition. In the longitudinal direction, the image acquisition time scales directly as the depth or length of the longitudinal axial scan necessary to image the desired structure.

1.8 IMAGE CONTRAST PENETRATION DEPTHS

The detection sensitivity determines the imaging performance of optical coherence tomography for different applications. It is helpful to consider OCT imaging in two limiting cases: (1) imaging in media with very weak scattering and (2) imaging in highly scattering media. When OCT is performed in very weakly scattering media, the imaging depth is not strongly limited, because there is very little attenuation of the incident beam. Instead, the sensitivity of the OCT detection establishes a limit on the smallest signals that can be detected. One example of this is in optical data storage applications that encode information using reflections from index mismatch [27]. In these applications it is desirable to use as small an index mismatch as possible. If an optical reflection is generated as the result of an index mismatch δn, then the magnitude of the intensity reflection is $\sim \delta n^2$. The high sensitivity of OCT means that extremely small reflections corresponding to small index mismatches can be measured. For example, if the detection sensitivity is $-100\,\text{dB}$, index mismatches in the range of $\delta n = 10^{-4}$–10^{-5} can be detected. The application of OCT for data storage is described in more detail in Chapter 14.

Another example of OCT imaging in structures with weak backscattering is ophthalmic imaging. Figures 6 and 7 show examples. In ophthalmic imaging, high sensitivity is essential in order to image structures such as the retina that are nominally transparent and have very low backscattering. In ophthalmic applications, the image contrast in OCT images arises because of differences in the backscattering properties of different tissues. Structures such as the retinal pigment epithelium (RPE) or retinal nerve fiber layer can be differentiated from other structures because of their different scattering amplitudes. Typical retinal images have signal levels within -50 to $-100\,\text{dB}$ of the incident signal. For retinal imaging, the ANSI standards govern the maximum permissible light exposure and set limits for both the sensitivity of OCT imaging and OCT imaging speeds [25,26,28]. The application of OCT for ophthalmic imaging is described in more detail in Chapters 17 and 18.

The second limiting case of OCT imaging is imaging in highly scattering media. Figure 8 shows an example. In this case, the detection sensitivity determines the maximum depth to which imaging can be performed. Most biological tissues are highly scattering. OCT imaging in tissues other than the eye became possible with the recognition that the use of longer optical wavelengths, for example, $1.3\,\mu\text{m}$ compared to 800 nm, can reduce scattering and increase image penetration depths [29–32]. Figure 9 shows an example of OCT imaging in a human epiglottis in vitro comparing 800 nm and 1300 nm imaging wavelengths. The dominant absorbers in most tissues are melanin and hemoglobin, which have absorption in the visible and near-infrared wavelength range. Water absorption becomes appreciable for wavelengths approaching 1.9–$2\,\mu\text{m}$. In most tissues, scattering at near-infrared wavelengths is one to two orders of magnitude higher than absorption. Scattering decreases for longer wavelengths, so OCT image penetration increases [33]. For example, if a tissue has a scattering coefficient in the range of $\sim 40\,\text{cm}^{-1}$ at 1300 nm, then the round-trip attenuation from scattering alone from a depth of 3 mm is e^{-24} or $\sim 4 \times 10^{11}$. Thus, if the detection sensitivity limit is $-100\,\text{dB}$, backscattered or backreflected signals are attenuated to the sensitivity limit when the image depth is 2–3 mm. Because the attenuation is exponential with depth, increasing the detection sensitivity by one order of magnitude would not appreciably increase the imaging depth.

The mechanisms of OCT image contrast in scattering media have been investigated and related to the optical properties of the medium [34]. The image contrast mechanisms for OCT are somewhat analogous to those of ultrasound. In order to visualize an internal feature in a highly scattering medium, it is necessary to detect light that is backscattered or backreflected from the internal feature. First, the OCT imaging beam is incident on the scattering medium and is attenuated by scattering and absorption during its forward propagation into the medium. The light is backscattered or backreflected by the internal feature and is further attenuated by scat-

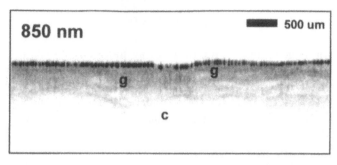

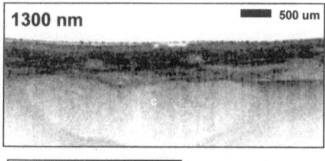

Figure 9 Wavelength dependence of OCT image penetration depth. Example of OCT images of human epiglottis in vitro acquired with light sources at 850 and 1300 nm. Attenuation from scattering is reduced by using longer wavelengths. Superficial glands (g) can be visualized at both wavelengths, but the underlying cartilage (c) can be imaged only with 1300 nm light. With 100 dB detection sensitivity, image penetration of 2–3 mm is possible in most scattering tissues. The ability to perform OCT imaging in scattering tissues opened up a wide range of medical applications. (From Ref. 32.)

tering and absorption during its reverse propagation out of the medium. Thus, the contrast for OCT imaging in scattering media is determined by a combination of attenuation from scattering and absorption during propagation and backscattering from the internal feature that is being imaged. The situation is different for OCT imaging in weakly scattering media, where there is negligible attenuation from scattering and absorption during propagation. In this case, image contrast is determined by the backscattering properties of the internal features that are being imaged. A detailed discussion of tissue optical properties and mechanisms of OCT image contrast is presented in Chapter 16.

1.9 RESOLUTION AND IMAGE PENETRATION DEPTHS OF OCT AND ULTRASOUND

Two of the most important parameters for characterizing imaging performance are image resolution and imaging depth. There are interesting comparisons between OCT, ultrasound, and microscopy as shown in Fig. 10. The resolution of ultrasound imaging depends directly on the frequency or wavelength of the sound waves that are used [1–5]. For typical clinical ultrasound systems, sound wave

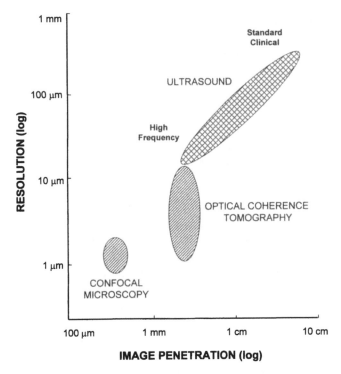

Figure 10 Resolution and penetration of ultrasound, OCT, and confocal microscopy. In ultrasound imaging, both image resolution and penetration are determined by the sound wave frequency. High axial resolutions are possible, but transverse resolutions are usually coarser. Ultrasonic attenuation limits penetration to a few millimeters. The image resolution in OCT is determined by the coherent length of the light source, and resolutions ranging from 1 to 15 μm can be achieved. In most scattering tissues, image penetration is limited to 2–3 mm. Confocal microscopy can have submicrometer transverse resolution, but axial resolution is coarser. The image penetration of confocal microscopy is typically limited to a few hundred micrometers in scattering tissues. Together these imaging modalities provide complementary performance.

frequencies are in the 10 MHz regime and yield spatial resolutions of up to 150 μm. Ultrasound imaging has the advantage that sound waves at this frequency are readily transmitted into most biological tissues and therefore it is possible to obtain images of structures up to several tens of centimeters deep within the body. High frequency ultrasound has been developed and investigated extensively in laboratory applications as well as in some limited clinical applications. Axial resolutions of 15–20 μm and higher have been achieved with frequencies of $\sim$ 100 MHz. It should be noted that the transverse resolution of ultrasound is governed by the dimension of the focused ultrasound beam. Although the sound frequency governs the focused spot size, it is difficult to achieve spot sizes on the order of the wavelength, and thus transverse resolutions are not as fine as axial resolutions. Another important limitation of high frequency ultrasound is that high frequencies are strongly attenuated in biological tissues, with attenuation increasing approximately in proportion to the frequency. Thus, high frequency ultrasound imaging is limited to depths of only a few millimeters.

As discussed previously, the axial and transverse resolutions of OCT imaging are governed by different processes. The axial resolution is determined by the coherence length of the optical source. Current OCT imaging technologies have resolutions ranging from 1 to 15 μm, approximately 10–100 times higher resolution than standard ultrasound B-mode imaging. The transverse resolution is governed by the focused spot size of the optical beam with a trade-off between transverse resolution and depth of field.

1.10 OPTICAL COHERENCE TOMOGRAPHY FROM THE SYSTEMS PERSPECTIVE

One of the advantages of optical coherence tomography is that it can be implemented using compact fiber-optic components and integrated with a wide range of medical instruments. Figure 11 shows a schematic of an OCT system using a fiber-optic Michelson-type interferometer with a scanning optical delay. A low coherence light source is coupled into the interferometer, and the interference at the output is detected with a photodiode. One arm of the interferometer emits a beam that is directed and scanned on the sample that is being imaged, and the other arm of the interferometer is a reference arm with a scanning delay line.

In a more general context, OCT systems can be considered from a modular viewpoint in terms of integrated hardware and software modules. Figure 12 shows a schematic of the different modules in an OCT imaging system. The OCT system can be divided into the imaging engine, low coherence light source, beam delivery and probes, computer control, and image processing.

The imaging engine is the heart of the OCT system. In general, the imaging engine can be any optical detection device that performs high resolution and high sensitivity ranging and detection of backreflected or backscattered optical echoes. Most OCT systems have employed a reference delay scanning interferometer using a low coherence light source. There are many different embodiments of the interferometer and imaging engine for specific applications such as polarization diversity (insensitive) imaging, polarization-sensitive imaging, and Doppler flow imaging. For example, Doppler flow imaging has been performed using imaging engines that detect the interferometric output rather than demodulating the interference fringes

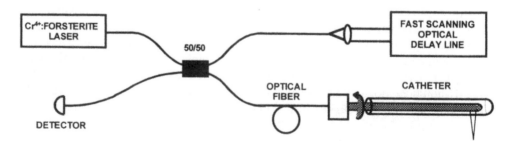

Figure 11 Schematic showing an example of an OCT instrument using a fiber-optic implementation of a Michelson interferometer with a laser low coherence light source. One arm of the interferometer is integrated with the imaging probe, and the other arm has a scanning delay line. The system shown is configured for high speed catheter-endoscope-based imaging.

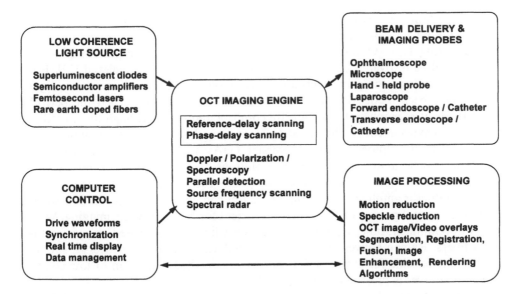

Figure 12   The systems perspective of OCT. OCT is a modular technology consisting of both hardware and software. The major submodules in the OCT system include the imaging engine, light source, delivery system and optical probes, computer control, and image processing. OCT draws upon a wide range of component technologies.

[35–38]. A comprehensive discussion of Doppler imaging using OCT is presented in Chapter 8. Polarization-sensitive detection techniques have been demonstrated using a dual channel interferometer [39–41]. These techniques permit imaging of the bire-fringence properties of structures. Collagen and other tissues are strongly birefrin-gent, and polarization-sensitive OCT can be a sensitive indicator of the tissue microstructural organization. Conversely, polarization diversity or polarization-insensitive interferometers can also be built using well-established polarization diver-sity detection methods from coherence heterodyne optical communication. A detailed discussion of techniques for OCT imaging and measurement of polarization is presented in Chapter 9. Finally, other imaging engine approaches have been demonstrated that are based on spectral analysis of broadband light sources as well as tunable narrow linewidth sources [42]. These imaging engines have the advan-tage that they do not require scanning an optical delay, and thus no moving parts are required. Discussions of these types of imaging techniques are presented in Chapters 12 and 13.

    The short coherence length light source determines the axial resolution of the OCT system. For research applications, short-pulse lasers are powerful light sources for OCT imaging because they have extremely short coherence lengths and high output powers, enabling high resolution, high speed imaging. Many studies have been performed using a short-pulse Cr^{4+} : forsterite laser. This laser produces output powers greater than 100 mW with ultrashort pulses of less than 100 fs at wavelengths near 1300 nm. By using nonlinear self-phase modulation in optical fibers, the spectral output can be broadened to produce bandwidths sufficient to achieve axial resolu-tions of 5–10 μm [43]. Image acquisition speeds of several frames per second are achieved with signal-to-noise ratios of 100 dB using incident powers in the 5–10 mW range. Short-pulse $Ti:Al_2O_3$ lasers operating near 800 nm have also been used to achieve high resolutions. Early studies demonstrated axial resolutions of $4\,\mu m$ [44]. Recently, using $Ti:Al_2O_3$ laser technology, which generates pulse durations of $\sim 5\,fs$ and bandwidths of over 300 nm, axial resolutions of $1\,\mu m$ were achieved [22]. For clinical applications, compact superluminescent diodes or semiconductor-based light sources have been used. Although these sources have not yet reached the performance levels of research systems, they are compact and robust enough to be used in the clinical environment. Ophthalmic OCT systems have employed commercially available (EG&G Optoelectronics) compact GaAs superluminescent diodes that operate near 800 nm and achieve axial resolutions of $\sim 10\,\mu m$ with output powers of a few milliwatts. Commercially available (AFC Technologies Inc.) sources based on semiconductor amplifiers operating at $1.3\,\mu m$ can achieve axial resolutions of $\sim 15\,\mu m$ with output powers of 15–20 mW, sufficient for real-time OCT imaging. With further development, other types of low coherence light sources based on rare-earth-doped fibers, Raman conversion, and other nonlinear conversion processes should also become feasible for clinical OCT systems. A detailed discussion of low coherence light sources is presented in Chapter 3.

In the reference delay scanning embodiments of OCT systems, the optical delay scanner determines the image acquisition rate of the system. The earliest scanning devices were constructed using galvanometers and retroreflectors [25,45]. These systems have scan ranges of up to a centimeter or more and have the advantage of simplicity. However, scan repetition rates are limited to approximately 100 Hz. A novel technique using PZTs to stretch optical fibers has been developed that can achieve scan ranges of a few millimeters with repetition rates of 500 Hz or more [46,47]. Many studies were performed using a high speed scanning optical delay line based on a diffraction grating phase control device [48]. This device is similar to pulse-shaping devices that are used in femtosecond optics [49]. The grating phase control scanner is attractive because it achieves extremely high scan speeds and also permits the phase and group velocity of the scanning to be independently controlled. Images of 250–500 transverse pixels can be produced at several frames per second [50]. A detailed discussion of high speed scanning techniques is presented in Chapter 4.

The OCT beam delivery and optical probes can be designed for specific applications. Because OCT imaging technology is based on fiber optics, it can be easily integrated with many standard optical diagnostic instruments, including instruments for internal body imaging. OCT imaging has been integrated with a slit lamp and fundus camera for ophthalmic imaging of the retina [25,51]. The OCT beam is scanned using a pair of galvanometric beam-steering mirrors and relay-imaged onto the retina. The ophthalmic OCT imaging instrument is relatively complex because it must image the retina (fundus) *en face* while showing the position of the tomographic scanning beam. The ability to register OCT images with *en face* features and pathology is an important consideration for many applications. Similar principles apply for the design of OCT using low numerical aperture microscopes. Low numerical aperture microscopes have been used for imaging in vivo developmental biological specimens as well as for surgical imaging applications [52–55].

Closely related beam delivery systems include forward imaging devices, which permit the delivery of a one- or two-dimensional scanned beam. Rigid laparoscopes are based on relay imaging using Hopkins-type relay lenses or graded index rod lenses. OCT may be readily integrated with laparoscopes to permit internal body OCT imaging with a simultaneous *en face* view of the scan registration [46,56]. Hand-held probes have also been demonstrated [56,57]. These devices resemble light pens and use piezoelectric or galvanometric beam scanning. Hand-held probes can be used in open field surgery to permit the clinician to view the subsurface structure of tissue by aiming the probe at the desired structure. These devices can also be integrated with conventional scalpels or laser surgical devices to permit real-time viewing as tissue is being resected.

Another class of imaging probes includes flexible miniature devices for internal body imaging. Because OCT beams are delivered using fiber optics, small-diameter scanning endoscopes and catheters can be developed. The first clinical studies of internal body imaging were performed using a novel forward-scanning flexible probe that could be used in conjunction with a standard endoscope or bronchoscope [46,57]. This device used a miniature galvanometric scanner to produce one-dimensional forward beam scanning in a 1.5–2 mm diameter probe. Transverse and linear scanning OCT catheter-endoscopes have also been developed [50,58,59]. Figure 13 shows an example of a transverse scanning OCT catheter-endoscope. The catheter-endoscope consists of a single-mode optical fiber encased in a hollow rotating torque cable coupled to a distal lens and a microprism that direct the OCT beam perpendicular to the axis of the catheter. The cable and distal optics are encased in a transparent housing. The OCT beam is scanned by rotating the cable to permit transluminal imaging, in a radarlike pattern, cross-sectionally through vessels or hollow organisms. The catheter-endoscope has a diameter of 2.9 French or 1 mm, comparable to the size of a standard intravascular ultrasound catheter. The development of even smaller diameter OCT catheter-endoscopes is possible.

Figure 13 also shows an example of an OCT catheter-endoscope image of the gastrointestinal trace and arterial imaging in the New Zealand White rabbit [60,61]. A short-pulse Cr^{4+}:forsterite laser was used as the light source to achieve high resolution with real-time image acquisition rates [43]. The two-dimensional image data were displayed using a polar coordinate transformation in gray scale and were recorded in both Super VHS and digital formats. OCT images of the esophagus permitted differentiation of the mucosal and submucosal layers of the esophageal wall. OCT images of the artery were performed with saline flushing to reduce scattering from blood.

These types of OCT imaging probes are small enough to fit in the accessory port of a standard endoscope or bronchoscope and permit an *en face* view of the area being scanned simultaneously with the tomographic image. Alternatively, they can be used independently, for example in intra-arterial imaging, where access to small arteries or other luminal structures is required. A comprehensive discussion of OCT imaging probes is presented in Chapter 5.

Image processing and display are performed by a software module of the OCT system. One of the advantages of electronic image data is that they can be processed using a wide range of techniques. Electronic image data are also amenable to electronic transmission, storage, and retrieval. There are several general categories of image processing techniques that can be applied to OCT images. These include motion correction algorithms, noise or speckle reduction algorithms, resolution enhancement algorithms, segmentation algorithms, and display algorithms. Perhaps the most widely used algorithms to date are the motion correction algo-

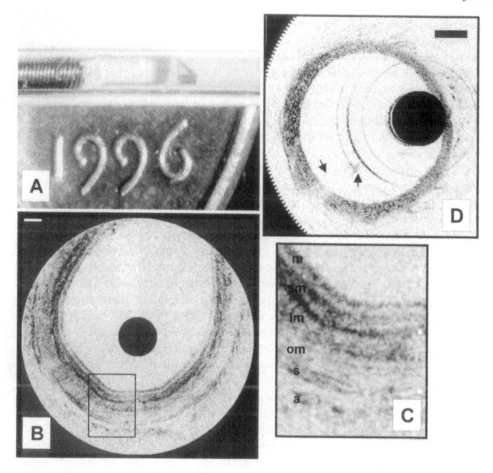

Figure 13 Examples of a miniature OCT catheter and images. (A) This 2.9 F (1 mm) diameter catheter is designed for transverse intraluminal imaging. A single-mode fiber is contained in a rotating flexible cable with distal beam optics that emit at 90° from the catheter axis. (B) In vivo OCT endoscopic image of the esophagus in a New Zealand White rabbit showing an example of internal body imaging. The image has $10\,\mu$m axial resolution and 512 circumferential pixels and was taken at 4 frames per second. (C) The mucosa, submucosa, inner muscularis, and outer muscularis are well differentiated. (D) OCT catheter image of arterial structure using saline flushing to reduce scattering from blood. The intima is less than $10\,\mu$m and is not resolved; the medium is visible as highly scattering. Small OCT probes enable a wide range of internal body imaging applications. (From Refs. 50 and 61.)

rithms that are used in ophthalmic imaging [28]. Because the resolution of OCT is extremely high, it is essential to compensate for motion of the eye during image acquisition. The dominant motion that blurs the image occurs in the axial (longitudinal) direction, because retinal structure in this direction has dimensions on the micrometer scale. Changes in the longitudinal position of the eye can be corrected for because the optical ranging measurement itself determines the long-itudinal position of the retina. The tomographic image is constructed by performing sequential axial scans at different transverse positions within the eye. The motion of the patient's eye in the axial direction can be measured by correlating adjacent axial data sets. Once the axial position of the patient's eye is known, the scans in the optical tomographic image can be displayed in the axial direction to align the microstructural features. Changes in the transverse position are not eliminated when this type of image processing is used; however, small changes in transverse position do not produce significant degradation in image quality, because typical features are larger in the transverse dimension than in the axial (longitudinal) direction.

Numerous other algorithms for OCT have also been developed or are currently being investigated. Techniques for resolution enhancement based upon deconvolution and iterative estimation have been demonstrated that can improve image resolution [62–64]. Deionising and speckle reduction algorithms have been applied in ultrasound and are very promising for OCT. Segmentation techniques have been used extensively in ophthalmic OCT for detecting the thickness of the retina and retinal nerve fiber layer [65,66]. Segmentation and rendering techniques have been used for surgical guidance applications as well as for studying composite materials. A detailed discussion of surgical imaging is presented in Chapter 23, and imaging in composite materials is presented in Chapter 15. A more detailed discussion of image processing techniques in general is presented in Chapter 6.

1.11   APPLICATIONS OF OPTICAL COHERENCE TOMOGRAPHY

The use of optical coherence tomography to perform two-dimensional measurements of optical backscattering or backreflection to image internal cross-sectional microstructure was demonstrated in 1991 [6]. OCT imaging was performed in vitro in the human retina and in atherosclerotic plaque as examples of imaging in transparent, weakly scattering media and highly scattering media. This study used a fiber-optic Michelson interferometer with reference arm scanning and a superluminescent diode low coherence light source at 800 nm with $10\,\mu$m axial resolution. Since that time, numerous applications of OCT for both materials and medical applications have emerged. At the same time, the performance specifications and capabilities of OCT imaging technology have improved dramatically.

A number of features make OCT attractive for a broad range of applications. First, imaging can be performed in situ and nondestructively. High resolutions are possible with typical image resolutions of 10–$15\,\mu$m and ultrahigh resolutions of up to $1\,\mu$m. High speed real-time imaging is possible with acquisition rates of several frames per second for 250–500 pixel images. OCT can be interfaced with a wide range of imaging delivery systems and imaging probes. OCT technology is based on fiber optics and uses components developed for the telecommunications industry. Image information is generated in electronic form, which is amenable to image processing and analysis as well as electronic transmission, storage, and retrieval. Finally, OCT systems can be engineered to be compact and low cost, suitable for applications in research, manufacturing, or the clinic.

Optical coherence tomography is a powerful imaging technology in medicine because it enables the real-time, in situ visualization of tissue microstructure without the need to excise and process a specimen as in conventional biopsy and histopathology. The concept of nonexcisional "optical biopsy" performed by OCT and the ability to visualize tissue morphology in real time under operator guidance can be used both for diagnostic imaging and to guide intervention. Coupled with catheter, endoscopic, or laparoscopic delivery, OCT promises to have a powerful impact on many medical applications ranging from improving the screening and diagnosis of neoplasia to enabling new microsurgical and minimally invasive surgical procedures. The next sections describe the use of OCT in examples of various medical applications. These examples review previous research, describe the characteristics of OCT technology that are important for given applications, and present scenarios where OCT imaging may have a significant impact. OCT also has many nonmedical applications, ranging from materials imaging to optical recording. These applications are described in more detail in Chapters 14 and 15.

1.11.1 OCT Imaging in Ophthalmology

Optical coherence tomography was first applied for imaging in the eye, and to date it has had the greatest clinical impact in ophthalmology. The first *in vivo* tomograms of the human optic disc and macula were demonstrated in 1993 [28,67]. Numerous clinical studies have been performed in the last few years. OCT enables the non-contact, noninvasive imaging of the anterior eye and retina [25,68,69]. It is helpful to review ophthalmic OCT because it is the most clinically advanced application and is a model for other clinical applications.

Figure 7 shows an example of an OCT image of the normal retina of a human subject. OCT provides a cross-sectional view of the retina with unprecedented high resolution and allows detailed structures to be differentiated. Although the retina is almost transparent and has extremely low optical backscattering, the high sensitivity of OCT imaging allows extremely small backscattering features such as interretinal layers to be differentiated. The retinal pigment epithelium, which contains melanin, and the choroid, which is highly vascular, are visible as highly scattering structures in the OCT image.

Optical coherence tomography has been demonstrated for the detection and monitoring of a variety of macular diseases [69], including macular edema [70], macular holes [71], central serous chorioretinopathy [72], age-related macular degeneration and choroidal neovascularization [73], and epiretinal membranes. The retinal nerve fiber layer thickness, a predictor for early glaucoma, can be quantified in normal and glaucomatous eyes and correlated with conventional measurements of the optic nerve structure and function [65,66,74,75]. In addition, OCT has been applied for the evaluation of choroidal tumors [76], congenital optic disc pits [77,78], and argon laser lesions [79]. Retinal OCT images have been correlated with histology [80], and OCT has been used to investigate microanatomy and retinal degeneration in the chicken [81].

Because it can provide quantitative information on retinal pathology, which is a measure of disease progression, OCT is especially promising for the diagnosis and monitoring of diseases such as glaucoma or macular edema associated with diabetic retinopathy. Images can be analyzed quantitatively and processed using intelligent algorithms to extract features such as retinal or retinal nerve fiber layer thickness [65,66,74,75,82]. Mapping and display techniques have been developed to represent the tomographic data in alterative forms, such as thickness maps, to aid interpretation. Figure 14 (see color plate) shows an example of an OCT topographic map of retinal thickness. The thickness map is constructed by performing six standard OCT scans at varying angular orientations through the fovea. The images are then segmented to detect the retinal thickness along the OCT tomograms. The retinal thick-

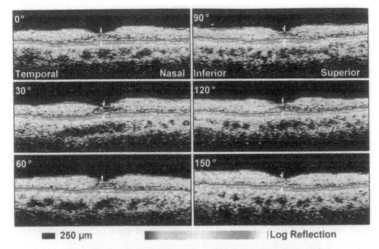

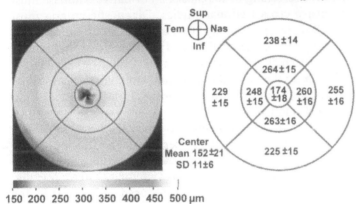

Figure 14 Topographical mapping of retinal thickness as an example of image processing and display. The topographical representation is constructed by performing six OCT tomograms at different angles through the fovea. The tomograms are processed to extract retinal thickness, and the thickness values are interpolated over the macular region. The retinal thickness is displayed using a false color scale. Quantitative data of retinal thickness in nine different zones are also shown. These values are from a normative database and are displayed as mean and standard deviation. Quantitative data are more useful for screening purpose, whereas images are necessary for specific diagnosis or treatment planning. (See color plate.) (From Ref. 82.)

ness is linearly interpolated over the macular region and represented in false color. Retinal thickness values between 0 and 500 μm are displayed by colors ranging from blue to red. The result is a color-coded topographic map of retinal thickness that displays the retinal thickness in an *en face* view corresponding to the macula. For quantitative interpretation, the macula was also divided into nine regions. Figure 14 shows the average retinal thickness measured from OCT imaging on 96 normal individuals with statistics including mean values and standard deviations (SDs) [82]. The SD provides a simple estimate of the measurement reproducibility.

The ability to reduce image information to quantitative form is important because it allows the construction of a normative database and calculation of statistics. The topographic thickness map demonstrates how OCT image information can be processed to yield different levels of detail. On the coarsest level, a single number, the foveal thickness, can provide a diagnostic indicator of macular edema in a patient. This type of information might be useful in a screening context, where high risk patient populations are screened in a primary care setting. On the next, more detailed level, the retinal thickness values in the nine regions can be used to more specifically localize the possible region where macular edema is present and improve the statistical accuracy of the measurement. The topographic false color map provides more graphic information that can be compared directly to the fundus image of the retina. Finally, the raw tomographic images contain the most detailed information and can be used to diagnose other retinal pathologies in addition to macular edema. This information would be useful for the ophthalmologist or specialist but would be excessively detailed for the primary care setting.

For the data to be used for screening or diagnosis, a normative database must be developed, requiring extensive cross-sectional studies. Diagnostic criteria must also be developed that will allow the OCT image or numerical information to be used to determine the presence or the stage of disease. The diagnostic criteria must have sufficient sensitivity and specificity. In many cases, screening or diagnosis is complicated by natural variations in the normal population. Ongoing clinical studies are investigating OCT for screening and diagnosis of diabetic macular edema and glaucoma, two leading causes of blindness.

Optical coherence tomgraphy has the potential to detect and diagnose early stages of disease before physical symptoms and irreversible loss of vision occur. Many thousands of patients have been examined to date, and numerous clinical studies are currently under way in many research groups and clinics internationally. OCT technology was transferred to industry and introduced commercially for ophthalmic diagnostics in 1996 (Humphrey Systems, Dublin, CA). With further development and clinical investigation, we expect that OCT will become a standard ophthalmic diagnostic tool within the next few years. For a more detailed discussion of OCT in ophthalmology, see Chapters 17 and 18.

1.11.2   Optical Coherence Tomography and Optical Biopsy

With recent research advances, OCT imaging of optically scattering, nontransparent tissues has become possible, enabling a wide variety of medical applications. One of the techniques that enables OCT imaging in nontransparent tissues has been the use of longer wavelengths, which reduces optical scattering [29–32]. By using $1.3\,\mu m$ wavelengths, image penetration depths of 2–3 mm can be achieved in most tissues. This imaging depth is not as great as that of ultrasound, but it is comparable to the depth over which many biopsies are performed. Many diagnostically important changes of tissue morphology occur at the epithelial surfaces of organ lumens. The capability to perform in situ, real-time imaging can be important in a variety of clinical scenarios, including (1) imaging tissue pathology in situations where conventional excisional biopsy would be hazardous or impossible, (2) guiding conventional biopsy to reduce false negative rates from sampling errors and the detection of early neoplastic changes, and (3) guiding surgical or microsurgical intervention.

Imaging Where Excisional Biopsy is Hazardous or Impossible

One class of applications where OCT could be especially powerful comprises those for which conventional excisional biopsy is hazardous or impossible. In ophthalmology, biopsy of the retina is not possible and OCT can provide high resolution images of retinal structure that cannot be obtained using any other technique. Another example of a scenario where biopsy is not possible is the imaging of atherosclerotic plaque morphology in the coronary arteries [32,83]. Recent research has demonstrated that most myocardial infarctions result from the rupture of small to moderately sized cholesterol-laden coronary artery plaques followed by thrombosis and vessel occlusion [84–87]. The plaques at highest risk for rupture are those that have a structurally weak fibrous cap [88]. These plaque morphologies are difficult to detect by conventional radiological techniques, and their microstructural features cannot be determined. Identifying high risk unstable plaques and patients at risk for myocardial infarction is important because of the high percentage of occlusions that result in sudden death [89]. OCT could be powerful for diagnostic intravascular imaging as well as for guidance of interventional procedures such as atherectomy and stenting.

Imaging studies of arterial lesions in vitro have been performed to investigate the correlation of OCT and histology [32,83]. Figure 15 shows an example of an unstable plaque morphology from a human abdominal aorta specimen with corresponding histology. Specimens were imaged by an OCT microscope prior to fixation. OCT imaging was performed at 1300 nm wavelength using a superluminescent diode light source with an axial resolution of $\sim 16\,\mu m$. The OCT image and histology show a small intimal layer covering a large atherosclerotic plaque that is heavily calcified and has a relatively low lipid content. The optical scattering properties of lipid, adipose tissue, and calcified plaque are different and provide contrast between different structures and plaque morphologies. The thin intimal wall increases the likelihood of rupture. Currently, these lesions can be accurately diagnosed only by postmortem histology, and therefore interventional techniques cannot be used effectively to treat them. The ability to identify structural detail such as the presence and thickness of intimal caps using catheter-based OCT imaging techniques could lead to significant improvements in patient outcome.

Conventional angiography, ultrasound, or magnetic resonance imaging (MRI) do not have sufficient resolution to identify these lesions or to guide the removal of plaque by catheter-based atherectomy procedures. High frequency (20–30 MHz) intravascular ultrasound (IVUS) can be used to measure arterial stenosis as well as to guide intervention procedures such as stent deployment [90,91]. However, the resolution of IVUS is limited to approximately $100\,\mu m$, and thus it is difficult to decisively identify high risk plaque morphologies [92]. Studies have been performed that compare IVUS and OCT imaging in vitro and demonstrate the ability of OCT to identify clinically relevant pathology [83]. *In vivo* OCT arterial imaging has also been performed in rabbits using a catheter-based delivery system [61]. Optical scattering from blood limits OCT imaging penetration depths, so saline flushing at low rates was required for imaging. These effects depend on vessel diameter as well as other factors, and additional investigation is required. A comprehensive discussion of OCT applications for cardiovascular imaging is presented in Chapter 26.

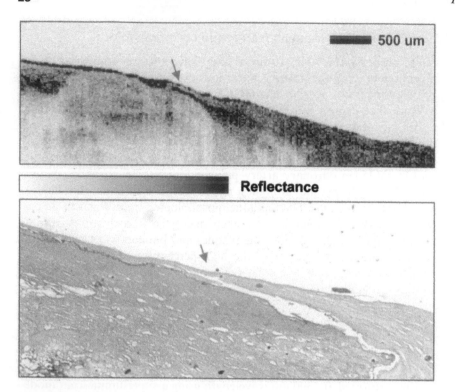

Figure 15 Optical coherence tomographic image showing atherosclerotic plaque in vitro and corresponding histology. This is an example of OCT imaging in tissues where standard excisional biopsy is not possible. The plaque is highly calcified with a low lipid content, and a thin intimal cap layer is observed. The high resolution of OCT can resolve small structures such as the thin intimal layer that are associated with unstable plaques. OCT could have important applications for diagnosis and interventional guidance in cardiovascular disease. (From Ref. 32.)

Detecting Early Neoplastic Changes

Another major class of OCT imaging applications applies in situations where conventional excisional biopsy has unacceptably high false negative rates due to sampling errors. This is the scenario in the detection of early neoplasia. OCT can resolve changes in architectural morphology that are associated with many early neoplasias. Studies have been performed in vitro to correlate OCT images with histology for pathologies of the gastrointestinal, female reproductive, pulmonary, and biliary tracts [60,93–101]. Preliminary studies in human subjects have also been performed using endoscopy- and laparoscopy-based OCT imaging [46,57,102].

One of the key issues for the use of OCT imaging in the detection of early neoplastic changes is the ability to differentiate clinically relevant pathologies with a given image resolution. Many early neoplastic changes are manifested by disruption of the normal glandular organization or architectural morphology of tissues. These changes can be imaged using standard 10–15 μm resolution OCT systems. Figure 16 shows an example of an in vitro OCT image of normal colon and ampullary carcinoma. The OCT image of the colon epithelium shows normal glandular organiza-

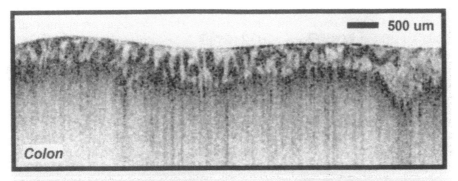

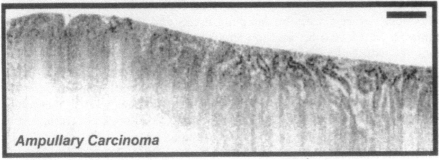

Figure 16 Imaging neoplastic changes. OCT images of gastrointestinal tissues in vitro showing normal colon and ampullary carcinoma. OCT can image differences in architectural morphology or glandular organization that are associated with neoplastic changes. The normal colon shows columnar epithelial morphology with crypt structures visible. The carcinoma, on the left of the image, is characterized by a loss of normal epithelial structure. Normal structure, visible on the right, has progressive disorganization of the crypts in the region nearing the cancer. Architectural morphology such as this can be imaged with standard OCT resolutions of $10-15\,\mu$m. (From Ref. 60.)

tion associated with columnar epithelial structure [60]. The mucosa and muscularis mucosa can be differentiated due to the different backscattering characteristics within each layer. Architectural morphology such as crypts or glands within the mucosa can be seen. The OCT image of ampullary carcinoma shows disruption of architectural morphology or glandular organization. The area on the right of the image is normal, while the carcinoma is on the left of the image. The crypt structures have become dilated and distorted in the middle of the image, with complete loss of structure in the carcinoma.

The ability to delineate tissue architectural morphology could increase the diagnostic capabilities of conventional endoscopy, allowing a wide range of clinical disorders to be addressed. Endoscopic ultrasound has recently been introduced as a new technology for high resolution endoscopic imaging [103–108]. Using ultrasound frequencies in the range of 10–30 MHz, axial resolutions in the range of 100 μm can be achieved [109–111]. Imaging of the esophagus or bowel requires filling the lumen with saline or using a liquid-filled balloon to couple the ultrasound into the tissue. Ultrasound can be used as an adjunct to endoscopy to diagnose and stage early esophageal and gastric neoplasms. Impressive results have been achieved using high frequency endoscopic ultrasound, which demonstrates the differentiation of mucosal and submucosal structures.

Using standard OCT, image resolutions of 10–15 μm are achieved, sufficient to enable the visualization of tissue architectural morphology. OCT can also be used to assess other features such as the integrity of the basement membrane. Ultrahigh resolution OCT with resolutions of 1–5 μm enables cellular level imaging and could expand the range of neoplastic changes that can be imaged [22,43,44,112]. The imaging depth of OCT is 2–3 mm, less than that of ultrasound. However, many diseases originate from or involve epithelial structures, and imaging the microscopic structure of small lesions is within the range of OCT.

Conventional excisional biopsy often suffers from high false negative rates because the biopsy process relies on sampling tissue, and the diseased tissues can easily be missed. OCT could be used to identify suspect lesions and to guide excisional biopsy to reduce the false negative rates. This would reduce the number of costly biopsies, and at the same time clinical diagnoses could be made using excisional biopsy and histopathology, which is the established clinical standard. In the future, after detailed clinical studies and more extensive statistical data become available, it may be possible to use OCT directly for the diagnosis of certain types of neoplasias or for determining the grade of dysplasias.

The development of miniature, flexible OCT imaging probes and high speed OCT imaging systems enables the acquisition of OCT images of internal organ systems. Imaging of the pulmonary, gastrointestinal, and urinary tracts and arterial imaging have been demonstrated in animals [50,61,100]. Preliminary OCT internal body imaging studies in patients have been performed in many different organ systems, including the gastrointestinal, urinary, pulmonary, and female reproductive tracts [46,57,113]. These studies demonstrate the feasibility of performing internal body OCT imaging and suggest a broad range of future clinical applications. More systematic studies that compare OCT imaging with histological or other diagnostic endpoints are needed. At present, several research groups are performing numerous clinical OCT imaging studies, and more detailed data should be available shortly. Comprehensive discussions of OCT imaging applications in different organ systems are presented in Chapters 21, 24, 25, 27, and 28.

1.11.3 Guiding Surgical Intervention

In another important class of applications, OCT is used for guiding surgical intervention. The ability to see beneath the surface of tissue in real time can guide surgery near sensitive structures such as vessels or nerves as well as assisting in microsurgical procedures [52,54]. Optical instruments such as surgical microscopes are routinely used to magnify tissue to prevent iatrogenic injury and to guide delicate surgical techniques. OCT can be easily integrated with surgical microscopes. Hand-held OCT surgical probes and laparoscopes have also been demonstrated [56].

One example of a surgical application for OCT is the repair of small vessels and nerves following traumatic injury. A technique capable of real-time, subsurface, three-dimensional, micrometer-scale imaging would permit the intraoperative monitoring of microsurgical procedures, giving immediate feedback to the surgeon that could improve outcome and enable difficult procedures. Studies have been performed in vitro that demonstrate the use of OCT imaging for diagnostically assessing microsurgical procedures using an OCT microscope delivery system [54]. Figure 17 shows OCT images of an arterial anastomosis of a rabbit inguinal artery, demonstrating the ability of OCT to assess internal structure and luminal patency. An artery segment was bisected cross-sectionally and then reanastomosed. For precise registration of the OCT images, the specimen was positioned on a computer-controlled, motorized translation stage in an OCT microscope. The specimen was also digitally imaged with a CCCD camera. Cross-sectional OCT images of a 1 mm diameter rabbit inguinal artery are shown. Figures 17A–D were acquired transversely at different positions through the anastomosis. The images of the ends of the artery clearly show arterial morphology corresponding to the intimal, medial, and adventitial layers of the elastic artery. The image from the site of the anastomosis shows that the lumen was obstructed by a tissue flap. By assembling a series of cross-sectional two-dimensional images, a three-dimensional dataset was produced. Arbitrary planes can be selected and sections displayed.

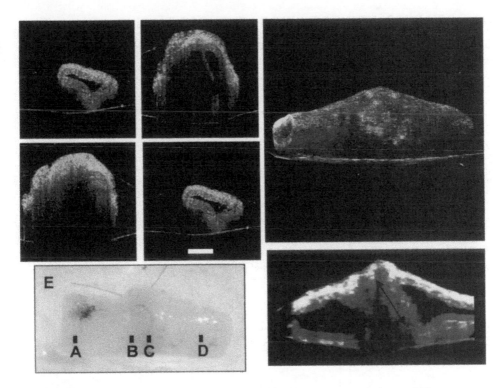

Figure 17 Microsurgical imaging. OCT images of an anastomosis in a rabbit artery as an example of microsurgical imaging. The 1 mm diameter rabbit artery was anastomosed with a continuous suture as seen in the digital image (D). The labels indicate the planes from which corresponding cross-sectional OCT images were acquired. (A,D) Opposite ends of the anastomosis show the multilayered structure of the artery with a patent lumen. (B) Partially obstructed lumen and the presence of a thrombogenic flap. (C) Fully obstructed portion of the anastomosis site. (E) Three-dimensional reconstruction of artery. (G) Virtual longitudinal section view constructed from three-dimensional image data sets shows the obstruction (o). OCT microscopy could be a powerful tool for many microsurgical procedures. (From Ref. 54.)

Because OCT imaging can be performed at high speeds, in real time, it can be integrated directly with surgery. The feasibility of using high speed OCT imaging to guide the placement and image the dynamics of surgical laser ablation has been investigated [55]. Figure 18 shows an example of real-time OCT imaging during laser ablation of a bovine muscle specimen. The laser exposure was 2 W from the argon laser. At 0.5 s changes in optical properties of the tissue are observed due to heating, and explosive ablation begins at 2.25 s. These studies were performed using a commercially available low coherence light source (AFC Technologies Inc., Hull, Quebec, Canada) with a wavelength at 1.3 µm and an axial resolution of 18 µm. Using 5 mW of incident power on the specimen, a signal-to-noise ratio of 115 dB was achieved. The acquisition rate was 8 frames per second for a 250 transverse pixel image. Optical coherence tomography should improve intraoperative diagnostics by providing high resolution, subsurface, cross-sectional imaging in real time. A comprehensive discussion of OCT applications for the guidance of intervention is presented in Chapter 23.

1.12   HIGH RESOLUTION CELLULAR LEVEL OCT IMAGING

The development of high resolution OCT is also an important area of active research. Increasing resolution to the cellular and subcellular levels is important

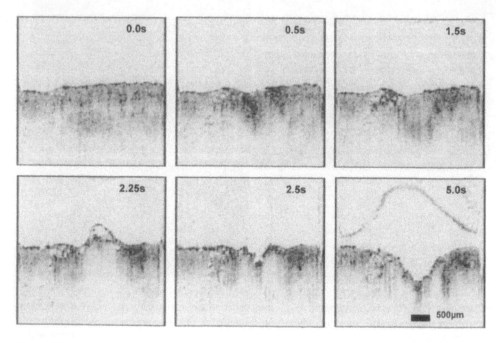

Figure 18   Real-time OCT imaging of laser ablation showing a series of OCT images taken at 8 frames per second during argon laser exposure of beef muscle. The exposure was 1 W with a 0.8 mm spot diameter on tissue. The times indicated are in seconds after exposure is initiated. At 2.25 s, the formation of a blister at the surface is observed. At 2.5 s, the blister explodes and a crater develops (5 s). These images show the ability of OCT to perform high speed, real-time imaging during interventional procedures. (From Ref. 55.)

for many applications, including the diagnosis of early neoplasias. As discussed previously, the axial resolution of OCT is determined by the coherence length of the light source used for imaging. Light sources for OCT imaging should have a short coherence length or broad bandwidth but also must have a single spatial mode to enable interferometry. Since the signal-to-noise ratio depends on the incident power, light sources with average powers of several milliwatts are typically necessary to achieve real-time imaging One approach for achieving high resolution is to use short-pulse femtosecond solid-state lasers as light sources [22,43,44,112].

High resolution OCT imaging has been demonstrated in vivo in developmental biology specimens [22,112]. Figure 19 shows an example of high resolution OCT images of a *Xenopus laevis* (African frog) tadpole. The OCT system in this study was a KLM femtosecond Ti : sapphire laser that emits sub-two-cycle pulses, corresponding to bandwidths of up to 350 nm (FWHM) around 800 nm. The ultrahigh resolution OCT system supported bandwidths up to 260 nm (FWHM), achieving a 1.5 μm longitudinal resolution in free space of $\sim$ 1 μm in tissue. To overcome the depth-of-field limitations associated with the high transverse resolution, a zone focus and image fusion technique was used. The figure was constructed by fusing multiple separate images recorded with different focal depths of the optics similar to C-mode scanning in ultrasound. OCT can image nuclear and intracellular morphology as well as identify cells in different stages of mitosis and visualize mitotic activity.

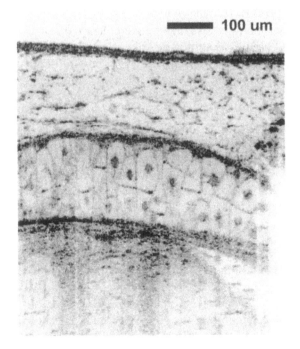

Figure 19 High resolution OCT images of a *Xenopus laevis* (African frog) tadpole in vivo performed with 1 μm axial and 3 μm transverse resolution. An image fusion technique is used to overcome depth-of-field limitations associated with the high transverse resolution. Individual cells and nuclei are clearly visible. Cellular level imaging has important implications for a variety of OCT applications. (See Refs. 112 and 22.)

The ability to image subcellular structure can be an important tool for studying mitotic activity and cell migration in developmental biology. The extension of these results to human cells has important implications. Because differentiated human cells are smaller than developing cells, additional improvements in resolution and performance are necessary. In ophthalmology, improving the resolution should improve morphometric measurements such as retinal thickness and retinal nerve fiber layer thickness, which are relevant for the detection of macular edema and glaucoma. High resolution imaging also has implications for diagnosis of neoplasia. Standard OCT image resolutions enable the imaging of architectural morphology on the 10–15 μm scale and can identify many early neoplastic changes. The extension of imaging to the cellular and subcellular levels would not only enhance the spectrum of early neoplasias and dysplasias that could be imaged but also improve sensitivity and specificity.

1.13 SUMMARY

Optical coherence tomography is a fundamentally new imaging modality with rapidly emerging applications spanning a range of fields. OCT can perform micrometer-scale imaging of internal microstructure in materials and biological tissues *in situ* and in real time. For medical imaging applications, OCT can function as a type of optical biopsy to obtain microstructural information with resolution approaching that of conventional histopathology. Image information is available immediately without the need for excise and histological processing of a specimen. The development of high speed OCT technology now permits real-time imaging with high pixel densities. A wide range of OCT imaging platforms and probes have been developed, including ophthalmoscopes, microscopes, laparoscopes, hand-held probes, and miniature, flexible catheter-endoscopes. These imaging probes can be used either separately or in conjunction with other medical imaging instruments such as endoscopes and bronchoscopes and can permit internal body imaging in a wide range of organ systems. There are numerous research applications of this technology in a broad range of fields as well as continuing development of the technology itself. More research remains to be done, and numerous clinical studies must be performed to identify the clinical situations in which OCT can play a role. However, the unique capabilities of OCT imaging suggest that it could have a significant impact on fundamental research as well as on health care.

ACKNOWLEDGMENTS

Our research would not have been possible without the long-term collaboration and support of a talented multidisciplinary research team. The invaluable contributions of Dr. Mark Brezinski of the Massachusetts General Hospital and Harvard Medical School, Dr. Joel Schuman and Dr. Carmen Puliafito of the New England Eye Center and Tufts University School of Medicine, and Eric Swanson of Coherent Diagnostic Technology are greatly appreciated. We acknowledge the contributions of visiting scientists, including Dr. Wolfgang Drexler of the University of Vienna, Dr. Juergen Herrmann of the University of Erlangen, and Stephan Kubasiak of the Laser Medical Center of Lubeck. Present and former group members—postdoctoral associates, MD/PhD students, and PhD students, including Dr. Stephen Boppart,

Dr. Brett Bouma, Ravi Ghanta, Dr. David Huang, Dr. Michael Hee, Christine Jesser, Dr. Xingde Li, Constantinos Pitris, and Dr. Gary Tearney—have made invaluable contributions. This research has been supported in part by the National Institutes of Health, contracts NIH-1-RO1-CA75289-02 and NIH-1-RO1-EY11289-13, the Medical Free Electron Laser Program, Office of Naval Research contract N000014-97-1-1066, and the Air Force Office of Scientific Research, contract F4920-98-1-0139.

REFERENCES

1. Kremkau FW. Diagnostic Ultrasound: Principles, Instrumentation, and Exercises. 2nd ed. Philadelphia: Grune and Stratton, 1984.
2. Fish P. Physics and Instrumentation of Diagnostic Medical Ultrasound. New York: Wiley, 1990.
3. Kremkau FW. Doppler Ultrasound: Principles and Instruments. Philadelphia: WB Saunders, 1990.
4. Zwiebel WJ. Introduction to Vascular Ultrasonography. 3rd ed. Philadelphia: WB Saunders, 1992.
5. Erbel R, Roelandt JRTC, Ge J, Gorge G. Intravascular Ultrasound. London: Martin Dunitz, 1998.
6. Huang D, Swanson EA, Lin CP, Schuman JS, Stinson WG, Chang W, Hee MR, Flotte T, Gregory K, Puliafito CA, Fujimoto JG. Optical coherence tomography. Science 254:1178–1181, 1991.
7. Duguay MA, Hansen JW. Optical sampling of subnanosecond light pulses. Appl Phys Lett 13:178–180, 1968.
8. Duguay MA, Mattick AT. Ultrahigh speed photography of picosecond light pulses and echoes. Appl Opt 10:2162–2170, 1971.
9. Duguay MA. Light photographed in flight. Am Sci 59:551–556, 1971.
10. Bruckner AP. Picosecond light scattering measurements of cataract microstructure. Appl Opt 17:3177–3183, 1978.
11. Park H, Chodorow M, Kompfner R. High resolution optical ranging system. Appl Opt 20:2389–2394, 1981.
12. Fujimoto JG, De Silvestri S, Ippen EP, Puliafito CA, Margolis R, Oseroff A. Femtosecond optical ranging in biological systems. Opt Lett 11:150–152, 1986.
13. Youngquist RC, Carr S, Davies DEN. Optical coherence-domain reflectometry: A new optical evaluation technique. Opt Lett 12:158–160, 1987.
14. Takada K, Yokohama I, Chida K, Noda J. New measurement system for fault location in optical waveguide devices based on an interferometric technique. Appl Opt 26:1603–1606, 1987.
15. Gilgen HH, Novak RP, Salathe RP, Hodel W, Beaud P. Submillimeter optical reflectometry. IEEE J Lightwave Technol 7:1225–1233, 1989.
16. Fercher AF, Mengedoht K, Werner W. Eye-length measurement by interferometry with partially coherent light. Opt Lett 13:1867–1869, 1988.
17. Clivaz X, Marquis-Weible F, Salathe RP, Novak RP, Gilgen HH. High resolution reflectometry in biological tissues. Optics Lett 17:4–6, 1992.
18. Schmitt JM, Knuttel A, Bonner RF. Measurement of optical properties of biological tissues by low-coherence reflectometry. Appl Opt 32:6032–6042, 1993.
19. Hitzenberger CK. Optical measurement of the axial eye length by laser Doppler interferometry. Invest Ophthalmol Vis Sci 32:616–624, 1991.

20. Huang D, Wang J, Lin CP, Puliafito CA, Fujimoto JG. Micro-resolution ranging of cornea and anterior chamber by optical reflectometry. Lasers Surg Med 11:419–425, 1991.

21. Schmitt JM, Lee SL, Yung KM. An optical coherence microscope with enhanced resolving power in thick tissue. Optics Commun. 142:4–6, 203–207, Oct. 1997.

22. Drexler W, Morgner U, Kaertner FX, Pitris C, Boppart SA, Li XD, Ippen EP, Fujimoto JG. In vivo ultrahigh resolution optical coherence tomography. Opt Lett 24:1221–1223, 1999.

23. Podoleanu AG, Dobre GM, Webb DJ, Jackson DA. Simultaneous en-face imaging of two layers in the human retina by low-coherence reflectometry. Opt Lett 22:1039–1041, 1997.

24. Podoleanu AG, Dobre GM, Jackson DA. En-face coherence imaging using galvanometer scanner modulation. Opt Lett 23:147–149, 1998.

25. Hee MR, Izatt JA, Swanson EA, Huang D, Schuman JS, Lin CP, Puliafito CA, Fujimoto JG. Optical coherence tomography of the human retina. Arch Ophthalmol 113:325–332, 1995.

26. American National Standards Institute. Safe Use of Lasers. New York: ANSI, 1993.

27. Chinn SR, Swanson EA. Multi-layer optical readout using direct or interferometric detection and broad-bandwidth light sources. Opt Memory Neural Networks 5:197–217, 1996.

28. Swanson EA, Izatt JA, Hee MR, Huang D, Lin CP, Schuman JS, Puliafito CA, Fujimoto JG. In vivo retinal imaging by optical coherence tomography. Opt Lett 18:1864–1866, 1993.

29. Schmitt JM, Knuttel A, Yadlowsky M, Eckhaus MA. Optical coherence tomography of a dense tissue: Statistics of attenuation and backscattering. Phys Med Biol 39:1705–1720, 1994.

30. Schmitt JM, Yadlowsky M, Bonner RF. Subsurface imaging of living skin with optical coherence tomography. Dermatology 191:93–98, 1995.

31. Fujimoto JG, Brezinski ME, Tearney GJ, Boppart SA, Bouma B, Hee MR, Southern JF, Swanson EA. Optical biopsy and imaging using optical coherence tomography. Nature Med 1:970–972, 1995.

32. Brezinski ME, Tearney GJ, Bouma BE, Izatt JA, Hee MR, Swanson EA, Southern JF, Fujimoto JG. Optical coherence tomography for optical biopsy: Properties and demonstration of vascular pathology. Circulation 93:1206–1213, 1996.

33. Parsa P, Jacques SL, Nishioka NS. Optical properties of rat liver between 350 and 2200 nm. Appl Opt 28:2325–2330, 1989.

34. Schmitt JM, Knuttel A. Model of optical coherent tomography of heterogeneous tissue. J Opt Soc Am A 14:1231–1242, 1997.

35. Izatt JA, Kulkami MD, Yazdanfar S, Barton JK, Welch AJ. In vivo bidirectional color Doppler flow imaging of picoliter blood volumes using optical coherence tomography. Opt Lett 22:1439–1441, 1997.

36. Chen Z, Milner TE, Dave D, Nelson JS. Optical Doppler tomographic imaging of fluid flow velocity in highly scattering media. Opt Lett 22:64–66, 1997.

37. Chen Z, Milner TE, Srinivas S, Wang X, Malekafzali A, van Gemert MJC, Nelson JS. Noninvasive imaging of in vivo blood flow velocity using optical Doppler tomography. Opt Lett 22:1119–1121, 1997.

38. Kulkarni MD, van Leeuwen TG, Yazdanfar S, Izatt JA. Velocity-estimation accuracy and frame-rate limitations in color Doppler optical coherence tomography. Opt Lett 23:1057–1059, 1998.

39. Hee MR, Huang D, Swanson EA, Fujimoto JG. Polarization-sensitive low-coherence reflectometer for birefringence characterization and ranging. J. Opt Soc Am B 9:903–908, 1992.

40. de Boer JF, Milner TE, van Gemert MJC, Nelson JS. Two-dimensional birefringence imaging in biological tissue by polarization-sensitive optical coherence tomography. Opt Lett 22:934–936, 1997.

41. Everett MJ, Schoenenberger K, Colston BW, Da Silva LB. Birefringence characterization of biological tissue by use of optical coherence tomography. Opt Lett 23:228–230, 1998.

42. Hausler G, Lindner MW. Coherent radar and spectral radar: New tools for dermatological diagnosis. J Biomed Opt 3:21–31, 1998.

43. Bouma BE, Tearney GJ, Bilinsky IP, Golubovic B. Self phase modulated Kerr-lens mode locked Cr:forsterite laser source for optical coherent tomography. Opt Lett 21:1839–1841, 1996.

44. Bouma B, Tearney GJ, Boppart SA, Hee MR, Brezinski ME, Fujimoto JG. High-resolution optical coherence tomographic imaging using a mode-locked Ti-Al$_2$O$_3$ laser source. Opt Lett 20:1486–1488, 1995.

45. Swanson EA, Huang D, Hee MR, Fujimoto JG, Lin CP, Puliafito CA. High-speed optical coherence domain reflectometry. Opt Lett 17:151–153, 1992.

46. Sergeev AM, Gelikonov VM, Gelikonov GV, Feldchtein FI, Kuranov REV, Gladkova ND, Shakhova NM, Snopova LB, Shakov AV, Kuznetzova IA. Denisenko AN, Pochinko VV, Chumakov YP, Streltzova OS. In vivo endoscopic OCT imaging of precancer and cancer states of human mucosa. Opt Express 1:432, 1997.

47. Tearney GJ, Bouma BE, Boppart SA, Golubovic B, Swanson EA, Fujimoto JG. Rapid acquisition of in vivo biological images by use of optical coherence tomography. Opt Lett 21:1408–1410, 1996.

48. Tearney GJ, Bouma BE, Fujimoto JG. High-speed phase- and group-delay scanning with a grating-based phase control delay line. Opt Lett 22:1811–1813, 1997.

49. Weiner AM, Heritage JP, Kirschner EM. High resolution femtosecond pulse shaping. J Opt Soc Am B 5:1563–1572, 1986.

50. Tearney GJ, Brezinski ME, Bouma BE, Boppart SA, Pitris C, Southern JF, Fujimoto JG. In vivo endoscopic optical biopsy with optical coherence tomography. Science 276:2037–2039, 1997.

51. Puliafito CA, Hee MR, Schuman JS, Fujimoto JG. Optical coherence tomography of ocular diseases. Thorofare, NJ: Slack Inc, 1996.

52. Brezinski ME, Tearney GJ, Boppart SA, Swanson EA, Southern JF, Fujimoto JG. Optical biopsy with optical coherence tomography, feasibility for surgical diagnostics. J Surg Res 71:32–40, 1997.

53. Boppart SA, Brezinski ME, Bouma BE, Tearney GJ, Fujimoto JG. Investigation of developing embryonic morphology using optical coherence tomography. Dev Biol 177:54–63, 1996.

54. Boppart SA, Bouma BE, Pitris C, Southern JF, Brezinski ME, Fujimoto JG. Intraoperative assessment of microsurgery with three-dimensional optical coherence tomography. Radiology 208:81–86, 1998.

55. Boppart SA, Herrmann J, Pitris C, Stamper DL, Brezinski ME, Fujimoto JG. High-resolution optical coherence tomography-guided laser ablation of surgical tissue. J Surg Res 82:275–284, 1999.

56. Boppart SA, Bouma BE, Pitris C, Tearney GJ, Fujimoto JG, Brezinski ME. Forward-imaging instruments for optical coherence tomography. Opt Lett 22:1618–1620, 1997.

57. Feldchtein FI, Gelikonov GV, Gelikonov VM, Kuranov RV, Sergeev A, Gladkova ND, Shakhov AV, Shakova NM, Snopova LB. Terent'eva AB, Zagainova EV, Chumakov YP, Kuznetzova IA. Endoscopic applications of optical coherence tomography. Opt Express 3:257, 1998.

58. Tearney GJ, Boppart SA, Bouma BE, Brezinski ME, Weissman NJ, Southern JF, Fujimoto JG. Scanning single-mode fiber optic catheter-endoscope for optical coherence tomography. Opt Lett 21:543–545, 1996.

59. Bouma BE, Tearney GJ. Power-efficient nonreciprocal interferometer and linear-scanning fiber-optical catheter for optical coherence tomography. Opt Lett 24:531–533, 1999.

60. Tearney GJ, Brezinski ME, Southern JF, Bouma BE, Boppart SA, Fujimoto JG. Optical biopsy in human gastrointestinal tissue using optical coherence tomography. Am J Gastroenterol 92:1800–1804, 1997.

61. Fujimoto JG, Boppart SA, Tearney GJ, Bouma BE, Pitris C, Brezinski ME. High resolution in vivo intraarterial imaging with optical coherence tomography. Heart 82:128–133, 1999.

62. Kulkarni MD, Thomas CW, Izatt JA. Image enhancement in optical coherence tomography using deconvolution. Electron Lett 33:1365–1367, 1997.

63. Schmitt JM. Restoration of optical coherence images of living tissue using the CLEAN algorithm. J Biomed Opt 3:66–75, 1998.

64. Schmitt JM, Xiang SH, Yung KM. Speckle in optical coherence tomography. J Biomed Opt 4:95–105, 1999.

65. Schuman JS, Hee MR, Puliafito CA, Wong C, Pedut-Kloizman T, Lin CP, Hertzmark E, Izatt JA, Swanson EA, Fujimoto JG. Quantification of nerve fiber layer thickness in normal and glaucomatous eyes using optical coherence tomography. Arch Ophthalmol 113:586–596, 1995.

66. Schuman JS, Hee MR, Arya AV, Pedut-Kloizman T, Puliafito CA, Fujimoto JG, Swanson EA. Optical coherence tomography: A new tool for glaucoma diagnosis. Curr Opin Ophthalmol 6:89–95, 1995.

67. Fercher AF, Hitzenberger CK, Drexler W, Kamp G, Sattmann H. In vivo optical coherence tomography. Am J Ophthalmol 116:113–114, 1993.

68. Izatt JA, Hee MR, Swanson EA, Lin CP, Huang D, Schuman JS, Puliafito CA, Fujimoto JG. Micrometer-scale resolution imaging of the anterior eye in vivo with optical coherence tomography. Arch Ophthalmol 112:1584–1589, 1994.

69. Puliafito CA, Hee, MR, Lin CP, Reichel E, Schuman JS, Duker JS, Izatt JA, Swanson EA, Fujimoto JG. Imaging of macular diseases with optical coherence tomography. Ophthalmology 102:217–229, 1995.

70. Hee MR, Puliafito CA, Wong C, Duker JS, Reichel E, Rutledge B, Schuman JS, Swanson EA, Fujimoto JG. Quantitative assessment of macular edema with optical coherence tomography. Arch Ophthalmol 113:1019–1029, 1995.

71. Hee MR, Puliafito CA, Wong C, Duker JS, Reichel E, Schuman JS, Swanson EA, Fujimoto JG. Optical coherence tomography of macular holes. Ophthalmology 102:748–756, 1995.

72. Hee MR, Puliafito CA, Wong C, Reichel E, Duker JS, Schuman JS, Swanson EA, Fujimoto JG. Optical coherence tomography of central serous chorioretinopathy. Am J Ophthalmol 120:65–74, 1995.

73. Hee MR, Baumal CR, Puliafito CA, Duker JS, Reichel E, Wilkins JR, Coker JG, Schuman JS, Swanson EA, Fujimoto JG. Optical coherence tomography of age-related macular degeneration and choroidal neovascularization. Ophthalmology 103:1260–1270, 1996.

74. Schuman JS, Noecker RJ. Imaging of the optic nerve head and nerve fiber layer in glaucoma. Ophthalmol Clin N Am 8:259–279, 1995.

75. Schuman JS, Pedut-Kloizman T, Hertzmark E, Hee MR, Wilkins JR, Coker JG, Puliafito CA, Fujimoto JG, Swanson EA. Reproducibility of nerve fiber layer thickness measurements using optical coherence tomography. Ophthalmology 103:1889–1898, 1996.

76. Schaudig U, Hassenstein A, Bernd A, Walter A, Richard G. Limitations of imaging choroidal tumors in vivo by optical coherence tomography. Graefe's Arch Clin Exp Ophthalmol 236:588–592, 1998.

77. Krivoy D, Gentile R, Liebmann JM, Stegman Z, Walsh JB, Ritch R. Imaging congenital optic disc pits and associated maculopathy using optical coherence tomography. Arch Ophthalmol 114:165–170, 1996.

78. Lincoff H, Kreissig I. Optical coherence tomography of pneumatic displacement of optic disc pit maculopathy. Br J Ophthalmol 82:367–372, 1998.

79. Toth Ca, Birngruber R, Boppart SA, Hee MR, Fujimoto JG, DiCarlo CD, Swanson EA, Cain CP, Narayan DG, Noojin GD, Roach WP. Argon laser retinal lesions evaluated in vivo by optical coherence tomography. Am J Ophthalmol 123:188–198, 1997.

80. Toth CA, Narayan DG, Boppart SA, Hee MR, Fujimoto JG, Birngruber R, Cain CP, DiCarlo CD, Roach WP. A comparison of retinal morphology viewed by optical coherence tomography and by light microscopy. Arch Ophthalmol 115:1425–1428, 1997.

81. Huang Y, Cideciyan AV, Papstergiou GI, Banin E, Semple-Rowland SL, Milam AH, Jacobson SG. Relation of optical coherence tomography to microanatomy in normal and rd chickens. Invest Ophthalmol Visual Sci 39:2405–2416, 1998.

82. Hee MR, Puliafito CA, Duker JS, Reichel E, Coker JG, Wilkins JR, Schuman JS, Swanson EA, Fujimoto JG. Topography of diabetic macular edema with optical coherence tomography. Ophthalmology 105:360–370, 1998.

83. Brezinski ME, Tearney GJ, Weissman NJ, Boppart SA, Bouma BE, Hee MR, Weyman AE, Swanson EA, Southern JF, Fujimoto JG. Assessing atherosclerotic plaque morphology: Comparison of optical coherence tomography and high frequency intravascular ultrasound. Br Heart J 77:397–404, 1997.

84. Falk E. Plaque rupture with severe pre-existing stenosis precipitating coronary thrombosis, characteristics of coronary atherosclerotic plaques underlying fatal occlusive thrombi. Br Heart J 50:127–134, 1983.

85. Davies MJ, Thomas AC. Plaque fissuring: The cause of acute myocardial infarction, sudden ischemic death, and crescendo angina. Br Heart J 53:363–373, 1983.

86. Richardson PD, Davies MJ, Born GVR. Influence of plaque configuration and stress distribution on fissuring of coronary atherosclerotic plaques. Lancet i:941–944, 1989.

87. Fuster VL, Badimon L, Badimon JJ, et al. The pathogenesis of coronary artery disease and the acute coronary syndromes. N Engl J Med 326:242–249, 1992.

88. Loree HM, Lee R. Stress analysis of unstable plaque. Circ Res 71:850, 1992.

89. Gillum RF. Sudden coronary death in the United States; 1980–1985. Circulation 79:756–764, 1989.

90. Nissen SE, Gurley JC, Booth DC, Demaria AN. Intravascular ultrasound of the coronary arteries: Current applications and future directions. Am J Cardiol 69:18H–29H, 1992.

91. Lee D-Y, Eigler N, Luo H, Steffen W, Tabak S, Seigel RJ. Intravascular coronary ultrasound imaging, is it useful? J Am College Cardiol Suppl: 241A, 1994.

92. Benkeser PH, Churchwell AL, Lee C, Aboucinaser DM. Resolution limitations in intravascular ultrasound imaging. J Am Soc Echocardiol 6:158–165, 1993.

93. Izatt JA, Kulkarni MD, Hsing-Wen W, Kobayashi K, Sivak MV Jr. Optical coherence tomography and microscopy in gastrointestinal tissues. IEEE J Selected Topics Quantum Electron 2:1017–1028, 1996.

94. Tearney GJ, Brezinski ME, Southern JF, Bouma BE, Boppart SA, Fujimoto JG. Optical biopsy in human urologic tissue using optical coherence tomography. J Urol 157:1915–1919, 1997.

95. Tearney GJ, Brezinski ME, Southern JF, Bouma BE, Boppart SA, Fujimoto JG. Optical biopsy in human pancreatobiliary tissue using optical coherence tomography. Dig Dis Sci 43:1193–1199, 1998.

96. Kobayashi K, Izatt JA, Kulkarni MD, Willis J, Sivak MV. High-resolution cross-sectional imaging of the gastrointestinal tract using optical coherence tomography: Preliminary results. Gastrointest Endosci 47:515–523, 1998.

97. Pitris C, Brezinski ME, Bouma BE, Tearney GJ, Southern JF, Fujimoto JG. High resolution imaging of the upper respiratory tract with optical coherence tomography: A feasibility study. Am J Respir Crit Care Med 157:1640–1644, 1998.

98. Pitris C, Goodman A, Boppart SA, Libus JJ, Fujimoto JG, Brezinski ME. High-resolution imaging of gynecologic neoplasms using optical coherence tomography. Obstet Gynecol 93:135–139, 1999.

99. Pitris C, Jesser C, Boppart SA, Stamper D, Brezinski ME, Fujimoto JG. Feasibility of optical coherence tomography for high resolution imaging of human gastrointestinal tract malignancies. J Gastroenterol. 35:87–92, 2000.

100. Jesser CA, Pitris C, Stamper DL, Boppart SA, Nielsen GP, Brezinski ME, Fujimoto JG. High resolution endoscopic evaluation of transitional cell carcinoma with optical coherence tomography. Br J Radiol. 72:1170–1176, 1999.

101. Boppart SA, Goodman A, Libus J, Pitris C, Jesser C, Brezinski ME, Fujimoto JG. High resolution imaging of endometriosis and ovarian carcinoma with optical coherence tomography: Feasibility for laparoscopic-based imaging. Br J Obstet Gynecol 1999.

102. Feldchtein FI, Gelikonov GV, Gelikonov VM, Iksanov RR, Kuranov RV, Sergeev AM, Gladkova ND, Ourutina MN, Warren JA, Reitze DH. In vivo OCT imaging of hard and soft tissue of the oral cavity. Opt Express 3:239–250, 1998.

103. Kimmey MB, Martin RW, Haggitt RC, et al. Histologic correlates of gastrointestinal ultrasound images. Gastroenterology 96:433–441, 1989.

104. Botet JF, Lightdale C. Endoscopic ultrasonography of the upper gastrointestinal tract. Radiol Clin N Am 30:1067–1083, 1992.

105. Hawes RH. New staging techniques: Endoscopic ultrasound. Cancer 71:4207–4213, 1993.

106. Furukawa T, Naitoh Y, Tsukamoto Y. New technique using intraductal ultrasound for diagnosis of disease of the pancreatobiliary system. J Ultrasound Med 11:607–612, 1992.

107. Rosh T. Endoscopic ultrasonography. Endoscopy 26:148–168, 1994.

108. Falk GW, Catalano MF, Sivak MV, Rice TW, Van Dam J. Endosonography in the evaluation of patients with Barrett's esophagus and high grade dysplasia. Gastrointest Endosc 40:207–212, 1994.

109. Hizawa K, Suekane H, Aoyagi K, Matsumoto T, Nakamura S, Fujishima M. Use of endosonographic evaluation of colorectal tumor depth in determining the appropriateness of endoscopic mucosal resection. Am J Gastroenterol 91:768–771, 1996.

110. Wiersema MJ, Wiersema LM. High-resolution 25-MHz ultrasonography of the gastrointestinal wall: Histologic correlates. Gastrointest Endosc 39:499–504, 1993.

111. Yanai H, Tada M, Karita M. Okita K. Diagnostic utility of 20-megahertz linear endoscopic ultrasonography in early gastric cancer. Gastrointest Endosc 44:29–33, 1996.

112. Boppart SA, Bouma BE, Pitris C, Southern JF, Brezinski ME, Fujimoto JG. In vivo cellular optical coherence tomography imaging. Nat Med 4:861–865, 1998.

113. Rollins AM, Chak A, Wong CK, Kobayashi K, Sivak MV, Ung-arunyawee R, Izatt JA. Real-time in vivo imaging of gastrointestinal ultrastructure using endoscopic optical coherence tomography with a novel efficient interferometer design. Opt Lett. Vol. 24, 19:1358–1360, 1999.

2

Optical Coherence Tomography: Theory

MICHAEL R. HEE

University of California, San Francisco, California

2.1 INTRODUCTION

In optical coherence tomography (OCT), the principles of interferometry with low temporal coherence light and optical heterodyne detection are combined to obtain both a high axial resolution and a high sensitivity to light that is weakly reflected from the sample being imaged. This chapter will describe the fundamental laws that govern the axial resolution and sensitivity of OCT. In particular, the axial resolution will be shown to be inversely related to the spectral bandwidth of the light source used for imaging. For the case of a sample that is free from optical dispersion, the system's axial point spread function (PSF) will be shown to be exactly the Fourier transform pair of the power spectrum of the light source. Chromatic dispersion degrades both the axial PSF and the detection sensitivity.

In addition, typical electronic circuits for detection and filtering will be presented. The fundamental noise characteristics of these circuits will be derived and used to discuss how the OCT system can be designed to achieve a detection sensitivity that approaches the quantum limit of a single photon. The four fundamental design parameters—axial resolution, sensitivity to weakly reflected light, optical power incident on the sample, and image acquisition time—will be shown to be linearly related and constrained by the quantum detection limit.

2.2 LOW COHERENCE INTERFEROMETRY AND AXIAL RESOLUTION

A schematic diagram of a simplified OCT system is shown in Fig. 1. Low coherence light is coupled into a fiber-optic Michelson interferometer and is divided at a fiber coupler into reference and sample paths. Light retroreflected from a scanning reference mirror is recombined in the coupler with light backscattered from the sample under interrogation. Time-of-flight information is contained in the interference signal between the reference and sample beams, which is detected by a photodiode followed by signal processing electronics and computer data acquisition.

A single axial profile of optical reflectivity versus distance into the sample is obtained by rapidly translating the reference arm mirror and synchronously recording the magnitude of the resulting interference signal. Interference fringes are evident only when the reference arm distance matches the length of a relative path through the sample to within the coherence length of the light source. Thus, the coherence length, which is a fundamental property of the light source, determines the axial ranging resolution. Cross-sectional images are constructed from a sequence of axial reflectivity profiles obtained while scanning the probe beam across the sample.

Low coherence interferometry allows the position of reflective boundaries within the sample to be precisely located. This section will derive the Fourier transform relationship between the power spectrum of the light source and the axial PSF. Chromatic dispersion will be shown to degrade this resolution by broadening the axial PSF in direct analogy to the case of short-pulse propagation through dispersive media.

2.2.1 Interferometer with Coherent Light

Consider the simplified schematic of the Michelson interferometer shown in Fig. 2, where the sample has been replaced by a perfectly reflecting mirror. Light from the source is divided at a beamsplitter into reference and sample beams. Light reflected

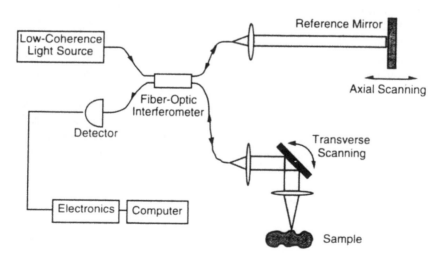

Figure 1   Schematic of the OCT system.

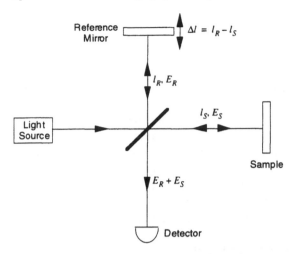

Figure 2 The Michelson interferometer.

from the reference and sample mirrors is recombined at the same beamsplitter and incident on a detector. The reference and sample mirrors are positioned at distances l_R and l_S, respectively, from the beamsplitter. If the light source is perfectly coherent (i.e., monochromatic), then reflection from the reference and sample mirrors produces a sum of two monochromatic electric field components E_S and E_R at the detector. These fields may be expressed by the phasors

$$E_R = A_R \exp\left[-j(2\beta_R l_R - \omega t)\right] \quad \text{and} \quad E_S = A_S \exp\left[-j(2\beta_S l_S - \omega t)\right] \quad (1)$$

where ω is the optical frequency of the light source and β is the propagation constant. The factors of 2 multiplying the propagation constants β_R and β_S arise from the round-trip propagation of light to and from the reference and sample mirrors.

Note that E_R and E_S represent the field components in the interferometer *after* reflection and recombination at the beamsplitter, which eliminates the necessity of considering the split ratio and phase shift of the beam splitter. In general, the time-averaged photocurrent I at the detector is given by

$$I = \left\langle \frac{\eta e}{h\nu}\left(\frac{|E_R + E_S|^2}{2\eta_0}\right)\right\rangle \quad (2)$$

where η is the detector quantum efficiency, e is the electronic charge, $h\nu$ is the photon energy, and η_0 is the intrinsic impedance of free space. For monochromatic fields, Eq. (2) can be written

$$I = \frac{\eta e}{h\nu}\left(\frac{1}{\eta_0}\right)\left[\frac{1}{2}|A_R|^2 + \frac{1}{2}|A_S|^2 + \text{real}\{E_S E_R^*\}\right] \quad (3)$$

where the term

$$\text{real}\{E_S E_R^*\} = A_R A_S \cos(2\beta_R l_R - 2\beta_S l_S) \quad (4)$$

describes the variation of the photocurrent with the positions of the reference and sample mirrors. In free space, the propagation constants are equal for the reference and sample fields, giving $\beta_R = \beta_S = 2\pi/\lambda$ and

$$\text{real}\left\{E_S E_R^*\right\} = A_R A_S \cos\left(2\pi \frac{\Delta l}{\lambda/2}\right) \tag{5}$$

where $\Delta l = l_S - l_R$ is the mismatch in distance between the reference and sample beam paths. Equation (5) shows that the photocurrent contains a sinusoidally varying term representing the interference between the reference and sample fields. The interference has a period of $\lambda/2$ relative to the length mismatch Δl.

Because all of the interference information is contained in the real part of the cross-spectral term $E_S E_R^*$, subsequent analysis of interferometry in the case of low coherence light source will focus on calculating this term only.

2.2.2 Interferometer with Low Coherence Light

A low coherence light source consists of a finite bandwidth of frequencies rather than just a single frequency. The analysis in Section 2.2.1 can be extended to account for partially coherent light by integrating the cross-spectral term $E_S E_R^*$ over the harmonic content of the light source. We allow the reference and sample fields to be functions of frequency:

$$E_R(\omega) = A_R(\omega)\exp^{\{-j[2\beta_R(\omega)l_R - \omega t]\}}$$

$$E_S(\omega) = A_S(\omega)\exp\left\{-j[2\beta_S(\omega)l_S - \omega t]\right\} \tag{6}$$

The interference signal at the photodetector is proportional to the sum of the interference due to each monochromatic plane wave component, according to

$$I \propto \text{real}\left\{\int_{-\infty}^{\infty} E_S(\omega)E_R(\omega)^* \frac{d\omega}{2\pi}\right\} = \text{real}\left\{\int_{-\infty}^{\infty} S(\omega)\exp\left[-j\Delta\phi(\omega)\right]\frac{d\omega}{2\pi}\right\} \tag{7}$$

where we have used the definitions

$$S(\omega) = A_S(\omega)A_R(\omega)^*) \tag{8}$$

and

$$\Delta\phi(\omega) = 2\beta_S(\omega)l_S - 2\beta_R(\omega)l_R \tag{9}$$

If the sample and reference arm fields have the same spectral components as the light source (i.e., if the reflectors in each arm and the fiber beamsplitter are spectrally uniform), then $S(\omega)$ is essentially equivalent to the power spectrum of the light source. $\Delta(\omega)$ expresses the phase mismatch at the detector of each frequency component. We will show that Eq. (7) expresses a fundamental inverse Fourier transform relation between the source spectrum and the detector photocurrent.

2.2.3 Nondispersive Medium

Consider the case where the sample and reference arms consist of a uniform, linear, nondispersive material. Let the spectrum of the light source $S(\omega - \omega_0)$ be band-limited with a center frequency of ω_0. We assume that the propagation constants

β in each arm are the same and rewrite them as first-order Taylor expansions around the center frequency:

$$\beta_S(\omega) = \beta_R(\omega) = \beta(\omega_0) + \beta'(\omega_0)(\omega - \omega_0) \tag{10}$$

Then the phase mismatch $\Delta\phi(\omega)$ in Eq. (9) is determined solely by the length mismatch $\Delta l = l_S - l_R$ between the reference and sample arms through

$$\Delta\phi(\omega) = \beta(\omega_0)(2\Delta l) + \beta'(\omega_0)(\omega - \omega_0)(2\Delta l) \tag{11}$$

The integral over the power spectral density in Eq. (7) becomes

$$I \propto \text{real} \left\{ \exp\left[-j\omega_0 \,\Delta\tau_p\right] \int_{-\infty}^{\infty} S(\omega - \omega_0) \exp\left[-j(\omega - \omega_0)\,\Delta\tau_g\right] \frac{d(\omega - \omega_0)}{2\pi} \right\} \tag{12}$$

where the phase delay mismatch $\Delta\tau_p$ and the group delay mismatch $\Delta\tau_g$ are defined as

$$\Delta\tau_p = \frac{\beta(\omega_0)}{\omega_0}(2\Delta l) = \frac{2\Delta l}{v_p} \tag{13}$$

and

$$\Delta\tau_g = \beta'(\omega_0)(2\Delta l) = \frac{2\Delta l}{v_g} \tag{14}$$

Thus, $v_p = \omega_0/\beta(\omega_0)$ corresponds to the center frequency phase velocity and $v_g = 1/\beta'(\omega_0)$ is the group velocity. Equation (12) is basically a statement of the familiar Wiener–Khintchin theorem: The autocorrelation function is equal to the inverse Fourier transform of the power spectral density. Equations (12)–(14) show that the interferometric term of the photocurrent consists of a carrier and an envelope. The carrier oscillates with increasing path length mismatch $2\Delta l$ at a spatial frequency of $\beta(\omega_0)$. The envelope, which determines the axial point spread function of the interferometer, is essentially the inverse Fourier transform of the source power spectrum $S(\omega - \omega_0)$.

Gaussian Power Spectrum and Nondispersive Medium

Assume that the light source has a Gaussian power spectral density given by

$$S(\omega - \omega_0) = \left(\frac{2\pi}{\sigma_\omega^2}\right)^{\frac{1}{2}} \exp\left[-\frac{(\omega - \omega_0)^2}{2\sigma_\omega^2}\right] \tag{15}$$

which has been normalized to unit power,

$$\int_{-\infty}^{\infty} S(\omega) \frac{d\omega}{2\pi} = 1 \tag{16}$$

and where ω_0 is defined as the center frequency and $2\sigma_\omega$ is the standard deviation power spectral bandwidth (radians per second). Substitution of this power spectrum into Eq. (12) gives the interferometric photocurrent.

$$I \propto \exp\left[-\frac{\Delta\tau^2}{2\sigma_\tau^2}\right] \exp\left[-j\omega_0 \Delta\tau_p\right] \tag{17}$$

where the real { } notation has been discarded for convenience. The photocurrent contains a Gaussian envelope with a characteristic standard deviation temporal width $2\sigma_\tau$ (seconds) that is inversely proportional to the power spectral bandwidth:

$$2\sigma_\tau = \frac{2}{\sigma_\omega} \tag{18}$$

Note that $\sigma_\tau \sigma_\omega = 1$ (i.e., the time–frequency uncertainty relation is minimized for a Gaussian waveform). The envelope falls off quickly with increasing group delay mismatch $\Delta\tau_g$ and is modulated by interference fringes that oscillate with increasing phase delay mismatch $\Delta\tau_p$. Thus, Eq.(17) defines the axial resolving properties of the OCT system. The detector sees interference fringes only when the reference and sample arm lengths are matched, so the group delay mismatch falls within the Gaussian envelope:

$$-\sigma_\tau < \beta'(\omega_0)(2\Delta l) < \sigma_\tau \tag{19}$$

The standard deviation axial resolution, or width of the axial point spread function (i.e., the $\pm\sigma_\tau$ width of the Gaussian envelope in units of length mismatch Δl) is, from Eqs. (14), (18), and (19),

$$\Delta l_{\mathrm{SD}} = \frac{1}{\beta'(\omega_0)\sigma_\omega} = \frac{v_g}{\sigma_\omega} \tag{20}$$

For propagation in free space, both the phase velocity and group velocity equal the speed of light c, and Eq. (20) reduces to

$$\Delta l_{\mathrm{SD}} = \frac{c}{\sigma_\omega} \tag{21}$$

showing that the axial resolution is inversely proportional to the bandwidth.

For measurements of bandwidth and resolution, a full-width at half-maximum (FWHM) criterion is more convenient than a standard deviation measure. For a Gaussian with standard deviation σ, the FWHM equals $2\sigma\sqrt{2\ln 2}$. Thus, for the interferometer in free space, the FWHM resolution Δl_{FWHM} is related to the FWHM wavelength bandwidth $\Delta\lambda$ for a Gaussian source by

$$\Delta l_{\mathrm{FWHM}} = \frac{2\ln 2}{\pi}\left(\frac{\lambda_0^2}{\Delta\lambda}\right) \tag{22}$$

where λ_0 is the center wavelength.

2.2.4 Group Velocity Dispersion

Group velocity dispersion (GVD) causes different frequencies to propagate with nonlinearly related velocities. A short pulse in dispersive media will broaden if significant dispersion is present. In analogy to the short-pulse case, the interferometric autocorrelation (i.e., the axial PSF) will also broaden if there is significant GVD mismatch between reference and sample arms. Both the fiber optics and the sample may have significant GVD.

To include GVD in the analysis, the propagation constants β_R and β_S are Taylor expanded to second order around the center frequency ω_0:

$$\beta(\omega) = \beta(\omega_0) + \beta'(\omega_0)(\omega - \omega_0) + \frac{1}{2}\beta''(\omega_0)(\omega - \omega_0)^2 \tag{23}$$

We assume that a GVD mismatch exists in a length L of the sample and reference paths. The frequency-dependent phase mismatch from Eq. (9) is then

$$\Delta\phi(\omega) = \beta(\omega_0)(2\Delta l) + \beta'(\omega_0)(\omega - \omega_0)(2\Delta l) + \frac{1}{2}\Delta\beta''(\omega_0)(\omega - \omega_0)^2(2L) \tag{24}$$

where Δl is defined as before and $\Delta\beta''(\omega_0) = \beta_S''(\omega_0) - \beta_R''(\omega_0)$ is the GVD mismatch between the reference and sample paths. Note that only the difference in GVD between the two interferometer arms enters Eq. (24). Thus, the deleterious effects of dispersion may be decreased by equalizing the GVD in the two interferometer arms.

Inserting $\Delta\phi(\omega)$ into the propagation equation Eq. (7), gives the photocurrent

$$I \propto \exp\left[-j\omega_0\Delta\tau_p\right] \int_{-\infty}^{\infty} S(\omega - \omega_0) \exp\left[-j\frac{1}{2}\Delta\beta''(\omega_0)(\omega - \omega_0)^2(2L)\right] \times$$
$$\exp\left[-j(\omega - \omega_0)\Delta\tau_g\right] \frac{d(\omega - \omega_0)}{2\pi} \tag{25}$$

where the phase delay mismatch $\Delta\tau_p$ and group delay mismatch $\Delta\tau_g$ have been defined in Eqs. (13) and (14). Again the real { } notation has been dropped for convenience. The GVD mismatch multiplies the source power spectral density $S(\omega - \omega_0)$ in a frequency-dependent quadratic phase term. The interferometric signal looks like a short pulse, with Fourier transform $S(\omega - \omega_0)$, which propagates through a length L of dispersive medium with second-order dispersion equal to the difference in GVD between the interferometer arms. Thus, just as a short pulse broadens and chirps after propagation through a dispersive medium, the interferometric signal should also broaden and chirp due to GVD mismatch in the two interferometer arms.

Gaussian Power Spectrum and Dispersive Medium

To establish the analogy further, assume that the source has a Gaussian power spectral density according to Eq. (15). Then, after substitution into Eq. (25), we obtain a modulated interferometric signal with a complex Gaussian envelope described by

$$I \propto \frac{\sigma_\tau}{\Gamma(2L)} \exp\left[-\frac{\Delta\tau_g^2}{2\Gamma(2L)^2}\right] \exp\left[-j\omega_0\Delta\tau_p\right] \tag{26}$$

where σ_τ is the standard deviation half-width from Eq. (18). The characteristic width of the axial point spread function in the presence of dispersion, $\Gamma(2L)$, is a complex parameter that depends on both the round-trip length of GVD mismatch $2L$ and σ_τ via

$$\Gamma(2L)^2 = \sigma_\tau^2 + j\Delta\beta''(\omega_0)(2L) \tag{27}$$

The real and imaginary components of $1/\Gamma(2L)^2$ describe the broadening and chirping, respectively, of the interferometric signal and are

$$\frac{1}{\Gamma(2L)^2} = \frac{\sigma_\tau^2}{\sigma_\tau^4 + \tau_{critical}^4} - j\frac{\tau_{critical}^2}{\sigma_\tau^4 + \tau_{critical}^4} \tag{28}$$

where we have defined the dispersion parameter

$$\tau_{\text{critical}} = \left[\Delta\beta''(\omega_0)(2L)\right]^{1/2} \tag{29}$$

Substituting the expression for $1/\Gamma(2L)^2$ into Eq. (26), we discover that the Gaussian envelope is broadened to the new standard deviation width $2\tilde{\sigma}_\tau$:

$$2\tilde{\sigma}_\tau = 2\sigma_\tau\left[1 + \left(\frac{\tau_{\text{critical}}}{\sigma_\tau}\right)^4\right]^{1/2} \tag{30}$$

The broadening factor becomes appreciable when the magnitude of the dispersion parameter τ_{critical} becomes greater than the unbroadened standard deviation temporal width σ_τ. For a typical fused silica fiber at 800 nm, $\beta'' = 350\,\text{fs}^2/\text{cm}$. For a typical resolution achieved by OCT, $\Delta l_{\text{FWHM}} = 10\,\mu\text{m}$, implying $\sigma_\tau = 28$ fs. Thus, dispersive broadening becomes a factor if the fiber arm lengths are mismatched by at least $L \approx 1$ cm.

The chirping of the interferometric signal with increasing path length mismatch Δl can be described by differentiating the phase in the exponent of Eq. (26), leading to

$$k = \frac{d\phi}{d\,\Delta l} = 2\beta(\omega_0) - \frac{\tau_{\text{critical}}^2}{\sigma_\tau^4 + \tau_{\text{critical}}^4}\left[4\Delta\beta''(\omega_0)^2\right]\Delta l \tag{31}$$

where k describes the spatial frequency of the interference fringes versus the distance measured Δl. For example, in the positive dispersion mismatch regime $\Delta\beta''(\omega_0) > 0$, as the reference arm path length is increased, Δl decreases, the wavenumber k increases, and interference fringes occur at the detector more often. It is important to note that GVD changes the phase but not the bandwidth of the interference signal.

Dispersion mismatch also degrades the peak height of the interferometric envelope, which reduces the system dynamic range. The degradation in the photocurrent amplitude is described by the multiplicative factor

$$\frac{\sigma_\tau}{|\Gamma(2L)|} = \frac{1}{\left[1 + (\tau_{\text{critical}}/\sigma_\tau)^4\right]^{1/4}} \tag{32}$$

The reduction of the signal amplitude peak scales as the square root of the broadening. Assuming that the dynamic range is measured in terms of reflected optical power, which is proportional to photocurrent power, then the loss in dynamic range scales linearly with the broadening.

2.2.5 Non-Gaussian Light Sources

If the light source has a non-Gaussian spectrum, then several abnormalities in the axial point spread function may occur that can be predicted using the inverse Fourier transform relation in Eq. (12).

Spectral Modulation

Modulation or ripples in the light source spectrum can cause echoes to appear in the axial point spread function. Assume that we may write the modulated spectrum $S_m(\omega)$ as a function of an ideal, unmodulated spectrum $S(\omega)$ in the form

$$S_m(\omega) = S(\omega)\left[1 + \frac{M}{2}\cos\left(\omega\frac{\lambda_0^2}{c\lambda_m}\right)\right] \tag{33}$$

where λ_0 is the center wavelength, M is the ratio of the peak-to-peak modulation height to the average spectral height, and λ_m is the approximate modulation period measured in the wavelength domain. Then by the inverse Fourier transform relation in Eq. (12) for a nondispersive medium, the photocurrent will consist of a main peak situation at $\Delta l = 0$ and two side peaks or echoes with a height of M/r relative to the main peak situated at

$$\Delta l = \pm\frac{\lambda_0^2}{2\lambda_m}\left(\frac{v_g}{c}\right) \tag{34}$$

Equation (34) reduces to $\Delta l = \pm\lambda_0^2/2\lambda_m$ in free space.

Blindness

Blindness occurs if the tails of the axial point spread function are sufficiently broad to prevent the observation of a weak reflection placed next to a strong reflection. The effect is a function of the light source spectrum according to the inverse Fourier transform relationship in Eq. (12). If the source has a Gaussian spectrum, then the axial point spread function is also Gaussian and its tails decay exponentially with the squared path length mismatch between reference and sample arms. However, if the source is non-Gaussian, then significant tails in the axial point spread function may occur, preventing the detection of a weaker reflector nearby. A Lorentzian line shape, for example, will only decay exponentially with the linear path length mismatch.

2.3 DETECTION ELECTRONICS

Section 2.2 showed that the interferometric photocurrent consists of an axial point spread function envelope superimposed on a carrier frequency. An electric circuit is used to extract the envelope of the detected signal in a manner similar to the demodulation of AM radio signals. In the actual OCT system, the reference mirror oscillates rapidly and travels at a velocity v_s during scanning. Therefore, the axial point spread function, which is a function of the path length mismatch Δl, is mapped into a function of time by the change of variables $\Delta l = -v_s t$ (where time $t = 0$ occurs when the two path lengths are matched, and t increases as the reference mirror is translated farther from the beamsplitter). From Eq. (13), the resulting electric signal has a carrier frequency of

$$\tilde{\omega}_D = \frac{2v_s}{v_p}\omega_0 \tag{35}$$

where ω_0 is, as before, the center frequency of the source spectrum, and the tilde denotes the electronic frequency counterpart of the corresponding optical frequency. If free space propagation is assumed, then Eq. (35) simplifies to

$$\tilde{f}_D = \frac{2v_s}{\lambda_0} \tag{36}$$

The carrier frequency $\tilde{f}_D$ can also be interpreted as the Doppler shift caused by the moving reference mirror, which creates a beat frequency at the photodetector after mixing with unshifted light returning from the sample mirror.

To extract this signal, the detection circuit consists of three main elements in succession after the photodetector, shown in Fig. 3: (1) a transimpedance amplifier with a gain of R that converts the interferometric photocurrent into a voltage; (2) a bandpass filter with a transfer function $H_{bp}(s)$ centered at the carrier frequency $\tilde{f}_D$ that separates the actual interferometric signal from the DC photocurrent and noise; and (3) an amplitude demodulator that extracts the envelope of the interferometric signal. The envelope is subsequently digitized and stored on a computer. As will be discussed later, the amplitude demodulator can be realized by mixing or by envelope detection. Mixing involves multiplication of the interferometric signal by a sinusoidal reference at the carrier frequency followed by low-pass filtering. Envelope detection entails rectification, for example, square-law detection, followed by low-pass filtering.

2.3.1   Correspondence Between Optical and Electrical Frequency

A one-to-one mapping may be established between the source power spectrum in the optical frequency domain and the interferometric photocurrent in the electrical frequency domain. Consider $\phi(\omega)$ given by Eq. (23) for the case of dispersive media. If we define a linear transformation $T(\omega)$ between optical frequencies and electrical frequencies $\tilde{\omega}$ such that

$$\tilde{\omega} = T(\omega) = \frac{2v_s}{v_g}\left[\omega - \omega_0\left(\frac{v_g}{v_p} - 1\right)\right] \tag{37}$$

then Eq. (35) is automatically satisfied, and the phase mismatch term in Eq. (24) can be rewritten as

$$\Delta\phi(\omega) = \Phi(\tilde{\omega}) - \tilde{\omega}t \tag{38}$$

In Eq. (38), $\tilde{\omega}t$ contains the entire linear component of the frequency dependence and

$$\Phi(\tilde{\omega}) = \frac{1}{2}\left[\Delta\beta''(\omega_0)(2L)\right]\left[\frac{v_g}{2v_s}(\tilde{\omega} - \tilde{\omega}_0)\right]^2 \tag{39}$$

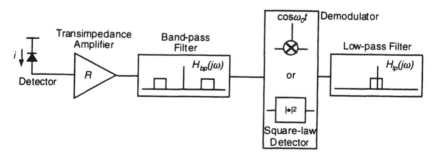

Figure 3   Block diagram of OCT electronics.

contains the quadratic phase variation. The propagation equation, Eq. (7), then reduces to an inverse Fourier transform relation between the time and electric frequency domains, described by

$$I \propto \frac{v_g}{2v_s} \int_{-\infty}^{\infty} S[T^{-1}(\tilde{\omega})] e^{-j\Phi(\tilde{\omega})} e^{j\tilde{\omega}t} \frac{d\tilde{\omega}}{2\pi} = \frac{v_g}{2v_s} F^{-1}\left\{ S[T^{-1}(\tilde{\omega})] e^{-j\Phi(\tilde{\omega})} \right\} \tag{40}$$

The Fourier transform $F\{I\}$ of the photocurrent from the time domain t to the electrical frequency domain $\tilde{\omega}$ simply reverses the inverse transform in Eq. (40):

$$F\{I\} \propto \frac{v_g}{2v_s} S[T^{-1}(\tilde{\omega})] e^{-j\Phi(\tilde{\omega})} \tag{41}$$

Equation (41) shows that the frequency domain representation of the photocurrent is simply a shifted and scaled version of the light source power spectrum that is multiplied by a quadratic phase factor that accounts for dispersion. In other words, in the case of nondispersive propagation, the shape of the frequency domain representation of the electronic signal is exactly the shape of the light source power spectrum. The mapping of optical frequencies f to electrical frequencies $\tilde{f}$ is given by Eq. (37), which, for the case of free space propagation, reduces to

$$\tilde{f} = \frac{2v_s}{\lambda} \tag{42}$$

where we have written the optical frequencies in terms of optical wavelengths λ. Note that Eq. (42) holds not only for the Doppler shift frequency $\tilde{f}_D$ corresponding to the center optical wavelength λ_0 but also for the other optical wavelengths within the source spectral bandwidth as well.

Equation (37) is particularly useful for calculating the bandwidth and quality factor of the photocurrent from the bandwidth and quality factor of the source spectrum because the mapping is independent of both the specific shape of the source spectrum and the particular definition of bandwidth. If $\Delta\tilde{f}$, Δf, and $\Delta\lambda$ are arbitrary but equivalent measures of electrical frequency bandwidth, optical frequency bandwidth, and optical wavelength bandwidth, respectively, then

$$\Delta\tilde{f} = \frac{2v_s}{v_g} \Delta f \approx \frac{2v_s}{v_g} \left(\frac{c}{\lambda_0^2} \right) \Delta\lambda \tag{43}$$

where λ_0 is the center optical wavelength. In free space, Eq. (43) becomes

$$\Delta\tilde{f} \approx \frac{2v_s}{\lambda_0^2} \Delta\lambda \tag{44}$$

Note that the scaling factor in Eq. (43) is the ratio between the round-trip mirror velocity $2v_s$ and the optical group velocity v_g. Because the scaling factor is constant, the mapping is linear, and the scaling factor cancels out of any ratios. Therefore, the quality factors Q in the optical and electrical domains are identical and are given by the simple relations

$$\frac{1}{Q} = \frac{\Delta\tilde{f}}{\tilde{f}_D} = \frac{\Delta f}{f_0} \approx \frac{\Delta\lambda}{\lambda_0} \tag{45}$$

where the subscript 0 denotes the center optical frequency or optical wavelength and the subscript D indicates the center (Doppler shift) electronic frequency. Equation (45) approximately gives the Q desired for the bandpass filter in terms of the wavelength bandwidth $\Delta\lambda$ of the light source.

2.3.2 Transimpedance Amplifier

The photodetector is followed by a transimpedance amplifier, shown in Fig. 4, which converts the photocurrent i into an output voltage v. For low frequencies, the output voltage is simply

$$v = iR \tag{46}$$

The capacitance C in parallel with the feedback resistance is necessary for amplifier stability and causes the amplifier to roll off at 20 dB per decade above the dominant pole at

$$\omega_c = \frac{1}{RC} \tag{47}$$

2.3.3 Bandpass Filter

A bandpass filter follows the transimpedance amplifier (after a simple single-pole RC circuit that removes the DC photocurrent) to separate the band-limited interferometric signal from noise. The filter is designed with a center frequency $\tilde{f}_D$ and quality factor Q given by Eqs. (36) and (45), respectively. In the discussion below, the tilde indicating electrical frequencies will be dropped. Design strategies for both an active and a passive filter will be given.

Active Sallen and Key Cascade Filter

An active bandpass filter is most useful for barrier frequencies below 100 kHz. For higher frequencies, active filters may be limited by the slew rate of the operational amplifier and passive network filters are required. An active bandpass filter may be created by cascading a low-pass Sallen and Key biquad filter followed by a high-pass one.

Figure 5 depicts the low-pass Sallen and Key filter in a unity gain configuration. The transfer function is given by the standard second-order form

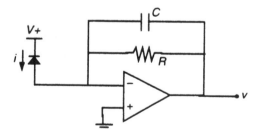

Figure 4 Transimpedance amplifier.

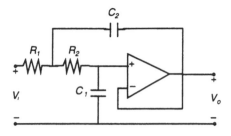

Figure 5 Sallen and Key low-pass filter.

$$H(s) = \frac{V_o(s)}{V_i(s)} = \frac{\omega_n^2}{s^2 + (\omega_n/Q)S + \omega_n^2} \tag{48}$$

where the undamped natural frequency ω_n is

$$\omega_n = \frac{1}{R\sqrt{C_1 C_2}} \tag{49}$$

and the quality factor Q is

$$Q = \frac{1}{2}\sqrt{\frac{C_2}{C_1}} \tag{50}$$

using the simplification $R = R_1 = R_2$.

The resonance frequency ω_n is chosen to be equal to the signal carrier frequency ω_D. In practice the quality factor Q is chosen to be smaller than the value given by Eq. (45) so that the filter bandwidth is larger than the signal bandwidth. A filter bandwidth that is too narrow will widen the signal in time and arbitrarily limit the axial point spread function. Section 2.5 will show that a filter bandwidth that is too large will let in more noise and reduce the minimum detectable reflectivity or dynamic range of the system.

The unity gain Sallen and Key high-pass filter is exactly the dual or the low-pass filter except that resistor are interchanged with capacitors (Fig. 6). The high-pass transfer function is

$$H(s) = \frac{V_o(s)}{V_i(s)} = \frac{\omega_n^2 s^2}{s^2 + (\omega_n/Q)s + \omega_n^2} \tag{51}$$

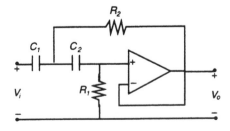

Figure 6 Sallen and Key high-pass filter.

where

$$\omega_n = \frac{1}{C\sqrt{R_1 R_2}} \tag{52}$$

and

$$Q = \frac{1}{2\zeta} = \frac{1}{2}\sqrt{\frac{R_1}{R_2}} \tag{53}$$

using the simplification $C = C_1 = C_2$. The resonance frequency and quality factor are chosen to match those for the low-pass filter.

The bandpass filter $H_{bp}(s)$ created by the cascade of the low-pass and high-pass filters has two sets of pole pairs at

$$P_{1,2} = -\frac{\omega_n}{2Q} \pm j\omega_n\left(1 - \frac{1}{4Q^2}\right)^{1/2} \tag{54}$$

Thus, the frequency response rolls off at 40 dB per decade in both directions outside of the resonance peak.

Passive Network Butterworth Filter

A passive network bandpass filter may be designed for high frequency operation using the standard techniques for broadband-matching network synthesis. The problem is formulated as follows in relation to Fig. 7: Given a Thevenin equivalent voltage source defined by V_t and R_t, synthesize a lossless two-port network that is matched to the load impedance R_2 and has the desired transfer function power gain characteristic $|H(j\omega)|^2 = |V_2(j\omega)/V_t(j\omega)|^2$.

The solution to the general problem has been explored in detail, and only one particular solution using resistive termination will be given here. A passive network bandpass filter can be designed easily by starting with a prototypical low-pass filter and then "frequency warping" this filter into the bandpass domain. The Butterworth low-pass filter works well for this purpose because an LC ladder can always be obtained to match a purely resistive source and load and achieve the nth order Butterworth low-pass characteristic given by

$$|H(j\omega)|^2 = \frac{K}{1 + (j\omega/j\omega_c)^{2n}} \tag{55}$$

The Butterworth filter with DC gain K and low-pass cutoff ω_c is maximally flat in the passband and has evenly spaced poles placed in the left half plane (LHP) on a circle centered at the frequency origin. Furthermore, explicit recursive formulas exist for

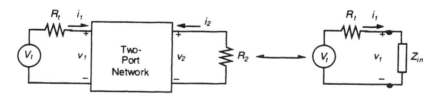

Figure 7 Network synthesis problem.

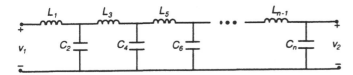

Figure 8 *LC* ladder network of order *n*.

the element values of the *LC* ladder, shown in Fig. 8, which simplifies the design process. (An odd-order filter is realized by removing the terminating capacitor.)

Under the condition of equal source and load resistances ($R_t = R_2$), a simple nonrecursive formula is applicable. Using this restriction, in order to realize a Butterworth filter of order *n* with cutoff frequency ω_c and a DC gain of unity, the *m*th component values of the *LC* ladder shown in Fig. 8 are given by the following definitions:

$$L_m = \frac{2R_t}{\omega_c} \sin\left[\frac{(2m-1)\pi}{2n}\right] \tag{56}$$

$$C_m = \frac{2}{R_t\omega_c} \sin\left[\frac{(2m-1)\pi}{2n}\right] \tag{57}$$

To realize a bandpass filter with low-pass cutoff ω_1 and high-pass cutoff ω_2, one first designs a normalized, prototype low-pass filter with a cutoff frequency of $\omega_c = 1$ rad/s. The following frequency transformation is then used to warp the filter from the low-pass domain *s*, with a passband of $-1 \leftrightarrow 1$ rad/s, to the bandpass domain $\tilde{s}$, with passbands $\omega_1 \leftrightarrow \omega_2$ and $-\omega_2 \leftrightarrow -\omega_1$:

$$s = \frac{\omega_m}{B}\left[\frac{\tilde{s}}{\omega_m} + \frac{\omega_m}{\tilde{s}}\right] \tag{58}$$

We have defined $B = \omega_2 - \omega_1$ as the desired bandpass filter bandwidth and $\omega_m = \omega_1\omega_2$ as the midband (geometric mean) frequency. It is straightforward to verify that the transformation described by Eq. (58) involves replacing inductors in the prototypical filter (Fig. 8) by an inductor and a capacitor in series and replacing capacitors in the prototypical filter by an inductor and a capacitor in parallel. The necessary component values for this low-pass to bandpass frequency warping are shown in Fig. 9. Resistors remain unchanged. The low-pass to bandpass frequency warping process doubles the number of poles in the system.

Figure 10 shows an example of a second-order prototypical Butterworth low-pass filter that is transformed into a four-pole bandpass filter. For $R_t = R_2 = 5\,\text{k}\Omega$ and design parameters of a center frequency of 400 kHz and a quality factor of 10,

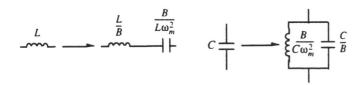

Figure 9 Low-pass to bandpass frequency warping.

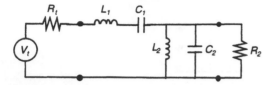

Figure 10 Second-order Butterworth bandpass filter.

the following component values are obtained: $L_1 = 28.1\,\text{mH}$, $C_1 = 5.64\,\text{pF}$, $L_2 = 141\,\mu\text{H}$, and $C_2 = 1.13$ nF. The frequency response of the resulting bandpass filter is shown in Fig. 11. The filter has two zeros located at the origin and two complex pole pairs located at

$$p_{1,2} = -0.092 \pm j2.60 \quad \text{and} \quad p_{3,4} = -0.086 \pm j2.42 \quad \text{rad/s} \times 10^6 \quad (59)$$

Thus, the frequency response rolls off at 40 db per decade in both directions off the main peak.

2.3.4 Demodulation

Amplitude demodulation can occur by either mixing or envelope detection. Both models will be briefly introduced here so that noise propagation through the electronics can be understood for both methods.

Mixing

Demodulation by mixing entails multiplication with a reference sinusoidal signal of the correct phase followed by low-pass filtering. Mixing is easily implemented by

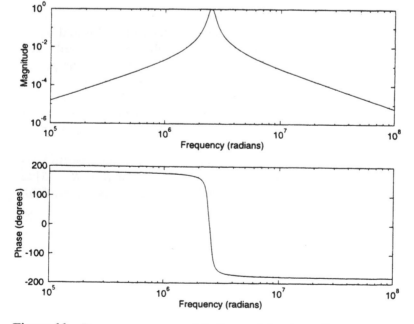

Figure 11 Frequency response of Butterworth bandpass filter.

using a lock-in amplifier. The reference frequency is chosen to match the Doppler shift carrier frequency ω_D, and the bandwidth of the low-pass filter is chosen to be slightly larger than approximately one-half the signal bandwidth $\Delta\omega$. In a typical lock-in amplifier, a single-pole RC time constant is used, giving a low-pass transfer function

$$H_{lp}(s) = \frac{H_0}{RCs + 1} \tag{60}$$

with a bandwidth of $1/RC$ rad/s.

The phase of the reference sine wave must be locked to the phase of the signal for adequate demodulation. If this is not possible, then the signal can be divided and correlated simultaneously in quadrature (i.e., with both a sine and a cosine). The sum of the squares of the two quadrature components accurately gives the signal power independent of the actual phase.

Envelope Detection

Envelope detection occurs by rectification followed by low-pass filtering. A single-chip implementation may be used that can provide either a linear or a logarithmic output. For ease of calculation, envelope detection can be modeled by a single-pole low-pass transfer function [e.g., Eq. (60)] operating on the square of the input voltage.

Envelope detection is more advantageous than mixing when the phase or frequency of the carrier has nonlinear variations (for example, due to nonlinear sweeping of the reference mirror).

2.4 NOISE SOURCES

In OCT, the principle of heterodyne detection is used to achieve a detection sensitivity that approaches the quantum limit of a single photon. This section will review thermal noise, shot noise, relative intensity noise, and amplified spontaneous emission noise, which are the dominant sources of noise that affect the OCT electronics.

The noise sources below can be described by wide-sense stationary (WSS) stochastic processes. A WSS stochastic process $p(t)$ has a constant mean

$$E\{p(t)\} = \langle p(t) \rangle = m_p \tag{61}$$

and a statistical autocorrelation

$$R_p(t_1, t_2) = E\{p(t_1)p(t_2)\} = \langle p(t_1)p(t_2) \rangle \tag{62}$$

that is a function of $\tau = t_2 - t_1$ alone. A description of the frequency content of a WSS stochastic process is given by the power spectral density

$$S_p(\omega) = \int_{-\infty}^{\infty} R_p(\tau) e^{-j\omega t}\, d\tau \tag{63}$$

which is simply the Fourier transform of the statistical autocorrelation.

The power spectral density $S_p(\omega)$ is defined for both positive and negative frequencies and is a real and even function of ω by definition. In practice, however, only positive frequencies are measured. For convenience we define a positive frequency or single-sided power spectral density

$$S_p^+(\omega) = S_p(\omega) + S_p(-\omega) = 2S_p(\omega) \tag{64}$$

which is valid for $\omega \geq 0$ and allows comparison of theory with experiment.

2.4.1 Thermal Noise

Thermal noise arises from random particle motion due to the thermal energy of a system. In electric circuits, resistors are the only passive elements that exchange energy with the environment. Thus, thermal noise is associated with the transfer of energy and the temperature equilibrium established between a resistor and its surroundings. A noisy resistor can be modeled as the parallel combination of an ideal resistor with resistance R and a noisy current source i_n that represents the thermal noise or energy provided by the environment. The noise current is approximated by zero-mean white noise with a double-sided power spectral density

$$S_{i_n}(\omega) = \frac{2kT}{R} \tag{65}$$

where T is the temperature and k is Boltzmann's constant.

2.4.2 Shot Noise

Shot noise arises from current fluctuations due to the quantization of light and charge. A photodetector will emit charge corresponding to a mean rate defined by the photocurrent; however, the time between specific emissions will be random. The photon arrival and electron emission times may be described by a Poisson distributed random variable. It can be shown that the shot noise associated with any photocurrent $\langle i \rangle$ is a white noise process with mean $\langle i \rangle$ and double-sided power spectral density

$$S_{i_n}(\omega) = e\langle i \rangle \tag{66}$$

The shot noise power is proportional to the electronic charge and the square root of the photocurrent power $\langle i \rangle^2$.

2.4.3 Relative Intensity Noise and Amplified Spontaneous Emission

Relative intensity noise (RIN) includes any noise source whose power spectral density scales linearly with the mean photocurrent power $\langle i \rangle^2$. Examples include fluctuations in optical power from the source and from the mechanical motion of optical mounts. With a superluminescent diode source using heterodyne detection, amplified spontaneous emission (ASE) also results in noise that scales linearly with the photocurrent power. The spectral density of RIN and ASE noise can be approximated as white over the frequency band of interest and can be modeled as

$$S_{i_n}(\omega) = e\gamma\langle i \rangle^2 \tag{67}$$

where the noise parameter γ must usually be determined by experiment.

2.5 SENSITIVITY

This section will give expressions for the expected sensitivity of the OCT system considering the noise sources described in Section 2.4. The sensitivity is a measure of the minimum detectable reflectivity of the OCT system. The sensitivity, or signal-to-noise ratio (SNR), for any system is defined simply as the signal power P_{signal} divided by the noise process variance var $\{n(t)\}$. If the noise process is zero-mean WSS, then

$$\text{SNR} = \frac{P_{signal}}{\text{var}\,\{n(t)\}} = \frac{P_{signal}}{R_n(0)} = \frac{P_{signal}}{\int_{-\infty}^{\infty} S_n(\omega)\,d\omega/2\pi} \tag{68}$$

which shows that the SNR is equal to the signal power divided by the mean noise power, where the noise power is the integral of its power spectral density $S_n(\omega)$ over all frequencies.

The signal-to-noise ratio will be derived below by propagating the various sources of noise described in Section 2.4 through the detection electronics described in Section 2.3. In the shot noise limit, the noise power is dominated by the shot noise of the reference beam, also termed the local oscillator. The signal power is given by the correlation of the power reflected from the sample with the power in the local oscillator. Weak reflections from within the sample are therefore multiplied by the local oscillator field to create a relatively strong interference signal at the detector. In this manner, a relatively high SNR can be achieved. Figure 12 displays the variables used for the noise process, power spectral densities, and noise equivalent bandwidths at various points in the system and will be helpful in the subsequent sections.

2.5.1 Photodetection Noise

From Eq. (3), the photodetector current is the sum of the DC power $P_R = |A_R|^2/2\eta_0$ returning from the reference path, the DC power $P_S = |A_S|^2/2\eta_0$ returning from the sample, and an interference term real $\{E_S E_R^*\}$ from the correlation of the signal and the local oscillator:

$$I = \frac{\eta e}{h\upsilon}\left[P_R + P_S + \frac{1}{\eta_0}\text{real}\,\{E_S E_R^*\}\right] + i_{dark} \tag{69}$$

We have also added a term i_{dark} that represents the dark current of the photodiode. The signal power is completely contained within the term real $\{E_S E_R^*\}$, which is separated from the DC components P_R and P_S by bandpass filtering and demodula-

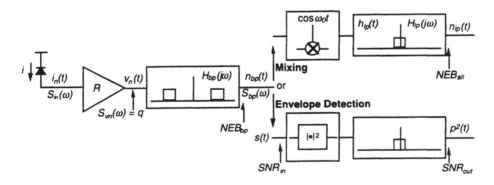

Figure 12 Noise variable definitions.

tion. The filtering and demodulation steps, however, do not eliminate the noise associated with these components, which may exist at all frequencies.

Both shot noise [Eq. (66)] and RIN [Eq. (67)] contribute to the photocurrent noise $i_n(t)$, which can propagate through the detection electronics. Therefore, the power spectral density $S_{i_n}(\omega)$ of this noise can be expressed as the sum of these two uncorrelated components:

$$S_{i_n}(\omega) = e\langle i \rangle + e\gamma \langle i \rangle^2 \tag{70}$$

where $\langle i \rangle$ is the mean photocurrent and contains contributions from the local oscillator beam, the sample beam, the signal, and the dark current.

2.5.2 Transimpedance Amplifier Noise

At the input to the transimpedance amplifier (Fig. 4), thermal noise [Eq. (65)] from the feedback gain resistor R is added to the photocurrent noise. Because all the noise sources are uncorrelated, the power spectral density of the noise current becomes

$$S_{i_n}(\omega) = e\langle i \rangle + e\gamma \langle i \rangle^2 + \frac{2kT}{R} \tag{71}$$

At the output of the transimpedance amplifier, the noise current $n_i(t)$ is transformed into a voltage $n_v(t)$ with a gain of R. Because the variance scales as R^2, the spectral density $S_{v_n}(\omega)$ of the output noise voltage is

$$S_{v_n}(\omega) = e\langle i \rangle R^2 + e\gamma \langle i \rangle^2 R^2 + 2kTR \tag{72}$$

Equation (72) can also be written in terms of the mean output voltage $\langle v \rangle = \langle i \rangle R$ as

$$S_{v_n}(\omega) = e\langle v \rangle R + e\gamma \langle v \rangle^2 + 2kTR = q \tag{73}$$

where a new variable q has been defined as representing the amplitude of the noise spectral density, which is constant across all frequencies. Equation (73) is useful because the voltage output of the transimpedance amplifier is more conveniently measured than the photocurrent.

2.5.3 Bandpass Filter Noise Equivalent Bandwidth

Let the bandpass filter have an impulse response $h_{bp}(t)$ and a transfer function $H_{bp}(s)$ given by one of the design procedures detailed in Section 2.3.3. The noise input to this filter is given by Eq. (73). Since the input noise is white with a constant spectral density, the output noise will be colored, or shaped according to the characteristics of the filter. Using the standard results for a WSS stochastic process through a linear time-invariant filter, we obtain the power spectral density $S_{bp}(\omega)$ of the noise process $n_{bp}(t)$ at the output of the filter:

$$S_{bp}(\omega) = q \left| H_{bp}(j\omega) \right|^2 \tag{74}$$

The corresponding autocorrelation $R_{bp}(\tau)$ can be found by taking the inverse Fourier transform:

$$R_{bp}(\tau) = q \int_{-\infty}^{\infty} \left| H_{bp}(j\omega) \right|^2 e^{j\omega\tau} \frac{d\omega}{2\pi} \tag{75}$$

The noise variance at the bandpass filter output is

$$\text{var}\{n_{bp}(t)\} = R_{bp}(0) = q \int_{-\infty}^{\infty} |H_{bp}(j\omega)|^2 \frac{d\omega}{2\pi}$$

$$= 2q \int_{0}^{\infty} |H_{bp}(j\omega)|^2 \frac{d\omega}{2\pi} = 2q \, \text{NEB}_{bp} \tag{76}$$

where the noise equivalent bandwidth (NEB) of the bandpass filter is defined as before and is a geometric measure of how much noise passes through the filter. The factor of 2 arises because the NEB is defined for positive frequencies only. Note that the bandpassed noise has zero mean, because the DC gain of the filter is zero.

2.5.4 Noise Equivalent Bandwidth for Demodulation by Mixing

The noise process $n_{bp}(t)$ at the output of the bandpass filter is then input to the demodulator. The NEB and resulting signal-to-noise ratio (SNR) of demodulation by mixing will be considered below and in Section 2.5.5. Demodulation by envelope detection will be considered separately in Section 2.5.6.

The discussion of the noise characteristics after demodulation by mixing is involved because the noise is not a WSS process after correlation with $\cos \omega_D t$. The demodulated noise process, however, is WSS. Therefore, the noise must be propagated through both the sinusoidal correlator and the low-pass filter in one step to compute the final power spectral density. Although the details of the calculation will not be repeated here, the final result is intuitively expected. In analogy to Eq. (76), the variance of the noise $n_{lp}(t)$ after mixing and low-pass filtering is given by

$$\text{var}\{n_{lp}(t)\} = 2q \, \text{NEB}_{all} \tag{77}$$

where the NEB of the entire circuit, NEB_{all}, including both bandpass filtering and demodulation by mixing, is defined by

$$\text{NEB}_{all} = \int_{0}^{\infty} |H_{lp}(j\omega)|^2 \left(\frac{1}{2}\right) \left[|H_{bp}(j\omega + j\omega_D)|^2 + |H_{bp}(j\omega - j\omega_D)|^2 \right] \frac{d\omega}{2\pi} \tag{78}$$

As expected, Eq. (78) gives the appealing result that the noise power of the entire circuit looks like the noise that would result from the bandpass and low-pass filters in succession, because the bandpass filter acts as if it were shifted to the frequency origin after demodulation by mixing. Thus, the NEB of the entire filtering and demodulation circuit is described by the frequency domain product of the low-pass and demodulated bandpass filters. One can see that for ideal rectangular filters the NEB of the entire system is determined by the NEB of the filter with the narrower bandwidth.

2.5.5 Signal-to-Noise Ratio for Demodulation by Mixing

The signal-to-noise ratio or sensitivity of OCT is defined by Eq. (68) and describes the minimum detectable reflection. To use Eq. (68), we define the signal power P_{signal} to be the peak voltage squared at the output of the filtering and demodulation circuit. Although other definitions could have been sued (e.g., the typical definition of signal energy is the integral of the signal squared over time), this particular definition is easily compared with experimental results.

To determine the output signal power, we propagate the interferometric signal through the detection and demodulation electronics. For simplicity, we will ignore the degradation in signal power caused by group velocity dispersion. Let $\bar{P}_S$ and $\bar{P}_R$ be the time-averaged optical powers returning from a perfectly reflective sample and the reference mirror, respectively, after recombination at the beamsplitter. From Eq. (69), the peak signal current after photodetection is given by the correlation of the reference arm and sample arm electric field as

$$i = \frac{\eta e}{h\upsilon} \sqrt{\bar{P}_S \bar{P}_R} \tag{79}$$

where η is the quantum efficiency of the photodetector, e is the electronic charge, and $h\upsilon$ is the photon energy. The transimpedance amplifier converts the current i into a voltage $v = iR$ with a gain of R. If we assume for simplicity that the signal power is preserved through bandpass filtering and demodulation, then the signal power as defined above is

$$P_{\text{signal}} = (iR)^2 = \left(\frac{\eta e}{h\upsilon}\right)^2 (\bar{P}_S \bar{P}_R) R^2 \tag{80}$$

which is proportional to the product of the reference and sample powers.

The noise variance is given by $2q$ NEB where q is the amplitude of the white noise input to the bandpass filter defined in Eq. (73) and NEB is the noise equivalent bandwidth defined in Eq. (78) for demodulation by mixing. In the shot noise limit, the white noise amplitude q is dominated by the shot noise from light reflected from the reference mirror. Section 2.6.1 will discuss the design considerations so that this limit can be achieved in practice. In the shot noise limit, the noise variance after filtering and demodulation is

$$\text{var}\left\{n_{lp}(t)\right\} = \frac{\eta e}{h\upsilon} 2e\bar{P}_R R^2 \text{ NEB} \tag{81}$$

Therefore, the signal-to-noise ratio in the shot noise limit is obtained by substituting Eqs. (80) and (81) into Eq. (68), resulting in

$$\text{SNR} = \frac{\eta}{h\upsilon}\left(\frac{\bar{P}_S}{2\,\text{NEB}}\right) \tag{82}$$

In the shot noise limit, the dynamic range does not depend on the reference arm power $\bar{P}_R$. The SNR scales linearly with the power $\bar{P}_S$ returning from a perfectly reflective sample and is inversely proportional to the noise equivalent measure of the detection bandwidth. Section 2.6.2 will discuss how Eq. (82) leads to design trade-offs between power, image acquisition time, and dynamic range.

2.5.6 Signal-to-Noise Ratio for Demodulation by Envelope Detection

Demodulation by envelope detection can be modeled as square-law detection followed by low-pass filtering as described in Section 2.3.4. Because the square-law detector is a nonlinear device, the output noise power will in general depend on both the input signal and the input noise power. Thus, a simple expression for the NEB that depends only on the input noise cannot be derived as in the case of demodulation by mixing. However, a fairly involved calculation eventually leads to a simple expression for the SNR at the output of the envelope detector in relation to the SNR at its input.

The results of this derivation can be summarized as follows. Let $s(t)$ denote the signal at the output of the bandpass filter and the input to the square-law detector. We assume that $s(t)$ has the form of a randomly amplitude modulated sine wave:

$$s(t) = p(t)\cos(\omega_D t + \theta) \tag{83}$$

where $p(t)$ is the modulating envelope (or axial reflectivity profile as a function of depth), ω_D is the electronic carrier frequency determined by the Doppler shift of the scanning reference mirror, and θ is a uniformly distributed random phase. In this case, with a low-pass filter bandwidth that is approximately twice the signal bandwidth, the SNR at the output of the square-law detector and low-pass filter can be written as

$$\mathrm{SNR_{out}} = \kappa \frac{(\mathrm{SNR_{in}})^2}{1 + 2\mathrm{SNR_{in}}} \tag{84}$$

where

$$\kappa = \frac{E\{p^4(t)\}}{E^2\{p^2(t)\}} \tag{85}$$

and $\mathrm{SNR_{in}}$ is the SNR at the input of the square-law detector. Note that κ is a function of only the form of the probability distribution of the signal envelope. For example, if $p(t)$ can be modeled as a Gaussian random variable, then $\kappa = 3$ exactly.

Equation (84) demonstrates that for an input SNR that is substantially greater than 1 the output SNR is linearly dependent on the input and is given by

$$\mathrm{SNR_{out}} \approx \frac{\kappa}{2} \mathrm{SNR_{in}} \tag{86}$$

Consideration of Eq. (82) shows that $\mathrm{SNR_{in}}$ can be defined in terms of the noise equivalent bandwidth of the bandpass filter $\mathrm{NEB_{bp}}$ and the sample arm power $\bar{P}_S$, leading to the relation

$$\mathrm{SNR_{out}} \approx \frac{\kappa}{2}\left(\frac{\eta}{h\nu}\right)\left(\frac{\bar{P}_S}{2\,\mathrm{NEB_{bp}}}\right) \tag{87}$$

Aside from the factor $\kappa/2$, demodulation by square-law detection is similar to demodulation by mixing except that only the NEB of the bandpass filter and not that of the final low-pass filter appears in the expression for the SNR. Although the derivation for Eq. (84) does assume that low-pass filter bandwidth is approximately twice the signal bandwidth [because the bandwidth of $s^2(t)$ is twice the bandwidth of $s(t)$], the exact form of the final low-pass filter is less important in the SNR for square-law detection than it is for demodulation by mixing. In addition, for square-law detection, the carrier $\cos(\omega_D t + \theta)$ is not required to have a constant phase (i.e., θ is a random variable). This property is advantageous when the velocity of the reference mirror is not perfectly linear. In this case, square-law detection is relatively insensitive to small variations in the phase of the Doppler shift or carrier frequency, which would otherwise cause problems for demodulation by mixing.

2.6 DESIGN ISSUES

2.6.1 Design for Shot Noise Limited Sensitivity

Equation (73) shows that the noise after photodetection and amplification can be represented as a zero-mean, white, WSS stochastic process that contains contributions from shot noise, thermal noise, and RIN and/or ASE noise. Quantum-limited operation is attained only when the shot noise dominates the other sources of noise. In the shot noise limit, described by Eq. (82), the detection sensitivity is approximately two photons per resolution element.

It is possible to design the system for shot noise limited sensitivity by using a spectrum analyzer to measure the noise $v_n(t)$ at the output of the transimpedance amplifier. Because the spectrum analyzer combines positive and negative frequencies, it effectively measures [from Eq. (73)] the positive frequency power spectral density

$$S\tilde{v}_n^+(\omega) = 2e\langle v\rangle R + 2e\gamma\langle v\rangle^2 + 4kTR = 2q \tag{88}$$

which contains, from left to right, the white noise contributions from shot noise, RIN and/or ASE noise, and thermal noise.

The transimpedance gain R and the reference arm power $\langle v\rangle$ are chosen such that the shot noise term is greater than the RIN and thermal noise. To ensure that shot noise eclipses the thermal noise, we require $2e\langle v\rangle R > 4kTR$, or

$$\langle v\rangle > \frac{2kT}{e} \approx 0.05\,\text{V} \qquad \text{for} \qquad T = 300\,\text{K} \tag{89}$$

This limit defines the absolute minimum reference arm power. Thus, in the absence of RIN or ASE noise, whenever the DC output of the reference arm power is greater than 50 mV, the system will be shot noise limited. The gain R must be chosen so that the shot noise dominates the RIN, or

$$R > \gamma\langle v\rangle \tag{90}$$

The upper limit of R is determined by the transimpedance amplifier stability and roll-off frequency in Eq. (47). Ideally the gain R should be as large as possible and the reference arm power $\langle v\rangle$ should be as small as possible to minimize the RIN and ASE noise (Section 2.4.3).

In practice, to construct the detector circuit, R is chosen before $\langle v\rangle$. Because the RIN parameter γ is usually unknown, given R, the optimal value of $\langle v\rangle$ must be determined experimentally. The procedure is to successively attenuate the reference arm power $\langle v\rangle$ and examine the noise spectral density on the spectrum analyzer until the white component equals the predicted shot noise value $2e\langle v\rangle R$. Attenuation of the reference arm intensity reduces the RIN as the square $\langle v\rangle^2$ of the intensity but affects the shot noise component only linearly with $\langle v\rangle$. If $\langle v\rangle$ needs to be decreased below the thermal noise limit of 0.05 V, then the amplifier gain R should be increased and the procedure repeated. If increasing R places the transimpedance amplifier roll-off frequency below the signal bandwidth, then other methods of reducing the RIN, such as dual-balanced detection, need to be considered.

2.6.2 Trade-Off Between Resolution, Power, Speed, and Sensitivity

The four fundamental design issues for OCT are the optical power, acquisition speed, signal-to-noise ratio, and axial resolution. Equation (82) establishes the linear relationship between the signal-to-noise, optical power incident on the sample, and noise equivalent bandwidth of the electronics:

$$\frac{\text{SNR} \times \text{NEB}}{\bar{P}_S} = \text{constant} \tag{91}$$

The NEB, however, is essentially equal to the electronic bandwidth $\Delta \tilde{f}$ used for detection of the interferometric signal. The electrical bandwidth is linearly related to the reference mirror scanning velocity v_s and the wavelength bandwidth $\Delta \lambda$ of the light source by Eq. (44). Therefore, we have

$$\text{NEB} \approx \Delta \tilde{f} \propto v_s \Delta \lambda \tag{92}$$

The axial resolution Δl is inversely proportional to the spectral bandwidth $\Delta \lambda$ of the light source, as seen in Eqs. (21) and (22), so we also may write

$$\text{NEB} \approx \Delta \tilde{f} \propto \frac{V_s}{\Delta l} \tag{93}$$

By combining Eqs. (91) and (93), we obtain the fundamental relationship between the four design parameters:

$$\frac{\text{SNR } v_s}{\bar{P}_S \, \Delta l} = \text{constant} \tag{94}$$

Equation (94), which is linear in all its parameters, expresses the basic idea that "you can't get something for nothing" and allows the major design issues to be easily considered in relation to one another.

The limitations expressed by Eq. (94) may be intuitively understood with an alternative interpretation of Eq. (82). The minimum detectable reflectivity $R_{\min}$ is equal to the reciprocal of the SNR. Equation (82) can then be rewritten as

$$\frac{2}{\eta} = \frac{P_S R_{\min}/\text{NEB}}{hv} \tag{95}$$

In Eq. (95), the quantity $P_s R_{\min}$ is equal to the power reflected from a minimally detectable point within the sample. The quantity 1/NEB is the inverse detection bandwidth or, equivalently, the time spent observing each resolution element within the sample. From Eq. (93) it is evident that this observation time is proportional to the longitudinal resolution Δl divided by the scanning velocity v_s. The right-hand-side numerator $P_s R_{\min}/\text{NEB}$ is therefore equal to the optical energy that returns from a minimally detectable resolution element during the observation period. By dividing this quantity by the photon energy hv, we obtain the number of photons returning from the resolution element. Equation (95) shows that the number of returning photons must be equal to or greater than $2/\eta$ in order to be detected. This requirement ensures that a minimum of one photon is detected by the photo-detector, because on average, only half of the reflected photons return to the detector through the beamsplitter and the probability that each returning photon is converted into a unit of electric charge is η.

The preceding discussion shows that the shot noise limit is directly related to the quantization of light. In summary, at least one (but actually $2/\eta$) photons need to be received for each resolution element in the OCT image in order for that resolution element to have a detectable reflectivity. Sensitivity can be increased only by increasing the number of incident photons, increasing the size of the resolution element, or increasing the time spent observing each element.

REFERENCE

1. Hee MR. Optical coherence tomography of the eye. PhD Thesis. Department of Electrical Engineering and Computer Science, Massachusetts Institute of Technology, February 1997.

3

Optical Sources

BRETT E. BOUMA and GUILLERMO J. TEARNEY

*Harvard Medical School and Wellman Laboratories of Photomedicine,
Massachusetts General Hospital, Boston, Massachusetts*

3.1 EVALUATING SOURCES FOR OPTICAL COHERENCE TOMOGRAPHY

The first demonstrations of low coherence ranging and OCT imaging in biomedicine were A-scans of the human eye and tomograms of the human retina. The light source used in these studies was a superluminescent diode (SLD) operating at 850 nm, a wavelength providing good penetration in both the vitreous and retina. Imaging the retina represents a unique case in the sense that exposure levels must be kept low, the tissues are highly transparent, and the primary structures of interest are morphological as opposed to cellular. In other human tissues, attenuation due to scattering is more significant and as a result other light sources have been shown to provide superior imaging compared with the prototype 850 nm SLD. This chapter will review issues relevant to the evaluation of sources for OCT and will summarize the progress that has been made to date.

3.1.1 General Source Criteria

Four primary considerations for evaluating optical sources for OCT imaging are wavelength, bandwidth, single-transverse-mode power, and stability. Folded into the last of these are issues such as portability, ease of use, and general compatibility with the application environment. In general, OCT imaging depth of penetration is limited by both absorption and scattering. Both of these sources of attenuation are wavelength-dependent. The red end of the visible spectrum is known as the therapeutic or diagnostic window, because it is the location of a relative minimum in the absorption of typical tissue constituents such as water and blood. Scattering, however, presents a nearly monotonic decrease with increasing wavelength over the visible and near-infrared spectral region. Maximizing OCT imaging depth of penetration therefore requires the use of a center wavelength that balances these two influences. Although no comprehensive study of the wavelength dependence of imaging contrast and depth of penetration in OCT has been published, theoretical treatments [1,2] and investigations of tissue optical properties [3–5] suggest that optimal image depth of penetration should occur near $1.3\,\mu m$ and near $1.65\,\mu m$.

Axial resolution in OCT imaging is determined by the bandwidth of the light source through the equation

$$\Delta L = \frac{2Ln2}{\pi}\left(\frac{\lambda^2}{\Delta\lambda}\right) \tag{1}$$

where λ is the source center wavelength and $\Delta\lambda$ is the full width at half-maximum (FWHM) spectral width. This equation determines the FWHM of the axial point spread function, ΔL, assuming a Gaussian spectral distribution. For a given source wavelength, an increase in bandwidth gives rise to a proportional increase in resolution. Although in frequency space relation (1) gives an inverse proportionality between bandwidth and resolution, the square law scaling in wavelength space points out a fundamental difficulty in using long-wavelength sources. For example, to achieve $10\,\mu m$ resolution at 800 nm requires a bandwidth of 28 nm, yet this same resolution requires a $1.6\,\mu m$ wavelength source to provide 113 nm of spectrum.

As described in Chapter 2, the power required from an optical source is constrained by the relation

$$\frac{\text{SNR}\ v_s}{P_s\ \Delta L} = \text{const} \tag{2}$$

where SNR is the signal-to-noise ratio (or sensitivity), v_s is proportional to the axial scanning acquisition rate, and P_s is the maximum source optical power that can reach the detector by way of the interferometer sample arm. This relation implies that to increase image acquisition rate and/or resolution while preserving sensitivity to weak sample reflections requires an increased source power. The derivation of this equation assumed that the source emitted all of its power into a single transverse mode. Spatially incoherent sources are difficult to use for OCT because the signal that is detected arises from interference between light returning from the sample and light returning from the interferometer reference arm. Unless both the sample and reference electric fields are returned to the detector with identical wave fronts, the interference will be washed out upon integration. In typical interferometers, the wave front transformations of the two pathways are not identical. When a single-transverse-mode source is used, spatial filters can be employed to remove any light that is scattered from the lowest order mode into higher order modes and thus preserve interference fringe contrast. The most common interferometer used in current OCT systems is based on single-mode optical fiber. In this case the fiber itself acts both to guide the light with minimal scattering into higher spatial modes and to spatially filter any higher order modes generated by the sample or other optics external to the fiber.

The derivation of Eq. (2) assumed shot noise limited detection. This is fairly straightforward to achieve using heterodyne detection and refers to a quantum-limited detection sensitivity. It is interesting to note that shot noise limited detection can be achieved using relatively low optical power ($\sim 10\,\mu$W) in the local oscillator (interferometer reference arm). Increasing the local oscillator power at the detectors above this level does not increase sensitivity. The most common interferometer design used for OCT, however, is a Michelson interferometer with a single beam splitter that is double-passed. In this case, 25% of the source power travels through the reference arm to the detector and 25% travels through the sample arm. Fully 50% of the source light is thrown away. In early OCT systems using superluminescent diodes, the available source power was only on the order of $100\,\mu$W so that the local oscillator power at the detectors was near the optimal value for shot noise limited detection. With the higher power sources currently available, the use of a Michelson interferometer has become extremely inefficient, because, in addition to the base 50% loss, nearly all of the reference arm light is superfluous. Recently a Mach–Zehnder interferometer with optical circulators was demonstrated that overcomes this inefficiency by biasing most of the source light into the sample arm of the interferometer [6]. This advancement will allow the efficient utilization of new higher power sources.

A final general criterion for evaluating optical sources for OCT is suitability to the application environment. Early studies demonstrating OCT imaging were performed in the laboratory, where the complexity of the system or source is not a critical issue. Many studies are now moving toward in situ and even in vivo imaging, for which a simple, compact, and robust system is essential. Unfortunately, the best sources in terms of resolution and image acquisition rate (femtosecond solid-state lasers) are the worst in terms of complexity, size, and environmental stability. Femtosecond lasers can already provide resolution near 1 μm and are available at several near-infrared wavelengths; the most exciting future advancements for OCT sources are likely to be reductions in the size, cost, and complexity of these sources.

3.1.2 Spectral Shape

In addition to the primary source criteria of wavelength, bandwidth, and power, it is important to recognize the significance of the specific shape or distribution of the source power spectrum. As was derived in Chapter 2, an OCT system free of unbalanced dispersion and wavelength-dependent loss provides an axial point spread function given by the Fourier transform of the source power spectrum:

$$G(\tau) = \int |E(t) + E(t + \tau)|^2 d\omega \approx \int P(\omega) e^{i\omega\tau} d\omega \tag{3}$$

where the delay coordinate is given by τ. This relationship provides a simple understanding of the effects of nonuniform spectral distributions. This section will describe some of the general implications of Eq. (3).

Because one of the primary distinguishing features of OCT is its high dynamic range, most applications under investigation and biomedical imaging in particular require an axial point spread function that has not only a narrow FWHM but also a well-behaved far-field dropoff. A spectral distribution that meets this criterion is the Gaussian

$$P(\lambda) = \exp\left[-4Ln2\left(\frac{\lambda - \lambda_0}{\Delta\lambda}\right)^2\right] \tag{4}$$

Another spectral distribution of interest is the hyperbolic secant:

$$P(\lambda) = \mathrm{sech}\left(1.76\frac{\lambda - \lambda_0}{\Delta\lambda}\right) \tag{5}$$

In both Eqs. (4) and (5) λ represents wavelength and $\Delta\lambda$ is the FWHM of the spectral distribution. To compare these distributions, Fig. 1 shows both the spectra and resulting point spread functions on linear and logarithmic scales. Also shown in this figure is a hyper-Gaussian distribution, a realistic approximation of a rectangle function. While the Gaussian (dots) and hyperbolic secant (solid) spectra give rise to rapidly extinguishing wings in the point spread function, the sharp vertical edges in the hyper-Gaussian spectrum (gray) gives rise to significant far-field ringing. The implications of this ringing for OCT imaging are most noticed near sharp discontinuities in the axial reflectivity or scattering profile, such as at the sample surface or cell or nuclear membranes. In these cases, the far-field wings can mask more weakly scattering adjacent structures. Examples of this artifact will be discussed in the sections on individual sources.

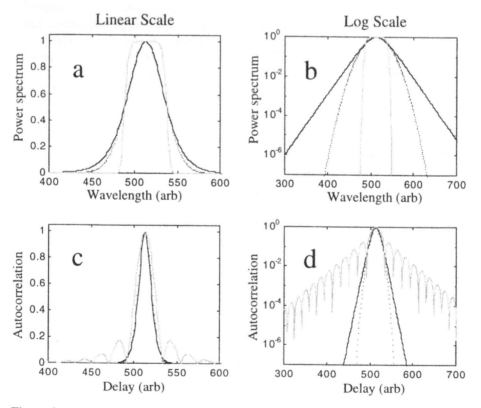

Figure 1   Power spectra (a,b) and autocorrelations (c,d) on linear (a,c) and logarithmic (b,d) scales for Gaussian, hyperbolic secant, and super-Gaussian functions.

Several manufacturers of superluminescent diodes have used multiple spectrally offset semiconductors in the attempt to synthesize broader spectra. Seemingly small distortions of the spectral distribution away from the well-defined Gaussian or hyperbolic secant shape, however, can significantly distort the OCT axial point spread function. As an example, two Gaussian spectra are combined in Fig. 2. The modified spectrum (solid line) was generated by combining a second, offset Gaussian with a narrower width with the Gaussian distribution of the previous figure. In the logarithmic plot of the spectra, this modification is barely discernible. In the logarithmic plot of the axial point spread function, however, the far-field wings are found to be substantial.

Noise superimposed onto a spectrum also has significant implications for OCT imaging. In Fig. 3 the Gaussian spectrum of the previous figures was modified by a multiplicative, random noise with a maximum amplitude of 10%. Although the noise appears small on the spectral plots, it acts to dramatically increase the apparent noise floor of the axial point spread function. In this case the noise was not periodic. In cases where the noise is oscillatory ripple, the point spread function develops discrete wings or echoes located at delay values determined by the period of the oscillation.

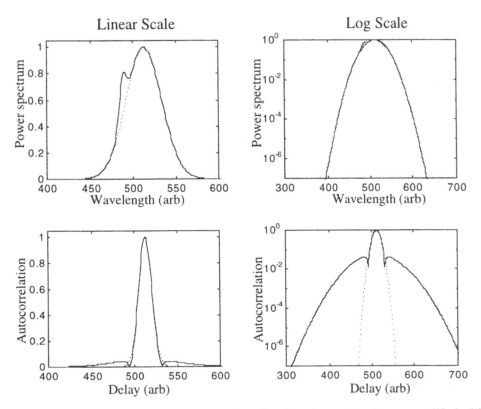

Figure 2 Power spectra and autocorrelations for Gaussian spectra that are modified with a second spectral peak. This is an example of the spectra that might result from combining two sources.

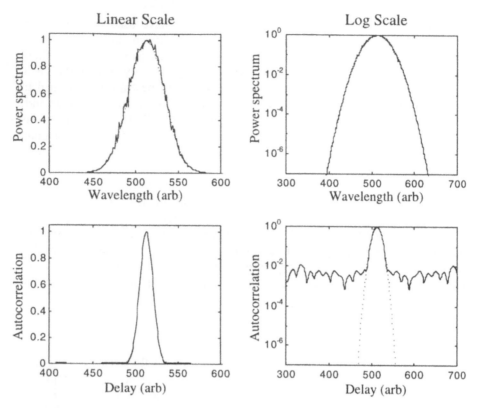

Figure 3 Power spectra and autocorrelations demonstrating the influence of noise or ripple superimposed on a Gaussian spectrum.

A final type of nonuniform spectrum frequently encountered in OCT system development is the clipped spectrum. This can arise from an element in the interferometer that acts as a notch, high-pass, or low-pass filter. In bulk optical systems, this type of filtering can be found in dielectric beamsplitters or mirrors. The phase control rapid scanning optical delay line [7] can also act to clip the spectrum, because this device uses a diffraction grating to spread the spectrum and a galvanometer mirror to reflect the spectrally dispersed light. In an effort to optimize the repetition rate of the galvanometer, the angular momentum of the mirror should be kept as small as possible, requiring minimization of the mirror width. If the mirror is not wide enough, however, a portion of the spectrum can either miss the mirror or be aberrated at the mirror edge. The influence of spectral clipping is shown in Fig. 4. In this case, the wings of the spectrum have been deleted below the 10% level. The resulting sharp edges give rise to weakly damped periodic oscillations in the wings of the point spread function and significantly increase the far-field response.

3.1.3 Amplitude Modulation

A final source characteristic that will be discussed is amplitude stability. In the most common implementation of OCT, light returning from the sample and reference interferometer paths is recombined at a photodiode and the electric current gener-

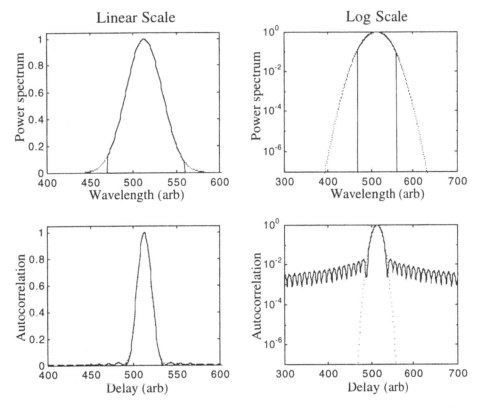

Figure 4 Power spectra and autocorrelation demonstrating the effect of spectral clipping.

ated by the photodiode is measured as a function of delay time. The idealized interferogram depicted in Fig. 5a consists of an envelope function modulated by a sinusoid. The radio-frequency spectrum is the Fourier transform of this and consists of a single-peaked, localized distribution (Fig. 5b). Prior to digitization of the interferogram, filtering electronics are used to reduce out-of-band noise. This can be done by using either bandpass filters or lock-in detection.

Frequently, optical sources generate noise in the form of amplitude modulation. In semiconductor sources, this can result from fluctuations in drive current.

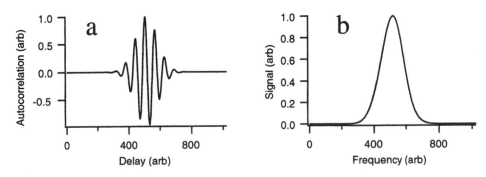

Figure 5 Autocorrelation function and spectrum of ideal Gaussian spectral shape.

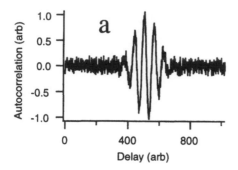

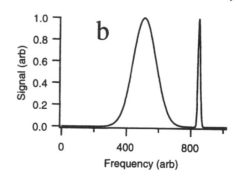

Figure 6 The effect of amplitude modulation either in the source or induced through mechanical instability in the interferometer. Periodic amplitude modulation appears as a discrete spike in frequency space (Fourier transform from interferogram).

Similarly, in solid-state sources, including doped fibers, amplitude modulation can result from fluctuations in pump laser power. Additional sources of light source amplitude instability are longitudinal mode beating and relaxation oscillations. Mechanical perturbations of the interferometer can also give rise to modulation in the photocurrent. The example of Fig. 6a depicts an interferogram that would result from a light source with amplitude modulation of a characteristic time constant. In the frequency domain (Fig. 6b), the modulation gives rise to a discrete peak that in this case is separated from the portion of the spectrum containing ranging information. Understanding the characteristic noise of the light source is important in OCT, because in most systems the heterodyne frequency can be chosen to optimize noise filtering.

The data of Fig. 7 were generated with an OCT system using a diffraction grating based rapid-scanning optical delay line [7]. The heterodyne frequency was adjusted to be 1.0 MHz, and the signal bandwidth was 500 kHz. In this spectrum, the primary contributions to noise are $1/f$ noise and a peak characteristic of the semiconductor light source of this system (Fig. 7a). Because the source noise peak occurring at 300 kHz is outside the information-containing band, a passive filter network (Butterworth filter) can be used to significantly improve the signal (Fig. 7b).

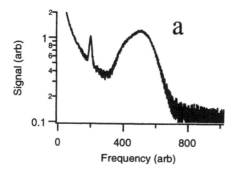

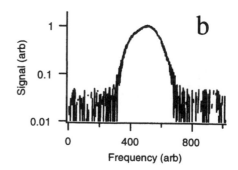

Figure 7 (a) Frequency distribution of OCT detector signal showing broad signal component, $1/f$ noise, and discrete frequency spike arising from amplitude modulation in the source. (b) Same signal after passive bandpass filter.

3.2 SEMICONDUCTOR SOURCES

The development of OCT technology has relied significantly on the availability of advanced devices developed for the telecommunications market. Perhaps the most influential telecom contributions have been in the area of broadband light source development. The first reports of coherence domain ranging and, later, OCT imaging were based on superluminescent diodes (SLDs). The primary advantages to the semiconductor sources are compactness, reliability, environmental stability, and ease of use. Until recently, however, the low power and bandwidth of these sources limited their application to slow acquisition and modest resolution imaging. This section will review typical characteristics of SLDs and the recently developed multiple quantum well semiconductor optical amplifier sources.

3.2.1 Superluminescent Diodes

As mentioned above, SLDs dominated the early work of OCT because of their simplicity and relatively low cost. Most of the early SLDs used for OCT imaging had center wavelengths near 850 nm and provided bandwidths of approximately 20 nm, supporting an OCT resolution of 15 μm. The total cost for these SLDs has been on the order of $5000–10,000 including the diodes, current sources, and thermo-electric cooler controllers. Typical powers for the early SLDs were below 1 mW. The smooth Gaussian spectra of these devices provided low noise, echo-free OCT imaging, but image acquisition times were typically several minutes.

Recent advances in SLD development have enhanced the power, bandwidth, and spectral coverable of available devices. Currently, broadband SLDs are available with center wavelengths near 670, 800, 980, 1300, and 1500 nm. The web site of one of the leaders in SLD development for OCT, Superlum, Ltd (http://www.superlum.ru/), provides complete specifications of some of the more advanced devices currently on the market.

3.2.2 Multiple Quantum Well Semiconductor Optical Amplifiers

A source developed in 1997 by AFC Inc. has become the de facto standard for clinical OCT imaging systems. The primary driving market behind this source was broadband telecommunications. The 1300 nm AFC source is based on a multiple quantum well semiconductor optical amplifier and uses proprietary filtering to achieve bandwidths of 50–80 nm and fiber-coupled powers of 9–30 mW.

At the core of the AFC source is a semiconductor chip containing several quantum wells with chirped periods. The varied confinement dimensions of the wells leads to a combined broad spectrum. The semiconductor chip is configured in a butterfly package with fiber-optic input and output. To further increase the power of the amplified spontaneous emission of these devices, one output direction can be spectrally filtered to precompensate for gain narrowing incurred during a second, amplifying pass through the waveguide. One potential drawback of this source is that its emission is unpolarized. Polarization-sensitive OCT imaging, which requires a polarized source, can therefore access only half of the available power.

An example image acquired using a 1300 nm AFC source is depicted in Fig. 8. This system used a nonreciprocal fiber-optic interferometer and a fiber-optic catheter

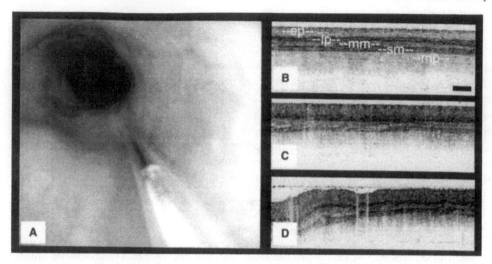

Figure 8   (A) Endoscope view showing linear scanning OCT catheter in human esophagus. (B–D) Although inter- and intrapatient variability of layer thickness and structure is noticed, five discrete layers are always observed in the normal esophagus. The OCT images were acquired using a semiconductor multiple quantum well optical amplifier emitting 10 mW at 1.3 μm.

to image the gastrointestinal tract of human patients [6]. Typical images of the human esophagus are shown.

3.3   DOPED FIBER SOURCES

The need for a high power, clinically viable low coherence source has motivated the investigation of diode-pumped rare-earth-doped single-mode fibers (REDFs). These single-mode, broad-bandwidth superfluorescent light sources are compact, relatively simple, and inexpensive. In addition to evaluating the capability of the REDFs as a high resolution, high power source for OCT, research using REDFs at different wavelengths has provided insight for the determination of appropriate wavelengths for OCT imaging in tissue.

If the excitation of the REDF is strong, the fluorescent light emitted from the fibers is amplified by stimulated emission. The pump energy is stored primarily as a population inversion, which in turn amplifies the guided fluorescence [8]. The wavelength dependence of the gain, however, leads to a narrowing of the emitted spectrum with amplification. In addition, if any backreflections are present in the fiber, either from a backscattering site within the device or from Rayleigh scattering from the fiber, lasing will commence and further reduce the spectral width [8]. For these reasons, many REDFs require spectral filtering to compensate for gain narrowing so that useful power levels can be achieved.

Figure 9 depicts several different fiber configurations used for creating REDF superfluorescent sources [9]. In order to suppress lasing, feedback from either one or both fiber ends can be eliminated by angle cleaving or polishing. The forward superfluorescent signal (SFS) configuration is the simplest to implement but reduces the

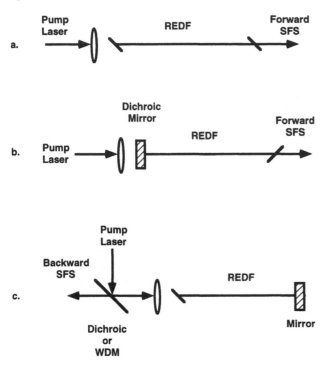

Figure 9 Rare-earth-doped single-mode fiber (REDF) pump and fiber configurations. (a) Single-pass forward SFS; (b) double-passed forward SFS; and (c) double-passed backward SFS.

useful superfluorescent power by 50% (Fig. 9a). In the single-pass forward SFS case, both fiber ends are cleaved and the superfluorescence is detected from the fiber face opposite the pump. Many of the REDF sources presented in this chapter use the single-pass forward SFS configuration because of its simplicity and complete elimination of feedback from both fiber ends. Figures 9b and 9c depict double-pass configurations. Double-pass SFS geometries enable the use of both forward- and backward-propagating superfluorescence.

One problem with REDF superfluorescent sources is the need for a high power ($\sim 500\,\text{mW}$) single-mode pump for optimal coupling into the doped single-mode core. Although some compact semiconductor diode sources produce a single-mode output with these powers, they are typically very expensive. Because of the need for an inexpensive and compact pump, a cladding-pumped geometry has been adopted to enable coupling into the fibers with less expensive multimode diodes (Fig. 10). The cladding-pumped REDF consists of an asymmetrical cladding surrounding the doped core [9]. The shape of the inner cladding can be tailored to match the geometry of the pump diode emissions. For a given dopant density, the length of the cladding-pumped fiber must be much greater than that of the single-mode doped fiber because the absorption of the pump light per unit length is much lower than for standard single-mode REDFs. For four-level systems, such as Nd : silica and Yb : silica, which exhibit little absorption in the emission band, the greater fiber length does not pose a prbolem. For three-level systems or quasi-four-level systems,

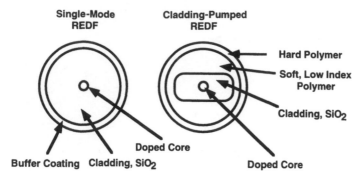

Figure 10   REDF cladding-pumped geometries.

however, such as Er : silica and Tm : silica, the increased length of the fiber causes increased absorption of the superfluorescence. For this reason, rare earth ions with three-level or quasi-four-level transitions have not been used in the cladding-pumped geometry.

3.3.1   Neodymium

Neodymium : silica excited at 800 nm has a strong four-level transition at 1060 nm and is therefore well suited as a dopant for the cladding-pumped fiber geometry. Initial experiments were performed using a double-clad fiber to evaluate the suitability of this source for OCT. Because optical scattering in tissue at 1060 nm is stronger than the scattering at 1300 nm, one would expect the penetration to be less. However, the absorption at 1060 is lower than the absorption at 1300 nm. One goal of the preliminary OCT studies with the Nd : silica fiber was to determine the significance of the differences in absorption and scattering in tissue.

Figure 11 depicts the fluorescence spectrum of a 10 m single-mode Nd : silica REDF pumped at 800 nm with 100 mW Ti : Al_2O_3 power. The Nd : silica REDF was obtained from J. Minelli, University of Southampton, UK. Although the shape of the fluorescence spectrum seems reasonable for OCT imaging without significant side lobes in the autocorrelation function, the total integrated power emitted was only 16 μW. At higher pump powers the amplified spontaneous emission exhibits significant narrowing. The Nd : silica REDF pumped with 600 mW produces 3.5 mW of SFS, but the spectrum contains significant gain narrowing at the dominant emission line, 1060 nm (Fig. 12). The width of the dominant peak is now only 8 nm, corresponding to a coherence length of 62 μm. If this peak narrowing can be suppressed, the wings of the SFS can be amplified and the REDF spectrum can be broadened. The next section describes the use of an in-line long-period Bragg grating to broaden the Nd : silica REDF SFS spectrum.

To decrease the gain narrowing in Nd : silica at high pump power, a Bragg grating filtered, cladding-pumped Nd : silica REDF has been developed. The Bragg grating filtered Nd : silica REDF was obtained from E. A. Swanson, Lincoln Laboratory, MA. A schematic of the system is shown in Fig. 13. This system uses 3.7 m of cladding-pumped Nd : silica fiber in a double-passed backward SFS configuration. To eliminate the spectral gain narrowing at 1060 nm, an in-line optical

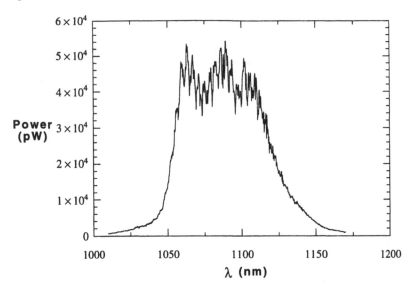

Figure 11 Spectrum of single-mode Nd : silica REDF pumped with 100 mW. The integrated emitted power was 16 μW.

notch filter is spliced between the REDF and the mirror. The notch filter is a long-period Bragg grating that is written into a single-mode optical fiber (Fig. 14). The Bragg grating flattens the spectrum by diminishing the peak at 1060 nm while allowing amplified spontaneous emission (ASE) to pass unfiltered outside of the bandwidth of the notch filter (Fig. 15). The output power from the filtered REDF is 7 mW, with a multimode diode pump power of 200 mW at 810 nm. The bandwidth of the filtered spectrum is 39 nm, corresponding to a measured FWHM coherence length of 16 μm.

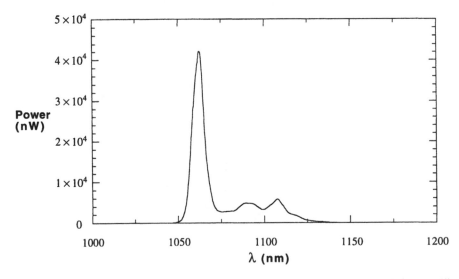

Figure 12 Gain-narrowed superfluorescent spectrum for a double-clad Nd : silica fiber pumped with 600 mW of 800 nm power. The total integrated power is 3.5 mW.

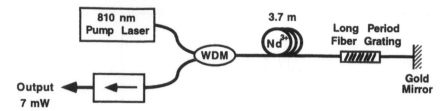

Figure 13   Schematic of the Nd:silica REDF superfluorescent source with the long-period Bragg fiber grating.

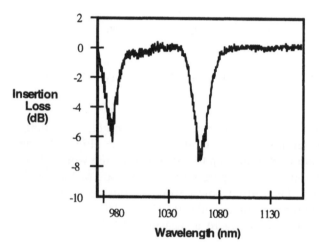

Figure 14   Long-period Bragg grating notch filter transmission spectrum.

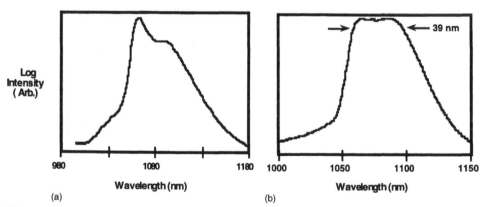

Figure 15   Double-clad SFS spectrum of Nd:silica REDF (a) without notch filter and (b) with notch filter.

The notch-filtered Nd : silica REDF effectively broadens the SFS spectrum to provide a FWHM coherence length that is comparable to the 1300 nm SLD coherence length. However, the filtered Nd : silica REDF spectral shape deviates significantly from Gaussian. The rectangular shape of the filtered Nd : silica REDF will cause side lobes of nonnegligible magnitude to appear in the autocorrelation function. The autocorrelation functions for both a 1300 nm SLD and the double-clad, filtered, Nd : silica-filtered REDF are shown in Fig. 16. The side lobes in the REDF autocorrelation function are only 15 dB down from the main peak.

After measurement of the spectra and autocorrelation functions, the filtered, double-clad Nd : silica source was coupled into an OCT system. Images of a calcified aortic plaque were compared to images of the same plaque taken with the 1300 nm SLD source. The source powers were adjusted so that the SNR of the OCT system was 105 dB for both sources. The images are shown in Fig. 17. In the REDF image, the side lobes in the autocorrelation function cause a blurred air/tissue interface at the top of the image. Because of the high reflectivity at this interface, the magnitude of the side lobes in the autocorrelation function is comparable to that of the tissue signal levels. This artifact can be perceived in all OCT images that have been acquired with a non-Gaussian source. In addition, the internal structures of the plaque, such as highly calcified foci, also appear blurred compared to the same features in the SLD image. Again, this artifact is due to side lobes caused by the rectangular shape of the filtered REDF spectrum. Finally, in this sample, the penetration is approximately the same for the two wavelengths. Possibly, the increase in scattering at 1060 nm may be offset by the decrease in water absorption at this wavelength. This result may indicate that the OCT imaging penetration depth at 1060 nm may be similar to the penetration depth at 1300 nm. These encouraging results suggest that further efforts to refine the Bragg filter and produce a more Gaussian spectrum are warranted.

3.3.2 Ytterbium

Ytterbium-doped silica has a broad emission spectrum ranging from 1000 to 1200 nm, with an absorption spectrum ranging from 850 to 1000 nm. Typically,

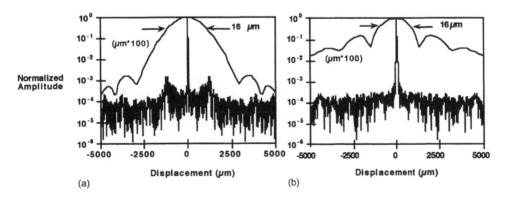

Figure 16 Autocorrelation functions for the (a) the 1300 nm SLD and (b) the filtered 1060 nm REDF. The top curve in both images represents a magnification of the displacement axis by 100×.

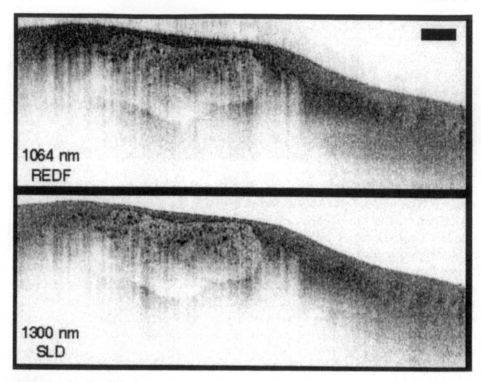

Figure 17   Optical coherence tomographic images of a calcified aortic atherosclerotic plaque taken with the 1064 nm filtered REDF and the 1300 nm SLD. Bar represents 500 μm.

Yb : silica is pumped at 980 nm because low cost, high power diodes are available at this wavelength. However, the gain-narrowed bandwidth for a cladding-pumped Yb : silica REDF in the single-passed SFS configuration is approximately 15 nm, which corresponds to a coherence length of only 35 μm (Fig. 18). The cladding-pumped Yb : silica REDF was obtained from M. Muendel, Polaroid Corporation, MA. Like the Nd : silica REDF, a shorter coherence length is desirable, and spectral notch filtering must be used to decrease peak narrowing at 1100 nm while allowing ASE to pass unfiltered outside the bandwidth of the notch filter.

   For comparison with the Bragg grating filtered Nd : silica REDF, a cladding-pumped Yb : silica REDF ASE source has been constructed that uses a cascade of custom wavelength division multiplexers (WDMs) to perform the spectral filtering. The WDM-filtered Yb : silica REDF was obtained from S. Chernikov, Imperial College, London. A schematic of the WDM-filtered Yb : silica source is shown in Fig. 19. The ASE source consists of two lengths of Yb : silica fiber pumped by using three separate 980 nm diodes in a double-passed SFS configuration.

   The spectrum of the WDM-filtered Yb : silica REDF source is shown in Fig. 20. The spectrum is very rectangular, which gives rise to severe artifacts in the autocorrelation. The autocorrelation function for this WDM-filtered Yb : silica REDF source is shown in Fig. 21. The 75 nm bandwidth centered at 1075 nm, produced by the Yb : silica REDF source, provides a FWHM coherence length of

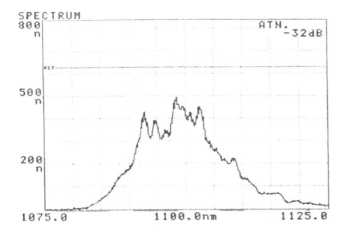

Figure 18 Spectrum of unfiltered Yb : silica fiber pumped at 980 nm. Pump power is 700 mW, total emission is 50 mW, bandwidth is 25 nm.

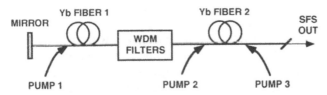

Figure 19 Schematic of the wavelength division multiplexer (WDM) filtered Yb : silica REDF ASE source.

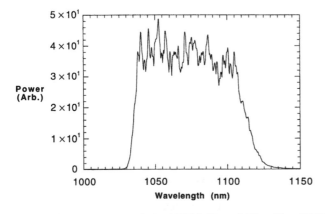

Figure 20 Spectrum of the WDM-filtered Yb : silica REDF source.

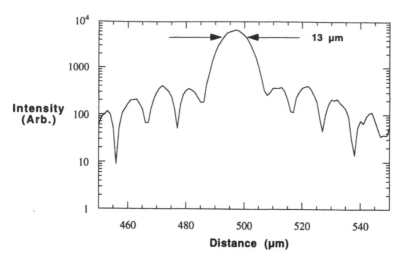

Figure 21 Autocorrelation function of the WDM-filtered Yb : silica REDF ASE source. The FWHM bandwidth is 13 μm.

13 μm with an output SFS power of 10 mW. Like the Bragg grating filtered Nd : silica REDF, the WDM-filtered Yb : silica source contains side lobes due to the rectangular shape of the spectrum. These side lobes are similar in magnitude to those of the Bragg grating filtered Nd : silica REDF.

Images of an in vitro human breast carcinoma were acquired with the WDM-filtered Yb : silica REDF ASE source (Fig. 22). Although some tissue features can be identified, such as adipose cells near the surface of the image, side lobes present in the autocorrelation function cause blurring of the surface and the internal structure. Because of these severe artifacts, a second-generation source must be designed that uses WDM filters to not only reduce gain peaking but also shape the spectrum to be more Gaussian.

3.3.3 Erbium

A very common single-mode doped fiber source used in telecommunications applications is the Er : silica REDF. The erbium fiber is pumped at 980 nm and has a

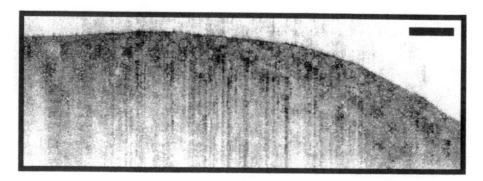

Figure 22 Optical coherence tomographic image of human breast carcinoma acquired using the WDM-filtered Yb : silica REDF. Bar represents 500 μm.

three-level transition with peak emission at 1550 nm and a bandwidth of approximately 50 nm [9]. The Er : silica REDF exhibits gain narrowing, so spectral filtering would be necessary to produce a sufficient coherence length. Because the Er : silica emission is a three-level transition, the cladding-pumped geometry cannot be used owing to absorption of the signal. In addition, although scattering is lower at 1550 nm that at any of the previous wavelengths, the erbium emission band overlaps with the high water absorption peak at 1480 nm. For this reason, it is expected that OCT imaging with Er : silica REDF ASE would have a lower penetration depth than imaging with other sources discussed in this chapter.

3.3.4 Praseodymium

Praseodymium-doped silica fiber has a gain-narrowed spectrum that is significantly broader than the gain-narrowed spectrum of Nd : silica REDF. A 590 nm pumped Pr : silica REDF ASE source has been reported to have a broad Gaussian spectrum with a FWHM at 25 nm [10]. With a pump power of 250 mW, the Pr : silica REDF produces 60 mW SFS at 1049 nm. The primary problem with the Pr : silica REDF is that there are no inexpensive high power single-mode diodes at 590 nm. Instead, Shi and Poulsen [10] used a dye laser to pump the Pr : silica REDF. Until an inexpensive diode source at 590 nm is available, the Pr : silica REDF is unlikely to become a clinically viable source for OCT.

3.3.5 Thulium

An intriguing spectral range for OCT imaging exists at wavelengths longer than the prominent water absorption band at 1480 nm. Between 1600 and 1800 nm, water absorption decreases, and near 2.0 μm it rises sharply again. Because of the inverse dependence of scattering on wavelength, the attenuation in tissue due to scattering in this wavelength range is low. Thus, sources between 1650 and 1800 nm could give rise to OCT imaging penetration depths equal to or greater than the penetration at 1300 nm.

Thulium-doped silica is an REDF with a quasi-four-level transition at 1800 nm. The maximum absorption peak is very narrow and is located at 785 nm. Figure 23 shows a plot of a single-mode Tm : silica REDF emission spectrum pumped at 785 nm in the single-passed SFS configuration. The Tm : silica REDF was obtained from L. Nelson and E. P. Ippen, Massachusetts Institute of Technology, Boston, MA. The single-mode doped fiber was 2 m long and was pumped with 500 mW of Ti : Al$_2$O$_3$ power at 785 nm. The SFS bandwidth is 80 nm, which gives rise to a FWHM coherence length of 18 μm. The gain-narrowed spectrum is asymmetrical but more Gaussian than the spectrally filtered ASE sources. The Tm : silica REDF produced a total integrated SFS output power of 4 mW. Figure 24 shows a comparison between an image of a calcified aortic plaque acquired using the Tm : silica source (Fig. 24a) and an image of the same plaque acquired with a 1300 nm SLD (Fig. 24b). Both OCT images were taken with the same SNR, 102 dB.

As can be seen in these images, the Tm : silica REDF shows sharp delineation of boundaries in the image, such as the calcified foci within the plaque. In addition, no blurring due to autocorrelation side lobes is seen at the surface. Finally, the penetration depth in this particular image of the heavily calcified aortic plaque seems to be at least equal to the penetration depth of the 1300 nm SLD image.

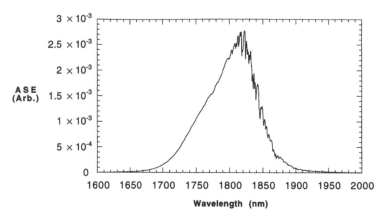

Figure 23   Superfluorescent spectrum of Tm : silica REDF.

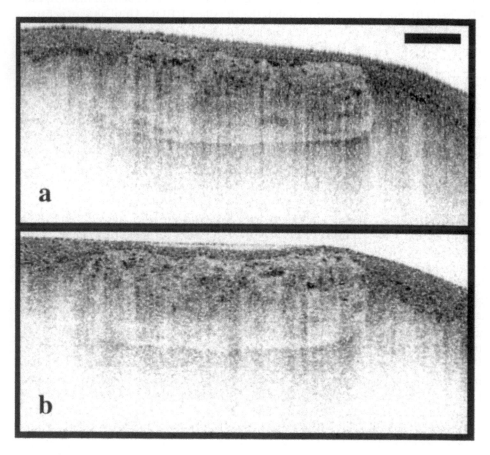

Figure 24   Optical coherence tomographic images of a calcified aortic atherosclerotic plaque taken with (a) the 1800 Tm : silica REDF source and (b) the 1300 nm SLD. Bar represents 500 μm.

One major disadvantage to Tm : silica is that it cannot be used in a cladding-pumped configuration because it is a quasi-four-level system. In a three-level or quasi-four-level system, the ground-state absorption of the SFS signal extinguishes the emission over a long length of fiber. Single-mode pumps at 785 nm are commercially available but expensive, and for this reason Tm : silica REDF ASE sources may not be as desirable as other less expensive, high power REDF ASE sources.

3.4 SOLID-STATE LASERS

Lasers that rely on a crystalline gain medium are one type of solid-state laser. Rare earth ions can be doped into the crystal, replacing one of the host ions at a specific lattice site. The choices of crystal host and rare earth ion allow many different possibilities of excitation and emission wavelengths. Over the last 15 years, several new laser crystals have been developed that take advantage of the vibrational interaction between the crystalline host and the dopant ion to significantly broaden the absorption and emission spectra [11]. The results have been quite impressive; these phonon-broadened sources provide greater spectral widths than any other laser sources.

The broad emission spectra of a solid-state laser can be used for OCT imaging in two ways, either as superluminescent sources [12] or through mode locking [13–15]. Because fluorescence is emitted isotropically in space and the laser crystal does not provide the light guiding and confinement of an optical fiber, it is difficult to produce more than a few microwatts of superluminescent light from solid-state sources. Mode locking provides a much more attractive alternative. By controlling the phase relationship of many longitudinal resonator modes, short duration pulses and therefore broad spectra can be produced. In addition, mode-locked solid-state lasers can produce hundreds of milliwatts of power and typically lower relative-intensity noise.

In this section, the application of two of the solid-state lasers through mode locking to OCT imaging will be reviewed. Both of these lasers rely on passive, Kerr lens mode locking and use similar resonator designs (Fig. 25). The resonator uses four mirrors, one of which is partially reflective to provide output coupling, and dispersion-compensating prisms. The laser crystal is mounted between two concave spherical mirrors and is excited longitudinally. Kerr lens mode locking takes advantage of the inherent nonlinearity of the laser crystal itself to provide a resonator loss that is dependent upon the intensity of the light in the cavity. This provides preferential gain for pulses of short temporal duration.

3.4.1 Ti : Al$_2$O$_3$

Mode-locked solid-state lasers have been used as high power and high resolution sources for OCT. Kerr lens mode locking (KLM) in Ti : Al$_2$O$_3$ oscillators (Fig. 25) has been shown to produce high average power near-infrared pulses with duration < 10 fs [16–18]. Ti : Al$_2$O$_3$ oscillators have been used for OCT imaging with outstanding resolution [13,15]. To maintain the high resolution of the Ti : Al$_2$O$_3$ source, dispersion imbalance between the interferometer arms must be precisely canceled [12]. To perform dispersion balancing, a fused silica prism pair with faces contacted and index matched to form a variable thickness window is inserted in the reference

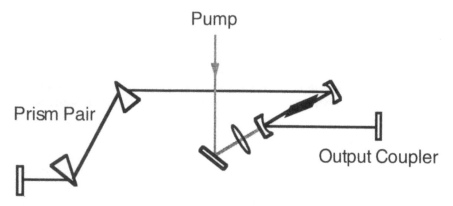

Figure 25 Schematic of KLM solid-state oscillator. This common, four-mirror design uses prisms for dispersion compensation. Excitation of the laser crystal is provided through longitudinal pumping.

arm (Fig. 26) [13]. The width of the autocorrelation function is minimized by translating the prisms along their contacted faces. This simple adjustment compensates for differences in fiber length, collimating lens, and microscope objectives between the interferometer arms. The Ti : Al_2O_3 laser has high amplitude noise relative to that of SLD sources. Thus, a dual balanced detection scheme is used to attain a shot noise limited signal-to-noise ratio (SNR) [13].

Optical coherence tomographic images of an onion performed with the standard resolution of 1300 nm SLD source system used in the tissue surveys and with the KLM Ti : Al_2O_3 system demonstrate a marked improvement in resolution provided by the Ti : Al_2O_3 laser (Fig. 27). In both images, the transverse resolution is approximately matched to the axial resolution. In the image acquired using the Ti : Al_2O_3 laser, the confocal parameter is $40\,\mu m$, corresponding to a spot size of $5\,\mu m$. Resolution degradation due to beam divergence becomes apparent at greater depths. The confocal parameter for the 1300 nm SLD image in Fig. 27 is $350\,\mu m$, correspond-

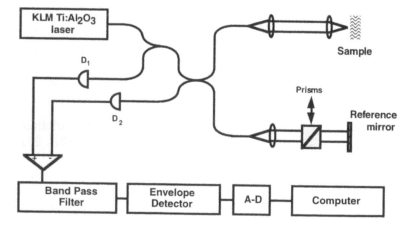

Figure 26 Schematic of Ti : Al_2O_3 oscillator coupled into the OCT system.

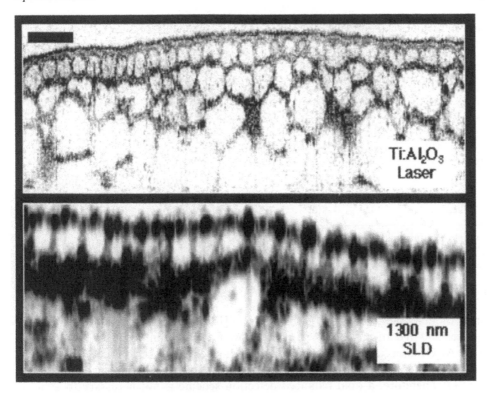

Figure 27 OCT images of an onion acquired with the 800 nm Ti : Al$_2$O$_3$ laser and the 1300 nm SLD source. Bar represents 100 μm.

ing to a spot size of approximately 17 μm. Both of these images have dimensions of 120 vertical and 360 horizontal pixels. The image acquisition time was 2.5 s.

The KLM Ti : Al$_2$O$_3$ laser coupled to an optimized OCT system enables high resolution, high power imaging of biological structures. Additionally, the application of KLM to other solid-state laser materials will provide high power, short coherence length source at wavelengths with greater penetration in tissue such as 1.3 μm from Cr^{4+} : forsterite and 1.5 μm from Cr^{4+} : YAG.

3.4.2 Cr^{4+} : Mg$_2$SiO$_4$

Although Ti : Al$_2$O$_3$ lasers can produce unrivaled resolution for OCT imaging, optical scattering in biological tissues near 800 nm limits imaging depth of penetration. Previous comparisons of imaging depth using 1.3 μm and 800 nm light from SLDs motivated the development of other solid-state lasers capable of providing broad spectra at longer wavelengths. Like Ti : Al$_2$O$_3$, Cr^{4+} : forsterite is a phonon broadened, tunable solid-state laser material that can be used for the generation of femtosecond optical pulses. Application of Kerr lens mode locking to a Nd : YAG-pumped Cr^{4+} : forsterite oscillator has been achieved with pulse duration as short as 25 fs [19,20].

A Cr^{4+} : forsterite laser has been constructed for use as a high power, high resolution OCT source by pumping Cr^{4+} : forsterite with 6.0 W of 1.06 mm light

Table 1 Summary of Relevant Parameters of Sources Demonstrated for OCT Imaging

Source	Pump λ (nm)	Pump power (W)	Emission λ (nm)	Bandwidth Δλ (nm) (Coherence length)		Emission power (mW)	Point spread function
Ti : Al$_2$O$_3$	514	6.0	800	300	(1 μm)	400	Good
Cr^{4+} : Mg$_2$SiO$_4$	1064	6.0	1280	200	(5 μm)	300	Fair
MQW SOA[a]			1300	80	(9 μm)	10	Excellent
Nd : silica	810	0.2[b]	1060	39	(16 μm)	7	Poor
Yb : silica	980	0.3[b]	1075	75	(13 μm)	10	Poor
Tm : silica	785	1.0[c]	1800	80	(18 μm)	4	Good

[a] Multiple quantum well semiconductor optical amplifier.
[b] Cladding pumped.
[c] Core pumped.

from a diode-excited Nd : YAG laser (Fig. 28) [14]. The KLM Cr^{4+} : forsterite laser produces 300 mW of mode-locked output power at 1280 nm. In addition, although the Ti : Al$_2$O$_3$ laser has a high relative intensity noise relative to that of SLD sources, the Cr^{4+} : forsterite amplitude fluctuations are much lower and comparable to that of the SLD. Therefore, a dual balanced detection scheme is not necessary to achieve shot noise limited detection. The single transverse mode output from this oscillator is well suited for coupling to standard single-mode optical fiber with sufficient power to enable rapid acquisition of OCT images while preserving high signal-to-noise ratios. The spectrum emitted from this laser has a FWHM bandwidth of 50 nm corresponding to a coherence length of 15 μm.

For high resolution imaging applications, the high peak power of the pulses from this laser have been used to nonlinearly broaden the laser spectrum

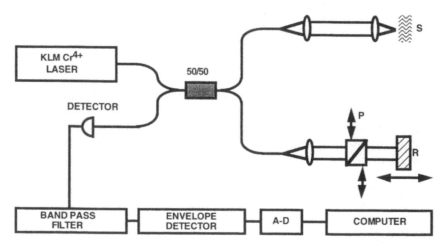

Figure 28 Schematic of the Cr^{4+} : forsterite laser coupled into the OCT system.

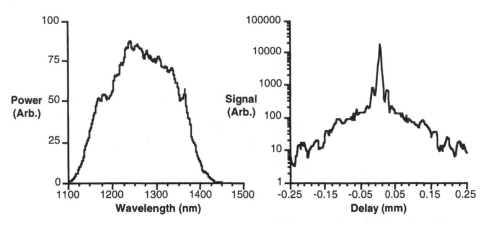

Figure 29 Spectrum and autocorrelation function for the self-phase-modulated Cr^{4+}:forsterite laser.

through self-phase modulation [14]. The mode-locked output of the Cr^{4+}:forsterite laser at 100 mW of average power was coupled into a single-mode Corning SMF/DS dispersion-shifted fiber (zero group velocity at $1.55\,\mu m$) as shown in Fig. 29. Figure 29 also displays the demodulated autocorrelation function corresponding to the spectrum. The FWHM coherence length produced from this source measures $5.7\,\mu m$. Side lobes in the autocorrelation function due to the rectangular shape of the spectrum are almost 20 dB lower than the maximum peak intensity.

A cross-sectional tomographic image of human adipose tissue generated in vitro with the Cr^{4+}:forsterite self-phase-modulated source is shown in Fig. 30. Again, the transverse resolution, determined by the spot size on the sample, was chosen to approximately match the axial resolution of the self-phase-modulated laser source, $6\,\mu m$. The power incident on the sample was 2 mW, corresponding to a measured signal-to-noise ratio of 115 dB. The image dimensions were 5.0 mm transverse (600 pixels) by 5 mm axial (200 pixels). The entire image was acquired in 30 s. The high resolution of this system permits the visualization of tissue microstructure including cell membranes and intercellular spaces.

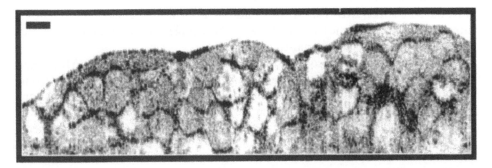

Figure 30 Optical coherence tomographic image of in vitro human adipose tissue acquired using the self-phase-modulated Cr^{4+}:forsterite source. Bar represents $100\,\mu m$.

3.4.3   Cr^{4+}:YAG

Neodymium:YAG-pumped Cr^{4+}:YAG KLM oscillators [21,22] can be mode locked over the range of 1.34–1.58 μm and have been shown to produce high intensity 70 fs pulses (37 nm bandwidth). Like the Cr^{4+}:forsterite sources, high peak intensity pulses from Cr^{4+}:YAG are capable of being spectrally broadened through self-phase modulation in optical fibers. Some degree of uncertainty exists about the utility of Cr^{4+}:YAG for OCT in tissue. Although tissue scattering in the wavelength range 1.34–1.58 μm is low, this range coincides with the water absorption peak at 1.48 μm. The increased tissue absorption at these wavelengths may decrease the imaging penetration of OCT systems using the KLM Cr^{4+}:YAG oscillator.

3.4.4   Optical Parametric Oscillator

An optical parametric oscillator (OPO) is a laser source that uses parametric frequency conversion as an amplifying medium [23]. Tunable synchronized pulses are generated simultaneously at two wavelengths, forming signal and idler branches of the parametric process. The wavelengths of the signal and the idler are constrained so that the sum of their photon energy is equal to the photon energy of the excitation light. Optical parametric oscillators configured for pumping with mode-locked Ti:Al$_2$O$_3$ lasers are commercially available and can produce pulse durations below 100 fs. In this case, tunability over the range of 1.1–2.2 μm can be achieved with output power over 100 mW in each branch.

   To investigate the use of an OPO as a source of tunable, low coherence light, an experiment was performed using a commercially available Ti:Al$_2$O$_3$ oscillator and OPO for OCT imaging of biological tissue.* The signal and idler branches of the OPO output were used to access wavelengths from 1.0 to 2.0 μm at intervals of approximately 50 nm. Light from the OPO was coupled into a fiber-optic interferometer, and a mechanically scanning reference arm was used to acquire axial scan information. Light from the sample arm of the interferometer was imaged through an aspheric lens pair so that identical focal spot sizes were achieved at each wavelength. The interferometer was composed of a single wavelength-flattened coupler with a transmission-to-reflection ratio of 50:50 from 1.2 μm to 1.5 μm with no more than 5% deviation. Outside of this wavelength range, the coupling ratio deviated from 50:50 by as much as 20%. Because as much as 100 mW of power could be coupled from the OPO into the fiber-optic interferometer, unbalanced coupling ratios could be compensated for by attenuation. At each wavelength in the study, one attenuator in the reference arm and one in the sample arm were used to achieve constant OCT sensitivity and signal-to-noise ratios.

   An example of the data acquired in this experiment is shown in Fig. 31. In this figure, images of human cadaver trachea are shown using center wavelengths from 1.3 μm to 1.9 μm. The specimen was held in a dish with saline to prevent dehydration during the experiment. The arc below the surface of the tissue is cartilage. At the center wavelengths 1350, 1450, and 1900 nm, the penetration depth is diminished,

---

* Bouma, BE, Pitris, C, Steinmeyer, G, Ripin, D, Ippen, EP, Fujimoto, JG. Unpublished. This study was performed in the laboratories of Professors Fujimoto and Ippen in the Research Laboratory of Electronics at MIT.

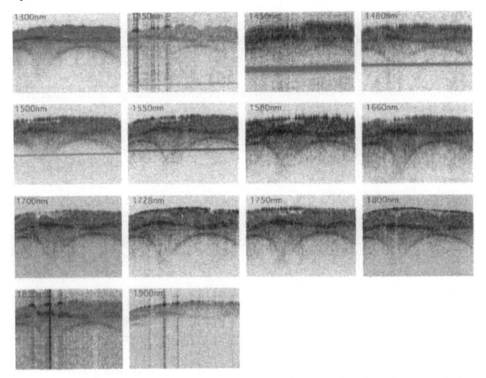

Figure 31 Images of human cadaver trachea at various wavelengths using an optical parametric oscillator.

most likely due to prominent water absorption bands. At other wavelengths, very little change is noticed in either contrast or depth of penetration.

In the images of Fig. 31, it is apparent that the axial point spread function of the OPO used in this study varied significantly both in width and in roll-off. The prominence of this artifact at wavelengths of 1350, 1450, 1850, and 1900 nm suggests that water vapor absorption in the OPO resonator may be responsible. If more efficient purging of the resonator can be used to significantly reduce this effect, the femtosecond OPO may become a more useful tool for OCT imaging. One application for a stable, tunable source of low coherence light would be the investigation of the wavelength dependence of optical properties in biological tissues [24].

3.5 SELF-PHASE MODULATION

Self-phase modulation is based on a third-order nonlinear effect known as the optical Kerr effect. The nonlinear polarization component at frequency ω produces a change in the susceptibility of the medium, $\Delta\chi$, such that

$$\Delta\chi = \frac{P_{\mathrm{NL}}(\omega)}{\epsilon_o E(\omega)} = \frac{3\chi^{(3)}|E(\omega)|^2}{\epsilon_o} = 6\chi^{(3)}\eta I \tag{6}$$

where

$$I = \frac{|E(\omega)|^2}{2\eta} \tag{7}$$

is the intensity of the incident optical wave and P_{NL} is the nonlinear polarization. Because the refractive index is determined by χ through the relation

$$n^2 = 1 + \chi \tag{8}$$

the Kerr nonlinearity gives rise to an intensity-dependent change in the refractive index:

$$\Delta n = \frac{\partial n}{\partial \chi} \Delta \chi = 3 \frac{\chi^{(3)}}{n} \eta I \tag{9}$$

Because of the optical Kerr effect, a pulse of light confined in an optical fiber is modulated in phase such that

$$\Delta \phi(t) = k \, \Delta n(t)l = k n_2 l I(t) \tag{10}$$

where l is the length of the optical fiber. The frequency is then modulated by

$$\Delta \omega(t) = -\frac{\partial}{\partial t} \Delta \phi(t) = -k n_2 l \frac{\partial}{\partial t} I(t) \tag{11}$$

For most glasses and laser host crystals, the magnitude of n_2 requires focused femtosecond pulses to generate appreciable frequency shifts. When these conditions are met, however, the rising edge of the pulse gives rise to a red-shifted spectrum while the falling edge creates a blue shift.

In typical media, the diffraction that results from tight focusing and normal dispersion acts to limit the integrated nonlinear frequency shift that can be achieved. In the work described Section 2.4.2 on $Cr^{4+}:Mg_2SiO_4$, femtosecond pulses at a wavelength of $1.3\,\mu m$ were focused into SMF-DS fiber for which dispersion is weak. This allowed the femtosecond pulses to travel a longer distance before dispersion reduced their intensity below the threshold for self-phase modulation by temporally broadening the pulses.

The generation of significant frequency broadening through self-phase modulation at a wavelength of 800 nm where standard optical fibers have large normal dispersion is not possible with unamplified laser pulses. A very exciting advancement in this area has recently come from Lucent Technologies, where a new type of optical fiber has been developed [25]. Lucent's fiber uses a microstructured cladding to induce a large difference between the index of refraction of the fiber core and the surrounding cladding (Fig. 32). This results in both stronger guiding and significant waveguide dispersion. Stronger guiding is advantageous for self-phase modulation, because as the cross-sectional area of the guide is reduced the power density of the light is increased. The anomalous waveguide dispersion of Lucent's fiber has been designed to balance the normal dispersion of bulk silica so that the net dispersion experienced by propagating pulses is zero near 800 nm. The combined result of strong confinement and dispersion-free propagation can lead to significant integrated nonlinearity and pronounced spectral broadening.

Using a 75 cm section of the microstructured fiber and 800 pJ, 100 fs pulses with a center wavelength of 790 nm, the Lucent researchers were able to generate a broadband continuum extending from 400 nm to 1600 nm (Fig. 33) [25]. Although it remains to be demonstrated as a source for OCT imaging, this spectrum could potentially provide submicrometer axial resolution. Perhaps more interesting, however, would be the use of this source for combined OCT imaging and spectroscopy.

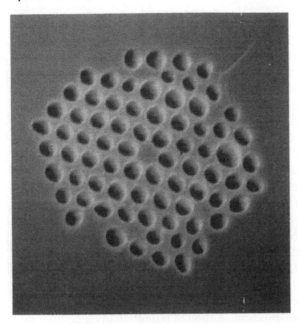

Figure 32 Air–silica microstructured fiber from Lucent Technologies.

3.6 SUMMARY

Solid-state lasers provide high power, broad-spectrum, low coherence light that enables both high speed and high resolution OCT. In their current state of development, they are valuable tools for performing preliminary OCT studies in vitro. However, the cost and size of these devices make their use impractical outside of a research setting. Development performed to miniaturize KLM solid-state lasers would greatly increase the likelihood that these sources could be integrated into a clinical setting. A second possibility for the use of femtosecond lasers in OCT would be as pulse sources for continuum generation in microstructured fiber. The exceptional bandwidth and potential for high power of this hybrid source will undoubtedly make it the focus of intense investigation in the next few years.

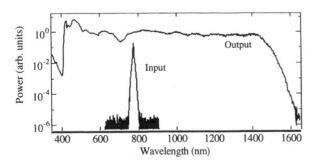

Figure 33 Spectrum generated through self-phase modulation of Ti : sapphire laser pulses in air–silica microstructured fiber.

The REDF ASE sources also require improvement. Both the filtered Nd : silica and the Yb : silica REDFs suffer from side lobes due to a rectangularly shaped emission spectrum. Distortions in the OCT images caused by autocorrelation side lobes should be improved in second generation ASE devices that not only diminish gain narrowing but also provide spectral shaping to avoid side lobes. Praseodymium : silica and Tm : silica REDF sources have broad enough gain bandwidths to be used without filtering, and their spectra are much closer to Gaussian. However, no 590 nm semiconductor diode is currently available to pump the Pr : silica ASE source. Although 785 nm diodes are available to pump the Tm : silica source, cladding-pumped geometries are impractical because the emission of 1800 for Tm : silica is not four-level. Although the shape of the Tm : silica REDF ASE spectrum and the optical properties of tissue at 1800 nm make the Tm : silica ASE source the most desirable of all of the REDFs, the cost of a single-mode pump may prohibit its widespread use. Most likely, the next generation clinically viable REDF source will be either a spectrally shaped Nd : silica or Yb : silica REDF with shaping that not only accounts for the spectral narrowing but also makes the spectrum more Gaussian.

Of all the sources investigated for OCT to date, semiconductors remain the only viable option for clinical implementation. Although potential advances in semiconductor source power and bandwidth are possible, they will require significant investment that may require a driving force in a much larger commercial sector such as the telecommunications industry.

REFERENCES

1. Schmitt JM, Kumar G. Optical scattering properties of soft tissue: A discrete particle model. Appl Opt 32:2788–2797, 1998.
2. Schmitt JM, Knuttel A, Yadlowsky M, Eckhaus MA. Optical-coherence tomography of a dense tissue: Statistic of attenuation and backscattering. Phys Med Biol 39:1705–1720, 1994.
3. Anderson RR, Parrish JA. The optics of human skin. J Invest Dermatol 77:13–19, 1981.
4. Matcher SJ, Cope M, Delpy DT. In vivo measurements of the wavelength dependence of tissue-scattering coefficients between 760 and 900 nm measured with time-resolved spectroscopy. Appl Opt 36:386–396, 1997.
5. Parsa P, Jacques SL, Nishioka NS. Optical properties of rat liver between 360 and 2200 nm. Appl Opt 28:2325–2330, 1989.
6. Bouma BE, Tearney GJ. Power-efficient nonreciprocal interferometer and linear-scanning fiber-optic catheter for optical coherence tomography. Opt Lett 24:531–533, 1999.
7. Tearney GJ, Bouma BE, Fujimoto JG. High-speed phase- and group-delay scanning with a grating-based phase control delay line. Opt Lett 22:1811–1813, 1997.
8. Monnom G, Dussardier B, Maurice E, Saissy A, Ostrovsky DB. Fluorescence and superfluorescence line narrowing and tunability of Nd^{3+} doped fibers. IEEE Quantum Electron 30:2361–2367, 1994.
9. Digonnet JF. Rare Earth Doped Fiber Lasers and Amplifiers. New York: Marcel Dekker, 1993.
10. Shi Y, Poulsen O. High-power broadband single mode Pr^{3+} doped fiber superfluorescence light source. Electron Lett 29:1945–1946, 1993.
11. Koechner W. Solid-State Laser Engineering. Springer Ser Opt Sci, Vol 1. New York: Springer-Verlag, 1998.

12. Clivaz X, Marquis-Weible F, Salthe RP, Novak RP, Gilgen HH. High-resolution reflectometry in biological tissues. Opt Lett 17:4–6, 1992.

13. Bouma BE, Tearney GJ, Boppart SA, Hee MR, Brezinski ME, Fujimoto JG. High resolution optical coherence tomographic imaging using a modelocked Ti:Al_2O_3. Opt Lett 20:1486–1488, 1995.

14. Bouma BE, Tearney GJ, Bilinsky IP, Golubovic B, Fujimoto JG. Self-phase-modulated Kerr lens mode-locked Cr:forsterite laser source for optical coherence tomography. Opt Lett 21:1839–1841, 1996.

15. Drexler W, Morgner U, Kartner FX, Pitris C, Boppart SA, Li XD, Ippen EP, Fujimjoto JG. In vivo ultrahigh-resolution optical coherence tomography. Opt Lett 24:1221–1223, 1999.

16. Zhou JZ, Taft G, Huang CP, Murnane MM, Kapteyn HC. Pulse evolution in a broad-bandwidth Ti:sapphire laser. Opt Lett 19:1149–1151, 1994.

17. Asaki MT, Huang CP, Garvey D, Zhou J, Kapteyn HC, Murnane MM. Generation of 11-fs pulses from a self-mode-locked Ti:sapphire laser. Opt Lett 18:977–979, 1993.

18. Morgner U, Kartner FX, Cho SH, Chen Y, Haus HA, Fujimoto JG, Ippen EP, Scheuer V, Angelow G, Tschudi T. Sub-two-cycle pulses form a Kerr-lens mode-locked Ti:sapphire laser. Opt Lett 24:411–413, 1999.

19. Yanovsky V, Pang Y, Wise F, Minkov BI. Generation of 25-fs pulses from a self-mode-locked Cr:forsterite laser with optimized group delay dispersion. Opt Lett 18:1541–1533, 1993.

20. Seas A, Petricevic V, Alfano RR. Generation of sub-100 fs pulses from a cw mode-locked chromium-doped forsterite laser. Opt Lett 17:937–939, 1992.

21. Conlon PJ, Tong YP, French MW, Taylor JR. Passive mode locking and dispersion measurement of a sub-100 fs Cr^{4+} laser. Opt Lett 19:1488–1490, 1994.

22. Senaroglu A, Pollock CR. Continuous-wave self-mode-locked operation of a femtosecond Cr^{4+}:YAG laser. Opt Lett 19:390–392, 1994.

23. Laenen R, Wolfrum K, Seilmeier A, Laubereau A. Tunable pulse generation with optical parametric amplification. Opt Soc Am B 10:2151–2155, 1993.

24. Tearney GJ, Brezinski ME, Southern JF, Bouma BE, Hee MR, Fujimoto JG. Determination of the refractive index of highly scattering human tissue by optical coherence tomography. Opt Lett 20:2258–2260, 1995.

25. Ranka JK, Windeler RS, Stentz AJ. Visible continuum generation in air-silica microstructure optical fibers with anomalous dispersion at 800 nm. Opt Lett 25:25–28, 2000.

4

Reference Optical Delay Scanning

ANDREW M. ROLLINS and JOSEPH A. IZATT

Case Western Reserve University, Cleveland, Ohio

4.1 INTRODUCTION

This chapter will review the field of scanning optical delay lines (ODLs), including essential theory and important features and parameters of ODLs for optical coherence tomography (OCT). Methods and devices that have been applied in OCT imaging systems will be emphasized. Scanning or adressable ODLs have been developed for many applications other than OCT. These include, for example, optical autocorrelation and frequency-resolved optical gating (FROG) for measurement and characterization of ultrafast laser pulses; optical coherence domain reflectometry (OCDR), also called optical low coherence reflectometry (OLCR), for high resolution, pathlength-resolved measurement of reflectivity; clocking and delay generation for time-division multiplexing in optical communications; and delay generation and addressing for optical computing and data storage. Most of these fields predate OCT; therefore, many of the delay lines used in OCT have their origins in other applications.

The ODLs that will be reviewed here can be loosely classified into four main categories:

1. ODLs that are based on linear translation of retroreflective elements
2. ODLs that vary optical pathlength by rotational methods
3. ODLs that are optical fiber stretchers
4. ODLs that are based on group delay generation using Fourier domain optical pulse shaping technology

All of the ODLs to be discussed in this chapter are retroreflecting, as opposed to transmissive. In other words, the light to be delayed is delivered to and collected from the ODL by the same optics. For a transmissive delay line, the light will be delivered to and collected from the ODL by separate optics. If a transmissive ODL is desired, many of the configurations to be presented here are adaptable to a transmissive mode, and the theoretical and design principles will still be applicable. The ODLs reviewed here will also be continuously scanning. Delay lines have been developed that scan pathlength in discrete steps, but these are seldom selected for OCT because in order to take advantage of heterodyne detection an additional phase modulation element would be required. If a continuously scanning ODL is used, the reference light is Doppler shifted, directly providing the needed phase modulation.

The appropriate ODL for a given OCT system depends on many factors, including imaging requirements, interferometer configuration, and available skills and resources. Some parameters and characteristics of ODLs that are important for OCT are

1. Working pathlength scan range
2. Pathlength scan velocity
3. Scan repetition rate
4. Pathlength scan duty cycle
5. Linearity of pathlength scan
6. Optical power loss
7. Polarization effects
8. Dispersion effects

The importance of these parameters will be discussed, and the ODLs discussed here will be characterized and compared according to these criteria.

4.1.1 Cross-Correlation and Autocorrelation

The essential theory will now be presented that relates the properties of the ODL to the OCT signal [1]. The basic measurement performed in OCT imaging is an interferometric cross-correlation, $\tilde{R}_{is}(\Delta l)$, of light returning from the reference and sample arms of the interferometer as a function of the optical pathlength difference Δl between the arms [2,3]. This cross-correlation measurement can be intuitively understood as a pathlength-resolved "gate" for the signal returning from the sample, set by a reference signal split off from the optical source. In other words, OCT probes a sample with light and uses an interferometer to localize backscatter sites in the sample. The straightforward way to obtain a measurement of the cross-correlation is to scan the optical pathlength difference by using a scanning optical delay line in the reference arm. The interferometric part of the photodetector current, $\tilde{i}_d(\Delta l)$, recorded as the ODL is scanned, is proportional to the interferometric cross-correlation:

$$\tilde{i}_d(\Delta l) = \rho \tilde{R}_{is}(\Delta l) \tag{1}$$

where ρ is the responsivity of the photodetector (in amperes per watt). The interferometric cross-correlation can be expressed as the product of the complex envelope of the interferometric cross-correlation, R_{is}, and a complex exponential carrier:

$$\tilde{R}_{is}(\Delta l_g, \Delta l_\phi) = R_{is}(\Delta l_g)e^{-jk_0 \Delta l_\phi} \tag{2}$$

Here Δl_g and Δl_ϕ are the group and phase delays, respectively, expressed as pathlength differences, and k_0 is the center wavenumber of the optical source. Note that the envelope, $R_{is}(\Delta l_g)$, is a function of group delay, whereas the carrier is a function of phase delay [4]. If dispersion in the sample and reference arms is not matched, then it is necessary to distinguish between group and phase pathlength difference. This is the case, for example, if the group delay and the phase delay effected by the delay line are not equal, as with the Fourier domain rapid scanning ODL to be described in Section 5.5. The complex envelope can be expressed as the convolution of the autocorrelation function of the optical source, $R_{ii}(\Delta l_g)$ and the amplitude backscatter profile of the sample, $r_s(\Delta l_g)$, which can be thought of as a set of impulses with various amplitudes representing discrete reflection or scattering locations in the sample [3]:

$$R_{is}(\Delta l_g) = R_{ii}(\Delta l_g) \otimes r_s(\Delta l_g) \tag{3}$$

An OCT system with a perfect mirror in the sample arm measures the interferometric autocorrelation of the source, $\tilde{R}_{ii}$, which can be expressed similarly to Eq. (2):

$$\tilde{R}_{ii}(\Delta l_g, \Delta l_\phi) = R_{ii}(\Delta l_g)e^{-jk_0\Delta l_\phi} \tag{4}$$

4.1.2 Phase Delay Scanning

When the pathlength difference is swept by a scanning delay line in the reference arm, the photodetector response is a time domain signal related to the interferometric autocorrelation by the speed of the scan of the delay. The center frequency of the detector response signal is related to the carrier of the autocorrelation by the phase delay scan speed, and hence the center frequency f_0 can be written in terms of the center of the optical source spectrum:

$$f_0 = \frac{V_\phi k_0}{2\pi} = v_0 \frac{V_\phi}{c} = \frac{V_\phi}{\lambda_0} \tag{6}$$

Here, V_ϕ is the scan speed of the phase delay, defined as the time derivative of the phase delay, $V_\phi = d\Delta l_\phi(t)/dt$, and v_0 and λ_0 are the center frequency and the center wavelength, respectively, of the optical source. The center frequency corresponds to the Doppler shift frequency of the center wavelength component of the reference arm light and equivalently to the beat frequency of the optical heterodyne detector response. In the case of a simple translating retroreflecting mirror, $V_\phi = 2s$, where s is the velocity of the mirror, and Eq. (6) becomes

$$f_0 = 2s/\lambda_0$$

which is the familiar Doppler shift equation. Note also that if the scan is linear (the translation speed is constant), then V_ϕ will be constant, and therefore f_0 will be constant. In the case of a nonlinearly scanning delay line, V_ϕ is a time-varying function; therefore, f_0 will also change with time correspondingly.

4.1.3 Group Delay Scanning

The frequency components of the detector response signal, expressed as offset from the carrier frequency $f' = (f - f_0)$, are related to the complex envelope of the autocorrelation by the scan speed of the group delay. They can thus be written in terms of the offset frequency $v' = (v - v_0)$ or wavelength components of the optical source:

$$f' = v' \frac{V_g}{c} = \left(\frac{1}{\lambda} - \frac{1}{\lambda_0} \right) V_g \tag{7}$$

Differentiating Eq. (7) gives the expression for the bandwidth of the detector response signal in terms of the optical source frequency bandwidth Δv or wavelength bandwidth $\Delta \lambda$:

$$\Delta f = \Delta v \frac{V_g}{c} = \frac{\Delta \lambda V_g}{\lambda_0^2} \tag{8}$$

The group delay scan speed is defined as the time derivative of the group delay:

$$V_g = \frac{d \, \Delta l_g(t)}{dt}$$

Note that the result expressed in Eq. (8) is independent of the optical source spectral shape [1]. In the case of a simple translating retroreflecting mirror, $V_g = V_\phi = 2s$, where s is the velocity of the mirror. When $V_\phi = V_g$, the familiar expression $\Delta f / f_0 = \Delta \lambda / \lambda_0$ holds true, which follows from Eqs. (6) and (8). Note also, as with phase delay, that if the scan is linear (the translation speed is constant), then V_g will be constant, and therefore Δf will be constant. In the case of a nonlinearly scanning delay line, V_g is a time-varying function; therefore, Δf will also change with time correspondingly. For most of the ODLs to be discussed here (except in Section 5.5), the phase delay scan speed and the group delay scan speed will be assumed to be identical.

4.1.4 Characteristics of Scanning Optical Delay Lines

Working Pathlength Scan Range

The working pathlength scan range (in meters per scan) is the portion of the delay sweep during which measurements can be made. In other words, this parameter refers to the depth range that will be imaged by the OCT system. It is important to note that group delay (as opposed to phase delay) sets the location of the coherence gate in OCT; therefore, this parameter specifically refers to the working scan range of the group delay. Typically 3 mm ($\sim$ 10 ps) is a sufficient depth scan range for OCT in turbid samples. The desired range depends on the application, however, and is determined by the scale of the features to be imaged and tissue attenuation. It is useful if this parameter can be varied continuously and easily.

Pathlength Scan Velocity

Pathlength scan velocity (in meters per second) is a parameter introduced in Sections 4.1.2 and 4.1.3. The scan velocity of the phase delay, V_ϕ, determines the Doppler shift of the reference light and therefore the center frequency of the detected signal. The scan velocity of the group delay, V_g, determines the bandwidth of the detected signal and relates to the imaging sweep. In the dispersionless case, which may be assumed for the first three categories of delay lines listed in the Introduction, V_ϕ and V_g are identical. The distinction becomes important only for category 4. This parameter also goes to the fundamental trade-off between imaging speed and sensitivity in OCT. Imaging speed obviously scales with pathlength scan velocity, and from Eq. (8) we see that the bandwidth Δf of the detected signal also scales with scan velocity. The detection bandwidth B must be broad enough to accept Δf. The signal-to-noise ratio (SNR) of an OCT system is inversely proportional to the detection bandwidth. Therefore, for a fixed image size and light intensity, SNR is inversely proportional to imaging speed.

Scan Repetition Rate

The scan repetition rate (in scans per second or hertz) is the number of pathlengths scans performed every second, or the inverse of the total scan period. This parameter depends on scan length and scan velocity and is important for determining the imaging frame rate (images per second) of the OCT system. A high scan repetition rate is necessary for real-time imaging and for eliminating motion artifact when living samples are being imaged. Motion artifact is the misalignment of adjacent depth scans in an OCT image due to motion in the sample that occurs during the course of the depth scan. Motion artifact can seriously degrade OCT images, requiring postprocessing to register or realign the adjacent depth scans, but it can be eliminated simply by imaging with a scan period much shorter than the time constant of the motion in the sample.

Pathlength Scan Duty Cycle

The pathlength scan duty cycle is defined as the usable fraction of the total scan period. This parameter can be calculated from the preceding three parameters as

$$\text{duty cycle} = \frac{\text{scan length (m/scan)} \times \text{rep rate(scans/s)}}{\text{scan velocity (m/s)}}$$

This parameter may not seem important at first, but it directly scales the power budget of the OCT system and therefore the SNR. In other words, if an OCT system uses an ODL with a 50% duty cycle, then it is imaging only half of the time, so it is effectively using only 50% of the light power provided by the optical source. An ideal ODL has a 100% duty cycle. Most of the ODLs reviewed here are actuated by "forward and back" motion. In other words, the delay is scanned in one direction, then the direction is reversed. Usually, imaging is performed on the forward stroke and the return stroke is minimized. We will refer to this technique as single-sided scanning. Alternatively, the actuator motion can be symmetrical on the forward and return strokes and images can be recorded during both. We will refer to this technique as double-sided scanning. Double-sided scanning requires that alternating data lines be reversed for display, because they were recorded during the "backward" scan stroke. If the "forward and back" actuator is driven at a frequency well below its mechanical resonance, a nearly 100% dutycycle can be realized. If the drive frequency is increased in order to increase the scan repetition rate, the duty cycle is compromised due to nonlinearity around the direction transitions. The extreme is the sinusoidal motion of a resonant scanner. A resonant scanner can move much faster than an equivalent linear scanner, but the duty cycle is decreased significantly. The trade-off must obviously be governed by the design requirements.

Linearity of Pathlength Scan

As discussed in Sections 4.1.1–4.1.3, the phase delay scan rate directly relates the measured interferogram center frequency to the carrier of the optical source autocorrelation, and the group delay scan rate directly relates the measured interferogram envelope to the envelope of the optical source autocorrelation. Therefore, any nonlinearity in the delay scan rate will result in variations in the measured interferogram center frequency f_0 and bandwidth Δf.

Several sources of scan nonlinearity are associated with various ODLs. One type of nonlinearity is quantization of the scan motion. This can occur if the ODL actuator is a stepper motor, for example. In this case, the motion of the ODL is in discrete steps, approximating a constant motion. The ODL may also move in discrete steps if the control waveform driving the actuator is synthesized with too few bits of resolution. Another source of scan nonlinearity is the jitter exhibited to some degree by many scanning devices used to actuate ODLs. Resonant devices can also be used to actuate some ODLs. In this case, instead of scanning at a constant rate, the ODL scans with a sinusoidally varying rate. This situation causes special problems, but resonant devices are sometimes desirable for fast scanning. If f_0 and Δf are not constant, then the bandwidth of the detection electronics must be broadened in order to capture all of the image information, decreasing the SNR. In the case of a resonant ODL, it is possible to avoid broadening the detection bandwidth by implementing a bandpass filter that tracks the variation of f_0. If the group delay (which determines depth of the coherence gate in the sample) is not scanned at a constant rate, the image may be warped if the data are sampled at a constant rate.

Insertion Loss

Insertion loss is defined as the fraction of optical power incident on the delay line that is lost and not returned to the interferometer. The typical implementation of OCT uses a Michelson interferometer with a single detector. In this configuration, the reference light is attenuated to improve the SNR by reducing excess photon noise. In this situation, optical power loss in the ODL is tolerable. If, however, a power-conserving interferometer configuration is used (as discussed in Chapter 6), then optical power loss in the ODL is undesirable. In any case, it is important that the ODL maintain a reasonably constant optical power throughput throughout the course of the scan in order to maintain a constant SNR.

Polarization Effects

Only those polarization components of the sample and reference light that are matched will interfere. The loss of fringe contrast due to polarization mismatch is called polarization fading. If the ODL changes the state of polarization (SOP) of the reference light in a way that does not change during the course of the delay scan or drift over the imaging time scale, then a simple polarization control can be used to realign the polarization state with that of the sample light. If the ODL causes a dynamic change in the SOP of the reference light, then further steps must be taken to reduce or reverse the change and avoid polarization fading.

Dispersion Effects

If dispersion in the reference arm of the interferometer is not matched with that of the sample arm, then the cross-correlation of the reference and sample light will be broadened, reducing the axial resolution of the OCT system. Even the dispersion mismatch due to a small difference in optical fiber length can significantly affect the resolution; therefore, it is good design practice to carefully account for dispersion in all elements of the sample and reference arms, including the ODL. If the ODL has dispersion that changes over the course of the delay scan, then it is very difficult to match the dispersion in the sample arm. Some ODLs allow dispersion to be adjusted easily, which is a useful feature.

4.2 LINEAR TRANSLATION

4.2.1 Linear Translator Mounted Retroreflector

The simplest scanning ODL is a retroreflector mounted on a linear translating stage (Fig. 1). The reference light is collimated and directed toward the retroreflector, which redirects the light back to the collimator, which recouples the light into the delivery fiber. The retroreflector is mounted on a linear translating stage in order to scan the delay. A mechanically translating stage will have more than enough translation range to provide a sufficient working pathlength scan. The major drawback of this type of ODL is a low scan velocity. Commercial linear translators can move at a speed of up to 100 mm/s (e.g., Newport model PM500-L). A linear translating ODL is very flexible, able to operate with a wide range of scan lengths and scan velocities. The scan repetition rate and duty cycle will depend on the selected scan range and velocity and on whether one-sided or two-sided scanning is used. Translating stages are commonly commercially available with several types of actuators such as dc motors, stepper motors, and linear motors. All will have some degree of nonlinearity in their motion due to jitter and/or because of motion taken in discrete steps. Care should be taken to choose a product that minimizes these nonlinearities, for reasons discussed in the preceding section. When necessary, mechanical damping can further

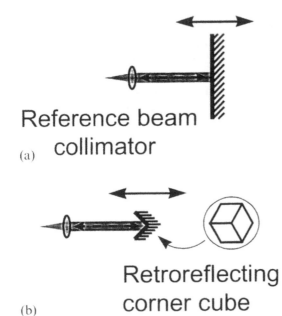

Figure 1 Schematic of an optical delay line consisting of a fixed delivery fiber and collimating lens plus a retroreflector mounted on a linear translating stage. A flat mirror (a) or a corner-cube retroreflector (b) can be used as the retroreflecting element. The corner-cube retroreflector is less alignment-sensitive than a flat mirror.

reduce scan nonlinearity. A PZT stack could also be used as the translating element, but it has a pathlength scan range of only a few tens of micrometers and it responds nonlinearly to the drive waveform. The collimator and retroreflector is the minimum configuration for a delay line, so the optical power loss will be minimum using this type of ODL. Loss will be caused by imperfect reflectivity of the retroreflector and imperfect coupling of light to and from the delivery fiber by the collimator and will typically be less than 50% (3 dB). This type of ODL should have no significant polarization or dispersion effects. From Eq. (6), using this ODL, the center frequency of the OCT signal will be given by

$$f_0 = 2s/\lambda_0 \tag{9}$$

where s is the velocity of the translating stage (the delay scan speed $V = 2s$). From Eq. (8) the bandwidth of the OCT signal is given by

$$\Delta f = \frac{\Delta\lambda\, 2s}{\lambda_0^2} = \frac{f_0\, \Delta\lambda}{\lambda_0} \tag{10}$$

4.2.2 Multipass Translating Retroreflectors

The scan range and velocity of a translating retroreflector can be amplified by allowing the reference light to make multiple passes off it. In other words, if the reference light reflects twice off a mirror moving at a scan velocity s, then the effective scan velocity is $2s$. One example [5] of a multipass ODL is illustrated in Fig. 2.

In this configuration, the pathlength scan range and velocity are scaled together by a factor $2m/(\cos\theta)$, where m is the number of reflections off mirror M1 and θ is the angle of incidence of the beam on mirror M1 (measured from the normal). Because of this amplification, a PZT stack can be used as the translating element, allowing a much higher delay scan velocity and repetition rate. Scans of 2–3 mm at repetition rates greater than 100 scans/s can be achieved with a high duty cycle. Higher repetition rates can be achieved at the expense of the duty cycle. The

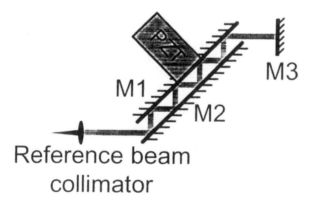

Figure 2 Schematic of an optical delay line consisting of a fixed delivery fiber and collimating lens, a parallel pair of mirrors, and a retroreflecting mirror. One of the parallel mirrors is translated with a piezoelectric actuator. (Adapted from Ref. 5.)

pathlength scan length is limited to 2–3 mm due to beam walk-off of mirror M1 and clipping by mirror M2. If high quality mirrors are used, optical power loss can be as little as 50%. Because of non-normal incidence, optical power loss due to mirrors M1 and M2 will have polarization dependence. This effect is also minimized with high reflectance (dielectric) mirrors. In addition, this effect does not change through the course of the scan, so the change in SOP should be correctable with a polarization controller. Using the amplification factor given above, the OCT signal center frequency and bandwidth can be obtained from Eqs. (9) and (10), respectively.

Another multipass design similar to the one illustrated in Fig. 2 is illustrated in Fig. 3. In this case, the mirrors face each other at a small angle β. The beam is incident on the system at an angle θ as shown in Fig. 3. The light reflects between the two mirrors multiple times, with the incidence angle decreasing by β on each reflection. If the angle of incidence is chosen such that $\theta = m\beta$, where m is an integer, then after m reflections the beam will strike the mirror at normal incidence and retroreflect. In this configuration, the pathlength scan range and velocity are approximately scaled together by a factor $2m/[\cos(\theta/2)]$, where $\theta/2$ is the average incidence angle. This system enjoys the advantage over the design in Fig. 2 that no external retroreflecting mirror is required. Performance in terms of loss and polarization-dependent loss should be equivalent to the case illustrated in Fig. 2. This ODL has been demonstrated to scan a 2 mm delay at 100 Hz with a duty cycle of 85% [6].

Figures 4 and 5 illustrate additional multipass translating retroreflector configurations [7,8]. These designs merit mention but will not be discussed in detail here.

4.2.3 Galvanometer-Mounted Retroreflector

An alternative to a linear stage actuator is a galvanometric scanner [2,9]. Although the galvanometer is a rotational actuator, an approximately linear translation can be effected by mounting a corner-cube retroreflector on a swing arm that is mounted on the galvanometer shaft, as illustrated in Fig. 6. A corner-cube retroreflector is used to ensure that the light is retroreflected independently of the angle of the swing arm. In many respects, this ODL is very similar to the linear stage mounted retroreflector, but this configuration is capable of higher scan velocities and therefore higher scan repetition rates. This ODL can scan several millimeters at up to 100 scans/s with a high duty cycle. The axial (translation) component of the retroreflector position is $d = r\sin\theta \cong r\theta$, where r is the length of the swing arm and θ is the angular position

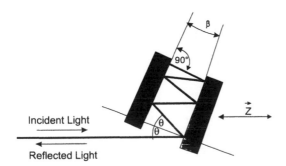

Figure 3   A multipass ODL design based on off-parallel facing mirrors. (From Ref. 6.)

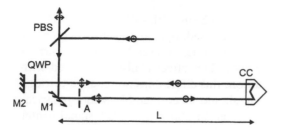

Figure 4 Schematic of an optical delay line that passes twice through the retroreflector. This ODL also demonstrates the use of polarization to use a retroreflecting delay line in a transmissive mode. PBS, polarizing beam splitter; QWP, quarter-wave plate; CC, corner cube; M1, M2, mirrors; A, aperture. (Courtesy of Optical Society of America.)

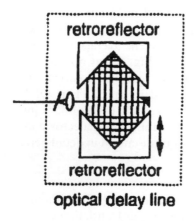

Figure 5 Schematic of a multipass optical delay line that uses facing retroreflectors instead of flat mirrors. The filled triangle represents a small flat mirror. (Courtesy of IEEE.)

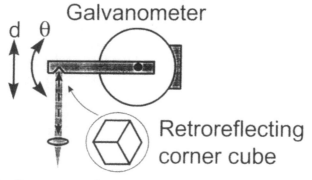

Figure 6 Schematic of an optical delay line consisting of a fixed delivery fiber and collimating lens and a corner-cube retroreflector mounted on a swing arm mounted on a galvanometer scanner.

of the galvanometer (Fig. 6 illustrates the $\theta = 0$ position.) The small-angle approximation is valid for configurations appropriate for OCT. For example, with a 4 cm swing arm, a scan range of 4 mm is effected with a rotation of less than $\pm 3°$. If the galvanometer is turning at a constant angular velocity ω, then the translation velocity is $s = r\omega \cos(\omega t) \cong r\omega$. The OCT signal center frequency and bandwidth are then given by Eqs. (9) and (10), respectively.

Figure 7 illustrates a scanning ODL very similar to the configuration just described, using rotational actuation but approximating linear translation [10]. This ODL is mechanically more sophisticated than the one described above but will not be discussed in detail here. This design has been commercialized (Clark-MXR Model ODL-150) and is capable of scan rates of more than 30 Hz.

4.3 ANGULAR SCANNING METHODS

4.3.1 Rotating Cube

The optical pathlength (OPL) that a beam traverses can be scanned rapidly by passing the beam through a glass cube that is rotating at a constant speed. As the glass cube rotates, the thickness of glass that the beam passes through changes, and therefore the OPL changes. An important motivation for this type of ODL is speed. A cube can be rotated rapidly, generating delay sweeps at repetition rates much higher than those of the ODLs described so far. Several configurations based on this principle have been implemented. The pathlength scan range depends on the size of the cube as well as the configuration (how many passes through the cube.) The pathlength scan range is easily adequate for OCT, even with a small cube, but the

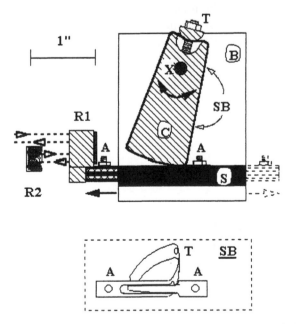

Figure 7 An ODL configuration similar to that of Fig. 6. The design is detailed in Ref. 10. (Courtesy of American Institute of Physics.)

scan range is not adjustable—it is fixed for a given cube size. The scan velocity depends on the configuration, the cube size, and the cube rotation speed. The cube can be rotated very fast, resulting in a high scan velocity and repetition rate. The duty cycle depends on the configuration. The insertion loss and polarization-dependent loss depend on the surface treatment of the cubes. For most configurations, the scan is not linear. In other words, the delay is not a linear function of the rotation angle. The other drawback of this design is the pathlength-dependent dispersion introduced by the glass cube. A fixed amount of dispersion can be compensated for by introducing a matching dispersive element into the sample arm. As the cube spins, however, and the pathlength within the dispersive glass changes, the amount of dispersion also changes. Whether or not this dynamic dispersion mismatch is significant depends on the cube material, the wavelength and bandwidth of the optical source, and the scan length.

Several ODL configurations have been implemented using rotating cubes. The following have been demonstrated in optical low coherence reflectivity measurements.

Single Pass, No Internal Reflections

Figure 8 illustrates the most straightforward rotating cube configuration. The index of refraction of the cube is higher than that of air (typically 1.5), so the beam is refracted as it enters and leaves the cube. As the cube rotates, the length of the path within the cube varies, but in a nonlinear way. The single-pass pathlength variation as a function of the incidence angle θ of the beam on the cube is given by

$$d = L\left[\sqrt{n^2 - \sin^2\theta} + 2\sin^2\left(\frac{\theta}{2}\right) - n\right]$$

where L is the dimension of the cube and n is the index of refraction of the cube [11,12]. When the cube is rotated at a fixed angular frequency ω, then $\theta = \omega t$ an the scan velocity $s = 2\,\partial d/\partial t$. The interferogram center frequency and bandwidth are

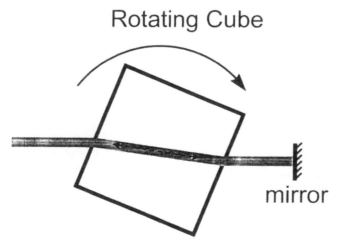

Figure 8 Rotating cube ODL that operates with a single pass, no internal reflections. (Adapted from Refs. 11 and 12.)

then given by Eqs. (9) and (10). The major drawback of this OPL is the nonlinearity of the scan. The scan velocity changes through the course of the scan, so the interferogram center frequency and bandwidth also change. This ODL configuration was demonstrated by rotating a 1.27 cm cube at 22 revolutions per second (rev/s), for a scan repetition rate of 88 Hz. Through the course of the 1.5 mm scan, the center frequency varied from 0 to 1000 kHz, corresponding to a varying scan velocity of 0–650 mm/s. The duty cycle was almost 50%, but if double-sided scanning were used the duty cycle would be almost 100%.

Single Pass, Two Internal Reflections

Figure 9 illustrates a configuration in which the reference beam is retroreflected inside the cube. Mirrors are deposited on portions of each face of the cube as illustrated in the inset of Fig. 10. This configuration was used to demonstrate the highest speed scanner yet implemented for OLCR. A $5 \times 5 \times 2$ mm^3 cube was turned at 7117 rev/s by an air turbine, resulting in a scan repetition rate of 28.5 kHz [13]. A pathlength variation of 2 mm was swept at 176 m/s. The scanning duty cycle was approximately 32%. The scan linearity and dispersion effects were not reported but should be comparable to those of the configuration described in the following subsection. The function describing pathlength scan as a function of the angular position of the cube given in the next section should be valid for this configuration if divided by a factor of 2. This ODL required custom deposition of mirrors on portions of each cube face and extremely precise mounting and alignment of the cube on the turbine shaft. At this high repetition rate, mechanically resonant instabilities resulted in cyclical variation in recoupling efficiency over the time scale of several scans. The OLCR system using this ultrahigh speed scanning ODL achieved a reflectivity sensitivity of only 36 dB, which is not sufficient for imaging in biological samples.

Double Pass, Four Internal Reflections

The configuration illustrated in Fig. 10 is similar to that of Fig. 9 except that it double-passes the reference beam through the cube, doubling the pathlength scan

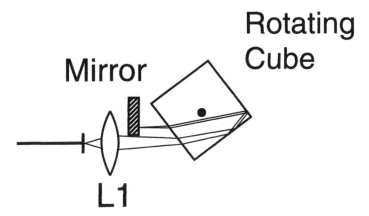

Figure 9   Rotating cube configuration with single pass, two internal reflections.

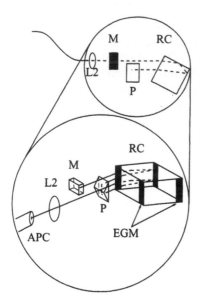

Figure 10 Optical pathlength configuration with double pass, four internal reflections. L2, lens; P, right-angle prism; M, mirror; EGM, reflecting gold layers; RC, rotating cube. (© Copyright 1998 IEEE.)

[14,15]. This configuration was demonstrated using a 12 mm × 12 mm × 4 mm cube rotated at 310 rev/s, resulting in a scan repetition rate of 1240 Hz. A pathlength of 11 mm was scanned at 42 m/s. The resultant duty cycle is approximately 32%. In most biological samples, only about 3 mm of pathlength scanning is useful, however, so this configuration would yield an effective duty cycle of about 9%. A smaller cube could be used to improve this. The (free space) pathlength variation as a function of angular position α of the cube is given by

$$d(\alpha) = L \left\{ 2n \left(-1 + \frac{1}{\cos[\sin^{-1}(\sin \alpha / n)]} \right) \right.$$

$$\left. + \left(\sin \alpha \left[1 + \tan \frac{\alpha}{2} - 2 \tan[\sin^{-1}(\sin \alpha / n)] \right] \right) \right\}$$

where L is the length of the side of the cube and n is the refractive index of the cube material. This function is obviously not linear, and a scan speed variation of ±17% was measured. When the cube is rotated at a fixed angular frequency ω, then $\alpha = \omega t$, and the scan velocity is $s = \partial d / \partial t$. The interferogram center frequency and bandwidth are then given by Eqs. (9) and (10). The autocorrelation width measured using this ODL was reported to be only 1% broader than the theoretical width (the source coherence length), so dispersion mismatch was apparently not significant. The type of glass that the cube was composed of was not specified. The optical sources used for this measurement had a center wavelength of 1310 nm and a bandwidth of 45 nm. This ODL required custom deposition of mirrors on portions of each cube face.

Double Pass for Sample and Reference Light, four Internal Reflections for Each path

The configuration illustrated in Fig. 11 is identical to the configuration in Fig. 10, but in this case both the reference and sample light beams are passed through the rotating cube [16]. In this way, the effective pathlength scan is doubled, and the scan nonlinearity is largely canceled. To optimize the nonlinearity cancellation, the incidence angle of the sample beam with respect to the reference beam must be carefully selected. The (free space) pathlength variation as a function of the angular position of the cube is given by

$$D(\alpha) = d(\alpha) - d(\alpha_0 - \alpha)$$

where $d(\alpha)$ is defined above and α_0 is the angle of incidence of the sample beam with respect to the reference beam, as illustrated in Fig. 11. This configuration was demonstrated by rotating a 60 mm cube at 76.25 rev/s, resulting in a scan repetition rate of 305 Hz. This ODL was designed for a long scan range of greater than 100 mm for OLCR measurements. The scan velocity was 95 m/s and the duty cycle was about 32%. The scan speed variation was only ±0.14%. In the reported demonstration, the OLCR using this ODL measured reflectivity with a sensitivity of 65 dB. This ODL requires the same type of custom cube as the previous configurations and obviously requires extremely careful alignment of both beams passing through the cube.

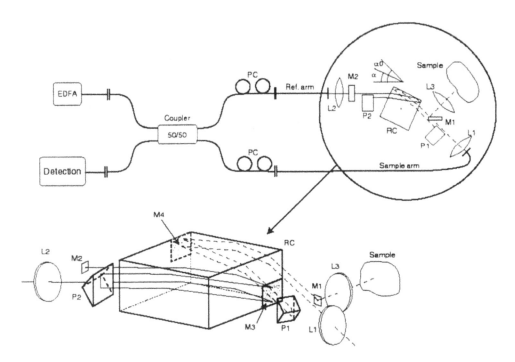

Figure 11 Double pass for sample and reference light, four internal reflections for each path. L1, L2, L3, lenses; Pc, polarization controllers; P1, P2, right-angle prisms; M1, M2, mirrors, M3, M4, reflecting gold layers; Rc, rotating cube.

4.3.2 Scanning Mirror

Another ODL based on the transformation of angular motion into pathlength variation is illustrated in Fig. 12 [17]. As with the rotating cubes and the galvanometer-mounted retroreflector, the motivation for using a rotational scanning element is speed. In addition to an angular scanning mirror, three additional mirrors and a lens are used. An examination of Figs 12a and 12b will instruct the reader as to the operation of this configuration, particularly the need to place the scanning mirror and mirror 2 one focal length from the lens. This configuration reflects the beam four times off the scanning mirror, amplifying the scan length and velocity by 4. It should be noted that 0 pathlength variation is effected by scanning the beam in a line across mirror 2. All of the pathlength variation arises from the beam being offset from the pivot of the scanning mirror so that there is an axial shift imposed on the beam in addition to the angular scan. In other words, if the beam were reflected from the pivot of the scanning mirror, then no pathlength variation would result from scanning the mirror. The pathlength variation d as a function of scan angle θ (referenced from the plane parallel to the lens) is given by $d = 4x \tan \theta \cong 4x\theta$ for small scan angles, where x is the distance that the beam is offset from the pivot of the scanning mirror. The scan velocity s is given by $s \cong 4x \, \delta\theta/\delta t$. For a constant angular velocity ω, $s \cong 4x\omega$. The interferogram center frequency and bandwidth will then be given by Eqs. (9) and (10). The pathlength variation achievable for a given configuration of this design will be limited by the need to keep the scanning mirror within the depth of focus of the lens and by the size of the lens and mirror 2. Optical power loss will be determined by the quality of the mirrors and the alignment. There should be no significant scan-dependent polarization or dispersion variation.

This ODL was demonstrated using a 1.2 kHz resonant scanner and 50 mm focal length lens. Pathlength was scanned by 3 mm at 1.2 kHz and a peak scan velocity of 11.3 m/s. Most likely the full 3 mm was not usable for imaging, because the motion of a resonant scanner is sinusoidal. The nonlinear pathlength variation with time would warp the image to an unacceptable degree near the extrema of the scan. A reasonable duty cycle for single-sided scanning using a resonant ODL is 33% (66% for double-sided scanning). In order to maintain a narrow detection bandwidth over the course of the scan (and prevent SNR degradation), the signal was bandpass filtered by a voltage-controlled oscillator that was controlled by the reso-

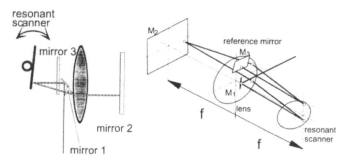

Figure 12 Schematic illustrations of an ODL based on the transformation of an angular mirror scan to pathlength variation. (© Copyright 1998, Taylor & Francis, Ltd.)

nant scan frequency control. This scheme does not compensate for image warping, however.

Figures 13 and 14 illustrate other ODLs based on pathlength variation due to rotation of reflective elements [18,19]. These designs have not been used for OCT and will not be discussed in detail here.

4.4 FIBER STRETCHING

Another method for scanning optical delay is stretching a long optical fiber [20,21,22]. This has been implemented in OCT by coiling a length of optical fiber on a piezoelectric plate or cylinder. With many fiber windings, the small expansion of the PZT actuator can create several millimeters of delay. For the case illustrated in Fig. 15, the pathlength change as a result of a change in the cylinder radius Δr is given by $\Delta d = 2\pi m \, \Delta r$, where m is the number of windings. The scan velocity is given by $s = 2\pi m \, \partial \Delta / \partial t$. The interferogram center frequency and bandwidth will then be given by Eqs. (9) and (10). This type of ODL has been demonstrated for OCT at scan rates of up to 1200 scans/s (600 Hz triangle drive waveform and double-sided scanning). This type of ODL resulted in the first demonstration of real-time imaging using OCT at 1 frame per second (fps) [20] and 4 fps [21]. The demonstrated duty cycle was 75% [22]. The fiber and air lengths in the reference and sample arms can easily be matched, so dispersion mismatch is not an issue. Optical power loss has not been reported but should be equivalent to linear translation ODLs. The major disadvantage of fiber-stretching ODLs is that there are polarization effects. The static effects of winding the fiber on the actuator can be compensated for by winding the matching length of fiber in the sample arm on a matching actuator. This second actuator can also be driven by the inverse of the reference delay waveform, generating a differential delay scan range of two times the range of a single scanner. As the fiber is stretched, dynamic stretch-induced birefringence will change the SOP of the light propagating through the fiber throughout the course of the scan stroke. This

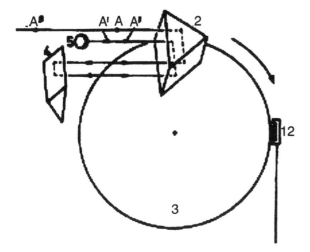

Figure 13   Schematic of an ODL based on a rotating roof prism.

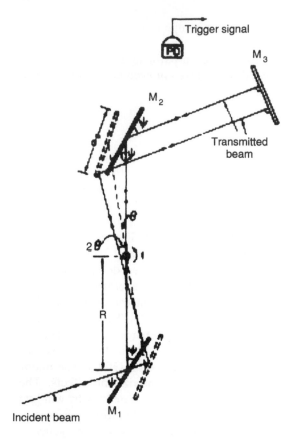

Figure 14   Schematic of an ODL based on a rotating pair of parallel mirrors. (Reprinted with permission from Elsevier Science.)

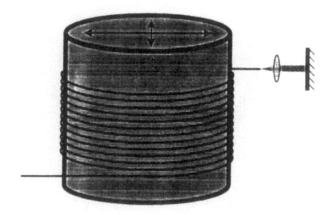

Figure 15   Schematic of an ODL based on optical fiber stretching. This design uses a cylindrical PZT element to uniformly stretch the fiber wound around the barrel of the cylinder.

effect can be compensated for by introducing 45° Faraday rotators (FRs) in the air gaps of the reference and sample arms so that on a double pass through the FRs, the SOP is conjugated and the return propagation through the fiber reverses the SOP change [23]. Alternatively, polarization-maintaining fiber can be used to minimize these effects. In addition, the temperature of the actuator should be carefully controlled in order to prevent temperature-dependent drift of the delay and SOP.

4.5 FOURIER DOMAIN RAPID SCANNING OPTICAL DELAY LINE

The Fourier domain rapid scanning optical delay line (RSOD) was developed for femtosecond pulse measurement [24–26] and has recently been applied to OCT [1,27,28]. The RSOD is based on Fourier transform pulse-shaping techniques, which have been demonstrated to also be capable of shaping the temporal properties of broadband incoherent light [29]. This delay line achieves scans of several millimeters at repetition rates of several kilohertz and also allows separation of group and phase delay, which provides an additional degree of control over the center frequency and bandwidth of the OCT signal.

The RSOD consists of a grating–lens pair in a folded, double-passed Fourier domain pulse-shaping configuration (Fig. 16). A flat mirror serves as a spatial phase filter, which imposes a linear phase ramp on the optical frequency spectrum. The delay line is based on the well-known property of the Fourier transform that a phase ramp in the frequency domain corresponds to a group delay in the time domain:

$$x(t - t_0) \overset{\mathfrak{J}}{\longleftrightarrow} X(\omega)e^{-j\omega t_0} \tag{11}$$

The angle of the incident light on the grating can be selected such that the center wavelength λ_0 of the diffracted beam is normal to the grating and the entire grating is in the focal plane of the lens. This is done to prevent introduction of group velocity dispersion (GVD), which varies throughout the course of the scan. If the distance from the grating to the lens is not one focal length, then GVD is introduced. Therefore, if the grating is at an angle not normal to the optical axis of the lens, then as light is laterally displaced on the grating by the scanning mirror it is also displaced from the focal plane of the lens, introducing GVD [30].

The mirror pivot can be offset from the center wavelength by an arbitrary distance x by a simple lateral translation of the scanning mirror. The phase shift ϕ (λ) as a function of wavelength λ for a given mirror tilt angle σ can be written as (refer to Fig. 16)

$$\phi(\lambda) = \frac{8\pi\sigma x}{\lambda} + \frac{8\pi\sigma l_f(\lambda - \lambda_0)}{p\lambda \cos\theta_0}$$

where l_f is the focal length of the lens, p is the pitch of the grating, and θ_0 is the first-order diffraction angle of the center wavelength from the grating (measured from the grating normal). Recall that in the configuration shown in Fig. 16, $\theta_0 = 0$, i.e., the grating is in the focal plane of the lens. In this case $\cos\theta_0$ evaluates to unity, so this factor will not be propagated further in the subsequent analysis.

The function $\phi(\lambda)$ was derived by using the grating equation and assuming that the small-angle approximation $\sin\theta \cong \theta$ holds for diffraction angles between different wavelengths off the grating and for small deflection angles effected by the scan-

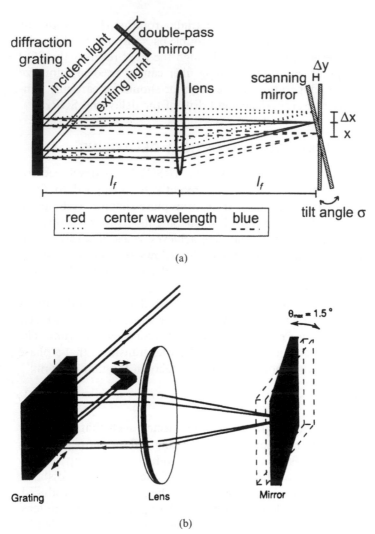

(a)

(b)

Figure 16 Schematics of the Fourier domain optical delay line. (a) View from above. The incident, collimated broadband light is diffracted from the grating and spectrally dispersed. The lens parallelizes the dispersed spectrum while focusing it to a line on the scanning mirror. The scanning mirror imposes a linear phase ramp on the spectrum and redirects the light back through the lens, which recollimates the beam and reconverges the spectrum onto the grating. The beam then diffracts in a reverse manner from the grating and propagates collimated and undispersed toward the double-pass mirror collinear with the incident beam. The double-pass mirror turns the light back through an identical path. Double passing is illustrated clearly in (b). (Courtesy of OSA.)

ning mirror [25]. The distance Δy that a wavelength component λ traverses as a function of scanning mirror tilt angle σ is calculated (taking into account the fact that the beam traverses the path Δy four times) and multiplied by $2\pi/\lambda$ to convert from displacement to phase shift. This phase shift can also be written as a function of angular optical frequency ω:

$$\phi(\omega) = \frac{4\sigma x \omega}{c} - \frac{8\pi\sigma l_f (\omega - \omega_0)}{p\omega} \tag{12}$$

where ω_0 is the center angular optical frequency. From Eq. (12) and the definition of phase delay, $t_\phi = \phi(\omega_0)/\omega_0$, the phase delay is given by $t_\phi = 4\sigma x/c$. This corresponds to the free-space phase pathlength difference Δl_ϕ (referenced from a zero scan angle),

$$\Delta l_\phi = 4\sigma x \tag{13}$$

From the definition of group delay, $t_g = \partial\phi(\omega)/\partial\omega|_{\omega=\omega_0}$, the group delay is given by

$$t_g = \frac{4\sigma x}{c} - \frac{4\sigma l_f \lambda_0}{cp}$$

which corresponds to the free-space group pathlength difference Δl_g,

$$\Delta l_g = 4\sigma x - \frac{4\sigma l_f \lambda_0}{p} \tag{14}$$

This expression for group pathlength difference can alternatively be derived by evaluating the change in pathlength experienced by the center wavelength as a result of an arbitrary mirror tilt angle. It can be seen that the group pathlength difference is equal to the phase pathlength difference plus an additional term that is a function of the properties of the lens, grating, and light source. Both the phase pathlength difference and the group pathlength difference are proportional to the tilt angle of the scanning mirror, so an angular scan of the mirror effects a scan of both phase and group pathlength differences. The second term in the expression for group pathlength difference is dominant in typical configurations; thus the group pathlength difference is much larger than the phase pathlength difference for a given angle σ. This feature is key to the value of this delay line. The mirror need be moved only a very small amount to generate a large scan of the group pathlength difference. It is also possible to adjust the offset x for a desired center frequency without significantly affecting the scan length of the group pathlength difference. If the center wavelength is located at the mirror pivot (i.e., $x = 0$), then the phase pathlength difference term Δl_ϕ vanishes and there is no phase pathlength scanning. This allows for the application of an external phase-modulating element that is truly independent of the group delay scanning if such a configuration is desired.

Differentiating Eq. (13) with respect to time and using Eq. (6), the center frequency of the interferogram measured using the Fourier domain scanning delay line is given as

$$f_0 = \frac{4x}{\lambda_0} \frac{\partial\sigma(t)}{\partial t} \tag{15}$$

Similarly, differentiating Eq. (14) with respect to time and using Eq. (8), the bandwidth of the interferogram measured using the Fourier domain scanning delay line is

$$\Delta f = \frac{2\,\Delta\lambda}{\lambda_0^2}\left(2x - \frac{2l_f \lambda_0}{p}\right)\frac{\partial\sigma(t)}{\partial t} \tag{16}$$

The design equations for the high speed OCT system using this delay line are Eqs. (14)–(16). Equation (14) is used to specify the grating pitch, the lens focal length, and the maximum angular excursion of the scanning mirror for a given source center wavelength and desired group delay scan. Equations (15) and (16) are used to calculate the center frequency and bandwidth, respectively, of the OCT signal for a given mirror offset x and mirror scan rate $\partial\sigma(t)/\partial t$. If the mirror is tilted at a fixed angular frequency ω, then $\sigma(t) = \omega t$ and $\partial\sigma(t)/\partial t = \omega$. Estimation of the signal bandwidth Δf from Eq. (16) can be simplified by recognizing that for a typical configuration, $2x \ll 2l_f\lambda_0/p$.

A resonant scanning mirror tilts as a sinusoidal function of time,

$$\sigma(t) = b\sin(2\pi f_m t)$$

where b is the maximum excursion of the tilt angle and f_m is the resonance frequency of the scanning mirror. Thus, from Eq. (15) the center frequency becomes

$$f_0(t) = \frac{4x}{\lambda_0} b2\pi f_m \cos(2\pi f_m t) \tag{17}$$

From Eq. (16) the interferogram bandwidth becomes

$$\Delta f(t) = \frac{2\Delta\lambda}{\lambda_0^2}\left(2x - \frac{2l_f\lambda_0}{p}\right) b2\pi f_m \cos(2\pi f_m t) \tag{18}$$

This sinusoidal variation of center frequency and bandwidth with time is the major disadvantage of using a resonant scanner in the delay line. The advantage is that resonant scanners can operate at much higher repetition rates than galvanometer-mounted scanners. Using a resonant scanner, a reasonable compromise between duty cycle and nonlinearity is to record the interferometric signal only during the middle two-thirds of the forward scan, resulting in an overall duty cycle of 33%. Double-sided scanning increases the duty cycle to 67%. A linear scanner can achieve a duty cycle of nearly 100% (at the expense of scan speed). Unless a tracking bandpass filter is used, as discussed in Section 5.2.3, the use of a resonant scanner with a reduced duty cycle requires the detection bandwidth to be increased compared to an equivalent linear scanner in order to accommodate the varying center frequency. This corresponds to degradation of the SNR. Thus, a resonant scanner is advantageous only in cases where the needed scan rate cannot be achieved with a linear scanner.

As discussed above, if the distance from the grating to the lens is not one focal length, then GVD is introduced. This requires careful alignment to prevent broadening of the cross-correlation due to dispersion mismatch. This property of the RSOD also provides a convenient means to compensate for dispersion mismatch due to dissimilar components in the reference and sample arms. For example, an endoscopic probe in the sample arm may not include an air gap to match the air gap in the RSOD. This dispersion mismatch requires compensation, which can be introduced by the RSOD [28,30,31].

This ODL has few disadvantages. Besides complexity, the major disadvantage is optical power loss. In a double-passed configuration, the light is diffracted into the first order four times. A grating blazed at the appropriate angle can increase the efficiency of diffraction into the first order, but the aggregate loss will be significantly greater than most of the other ODLs reviewed here. In the typical OCT configuration using a Michelson interferometer, the reference ODL must be attenuated to optimize imaging sensitivity. In this case, a lossy ODL is no disadvantage. If a power-conserving interferometer design is used (as detailed in Chapter 6) then any loss is undesirable. Even in this case, however, if the optical power incident on the ODL is low, the actual amount of power lost may not be significant.

Figure 17 illustrates an ODL similar to the RSOD described above [32]. In this configuration the Fourier domain pulse shaper is unfolded and an acousto-optic modulator is used as the scanning phase ramping element. This ODL was not developed for OCT or OLCR, but in principle it could be used for these applications. This design holds the potential to provide high speed, linear optical delay scanning without moving parts. Potential disadvantages include very high (radio-frequency) heterodyne frequency, optical power loss due to poor diffraction efficiency, and incompatibility with very broad optical bandwidths.

4.6 CONCLUSION

A review of scanning optical delay lines for OCT has been presented. Relevant theoretical background has been presented to relate ODL properties to the OCT signal generated by scanning the ODL. Operating principles and design equations have been described to facilitate the selection and design of ODLs for OCT. Selection and design criteria for an ODL depend on the requirements of the imaging application such as sample size, necessary frame rate, necessary dynamic range, and available resources.

Although several excellent optical delay lines have been demonstrated for OCT and similar technologies, even state-of-the-art designs have drawbacks. We expect that improvements will be made to existing optical delay scanning methods and that new approaches will continue to be developed. Potential areas of improvement include, but are not limited to, scan speed, scan linearity, and optical power through-put. Future innovations will likely yield optical delay lines that are broadband, efficient, and polarization-insensitive and that scan rapidly without moving parts or bulky components.

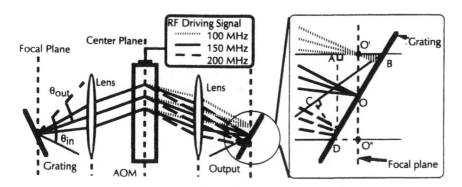

Figure 17 Schematic of another ODL based on the Fourier domain pulse shaper configuration. In this case the configuration is unfolded and an acousto-optic modulator is used to generate a scanning phase ramp.

REFERENCES

1. Rollins AM, Kulkarni MD, Yazdanfar S, Ung-arunyawee R, Izatt JA. In vivo video rate optical coherence tomography. Opt Express 3:219–229, 1998.
2. Izatt JA, Kulkarni MD, Wang H-W, Kobayashi K, Sivak MV. Optical coherence tomography and microscopy in gastrointestinal tissues. IEEE J Selected Topics Quantum Electron 2:1017–1028, 1996.
3. Kulkarni MD, Thomas CW, Izatt JA. Image enhancement in optical coherence tomography using deconvolution. Electron Lett 33:1365–1367, 1997.
4. Siegman AE. Lasers. Mill Valley, CA: Univ Sci Books, 1986.
5. Pan Y, Welzel J, Birngruber R, Engelhardt R. Optical coherence-gated imaging of biological tissues. IEEE J Selected Topics Quantum Electron 2:1029–1034, 1996.
6. Koch P. A novel approach to optical delay lines. Personal communication, 1999.
7. Klovekorn P, Munch J. Variable optical delay line with diffraction-limited autoalignment. Appl Opt 37:1903–1914, 1998.
8. Takada K, Yamada H, Hibino Y, Mitachi S. Range extension in optical low coherence reflectometry achieved by using a pair of retroreflectors. Electron Lett 31:1565–1567, 1995.
9. Swanson EA, Huang D, Hee MR, Fujimoto JG, Lin CP. Puliafito CA. High-speed optical coherence domain reflectometry. Opt Lett 17:151–153, 1992.
10. Edelstein DC, Romney RB, Scheuermann M. Rapid programmable 300 ps optical delay scanner and signal-averaging system for ultrafast measurements. Rev Sci Instrum 62:597–683, 1991.
11. Chavanne P, Gianotti P, Salathe RP. High speed, high precision broad band reflectometer. Presented at Applied Optics and Optoelectronics, York, UK, 1994.
12. Su CB. Achieving variation of the optical path length by a few millimeters at millisecond rates for imaging of turbid media and optical interferometry: A new technique. Opt Lett 22:665–667, 1997.
13. Szydlo J, Delachenal N, Gianotti R, Walti R, Bleuler H, Salathe RP. Air-turbine driven optical low-coherence reflectometry at 28.6-kHz scan repetition rate. Opt Commun 154:1–4, 1998.
14. Ballif J, Gianotti R, Chavanne P, Walti R, Salathe RP. Rapid and scalable scans at 21 m/s in optical low-coherence reflectometry. Opt Lett 22:757–759, 1997.
15. Lindgren F, Gianotti R, Walti R, Salathe RP, Haas A, Nussberger M, Schmatz ML, Bachtold W. 78-dB shot-noise limited optical low-coherence reflectometry at 42-m/s scan speed. IEEE Photon Technol Lett 9:1613–1615, 1997.
16. Delachenal N, Gianotti R, Walti R, Limberger H, Salathe RP. Constant high-speed optical low-coherence reflectometry over 0.12m scan range. Electron Lett 33:2059–2061, 1997.
17. Windecker R, Fleischer M, Franze B, Tiziani HJ. Two methods for fast coherence tomography and topometry. J Mod Opt 44:967–977, 1997.
18. Xinan G, Lambsdorff M, Kuhl J, Biachang W. Fast-scanning autocorrelator with 1-ns scanning range for characterization of mode-locked ion lasers. Rev Sci Instrum 59:2088–2090, 1988.
19. Yasa ZA, Amer NM. A rapid-scanning autocorrelation scheme for continuous monitoring of picosecond pulses. Opt Commun 36:406–408, 1981.
20. Gelikonov VM, Sergeev AM, Gelikonov GV, Feldchtein FI, Gladkova ND, Ioannovich J, Fragia K, Pirza T. Compact fast-scanning OCT device for in vivo biotissue imaging. Presented at Conference on Lasers and Electro-Optics, 1996.
21. Tearney GJ, Bouma BE, Boppart SA, Golubovic B, Swanson EA, Fujimoto JG. Rapid acquisition of in vivo biological images by use of optical coherence tomography. Opt Lett 21:1408–1410, 1996.

22. Feldchtein F. Personal communication, 1999.
23. Ferreira LA, Santos JL, Farahi F. Polarization insensitive fiber-optic white-light interferometry. Opt Commun 114:386–392, 1995.
24. Weiner AM, Leaird DE, Patel JS, Wullert JR. Programmable femtosecond pulse shaping by use of a multielement liquid-crystal phase modulator. Opt Lett 15:326–328, 1990.
25. Kwong KF, Yankelevich D, Chu KC, Heritage JP, Dienes A. 400-Hz mechanical scanning optical delay line. Opt Lett 18:558–560, 1993.
26. Chu KC, Liu K, Heritage JP, Dienes A. Scanning femtosecond optical delay with 1000× pulse width excursion. Presented at Conference on Lasers and Electro-Optics, 1994.
27. Tearney GJ, Brezinski ME, Bouma BE, Boppart SA, Pitris C, Southern JF, Fujimoto JG. In vivo endoscopic optical biopsy with optical coherence topography. Science 276:2037–2039, 1997.
28. Tearney GJ, Bouma BE, Fujimoto JG. High speed phase- and group-delay scanning with a grating-based phase control delay line. Opt Lett 22:1811–1813, 1997.
29. Binjrajka V, Chang C-C, Emanuel AWR, Leaird DE, Weiner AM. Pulse shaping of incoherent light by use of a liquid-crystal modulator array. Opt Lett 21:1756–1758, 1996.
30. Martinez OE. 3000 times grating compressor with positive group velocity dispersion: Application to fiber compensation in 1.3–1.6 μm region. IEEE J Quantum Electron QE-23:59–64, 1987.
31. Rollins AM, Ung-arunyawee R, Chak A, Wong RCK, Kobayashi K, Sivak MV Jr, Izatt JA. Real-time in vivo imaging of human gastrointestinal ultrastructure by use of endoscopic optical coherence tomography with a novel efficient interferometry design. Opt Lett. 24:1358–1360, 1999.
32. Yang W, Keusters D, Goswami D, Warren WS. Rapid ultrafine-tunable optical delay line at the 1.55-μm wavelength. Opt Lett 23:1843–1845, 1998.

5

Design of OCT Scanners

FELIX I. FELDCHTEIN, V. M. GELIKONOV, and G. V. GELIKONOV

Institute of Applied Physics, Nizhny Novgorod, Russia

5.1 INTRODUCTION

It is well known that OCT is essentially similar to ultrasound echography. In line with this analogy, one can say that the difference between OCT and optical low coherence reflectometry is the same as that between B-scan and A-scan in ultrasound—two dimensional cross-sectional imaging versus one-dimensional in-depth scanning only. With some rare exceptions, lateral scanning is performed slowly in comparisons with in-depth scanning. In particular, because of the constant velocity in-depth scanning and bandpass filtering of the interference signal, the most advanced implementation of OCT requires that the in-depth scanning be performed first. All known OCT lateral scanning systems are substantially mechanical. In the simplest case they provide linear translation of a sample or probing head as a whole. More advanced devices include means for lateral scanning within the probing head. Because the implementation of a scanner depends strongly on the probing head size and consequently on the space allowable for the scanning mechanism, existing scanners can be divided into three types: benchtop (virtually unlimited space), hand-held (available space of the order of several tens of cubic centimeters) and endoscopic (available space of the order of or less than $1\,cm^3$). On the other hand, one can classify lateral scanners that rely on the scanning principle into circumferential, deflecting, and translational.

All of the above discussion refers to the mechanical aspects of the scanning probe design. From the point of view of optical design, the probe should perform image relaying from the fiber tip to the tissue surface and scanning along the sample surface. The optical system may consist of a single lens, a series of lenses, or a gradient index (GRIN) lens.

5.2 GENERAL REQUIREMENTS AND APPROACHES TO SCANNER DESIGN

A lateral OCT scanner is a complex optomechanical system that satisfies certain engineering requirements. Because it is intended mainly for clinical use, several additional medical requirements are imposed such as safety, sterilizability, and convenience in application. In this section we discuss these issues.

5.2.1 Optical System

The main purpose of the scanner optical system is to deliver and focus the probing light onto the tissue surface and collect the scattered radiation back to the interferometer. In the case of a bulk mirror-based interferometer, it provides focusing of the collimated probing beam into a tissue sample. For a single-mode fiber interferometer, the optical system additionally relays the fiber tip image with a certain magnification to the tissue.

The lateral displacement of the probing beam at the sample surface depends on the optical system magnification M. The magnification in all existing OCT systems is typically chosen as a trade-off between the lateral resolution and the scanning depth. To preserve the resolution one usually scans within the range limited by the double Rayleigh length. If the probing beam has a diameter D and a nearly Gaussian intensity profile (which is a quite realistic assumption taking into account that the beam is coupled from a single-mode fiber), the Rayleigh length is $\pi D^2 / 4\lambda$. At the magnification value $M = 4$ for a fiber with a $5\,\mu$m mode diameter and a probing wavelength of $1.3\,\mu$m, the Rayleigh length is $\sim 250\,\mu$m.

The above numbers mean that a numerical aperture (NA) of a typical scanner optical system should be ~ 0.05 from the output (sample) side and 0.15 from the input (fiber) side. These NA values, although moderate, require aspherical optics to provide acceptable image quality. In most cases, aspherical or GRIN lenses are used; however, microscope objectives are also applicable in optical systems where space and cost are not critical.

5.2.2 Mechanical System

Generally, a mechanical system should provide scanning of the focused beam position along the sample surface. The main mechanical requirements for a scanner are size, scanning rate, and safety. Because the allowable size greatly affects a concrete implementation, some features are discussed separately in Section 5.2.3 for benchtop, hand-held, and endoscopic scanners.

The scanning rate is one of the most important issues. The ultimate values for different scanning methods are not clear yet, but there are no principal limitations to acquiring images at a rate of several frames per second (fps) with any of them. Circumferential and galvanometric scanners have already demonstrated high (up to 30 fps) acquisition rate capability [1,2]. Certainly, fast lateral scanning should be matched to the depth scanning rate employed to provide optimal sampling. This means that the lateral displacement during one period of the in-depth scanning should be kept 1.5–2 times less than the lateral resolution (focused beam diameter). Another limitation is the optical power needed to keep an acceptable signal-to-noise ratio as the image acquisition rate is increased. Taking into account that the power level affordable today in a clinical OCT device is around a few milliwatts, the optical scanning rate is typically 1–8 fps.

From the safety point of view, a low voltage supply is preferable for a scanner, especially for an endoscopic one. This requirement is met for all designs except for piezoceramic bimorph actuators. However, due to the high electrical resistance of piezoceramic elements it might be easy to keep a current through the probe head at the safe level. Another safety requirement (at least for endoscopic probes) is sterilizability. All known designs can be produced hermetically sealed and hence allow cold sterilization.

5.2.3 Classification of OCT Scanners in Size: Benchtop, Hand-Held, and Endoscopic Embodiments

The first published OCT experiments with benchtop scanners [3,4] performed linear translation of a probing head or angular rotation of a sample (eye). This approach, being the simplest one, has a number of advantages (e.g., absence of geometrical aberrations) and is still applied in the laboratory studies. An evident alternative is angular scanning of a probing beam in front of an objective lens that is focusing probing radiation on a sample. For instance, Ref. 5 reports lateral scanning performed by mirrors attached to a galvo scanner.

One of the most popular ways to scan laterally with a benchtop-size scanner with a fiber interferometer is to deflect a fiber tip in front of an optical lens system. Working in fact, in all spatial scales from benchtop to tiny endoscopic systems, this proves to be a quite universal solution. Because the same scanning principle is also applicable in various other fields (optical storage devices, lidars, etc.), it has been well known since the 1960s [6], and a number of embodiments were known in the 1970s [7]. They include various systems driving a fiber tip: galvanometric movers, piezoelectric bimorph (or polymorph) plates, magnetostrictive elements, and thermal expansion bimorph plates. In early OCT experiments [8,9] a fiber tip was attached to a needle of a usual microammeter head and the lateral scanning was performed by changing the current through the microammeter.

The most important feature of hand-held scanners in comparison with benchtop scanners is to provide convenient access to examined tissue in a clinical environment. This imposes certain constraints on the size and shape of the instrument while the basic methods of scanning are inherited from the benchtop scanner family. To examine the tissue in the oral cavity, L-shaped hand-held probes were developed that employ either translational [10–12] or galvanometric beam deflection [13] techniques. A straight hand-held scanner with a similar galvanometric actuator was constructed and used in skin research [14]. Another approach based on bimorph or polymorph plate actuators was proposed in Refs. 7 and 15.

Most challenging are the requirements for endoscopic OCT scanners. The diameter of a probe and its flexibility are crucial parameters here to comply with existing medical standards. For example, when examining human internal organs it is necessary for an OCT probe to fit a millimeter-size-diameter operating channel of a corresponding endoscope to provide an approach to the tissue and parallel visual and tomographic observation. As the first attempt to build an endoscopic OCT scanner, replication of an ultrasound intravascular instrument with a rotating distal part was undertaken [16]. This scanner, with a 1.1 mm diameter, was tested in experiments with animals to image narrow-diameter channels in the respiratory and gastrointestinal tracts. The first microscanner used in clinical experiments with humans [17] to image the gastrointestinal, respiratory, urinary, and genital tracts and the abdominal cavity during laparoscopy was based on an original galvanometric design and had a 2.8 mm diameter. The only moving part in this instrument is a tiny electromagnetic coil with the attached tip of the optical fiber. Another novel design of the endoscopic scanner was implemented [18] in which a remote mechanical actuator produced linear displacement that was conveyed through a cable to the distal end inside the human body. The probe diameter was small enough to fit the operating channel of a fibrogastroscope. Finally, one more type of OCT scanner constructed and tested in clinics [1] is similar to a commercial high frequency endoscopic ultrasound system with rotating probe shaft In general, a variety of endoscopic scanner designs demonstrated recently reflect the deep interest of researchers and clinicians in the potentialities provided by OCT in imaging internal organs.

5.3 IMPLEMENTATION OF OCT SCANNERS

5.3.1 Circumferential Scanners

Design of circumferential OCT scanners employs the principle of image construction analogous to that in ultrasonography. The probing beam rotates about the OCT probe axis, imaging cross-sectionally through the structure into which the probe is inserted. A recorded tomogram is then presented in polar coordinates; this has also been adopted from ultrasonography and hence is quite common for physicians. Apparently, this approach is adequate if the imaging depth is of the order of or more than the transverse size of the lumen of a hollow organ under observation. Otherwise, A-scans at different polar angles occur under unequal conditions, which leads to narrowing of the sector of quality image acquisition. This requirement is usually met in ultrasound echography with a centimeter-range penetration depth. Having in mind that OCT imaging is limited to 2–3 mm in depth, circumferential scanning is preferable for intravascular examination or investigation of comparatively narrow ducts such as those in the urinary or low respiratory systems.

The first prototype of a circumferential microscanner referred to by the authors as a catheter-endoscope was designed and constructed by the OCT group at MIT in 1996 [16]. It inherits several important features for an intravascular ultrasound probe supplemented with optical delivery and focusing systems. A schematic of the scanner is shown in Fig. 1. It consists of a fixed optical coupling element at the proximal end to introduce light from the main interferometer and a rotating body to direct, focus, and scan the optical beam and collect the backscattered radiation.

Coupling of the incident light from the stationary single-mode fiber to the rotating one is performed through a small air gap without any lens system. It is the most sensitive part of the optical layout, requiring both high precision, face-to-face alignment of the optical fiber apertures and high mechanical stability of the rotary motion. Variation in optical coupling during rotation results in overall losses and a dependence of the probing power on the polar angle (up to 3 dB losses were measured by the authors with the optimal alignment of the scanner). To drive the rotating body, which comprises an optical connector, a hollow cable with the fiber inside and a focusing unit at the distal end (see Fig. 1), a DC motor and a standard

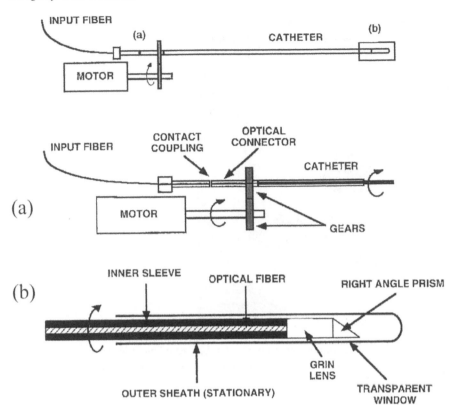

Figure 1 Schematic of catheter-endoscope. (a) Proximal end; and (b) body and distal end. (From Ref. 16.)

gear mechanism are used. The whole rotating assembly is inserted into an exchangeable stationary outer sheath protecting the surrounding tissue against mechanical irritation and biologically hazardous agents. The body of the catheter is flexible to allow bending during the passage of the scanner through channels of the human body to the area to be examined.

The micro-optical system focusing and directing the probing beam is located at the distal end of the catheter-endoscope. It includes a gradient index (GRIN) lens and a right-angle microprism. Attached to each other and to the optical fiber with ultraviolet-curing optical cement, they form a single unit with the rotating body of the catheter. Parameters of the GRIN lens are chosen based on the required working distance in the tissue being imaged (1–3 mm) and spot size comparable with the in-depth resolution (15–30 μm).

In the first prototype of a device operating at 1.3 μm wavelength, a single-mode isotropic fiber with the 9 μm core diameter was used in the scanner body to deliver light to a GRIN lens of 0.7 mm diameter and a 0.5 mm microprism. The outer diameter of the catheter was a small as 1.1 mm. An acquisition rate of 4 fps was demonstrated in the first in vivo studies with animals using this circumferential scanner. In Fig. 2 an OCT image of rabbit esophagus is shown as an example demonstrating the performance of the MIT OCT system with the above-described catheter-endoscope probe [19].

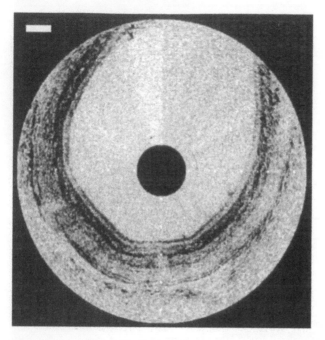

Figure 2 Optical coherence tomographic image of rabbit esophagus in vivo [19] obtained with catheter-endoscope [16] allows distinct visualization of different mucosa layer. Bar, 500 μm.

The basic design of the circumferential scanner described above has recently undergone several improvements introduced by the OCT group of Case Western Reserve University (CWRU) for development of a gastrointestinal imaging device [1]. At the distal end of the catheter, a Faraday rotator is placed between the GRIN lens and the right-angle prism (see Fig. 3). According to the well-known idea of optical fiber interferometry [20], it provides compensation for birefringence induced in the isotropic fiber due to bending of the sample arm inside the human body. The ultimate result is utilization of the optical power in both orthogonal wave polarizations and the elimination of dynamic polarization distortions caused by fiber bending and temperature drift. At the proximal end of the catheter, a second microsize GRIN lens is added to facilitate the image relay from the fixed optical fiber to the rotating one. Better and less angle-dependent coupling of light to the catheter body is

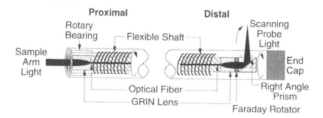

Figure 3 Schematic illustration of the circumferential endoscopic OCT probe suitable for passage through the biopsy channel of a standard fibrogastroscope. (From Ref. 1.)

expected with this arrangement when the drive shaft rotates. Using these modifications, a catheter probe suitable for passage through the accessory channel of a standard gastrointenstinal endoscope has been constructed and tested during examinations of human patients at the CWRU hospitals. Figure 4 is an individual OCT frame captured at the 4 fps rate in a normal human esophagus using the CWRU OCT system [1] with the described probe design.

To conclude this section, the advantages and limitations of the circumferential design of OCT scanners can be summarized. First of all, the rotational principle is promising due to its potentiality to accelerate the scanning speed. Regular rotary motion is less sensitive to undesirable inertial and hysteresis effects that occur with high speed oscillating motion. Real-time OCT imaging with a video rate of 20–30 fps is feasible with circumferential scanning when fast enough in-depth scanning and high sources of superluminescent radiation of enough power are at hand. Second, rotation does not prevent the OCT probe from being flexible, which is an important feature for an endoscopic OCT device. The described OCT probes directly employ this property from the standard ultrasound catheter design. Third, the circumferential scanning mode is favorable for the examination of organs with a narrow lumen and is especially suitable for intravascular imaging. On the other hand, there are several problems inherent to this approach. One of them is the difficulty in alignment

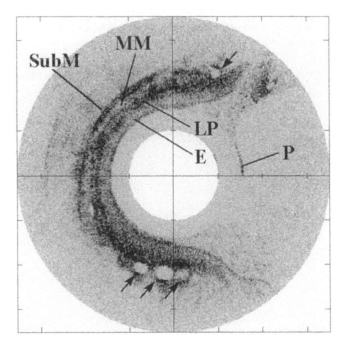

Figure 4 Optical coherence tomographic image of normal human esophagus in vivo obtained with circumferential endoscopic OCT probe. Scale markers represent 1 mm. P is the outer surface of the probe sheath. The substructure of the mucusal layer is differentiable, with the squamous epithelium (E), lamina propria (LP), and muscularis mucosae (MM). Light gray-scale ("echo-poor") inclusions (arrows) can be seen in the submucosa (SubM) that correspond to blood vessels and glands. (From Ref. 1.)

of the optical rotary junction, which results in high insertion losses and dependence of the probing power on the rotation angle. The circumferential scanners are also much less appropriate for large lumen channels or hollow organs where it is desirable to probe at different viewing angles to the scanner axis. For these purposes, apparatuses described in the following sections appear to be more attractive.

5.3.2 Deflecting Scanners

Design of deflecting OCT scanners employs the principle of beam motion that is similar to that in scanning microscopy. A probing beam is deflected transversely to the direction of its incidence on a stationary lens system that further guides it to the distal end and focuses it on tissue. Deflection is produced either by moving the tip of the optical fiber delivering the probing light from the main interferometer or by an oscillating (rotating) lens or a mirror that directs the beam coming out of the fiber to the stationary lens system. Several mechanisms for scanning the probe beam by moving optical components at the proximal end, including motor-driven galvano-metric, and piezoelectric techniques, have already been demonstrated in OCT devices.

Moving the fiber tip in the image plane of the stationary lens system appears to be the most universal and applicable technique for scanners of different sizes and functions. One of the first OCT systems comprising a scanner of this type was demonstrated by the OCT group of the Institute of Applied Physics (Nizhny Novgorod, Russia) [21]. The schematic of this hand-held probe capable of two-dimensional lateral scanning of the beam is presented in Fig. 5.

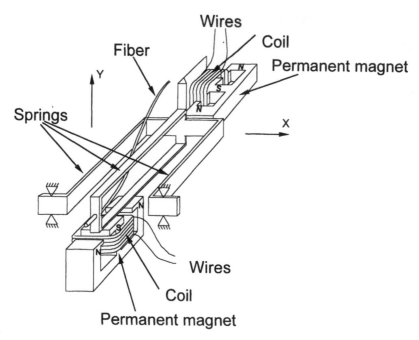

Figure 5 Schematic of deflecting OCT scanner with suspension arrangement in the form of embedded parallelograms. (From Ref. 8.)

The key mechanical feature in this design is a suspension arrangement in the form of embedded parallelograms formed by thin spring plates that provide independent orthogonal movement of a fiber in two directions relative to the probe case. The lens system and two permanent magnet units are fixed to the case, whereas two coils are attached to the spring frame and impart a deflecting torque whose components are controlled by the current magnitude in the coils. The magnetic field in the magnet bores reaches the value of 4.5–5 kG and produces a deflecting driving force of ~ 0.15 N at a current value of 50–70 mA. With a spring length of 50 mm the swing of transverse scanning in both directions is 2 mm. The image of the fiber tip is relayed by the lens system onto tissue with variable magnification that is controlled by the position of the lenses in the optical assembly and is dependent on the application (skin, eye, or teeth imaging).

As in any other mechanical system, hysteresis takes place when the direction of movement is being reversed. In this design, at the fiber tip with a swinging amplitude of 3 mm and a scanning rate of about 1 scan/s, hysteresis of the fiber position is significantly lower than that obtained with piezoceramic actuators and usually does not exceed 3%. To provide easily controlled periodic motion of the scanner it is important that higher harmonic components in the spectrum of the driving force for each orthogonal displacement do not enter domains of eigenresonances. In the described OCT probe, due to the appropriate choice of the spring material and geometry, the suspension has a lower resonance frequency of 62.5 Hz at a Q factor of 7 along the x coordinate and 30 Hz at a Q factor of 14 along the y coordinate. Eigenoscillations of the suspension are suppressed due to electromagnetic damping by means of a power amplifier with low output resistance. As a result, the mechanical movement of the scanner was practically free from hysteresis and oscillations when scanner was driven by isosceles triangle voltage waveform with 1 s period. Of course, to operate at scanning frequencies of the order of 10 Hz it is necessary to either increase the resonance frequency of the suspension or introduce certain predistortions in the driving current.

One of the scanners of this family, designed in an L-shaped form for better access to the tissue in the oral cavity, is shown in Fig. 6. The magnification of the optical system was 5, thus providing imaging of an area ~ 5 mm wide [14]. For skin imaging where the probe size does not cause a real limitation, lateral beam swinging as large as 15 mm was achieved on the tissue surface using another scanner of this kind. A typical tomogram of a skin nevus recorded with the aid of this scanner is shown in Fig. 7.

To study mucosa of human internal organs, the OCT group from the IAP developed in 1997 a one-dimensional lateral microscanner [17] using the principle of electromagnetic displacement of the fiber described above. It is small enough to be inserted into biopsy channels of standard endoscopic instruments such as fibrogastroscopes, hysteroscopes, laryngoscopes, and laparoscopic trocars. For instance, the diameter of a biopsy (instrumental) channel of many commercial endoscopes does not exceed 2.8 mm. There is also a limitation on the length of the rigid part of the scanner body. It should be short enough to allow penetration of the probe head into slightly curved endoscopic channels. Later in this section we describe the design and performance of such a small electromagnetic microscanner for endoscopic OCT.

In the microscanner design, the internal volume is used with maximal efficiency and the number of instrumental elements is minimal. In construction of a suspen-

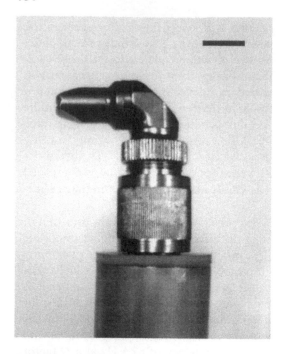

Figure 6 Photograph of L-shaped tip of deflecting scanner (Fig. 5) for examination of oral cavity. Bar = 1 cm.

sion, for instance, the elastic properties of the distal part of a quartz fiber itself are used when it is made an end part of the sample arm of the interferometer. The protective plastic coating is peeled off the optical fiber to reduce hysteresis effects caused by nonelastic deformations in the plastic when it is bent. Whereas at the proximal end of the microscanner the fiber is fixed to a base, the free end of the fiber serves as a console to which a coil of an electromagnetic system is attached (Fig. 8). The console part of the fiber is surrounded by the body of a permanent magnet, with a through-hole being formed by the facing grooves. The magnet is composed of two halves pressed together Their similar poles are aligned to produce fanlike magnetic force lines distributed in the plane of the coil. The coil is made of a thin wire and has thin input leads, which insignificantly increase the hysteresis effects of the mechanical suspension. The driving current applied to the coil causes it to interact

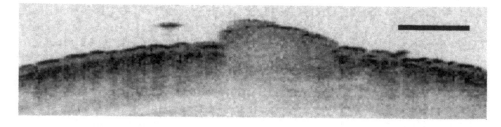

Figure 7 Image of skin nevus obtained with deflecting OCT scanner. Bar = 1 mm.

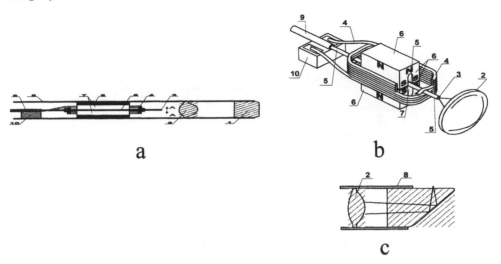

Figure 8 (a,b) Schematics of endoscopic microprobe. *1*, Output window, *2*, focusing lens; *3*, fiber tip; *4*, coil; *5*, fiber; *6*, permanent magnet; *7*, through-hole in magnet; *8*, probe sheath; *9*, fiber; *10*, fiber basement. (From Ref. 17.) (c) For side-view imaging, output glass window is made in the form of a prism directing the beam at a certain angle to the probe axis.

with the permanent magnet field and a deflecting torque to occur that deviates the fiber from equilibrium. When the current is about 100 μA, deviation of the fiber tip is about 0.3–0.5 mm, which is enough to move a focused beam with a swing of 2 mm at a magnification of the lens system of about 4–5.

At its distal end, the microscanner used for *en face* imaging has an output glass window inclined at an angle of 5–6°. The inclination decreases parasitic reflections of the probing light back into the fiber mode from both window surfaces; the inner surface is also antireflectively coated for the same purpose. The outer surface of the window touches a wet mucosa and becomes almost antireflective due to the refractive index matching. For side-view imaging, an output glass window is made in the form of a prism (see Fig. 8c) directing the beam at a certain angle to the probe axis. A single aspheric lens of a lens system focuses the light beam into the spot positioned near the tissue surface. Thus, operation of the microscanner requires neither an additional alignment of the optical system nor adjustment of the reference arm of the interferometer. As an example, in Fig. 9 an EOCT tomogram of healthy human esophagus is presented that was acquired with a portable IAP OCT device equipped with the microscanner inserted in the operating channel of a standard fibrogastroscope.

An alternative method of moving the fiber is based on the use of piezoelectric actuators. In 1997 the OCT group of MIT [15] demonstrated such scanner designs with piezoelectric cantilevers. The displacement of a cantilever made of a bimorph or polymorph plate several centimeters long can reach 1 mm at an applied voltage of several hundred volts. If a fiber is adhered to the cantilever, a deflecting torque is imparted to the optical system, thus producing scanning of the probe beam according to the applied voltage variation.

A schematic of a hand-held probe of this type is presented in Fig. 10. A 6.4 mm × 38 mm lead zirconate titanate piezoelectric cantilever was used with a 38 mm

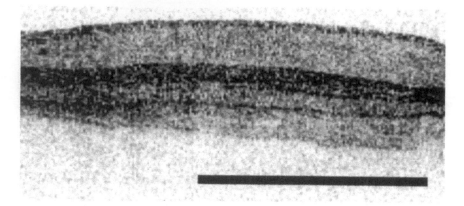

Figure 9 Endoscopic OCT image of healthy human esophagus that was obtained with deflecting endoscopic scanner. Bar = 1 mm (From Ref. 17.)

extension tube to double the cantilever arm length for transverse scanning. Total displacement of 2 mm was achieved at 300 V applied voltage. A single-mode optical fiber running along the tube was coupled to a GRIN lens through a narrow air gap. The faces of the GRIN lens and the fiber tip were slightly angled to reduce back-reflection to the interferometer and oriented parallel to each other to maximize optical coupling. The focal spot, about 30 μm in diameter, was positioned at work-ing distance of 3 mm from the lens. An OCT system with this scanner was tested in in vitro experiments to record images of human ovary and lung (Fig. 11).

Because of the rigid fixing of the GRIN lens to the oscillating tube, the described design possesses some features of translational scanners that are consid-ered in the next section. A similar design without an extension tube and a GRIN lens, employing a stationary telescope system to focus the beam, has some advan-tages over the one diagrammed in Fig. 10. It includes low mass (the fiber only) attached to the cantilever, allowing higher oscillation rates, and variable magnifica-tion of the optical system achieved by repositioning or changing lenses.

In general, evaluating the piezoelectric OCT scanner design, its simplicity and low cost are rather attractive. At the same time, it has a number of drawbacks in comparison with electromagnetically driven suspensions. Among them the use of high voltage to attain the same displacement magnitudes and a pronounced hyster-esis effect inherent to polymorph piezoactuators are the most important.

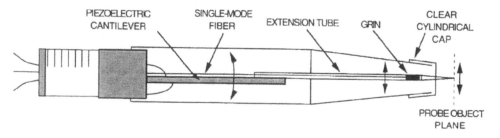

Figure 10 Schematic of hand-held probe with a piezoelectric cantilever. (From Ref. 15.)

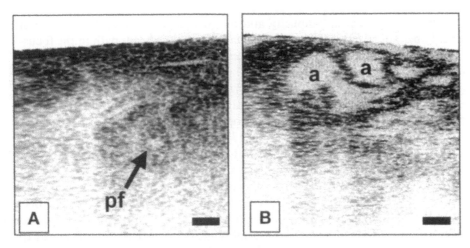

Figure 11 Optical coherence tomographic images of human ovary (A) and lung (B) obtained in vitro using hand-held probe with piezoelectric cantilever. pf, primordial follicle; a, lung alveoli.

The probe beam in deflecting OCT scanners can also be swung with galvanometer-driven mirrors or lenses. This method permits high acquisition rates and three-dimensional imaging but at the expense of increased size, cost, and complexity. This design was implemented in the first commercial OCT devices for ophthalmology produced by Zeiss Humphrey Systems, Dublin, CA. Another working prototype of a hand-held scanner of this type has recently been demonstrated by the OCT group of MIT [22]. A schematic of this design is given in Fig. 12. It contains a galvanometer-driven mirror changing the angle of incidence of the probe beam on a stationary assembly of relay lenses (Hopkins type).

5.3.3 Translational Scanners

The main distinctive feature of the design of this scanner family is the linear translational motion of the optical assembly as a whole with a remotely motor-driven

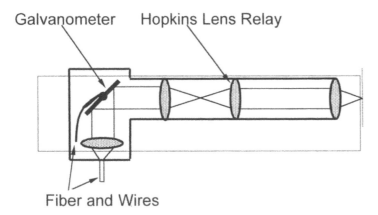

Figure 12 Schematic of galvanometer-based hand-held probe. (From Ref. 22.)

carriage. Due to its technical simplicity and an obvious advantage, the absence of geometrical aberrations caused otherwise by variation of the beam path in the focusing system, this approach is quite convenient in bench-top experiments without volume limitation on the layout of an OCT probe. It was the reason why in the very first OCT experiments the translational principle of scanning, applied to a probe or to an object, was implemented. Recently, translational scanners have been demonstrated in hand-held [11,12] and even endoscopic [18] designs.

One of these scanning devices (see Fig. 13) was developed by the OCT group of Lawrence Livermore National Laboratory (LLNL) to image the human oral cavity, primarily the hard dental tissue. A traveling stage with an optical system is displaced by a DC-motor-driven screw along the surface of the tissue. The scan direction (up or down) is set by depressing the appropriate switch and applying the necessary bias to the motor. Terminal switches restrict the range of lateral motion to the desired transverse scan dimension. The optical assembly includes a GRIN lens attached to the tip of a single-mode fiber with an index-matching UV-curable epoxy. The distance from the end of the GRIN lens to the tissue is adjusted by means of a screw-type mechanism, and a removable sterilizable cap is in contact with tissue.

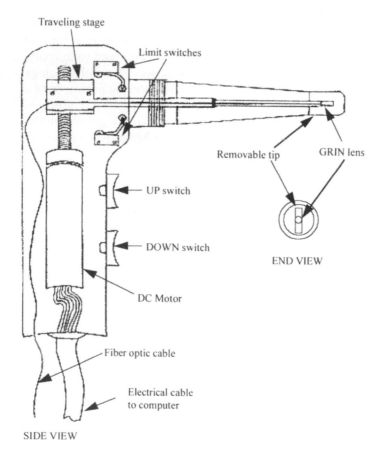

Figure 13 Schematic of translational hand-held OCT scanner [10] for examination of dental tissue.

The described device permits the recording of two-dimensional OCT images that are free of geometrical aberrations over the entire scanning range with a lateral size as large as several millimeters. The main drawback is the long time needed for image acquisition (several tens of seconds) because of the inertia of the displaced assembly and in part the low power of the light source. Figure 14 shows a typical tomogram of periodontal tissue taken with this scanner at a wavelength of 1.3 μm.

Another interesting design of translational scanners has recently been implemented by the OCT group of Harvard Medical School [18]. A narrow diameter, flexible endoscopic OCT probe has been constructed where scanning is conveyed

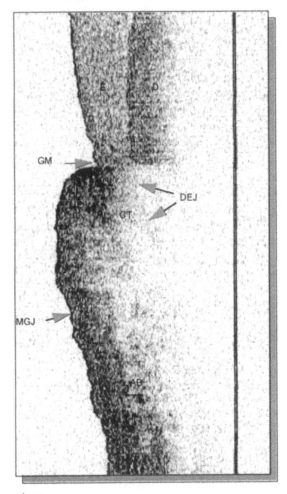

1 mm

Figure 14 Optical coherence tomographic images of the human periodontium acquired with translational scanner. Scales are represented in terms of optical distance. E, Enamel; D, dentin; GM, gingival margin; DEJ, dentoepithelial junction; CT, connective tissue; JE, junctional epithelium; MGJ, mucogingival junction; AM, alveolar mucosa; AB, alveolar bone. (From Ref. 10.)

mechanically to the distal end of the probe from a drive situated outside the human body. In contrast with the circumferential scanners described in Section 3.1, the body of the probe linearly translates within a static outer sheath. This construction eliminates the problem of transferring optical power from a stationary to rotating optical fiber, which is a weak point in the circumferential design. From the viewpoint of application areas, this design is more suitable for imaging internal organs with large lumens and hence to some extent is complementary to an MIT-type catheter-endoscope.

A schematic of the translational endoscopic scanner is shown in Fig. 15. As a mechanical actuator of scanning, a linearly displaced carriage driven by a rotating galvanometer at the proximal end of the probe is used. The translational motion is conveyed via a wound multiplayer cable that is attached to the carriage and houses an optical fiber inside. The helicity of the cable is reversed between layers to avoid rotation of the distal end while the cable is stretched or compressed. The sampling arm of the interferometer terminates with a 1.0 mm diameter gradient index lens and a 750 μm wide prism fixed to the distal tip of the cable. The optical system directs light transversely to the axis of the scanner and focuses it to a spot of 30 μm diameter at a distance of $\sim$ 700 μm from the outer wall of the catheter. This distance provides optimal imaging if the catheter is placed in contact with the tissue. To isolate the optical components from the tissue, a transparent disposable sheath is placed over the catheter cable during OCT examination.

A typical image of the normal human esophagus that was acquired in vivo with an OCT system equipped with the translational endoscopic scanner is presented in Fig. 16. This tomogram, recorded at a rate of 4 fps, demonstrates the high and constant quality of image acquisition over the entire lateral scanning range, which exceeded 5 mm. It is an impressive manifestation of the main advantage of the translational technique—the absence of image aberration due to invariable probing beam with respect to the moving optical system.

5.4 CONCLUSION

In this chapter, we have surveyed various types of OCT scanners. Their designs meet the main requirements for this instrument: to deliver and focus the probing light on the tissue, collect the scattered radiation, and provide beam motion along the sample surface at a rate adequate to that used for in-depth scanning. According to the

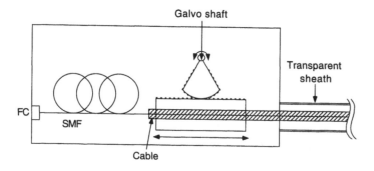

Figure 15   Schematic of translational endoscopic scanner. (From Ref. 18.)

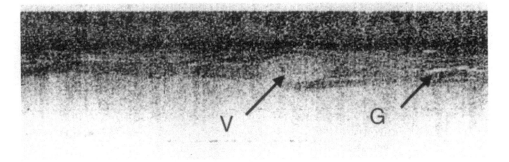

Figure 16 Optical coherence tomographic images of normal human esophagus obtained with translational endoscopic scanner. The image size is 5.5 mm horizontal and 1.8 mm vertical. A vessel (V) and several glands (G) are distinguishable. (From Ref. 18.)

character of beam motion in the scanner, we have classified them into three families: circumferential, deflecting, and translational scanners. In the first case, scanning is produced by beam rotation in the plane transverse to the instrument axis and image presentation is similar to that in ultrasonography. In the second case, a scanning mechanism deflect the beam before it is incident on the focusing system; this deflection can be in the form of 1-D oscillation or 2-D motion along an arbitrary trajectory in the transverse plane. In the third case, scanning is caused by the linear translation of the optical system itself while the beam position relative to the optical components remains invariable.

All these scanner designs have already been tested during in vivo experiments, including endoscopic OCT studies. Owing to specific advantages, each of the designs may be expected to find a niche in future OCT modalities. Apparently, circumferential scanning is more suitable for examination of organs with a narrow lumen, especially for intravascular imaging. Deflecting scanners are superior for *en face* imaging and suitable for 3-D image acquisition. A translational instrument is convenient for covering large surface area with minimal geometrical aberration of acquired images. All the designs discussed have the potentiality to operate at video rate provided powerful enough sources of the probing light are at hand and a fast enough in-depth scanning mechanism is employed.

Appreciating the progress in OCT scanner design, it would be unfair to conclude that the problem has been completely solved. A considerable upgrade of existing instruments and better design ideas are possible and desirable. This area of optical engineering as well as the OCT technique in general remain open and fruitful fields for competition of new ideas and approaches.

REFERENCES

1. Izatt JA, Rollins AM, Amitabh C et al. Real-time endoscopic optical coherence tomography in human patients. In: Conference on Lasers and Electro-Optics. Baltimore, MD: Opt Soc Am 1999, p 336.
2. Rollins AM, Kulkarni MD, Yazdanfar S et al. In vivo video rate optical coherence tomography. Opt Express 3(6):219–229, 1998.

3. Huang D, Swanson EA, Lin CP et al. Optical coherence tomography. Science 254:1178–1181, 1991.

4. Fercher AF, Hitzenberger CK, Drexler W et al. In vivo optical coherence tomography. Am J Ophthalmol 116:113–115, 1993.

5. Swanson EA, Izatt JA, Hee MR et al. In-vivo retinal imaging by optical coherence tomography. Opt Lett 18:1864, 1993.

6. Pike CA, Woodland NJ. Fibre deflection means. US Patent 3470320 (1969).

7. Russell JT. Optical fiber deflection device. US Patent 3941927 (1976).

8. Sergeev AM, Gelikonov VM, Gelikonov GV et al. In vivo optical coherence tomography of human skin microstructure. Proc SPIE 2328:144–150, 1994.

9. Gelikonov VM, Gelikonov GV, Kuranov RV et al. Coherent optical tomography of microscopic inhomogeneities in biological tissues. Pis'ma Zh Eksp Teor Fiz 61:149–153, 1995.

10. Everett MJ, Colston BW, Da Silva LB et al. Fiber optic-based optical coherence tomography (OCT) for dental applications. Proc SPIE 3489:53–59, 1998.

11. Colston BW, Everett MJ, Da Silva LB et al. Imaging of hard and soft tissue structure in the oral cavity by optical coherence tomography. Appl Opt 37:3582–3585, 1998.

12. Colston BW, Sathyam US, Da Silva LB et al. Dental OCT. Opt Express 3:230–238, 1998.

13. Feldchtein FI, Gelikonov GV, Gelikonov VM et al. In vivo OCT imaging of hard and soft tissue of the oral cavity. Opt Express 3:239–250, 1998.

14. Gelikonov VM, Sergeev AM, Gelikonov GV et al. Characterization of human skin using optical coherence tomography. Proc SPIE 2927:27–34, 1996.

15. Boppart SA, Bouma BE, Pitris C et al. Forward-imaging instruments for optical coherence tomography. Opt Lett 22:1618–1620, 1997.

16. Tearney GJ, Boppart SA, Bouma BE et al. Scanning single-mode fiber optic catheter-endoscope for optical coherence tomography. Opt Lett 21:543–545, 1996.

17. Sergeev AM, Gelikonov VM, Gelikonov GV et al. In vivo endoscopic OCT imaging of precancer and cancer states of human mucosa. Opt Express 1:432–440, 1997.

18. Bouma BE, Tearney GJ. Power efficient, non-reciprocal interferometer and linear scanning fiber-optic catheter for optical coherence tomography. Opt Lett 24:531–533, 1999.

19. Tearney GJ, Brezinski ME, Bouma BE et al. In vivo endoscopic optical biopsy with optical coherence tomography. Science 276:2037–2039, 1997.

20. Gelikonov VM, Gusovsky DM, Leonov VI et al. Birefringence compensation in single-mode optical fibers. Pis'ma Zh Tech Fiz 13:775–779, 1987.

21. Gelikonov VM, Sergeev AM, Gelikonov GV et al. Compact fast-scanning OCT device for in vivo biotissue imaging. In: Conference on Lasers and Electro-Optics. OSA Tech Dig Ser. Baltimore, MD: Opt Soc Am 1996, Vol 16, p. 58.

22. Li X, Drexler W, Pitris C et al. Imaging of osteoarthritic cartilage with optical coherence tomography: Micron-structure and polarization sensitivity. In: Conference on Lasers and Electro-Optics. Baltimore, MD: Opt Soc Am, 1999, CWP5.

6

System Integration and Signal/Image Processing

JOSEPH A. IZATT, ANDREW M. ROLLINS, RUJCHAI UNG-ARUNYAWEE, and SIAVASH YAZDANFAR

Case Western Reserve University, Cleveland, Ohio

MANISH D. KULKARNI

Zeiss Humphrey Systems, Dublin, California

6.1 INTRODUCTION

This chapter addresses the integration of the component technologies of OCT, described in the preceding chapters, into a complete imaging system (see Fig. 1). This includes both hardware considerations such as optimal interferometer topologies and scan synchronization dynamics and such software issues as image acquisition, transformation, display, and enhancement. A limited discussion of first-generation slow-scan systems (< 1 image/s) is included where it is illustrative; however, most of the discussion centers on state-of-the-art OCT systems acquiring images in real time or nearly so.

6.2 HARDWARE IMPLEMENTATION

6.2.1 Interferometer Topologies for Optimal SNR

The original and most common interferometer topology used in OCT systems is a simple Michelson interferometer, as depicted in earlier chapters. In this design, low coherence source light is split by a 50/50 beamsplitter into sample and reference paths. A retroreflecting variable optical delay line (ODL) forms the reference arm, and the sample specimen together with coupling and/or steering optics make up the sample arm. Light retroreflected by the reference ODL and light reflected by the sample are

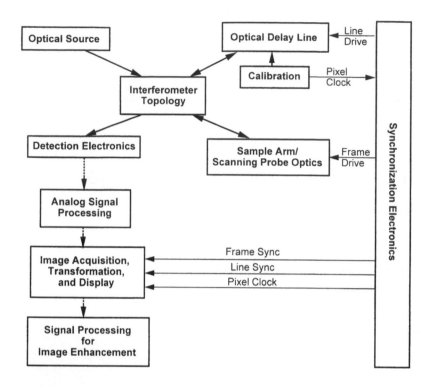

Figure 1 Optical coherence tomographic system components and synchronization requirements. Thick lines represent optical signals, dashed lines represent electronic signals, thin lines represent synchronization signals.

recombined at the beamsplitter and half is collected by a photodetector in the detection arm of the interferometer. Heterodyne detection of the interfering light is achieved by Doppler shifting of the reference light with a constant-velocity scanning ODL, or by phase modulating either the sample or reference arm. Single-mode fiber implementation of the interferometer has the advantage of simplicity and automatic assurance of the mutual spatial coherence of the sample and reference light incident on the detector. Although this design is intuitive and simple to implement, it is apparent that due to the reciprocal nature of the beamsplitter, half of the light backscattered from the sample and from the reference ODL is returned toward the source. Light returned to the source is lost to detection and may also compromise the modal stability of the source. Further, a detailed analysis of the signal-to-noise ratio (SNR) in low coherence interferometery [1,2] mandates that in order to optimally approach the shot noise detection limit for the Michelson topology, the reference arm light must be attenuated by several orders of magnitude (depending upon the source power level and the detector noise figure). Thus, in typical OCT implementations, up to 75% (or 6 dB) of the optical power supplied by the source does not contribute to image formation. Because light sources with high spatial coherence and low temporal coherence suitable for high speed OCT imaging in very low backscattering samples such as biological tissue are very expensive, optical power is a commodity well worth conserving in OCT systems.

Using optical circulators, unbalanced fiber couplers, and balanced heterodyne detection, two authors have recently demonstrated a new family of power-efficient fiber-optic interferometer topologies that recover most or all of the light lost in the Michelson configuration [2,3]. The three-port optical circulator is a nonreciprocal device that couples light incident on port I to port II and light incident on port II to port III. Current commercial fiber-coupled devices specify insertion losses of less than 0.7 dB (I to II, II to III) and isolation (III to II, II to I) and directivity (I to III) greater than 50 dB. Single-mode wideband fiber-optic couplers are commercially available with arbitrary (unbalanced) splitting ratios. Balanced heterodyne reception is an established technology in coherent optical communication [4,5] and has previously been used in OCDR [6] and in OCT [3,7–9].

Three types of new interferometer designs described by Rollins and Izatt [2] using these enabling technologies are illustrated in Fig. 2. The first design (A, including Ai and Aii) uses a Mach–Zehnder interferometer with the sample located in one arm and the reference ODL in the other arm. The first coupler is unbalanced, with a splitting ratio chosen to optimize the SNR by directing most of the source light to the sample. Light is coupled to the sample through an optical circulator so that the backscattered signal is collected by the delivery fiber and redirected to the second coupler. The reference ODL may be transmissive, or, alternatively, a retroreflecting ODL may be used with a second circulator. Design Aii of Fig. 2 is similar to Ai except that instead of balanced heterodyne detection, a second unbalanced splitter is used to direct most of the ample light to a single detector. The single-detector version is less expensive and easier to implement. For optical sources with high relative

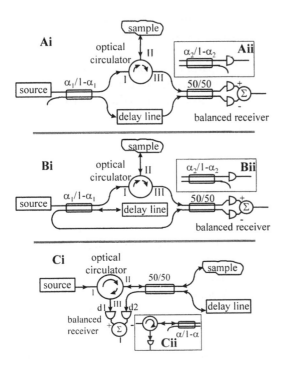

Figure 2 Schematics of optical power-conserving interferometer configurations. (From Ref. 2.)

intensity noise, and for sample probe designs from which there is appreciable back-reflection from the optics, shot noise limited detection may not be possible with a single detector. In these cases, dual balanced detection can provide a significant advantage by suppressing excess intensity noise and permitting near-shot-noise-limited detection.

Interferometer design B is similar to design A, as shown in the schematics labeled Bi and Bii in Fig. 2. In this case, a retroreflecting ODL is used without the need for a second optical circulator. Configuration Bii has recently been demonstrated for endoscopic OCT [3].

Design C uses a Michelson interferometer efficiently by introducing an optical circulator into the source arm instead of the sample arm, as in designs A and B. Configuration Ci uses a balanced receiver. Although configuration Ci does not make optimal use of optical source power by directing most light to the sample as the other efficient configurations do, this design has the significant advantage that an existing fiber-optic Michelson interferometer OCT system can be easily retrofitted with a circulator in the source arm and a balanced receiver, with no need to disturb the rest of the system. One drawback of configuration Ci is that more light is incident on the detectors than in the other configurations. Although the balanced receiver is effective in suppressing excess photon noise, a lower gain receiver is necessary to avoid saturation of the detectors. In a high speed OCT system, however, a lower gain receiver is necessary to accommodate the broad signal bandwidth. Design Ci has also recently been demonstrated for use in endoscopic OCT [9]. Design Cii uses an unbalanced splitter and a single detector.

An analysis of the signal-to-noise ratio for all of the designs illustrated in Fig. 2 reveals an SNR advantage of up to 6 dB compared to shot-noise-limited Michelson topology [2]. The balanced detection configurations can provide an SNR advantage in excess of 6 dB because of the additional capability of balanced reception to suppress excess intensity noise [6]. Maximum benefit is realized by optimizing the splitting ratio of the unbalanced couplers. An optimization procedure is provided in Ref. 2.

6.2.2 Analog Signal Processing

The critical function of the analog signal processing electronics in an OCT system is to extract the interferometric component of the voltage or current signal provided by the detection electronics with high dynamic range and to prepare it for analog-to-digital conversion. Other functions that could potentially be performed at this stage include signal processing operations for image enhancement, such as deconvolution, phase contrast, polarization-sensitive imaging, or Doppler OCT. Although to date almost all such image enhancement processing has been performed in software, as high speed imaging systems become more prevalent, predigitization time domain processing will inevitably become more sophisticated. For example, a recent demonstration of real-time signal processing for Doppler OCT used an analog approach [10].

Demodulation of the interferometric component of the detected signal may be performed using either an incoherent (i.e., peak detector) or coherent (quadrature demodulation) approach. Many early low speed OCT systems for which the Doppler shift frequency did not exceed several hundred kilohertz used a simple custom circuit employing a commercially available integrated-circuit RMS detector in conjunction with a one- or two-pole bandpass filter for incoherent demodulation [11,12]. Even more simply, satisfactory coherent demodulation can be accomplished by using a commercial dual-phase lock-in amplifier without any other external components [13,14]. By supplying the lock-in amplifier with a reference sine wave at the calculated reference arm Doppler shift frequency and using the lock-in time constant as a good quality high-order low-pass filter, the amplitude of the sum of the squares of the in-phase and quadrature outputs provides a high dynamic range monitor of the interferometric signal power. In more recent high speed OCT system implementations employing modulation frequencies in the megahertz range, more sophisticated electronics based on components designed for the ultrasound and cellular radio communications markets have been employed [3,9,15–18].

Dynamic Range Compression

As discussed in previous chapters, typical OCT systems routinely achieve sensitivity (defined as the minimum detectable optical power reflectivity of the sample) well below $-100\,\text{dB}$. Because the electronic interferometric signal amplitude (current or voltage) is proportional to the product of the reference and sample arm electric fields and thus to the square root of the sample power reflectivity, the signal-to-noise ratio of the electronic signal amplitude usually exceeds 50 dB. This value exceeds the dynamic range of the human visual system (which can sense brightness variations of only about 3 decades in a particular scene) and also approaches the dynamic range limit of many of the hardware components that make up the signal detection–processing–digitization chain. For example, the dynamic range of an A/D converter is given by $2^{2N}(\cong 6N\,\text{dB})$, where N is the number of bits of conversion; thus an 8-bit converter has a dynamic range of only 48 dB. For early OCT systems employing slow pixel digitization rates of only a few hundred kilohertz, this latter issue was not a limiting factor, because high dynamic range A/D converters (i.e., up to 16 bits) are common and inexpensive at these data rates. For high speed OCT imaging, however, megahertz digitization rates are required, and the dynamic range of the digitization step becomes an increasingly important factor in terms of both digitizer cost and downstream computation speed.

In order for an OCT image to be rapidly digitized and meaningfully observed, a means of hardware or software dynamic range compression is often employed. This is accomplished by transforming the detected sample reflectivity values with a nonlinear operation that has a maximum slope for low reflectivity values and a decreasing slope for increasing reflectivity values. The obvious and convenient method is to display the logarithm of reflectivity in units of decibels. The logarithm operation demonstrates the desired transform characteristic, and decibels are a meaningful, recognizable unit for reflectivity. The logarithm is not the only possible dynamic range compression transform. For example, the μ-law transform of communications systems or a sinusoidal transform could be used, but up to the present time, logarithmic compression is universal in display of OCT images.

Since the first report of OCT, images have conventionally been displayed in logarithmic format, usually having been transformed in software [19]. Although plots of A-scan data can be well visualized on a linear scale, in two-dimensional images displayed with a linear intensity scale only the brightest features are perceived (see, for example, Ref. 20). It is notable that the common definition of axial resolution in OCT as being given by half the coherence length of the light source is valid only when the data are presented on a linear scale; the 3 dB point of a sharp reflection in a logarithmically transformed image depends upon the dynamic range of the image data and is thus not well defined but is clearly wider than the half-coherence length.

Several options for hardware analog dynamic range compression are available. An approach that has been followed in several OCT implementation compresses the dynamic range of the signal before sampling by using an amplifier with a nonlinear gain characteristic [9,11]. In this way, commonly available data acquisition boards and frame grabbers with linear quantum levels can still be used for digitization. Demodulating logarithmic amplifiers are commercially available that compress the dynamic range of the OCT signal and also perform envelope detection. Alternatively, A/D converters are available with nonlinearly spaced quantum levels, for example following the μ-law transform. This would allow the low-reflectivity range to be sampled with high A/D dynamic range while sacrificing A/D dynamic range when sampling the high-reflectivity range, where it is not needed. Devices are also available that perform sinusoidal transformations.

6.2.3 Synchronization Electronics

As illustrated in Fig. 1, every OCT system implementation includes at least some form of optical delay line, sample scanning optics, and digitization/display electronics whose dynamic functions must be coordinated to acquire meaningful image data. In addition to the synchronization of these elements, which is common to all OCT systems, specially designed systems may also require coordination of dynamic properties of the optical source (e.g., frequency-tunable source implementations [21]), detection electronics, or analog signal processing electronics (e.g., frequency-tracking demodulators [22]).

A diagram illustrating the timing relationships between the elements in a standard minimal system is presented in Fig. 3. For most common systems that employ depth-priority scanning (i.e., in which depth A-scans are acquired more rapidly than lateral scans), individual image pixels are acquired in the 1 kHz–10 MHz range, the reference optical delay has a repetition rate in the 10 Hz–10 kHz range, and the lateral sample scanning optics repeat at 0.1–10 Hz frequencies. The optical delay line is driven by a waveform that is optimally a triangle or sawtooth to maximize the duration of the linear portion of the scan and thus the usable scan duty cycle, although harmonic and other nonlinear delay waveforms have been used for the fastest delay lines yet reported [18,23]. In either case, the synchronization electronics provide a frame sync signal synchronized to the sample lateral scan to signal the image acquisition electronics to start image frame acquisition. Similarly, the synchronization electronics provide a line sync signal synchronized to the depth scan to signal the image acquisition electronics to start A-scan digitization. In most OCT system implementations described to date, a pixel clock is generated by a synthesized source (i.e. by a function generator or on-board A/D conversion time) at a digitization rate given by the linescan rate multiplied by the number of desired pixels per line. However, an OCT system specially designed for coherent signal processing (used for both OCT image deconvolution [24] and

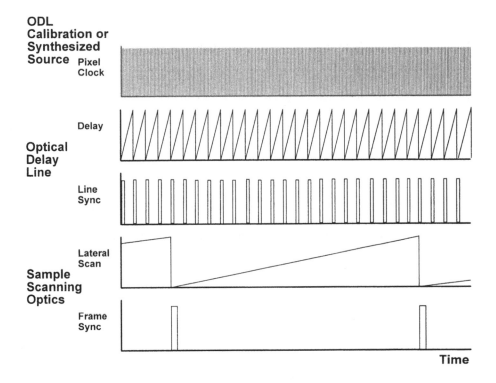

ODL
Calibration or
Synthesized
Source — Pixel Clock

Optical Delay Line — Delay, Line Sync

Sample Scanning Optics — Lateral Scan, Frame Sync

Time

Figure 3 Timing diagram for OCT synchronization electronics.

spectroscopic OCT [25]) has been reported that employed a helium-neon laser–based reference arm calibration interferometer to provide a pixel clock sync signal coordinated to the actual reference optical delay with nanometer accuracy. Lateral-priority scanning OCT systems have also been reported; in this case the timing of the depth and lateral scans is reversed [13,26–28].

The hardware comprising the synchronization and image acquisition electronics may be as simple as a multifunction data acquisition board (analog-to-digital, digital-to-analog, plus timer) residing in a personal computer. Alternatively, as described in the next section, a standard video frame grabber board may be programmed to perform the same functions at much higher frame rates.

6.2.4 Example of an Integrated OCT System

As an example of an integrated OCT system, a block diagram of a rapid-scan system designed for endoscopic evaluation of early cancer is provided in Fig. 4 [9]. The high speed OCT interferometer is based on a published design [18]. It includes a high power (22 mW), 1.3 μm center wavelength, broadband (67 nm FWHM) semiconductor amplifier-based light source and a Fourier domain rapid-scan optical delay line based on a resonant optical scanner operating at 2 kHz. Both forward and reverse scans of the optical delay line are used, resulting in an A-scan acquisition rate of 4 kHz. Image data are digitized during the center two-thirds of the forward and reverse scans, for an overall scanning duty cycle of 67%.

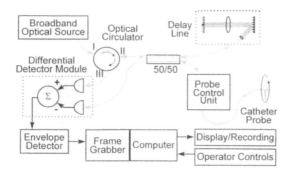

Figure 4 Block diagram of an endoscopic OCT (EOCT) system. Light from a high power broadband source is coupled through an optical circulator to a fiber-optic Michelson interferometer. The EOCT catheter probe and probe control unit constitute one arm of the interferometer, and a rapid-scanning optical delay line constitutes the other arm. Gray lines represent optical paths, and black lines represent electronic paths. (From Ref. 9.)

In this system, OCT probe light is delivered to the region of interest in the lumen of the GI tract via catheter probes that are passed through the accessory channel of a standard GI endoscope. A specialized shaft, which is axially flexible and torsionally rigid, mechanically supports the optical elements of the probe. The probe beam is scanned in a radial direction nearly perpendicular to the probe axis at 6.7 revolutions per second (the standard frame rate in commercial endoscopic ultrasound systems) or 4 rev/s. The converging beam exiting the probe is focused to a minimum spot of approximately 25 μm.

Optical signals returning from the sample and reference arms of the interferometer are delivered via the nonreciprocal interferometer topology (Fig. 2, Ci) to a dual-balanced InGaAs differential photoreceiver. The photoreceiver voltage is demodulated and the dynamic range compressed using a demodulating logarithmic amplifier. The resulting signal is digitized using a conventional variable-scan frame grabber residing in a Pentium II PC. The line sync signal for the frame grabber is provided by the resonant scanner controller, the frame sync signal is derived from the catheter probe rotary drive controller (one sync signal per rotation), and the pixel clock is generated internally in the frame grabber.

The PC-based endoscopic OCT (EOCT) imaging system is wholly contained in a single mobile rack appropriate for use in the endoscopic procedure suite. The system is electrically isolated, and the optical source is under interlock control of the probe control unit. The system meets institutional and federal electrical safety and laser safety regulations. The data capture and display subsystem acquires image data at a rate of 4000 lines per second using the variable-scan frame grabber. Alternate scan reversal is performed in software in order to use both forward and reverse scans of the optical delay line, followed by rectangular-to-polar scan conversion suing nearest-neighbor interpolation (see below). Six hundred (or 1000) A-scans are used to form each image. A software algorithm performs these spatial transformations in real time to create a full-screen (600 × 600 pixels) radial OCT image updated at 6.7 (or 4) fps. Endoscopic OCT images are displayed on the computer monitor and also digitally streamed to disk or archived to S-VHS video tape. Foot pedals controlling freeze-frame and frame capture commands are provided, allowing the endoscopist to quickly and effectively acquire data using the system.

6.3 IMAGE ACQUISITION AND DISPLAY

6.3.1 High Speed Data Capture and Display

Frame Grabber Technology

Frame grabbers are designed to digitize video signals, such as those from CCD cameras, CID cameras, and vidicon cameras. If each frame of video signals is 640 × 480 pixels, the amount of memory needed to store it is about 0.25 Mbyte for a monochrome image having 8 bits per pixel. Color images require three times this amount. Without a frame grabber, most inexpensive general-purpose personal computers cannot handle the bandwidth necessary to transfer, process, and display this much information, especially at the video rate of 30 fps. As a result, a frame grabber is always needed in an imaging system when images are displayed at or approaching video rate.

A block diagram of a simple frame grabber is shown in Fig. 5. Typical frame grabbers functionally comprise four sections: an A/D converter, a programmable pixel clock, an acquisition and window control unit, and a frame buffer. Video input is digitized by the A/D converter with characteristics such as filtering, reference and offset voltages, gain, sampling rate, and the source of sync signals controlled programmatically by the programmable pixel clock and acquisition and window control circuits. The frequency of the programmable pixel clock determines the video input signal digitization rate or sampling rate. In addition, the acquisition and window control circuitry also controls the region of interest (ROI), whose values are deter-

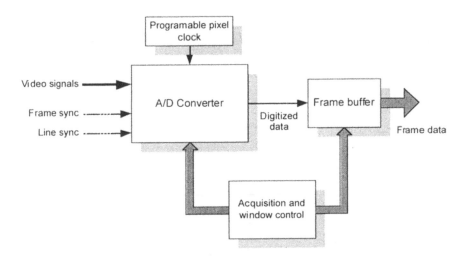

Figure 5 Block diagram of a simple frame grabber. Video signals can be either composite or noncomposite. External sync signals are selected by the acquisition and window control circuitry.

mined by the user. Image data outside of the ROI are not transferred to the frame buffer and are not displayed on the screen.

To use a frame grabber for general-purpose high speed data acquisition, it is important to understand the nature of video signals and how their acquisition is controlled by frame grabber driver software. A video signal comprises a sequence of different images, each of which is referred to as a frame. Each frame can be constructed from either one (noninterlaced) or two (interlaced) fields, depending upon the source of the signal. Most CCD cameras generate interlaced frames. The even field in an interlaced frame would contain lines 0, 2, 4, ..., the odd field would contain lines 1, 3, 5, and so on.

Figure 6 illustrates the components of a single horizontal line of noninterlaced video as well as the visual relationship between the signal components and the setting of the corresponding input controls. On the same basis, Fig. 7 shows the components of a single vertical field of video as well as the relationship between the signal and the setting of the corresponding input controls.

False Color and Gray-Scale Mapping

Once digitized by a conventional A/D converter or frame grabber, two-dimensional OCT image data representing cross-sectional or *en face* sample sections are typically represented as an intensity plot using gray-scale or false color mapping. The intensity plot typically encodes the logarithm of the detected signal amplitude as a gray-scale value or color that is plotted as a function of the two spatial dimensions. The choice of the color mapping used to represent OCT images has a significant effect on the perceived impact of the images and on the ease (and expense) with which images can be reproduced and displayed.

Many authors [13,14,18,21,29–31] have used the standard linear gray scale for OCT image representation, with low signal amplitudes mapping to black and strong reflections appearing as white. Some groups [3,32,33] have opted for a reverse gray scale, with strong reflections appearing as black on a white

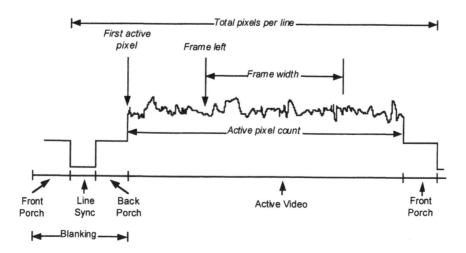

Figure 6   Signal components (normal) and input controls (italic) of the horizontal video signal.

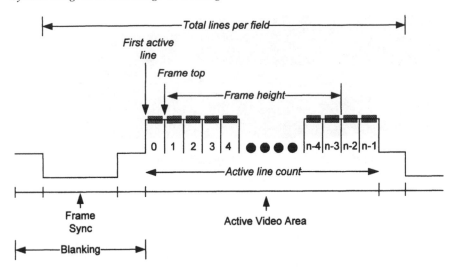

Figure 7 Signal components (normal) and input controls (italic) of the vertical video signal.

background, primarily motivated by the relative ease of printing and reproducing such images compared to the standard gray scale. A large variety of false color maps have been applied to OCT images, the most widely used being the original blue-green-yellow-red-white "retina" color scale designed by David Huang at MIT in 1991 [19]. This color map was adopted by Humphrey Systems Inc. as the primary map for their OCT retinal scanner and has also been used in some presentations of nonophthalmic data [19]. A plot of the retinal false color scale in red-green-blue (RGB) color space is reproduced in Fig. 8 (see color plate), and a comparison of an in vivo human retinal OCT image in each of the three color scales provided in Fig. 9 (see color plate).

Recent innovations in OCT technology that enhance structural or morphological imaging by the addition of functional information (e.g., Doppler flow imaging [34,35], polarization-sensitive OCT [36], spectroscopic OCT [25,37]) face

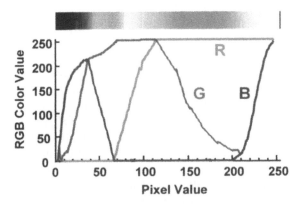

Figure 8 Plot of the retinal false color scale represented in RGB color space. Green and blue color values are identical between pixel values of 209 and 255. (See color plate.)

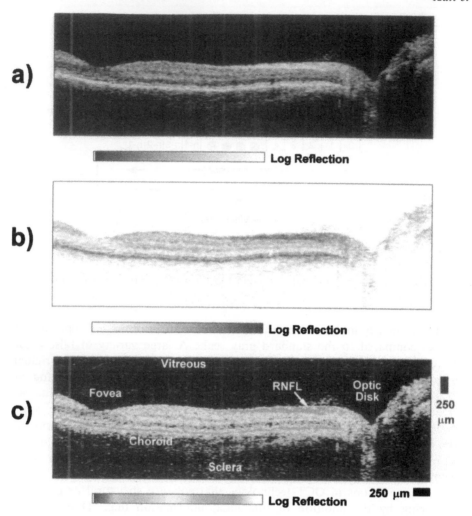

Figure 9 Comparison of an in vivo human retinal OCT image along the papillomacular axis represented in (a) linear gray scale, (b) reverse linear gray scale, and (c) retinal false color scale (with labels) (See color plate.). [Figure (c) reproduced from Ref. 57.]

a difficult problem in representing all of the resulting information in a single image. To date, two different pseudocolor image coding schemes have been employed to combine depth-resolved blood flow imaging or spectroscopy with conventional OCT reflectivity imaging. These are based on two standard color models described in image processing texts [38]. Briefly, these are the RGB (red, green, blue) and HSL (hue, saturation, luminance) models. Hue is associated with the perceived dominant wavelength of the color; saturation is its spectral purity, or the extent to which the color deviates from white; and luminance is the intensity of color. In the RGB model, the relative contributions from red, green, and blue are used to describe these properties for an arbitrary color. In the HSL model, color intensity is controlled independently from the hue and saturation of the color.

Published reports of Doppler OCT imaging [34,35] have adapted an RGB color map to simultaneously indicate reflectivity and Doppler shifts. Blood flow data are thresholded to remove noise and superimposed on the reflectivity image. The standard linear gray scale is used to represent backscatter amplitude, whereas blood flow direction is indicated with hue (red or blue for positive or negative Doppler shifts, respectively). Higher luminance indicates increased flow magnitude.

Recently, a variation of the HSL color map was introduced [37] for combining backscatter intensity and depth-resolved spectral shifts in tissue. As with the previous scheme, hue denotes a shift in the backscatter spectrum, where red, green, and yellow designate positive, negative, and no spectral shift, respectively. Saturation of each hue indicates tissue reflectivity, and the image contains constant luminance.

6.3.2 Image Transformations

In general, images may be defined in terms of two elementary sets: a *value* set and a *point* set [39]. The value set is the set of values the image data can assume. It can be a set of integers or real or complex numbers. The point set is a topological space, a subset of n-dimensional Euclidean space that describes the spatial location to which each of the values in the point set is assigned.

Given a point set X and a value set F, an image I can be represented in the form

$$I = \{(x, a(x)) : x\epsilon\ X, a(x)\epsilon F\} \tag{1}$$

An element of the image, $(x, a(x))$, is called a pixel, x is called the pixel location, and $a(x)$ is the pixel value at location x.

Two types of image transformations are of interest in the processing of OCT images. Spatial transformations operate on the image point set and can accomplish such operations as zooming, dewarping, and rectangular-to-polar conversion of images. Value transformations operate on the value set and thus modify pixel values rather than pixel locations. Examples of useful value transformations include modifying image brightness or contrast, exponential attenuation correction, and image despeckling.

Spatial Transformations

A spatial transformation defines a geometric relationship between each point in an input point set before transformation and the corresponding point in the output point set. A forward mapping function is used to map the input onto the output. A backward mapping function is used to map the output back onto the input (see Fig. 10). Assuming that $[u, v]$ and $[x, y]$ refer to the coordinates of the input and output pixels, the relationship between them may be represented as

$$[x, y] = [X(u, v), Y(u, v)] \quad \text{or} \quad [u, v] = [U(x, y), V(x, y)] \tag{2}$$

where X and Y are the forward mapping functions and U and V are the backward mapping functions.

Spatial Transformation Matrices

In a rectangular coordinate system, forward linear spatial transformations (e.g., translation, rotation, scaling, shearing) can be expressed in matrix form using a transformation matrix T_1 [39],

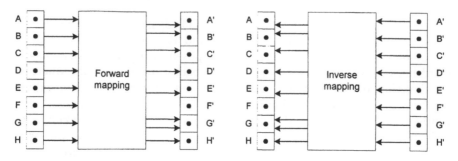

Figure 10   One-dimensional forward and inverse mappings.

$$
\begin{bmatrix} x \\ y \\ 1 \end{bmatrix} = T_1 \begin{bmatrix} u \\ v \\ 1 \end{bmatrix}, \quad \text{where } T_1 = \begin{bmatrix} a_{11} & a_{12} & a_{13} \\ a_{21} & a_{22} & a_{23} \\ a_{31} & a_{32} & a_{33} \end{bmatrix}
\tag{3}
$$

The 3×3 transformation matrix T_1 can be best understood by partitioning it into four separate submatrices. The 2×2 submatrix

$$
\begin{bmatrix} a_{11} & a_{12} \\ a_{21} & a_{22} \end{bmatrix}
$$

specifies a linear transformation for scaling, shearing, and rotation. The 2×1 submatrix $[a_{13}\ a_{23}]^T$ produces translation. The 1×2 submatrix $[a_{31}\ a_{32}]$ produces perspective transformation. The final 1×1 submatrix $[a_{33}]$ is responsible for overall scaling and usually takes a unity value. Note that the superscript T denotes matrix transposition, whereby rows and columns are interchanged. Examples of simple useful transformation matrices in rectangular and polar coordinates are provided in Table 1.

Mapping Arrays

Nonlinear spatial transformations that cannot be performed using transformation matrices (e.g., coordinate system conversions) can be performed using a mapping array. Specification of a mapping array is also a useful and necessary step in the computer implementation of linear spatial image transforms. A mapping array has the same dimensions as an expected output image. This array represents the point set of an output image in which each element contains the location of an input pixel. With the mapping array, the value set of the output image can be obtained by backward mapping to the input image. In a software implementation of image transformations, the required mapping array needs to be created only once and stored in memory. This approach minimizes computation time while imaging compared to iterative formula-based calculation of image transformations in real time.

Image Rotation

Image rotation is a commonly used image transformation in high speed OCT systems in which depth-priority OCT images (those acquired using a rapid z-scan and slower lateral scan) are captured using a frame grabber (which expects video images

Table 1   Some Useful Spatial Transformation (Point-Set Operation) Matrices

Translation

$$T_i = \begin{bmatrix} 1 & 0 & T_u \\ 0 & 1 & T_v \\ 0 & 0 & 1 \end{bmatrix}$$

Rotation

$$T_1 = \begin{bmatrix} \cos\theta & \sin\theta & 0 \\ -\sin\theta & \cos\theta & 0 \\ 0 & 0 & 1 \end{bmatrix}$$

Scaling

$$T_i \begin{bmatrix} S_u & 0 & 0 \\ 0 & S_v & 0 \\ 0 & & 1 \end{bmatrix}$$

Shearing

$$T_1 = \begin{bmatrix} 1 & H_v & 0 \\ 0 & 1 & 0 \\ 0 & 0 & 1 \end{bmatrix}$$

Radial translation

$$\begin{bmatrix} l \\ \alpha \\ 1 \end{bmatrix} = \begin{bmatrix} 1 & 0 & \Delta L \\ 0 & 1 & 0 \\ 0 & 0 & 1 \end{bmatrix} \begin{bmatrix} r \\ \theta \\ 1 \end{bmatrix}$$

Angular rotation

$$\begin{bmatrix} l \\ \alpha \\ 1 \end{bmatrix} = \begin{bmatrix} 1 & 0 & 0 \\ 0 & 1 & \Delta\Theta \\ 0 & 0 & 1 \end{bmatrix} \begin{bmatrix} r \\ \theta \\ 1 \end{bmatrix}$$

that have a rapid lateral scan). The image rotation transformation is illustrated in Fig. 11. A 90° rotation mapping array is created to reconstruct an image of the sample from the frame buffer of the frame grabber.

In this case, the backward spatial transformation used for creating the mapping array is

$$\begin{bmatrix} m \\ n \\ 1 \end{bmatrix} = \begin{bmatrix} 0 & 1 & 0 \\ -1 & 0 & I \\ 0 & 0 & 1 \end{bmatrix} \begin{bmatrix} i \\ j \\ 1 \end{bmatrix} \tag{4}$$

where

$$i = (0, 1, \ldots, I), \qquad j = (0, 1, \ldots, J)$$
$$m = (0, 1, \ldots, M), \qquad n = (0, 1, \ldots, N), \qquad I = N; \ J = M$$

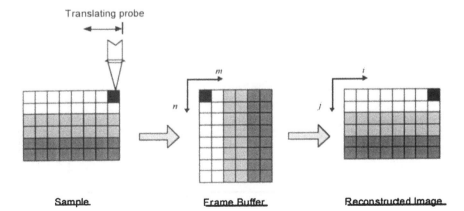

Figure 11   Image rotation transformation.

Rectangular-to-Polar Conversion

Rectangular-to-polar conversion is a nonlinear spatial transformation which is necessary when image data are obtained using a radially scanning OCT probe, such as an endoscopic catheter probe [9,40]. The A-scans will be recorded, by a frame grabber for example, sequentially into a rectangular array but must be displayed in a radial format corresponding to the geometry of the scanning probe, as illustrated in Fig. 12. The forward mapping operations are

$$x(r, \theta) = r\cos(\theta), \qquad y(r, \theta) = r\sin(\theta) \tag{5}$$

where x and y are the rectangular (Cartesian) coordinates and r and θ are the polar coordinates. The inverse mapping operations are

$$r(x, y) = \sqrt{x^2 + y^2}, \qquad \theta(x, y) = \tan^{-1}\left(\frac{y}{x}\right) \tag{6}$$

In the calculation of θ, an additional conditional is necessary because of ambiguity between the first and third and between the second and fourth quadrants of the polar coordinate system.

Double-Sided Scan Correction

When an OCT system uses double-sided scanning (i.e., A-scan acquisition during both directions of the reference arm scan), a transformation is necessary to rectify the alternate, reversed A-scans (Fig. 13). Again, a mapping array can be constructed to transform the acquired image array into the image array to be displayed. When implementing double-sided scanning correction, it is necessary that consecutive A-scans be registered with respect to one another. Depending upon the OCT system configuration, the scan registration can be accomplished by adjusting the delay line optics or line sync phase. In a clinical setting, however, where the hardware is closed, it may be more desirable to implement a software registration mechanism. This could be accomplished by allowing manual adjustment by the operator or by an automatic registration algorithm.

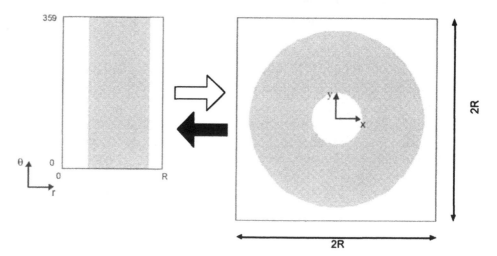

Figure 12   Rectangular-to-polar coordinate transformation.

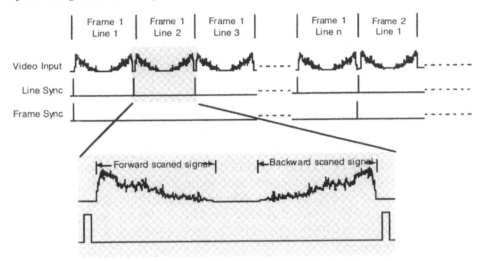

Figure 13 Timing diagram for double-sided line acquisition.

Image Dewarping

An acquired OCT image will be warped if the spatial distribution of the acquired data does not directly correspond to the spatial distribution of scattering profile of the sample. This occurs in OCT imaging when the image data are not sampled at regular intervals in space. For example, if the scanning motion of the OCT probe or delay line is not linear with time and the data are sampled at regular intervals in time, then the image will be warped. If the scan nonlinearity is a known function of time, however, the image can be "dewarped" by an appropriate spatial transformation. This is the case, for example, for the sinusoidal motion of a resonant scanning device. In this case, the coordinate corresponding to the resonant scanner can be transformed by a sinusoidal function with a period corresponding to the period of the scan in image space. Alternatively, if an accurate reference signal is available, a corresponding sampling trigger signal could be generated to sample nonlinearly in time such that the image is sampled linearly in space. This latter technique is common in Fourier transform spectrometers and has previously been applied in high accuracy interferogram acquisition in OCT [24].

Motion Artifact Reduction by A-Scan Registration

In OCT imaging of living human or animal subjects, motion artifact is a serious concern because the inherent spatial resolution of OCT imaging often exceeds the extent to which the subject is capable of remaining motionless under voluntary control. The most straightforward approach to eliminating this problem is to acquire images more rapidly, and the recent advent of high speed scanning systems has in large part alleviated this concern [18,33]. However, in cases where the available signal-to-noise ratio precludes high speed imaging (as, for example, in retinal imaging where high power sources cannot be used), image processing techniques can be applied.

The technique of cross-correlation scan registration for retinal image motion artifact reduction was developed by Hee, Izatt and coworkers in 1993 [12,41]. In this technique, an estimate of the patient's axial eye motion during image acquisition was formed from the peak of the cross-correlation $R_i(k)$ of each A-scan in the image with respect to its neighbor:

$$R_i(k) = \sum_i F_i(j)F_{i+1}(j-k) \tag{7}$$

Here, the $F_i(j)$ are the longitudinal scan data at the transverse scan index i, where j is the longitudinal pixel index. The profile of the motion estimated from the locus of the peaks of $R_i(k)$ was then low-pass-filtered to separate motion artifacts (which were assumed to occur at relatively high spatial frequency) from real variations in the patient's retinal profile (which were assumed to occur at relatively low spatial frequency). The smoothed profile was then subtracted from the original profile to generate an array of offset values that were applied to correct the positions of each A-scan in the image. An illustration of this procedure and its results is provided in Fig. 14 (see color plate).

It is worth noting that the position of the peak of the cross-correlation function in retinal images appears to depend heavily on the position of the retinal pigment epithelium (RPE). In images in which the strong RPE reflection is absent from some A-scans (for example, underneath strongly attenuating blood vessels), the cross-correlation technique is subject to registration errors. In such cases, a motion profile may alternatively be obtained by thresholding the A-scan data to locate the position of a strong reflectivity transition within the tissue structure, such as occurs at the inner limiting membrane. Thresholding at this boundary has recently been applied for A-scan registration of Doppler OCT images in the human retina [42]. In this case, the velocity data were also corrected by estimating the velocity of the patient motion from the spatial derivative of the scan-to-scan motion estimate and from knowledge of the A-scan acquisition time.

Value Set Operations

In contrast to spatial transformations, value set operations modify pixel values rather than pixel locations. Spatial filtering using convolution kernels are fundamental to image processing and can of course be applied to OCT images. Examples of useful convolution kernels include smoothing filters and edge detectors. OCT technology is relatively young, however, and extensive use has not yet been made of standard image processing techniques.

Exponential Correction

A value set operation that is not linear and cannot be implemented using a convolution kernel is exponential correction. In the single-scattering approximation [28], the detected OCT photodetector power from a scattering medium attenuates with depth according to:

$$\langle i_s \rangle^2 \propto F(z) \exp[-2\mu_t z] \tag{8}$$

Here $F(z)$ is a function of the focusing optics in the sample arm, μ_t is the total attenuation coefficient of the sample (given by the sum of the absorption and scattering coefficients), and z is the depth into the sample. If the depth of focus of the sample arm optics is greater than several attenuation mean free paths (given by $1/\mu_t$) in the sample, then the function $F(z)$ is relatively smooth over the available imaging

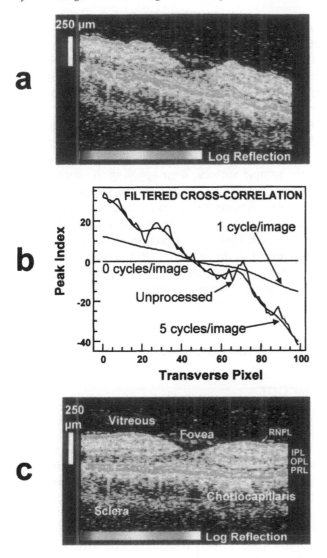

Figure 14 Motion artifact reduction by cross-correlation scan registration. Patient axial motion during acquisition of the original retinal image (a) was estimated from a profile built up from the peak of the cross-correlations of each A-scan with respect to its neighbor (b). The resulting profile was then high-pass-filtered to preserve the real retinal profile and used to reregister each individual A-scan in the image (c). (See color plate.) (From Ref. 12.)

depth and the attenuation can be considered to be dominated by the exponential term. If this condition is not met (i.e., for imaging with high numerical aperture), then the complete form of Eq. (8) must be taken into account. Equation (8) has been experimentally verified in model scattering media [28]. Thus, the reflectivity profile measured by OCT in a typical imaging situation is scaled by an exponential decay with depth. Because this decay is intuitively understood and expected, it is typically not corrected. It is possible, however, to correct the data such that a direct map of sample reflectivity is displayed. The analogous decay in ultrasound imaging is commonly corrected by varying the amplifier gain as a function of time by an amount corresponding to the decay [time-gain compensation (TGC).] In principle, this approach could also be used in OCT by varying the gain with an exponential rise corresponding to the inverse of the expected exponential decay: $e^{2\mu_t t/v}$, where v is the speed of the depth scan. This approach can also be implemented after sampling by simply multiplying each A-scan point by point with an exponential rise, $e^{2\mu_t z}$. This correction assumes, however, that the sample surface exactly corresponds to the first pixel of the A-scan. When not true, this assumption will produce error, especially when the location of the tissue surface varies from one A-scan to another. This error can be mitigated by first locating the sample surface, then applying the correction from that location on: $e^{2\mu_t [z-z(0)]}$, where $z(0)$ is the location of the sample surface. Alternatively, it can be noted that the error amounts to a scaling error and the index of the surface location can be used to correct the scale. It should be noted that if the data have been logarithmically compressed, then the correction is simply a linear rise. It is clear that information is not added to the image by application of this type of correction, noise is scaled together with signal, and the deeper sample regions become extremely noisy. Therefore, it is a subjective matter whether exponential correction improves or worsens the image viewability.

6.4 SIGNAL PROCESSING APPROACHES FOR IMAGE ENHANCEMENT

6.4.1 Systems Theory Model for OCT

To make use of signal and image processing concepts that are well known and have been extensively used in other medical imaging modalities, it is useful to describe OCT from a systems theory point of view. Fortunately, several authors have noted that since the low coherence interferometer at the heart of OCT is basically an optical cross-correlator, it is straightforward to construct a simple transfer function model for OCT that treats the interaction of the low coherence interferometer with the specimen as a linear time-invariant system [24,43–45].

As the basis for the following sections on coherent signal processing in OCT, the model developed by Kulkarni and Izatt [24,45] is summarized here. In this model, an optical wave with an electric field expressed using complex analytic signal representation as

$$2\tilde{e}_i = 2e_i(ct - z)\exp[j2\pi k_0(ct - z)]$$

is assumed to be incident on a Michelson interferometer, as illustrated in Fig. 15. We adopt a notation wherein variables with a tilde ($\sim$) represent modulated quantities, whereas identical variables not so marked represent their complex envelopes. Thus, $e_i(ct - z)$ is the complex envelope of the electric field, k_0 is the central wave number of the source spectrum, and c is the free-space speed of light. The quantities t and z represent the time and distance traveled by the wave, respectively. It is assumed for the purpose of this model that the dispersion mismatch between the interferometer arms is negligible. By setting $z = 0$ at the beamsplitter, the field returning to the beamsplitter from the reference mirror is given by

$$\sqrt{2}\tilde{e}_i(t, 2l_r) = \sqrt{2}e_i(ct - 2l_r)\exp[j2\pi k_0(ct - 2l_r)] \tag{9}$$

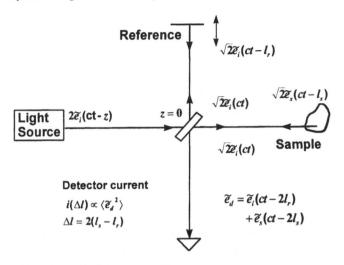

Figure 15 Schematic of systems theory model for OCT.

where l_r is the reference arm optical path length. In the sample arm, the light back-scattered from the sample with optical path length l_s reaching the beamsplitter is given by

$$\sqrt{2}\tilde{e}_s(t, \, 2l_s) = \sqrt{2}e_s(ct - 2l_s)\exp[j2\pi k_0(ct - 2l_s)] \tag{10}$$

Here $e_i(ct - 2l_s)$ is the complex envelope of the backscattered wave. The fields returning from the reference and sample arms interfere at the detector to provide the superposition field $\tilde{e}_d = \tilde{e}_i + \tilde{e}_s$. The alternating component of the detector current is given by

$$\tilde{i}(\Delta l) \propto \langle \tilde{e}_i(ct - 2l_r)\tilde{e}_s^*(ct - 2l_s)\rangle + \langle \tilde{e}_i^*(ct - 2l_r)\tilde{e}_s(ct - 2l_s)\rangle \tag{11}$$

where the angular brackets indicate temporal integration over the response time of the detector and $\Delta l = 2(l_r - l_s)$ is the round-trip path length difference between the interferometer arms.

The source autocorrelation can be measured by monitoring the interferometric signal when a perfect mirror is used as a specimen in the sample arm. We define the source interferometric autocorrelation function as

$$\tilde{R}_{ii}(\Delta l) \equiv \langle \tilde{e}_i(ct - 2l_r)\tilde{e}_i^*(ct - 2l_s)\rangle = R_{ii}(\Delta l)\exp(j2\pi k_0 \, \Delta l) \tag{12}$$

where $R_{ii}(\Delta l)$ is the autocorrelation of the complex envelopes of the electric fields. The autocorrelation function $R_{ii}(\Delta l)$ is experimentally measured by demodulating the detected interferogram at the reference arm Doppler shift frequency and recording the in-phase and quadrature components of this complex signal. According to the Wiener–Khinchin theorem [46], the source spectrum is given by the Fourier transform of the interferometric autocorrelation function:

$$\tilde{S}_{ii}(k) = \int_{-\infty}^{\infty} \tilde{R}_{ii}(\Delta l)\exp[-j2\pi k \, \Delta l]\,d(\Delta l) \tag{13}$$

For an arbitrary specimen in the sample arm, the interferometric cross-correlation function is defined as

$$\tilde{R}_{is}(\Delta l) \equiv \langle \tilde{e}_i(ct - 2l_r)\tilde{e}_s^*(ct - 2l_s)\rangle = R_{is}(\Delta l)\,\exp(j2\pi k_0\,\Delta l) \tag{14}$$

where $R_{is}(\Delta l)$ is the cross-correlation of the complex envelopes of the electric fields [46]. The cross-power spectrum $\tilde{S}_{is}(k)$ also follows by analogy:

$$\tilde{S}_{is}(k) = \int_{-\infty}^{\infty} \tilde{R}_{is}(\Delta l)\,\exp[j2\pi k(\Delta l)]\,d(\Delta l) \tag{15}$$

Sample Impulse Response

It is useful to represent the interaction between the specimen under study and the incident sample arm light as a linear shift-invariant (LSI) system characterized by a frequency-dependent transfer function [46–48]. The key insight this provides is that the transfer function $H(k)$ and its inverse Fourier transform, the sample impulse response $h(z)$, are physically meaningful quantities describing the backscatter spectrum and electric field reflection coefficient profile of the sample, respectively. We denote the impulse response experienced by the electric field $\tilde{e}_i$ by $\tilde{h}(z)$ and that experienced by the complex envelope field e_i by $h(z)$. This LSI model is valid when the contribution to e_s from multiply scattered light is not significant.

The impulse response $h(z)$ describes the actual locations and reflection coefficients of scattering sites within the sample and convolves with the source electric field envelope to create the scattered electric field envelope:

$$e_s(-z) = e_i(-z) \otimes h^*(z) \tag{16}$$

Here $\otimes$ represents the convolution operation, and the negative sign implies scattering in the negative direction (backscattering). Taking the Fourier transform of both sides of Eq. (16) provides

$$E_s(k) = E_i(k)H^*(k) \tag{17}$$

where $E_s(k)$, $E_i(k)$, and $H(k)$ are the Fourier transforms of $e_s(z)$, $e_i(z)$, and $h(z)$, respectively. The assumption of shift invariance ensures that

$$e_s(ct - 2l_s) = e_i(ct - 2l_s) \otimes h^*(-(ct - 2l_s)) \tag{18}$$

Substituting Eq. (18) in the definition of the correlation functions [Eqs. (12) and (14)] provides

$$R_{is}(\Delta l) = R_{ii}(\Delta l) \otimes h(\Delta l) \tag{19}$$

The source autocorrelation function, $R_{ii}(\Delta l)$ and the cross-correlation function of the sample and reference arm electric fields, $R_{is}(\Delta l)$ thus constitute the input and measured output, respectively, of an LSI system having the impulse response $h(z)$. Therefore, the impulse response that describes the electric field–specimen interaction as a function of z is exactly the same as that which connects the auto- and cross-correlation functions of the interferometer as a function of the pathlength difference Δl. Thus, this model provides access to understanding the fundamental properties of the interaction of the sample with the sample arm electric fields by using simple correlation function measurements.

Equation (19) also leads directly to a simple, albeit naive, approach for OCT image resolution improvement by deconvolution. Taking the Fourier transform of Eq. (19) and solving for the impulse response gives

$$h(\Delta l) \equiv h(z) = F^{-1} \left\{ \frac{S_{is}(k)}{S_{ii}(k)} \right\} \tag{20}$$

where F^{-1} denotes the inverse Fourier transform and $S_{is}(k)$ and $S_{ii}(k)$ are the complex envelopes of the cross- and auto-power spectra, respectively.

Depth-Resolved Spectral Estimation

The sample transfer function $|H(k)|^2$ that may be obtained from the Fourier transform of Eq. (19) describes the backscatter spectral characteristic of the sample, i.e., the ratio of the backscattered power spectrum to the spectrum that was incident. However, because the coherence length in an OCT system is short, it is possible to use an analog of time–frequency analysis methods [49] to extract the backscatter characteristic with depth discrimination. This can be accomplished by limiting the detected transfer function data to the region of interest in the sample by digitally windowing the auto- and cross-correlation data used to calculate $H(k)|^2$. This is the short-time Fourier transform [50] technique; wavelet transform [51] approaches can also be used.

All information regarding the spatial and frequency dependence of scattering within the sample is contained in the complex space domain function $h(z)$ and its Fourier transform $H(k)$. If the windowed region contains only a single scatterer, then $H(k)|^2$ is straightforwardly interpreted as the wavenumber-dependent backscatter characteristic of that scatterer, denoted $C(k)|^2$. In a medium containing many identical scatterers, the impulse response $h(z)$ windowed to the region of interest may be modeled as being a convolution of two new functions: $h(z) = b(z) \otimes c(z)$. Here, $b(z)$ describes the spatial distribution of scatters along the sample axis z, and $c(z)$ is the inverse Fourier transform of $C(k)$. Under the assumption that $b(z)$ is a white stoachastic process (i.e., the scatterer locations are uncorrelated), the expectation value of $H(k)|^2$ is then given by

$$E\left\{ |H(k)|^2 \right\} = E\left\{ |B(k)|^2 \right\} |C(k)|^2 = |C(k)|^2 \tag{21}$$

where $B(k)$ is the Fourier transform of $b(z)$. Thus, the backscatter characteristic of the individual scatters in a sample can be obtained directly within a user-selected region of the sample by appropriate Fourier domain averaging of coherently detected windowed interferogram data. This analysis is readily extended to the case of a medium containing a heterogeneous mixture of scatterers, each having its own backscatter characteristic. In this case, a similar signal processing algorithm produces an estimated spectrum corresponding to a weighted average of the individual backscatter spectra [45].

One final step allows for estimation of the actual backscattered spectrum of light returning from the sample rather than the backscatter transfer characteristic of the scatterers. Because the spectrum of light in the sample arm is defined as $\tilde{S}_{ss}(k) = \tilde{E}_s(k)\tilde{E}_s^*(k)$, using $\tilde{E}_s(k) = \tilde{E}_i(k)\tilde{H}^*(k)$ [the modulated analog of Eq. (17)] gives $\tilde{S}_{ss}(k) = |\tilde{S}_{is}(k)|^2/\tilde{S}_{ii}(k)$. Similar to the previous paragraph, ensemble averaging must be used to average out apparent spectral features that are really due to the spatial structure of the scatter distribution:

$$\tilde{S}_{ss}(k) = \frac{E\left\{\left|\tilde{S}_{is}(k)\right|^2\right\}}{\tilde{S}_{ii}(k)} \tag{22}$$

6.4.2 OCT Image Deconvolution

Straightforward Approach

The systems theory model described in the previous section predicts that the optical impulse response of tissue, $h(z)$ or $\tilde{h}(z)$, is calculable if the complete cross-correlation sequence making up the OCT signal is acquired with interferometric accuracy. The impulse response is interpreted as describing the actual locations and amplitudes of scattering sites within the sample arising from index of refraction inhomogeneities and particulate scatterers.

An example of the application of Eq. (20) for direct deconvolution of unde-modulated OCT A-scan is provided in Fig. 16. These data were acquired using a data acquisition system with interferometric calibration capable of capturing the cross-correlation sequence with nanometer spatial resolution [24]. An interferogram segment obtained with this system that includes several discrete reflections is plotted in the figure. Also plotted in the figure are the autocorrelation sequence from a mirror reflection and the impulse response calculated using the modulated analog of Eq. (20). An increase in resolution by a factor of > 2 was obtained between the original interferogram and the calculated impulse response profile. The improvement obtained using this simple, no-cost algorithm is quite striking when it is executed

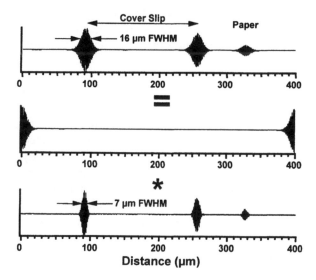

Figure 16 Example of digital deconvolution of low coherence interferometry data. Top, observed interferogram of a cover slip resting on a piece of paper. Middle, interferogram obtained with a mirror in the sample arm. Bottom, deconvolved impulse response file.

on two-dimensional data sets, as illustrated in Fig. 17. In this figure, digital deconvolution of magnitude-only demodulated A-scan data was used to improve image sharpness in the axial (vertical) direction of a cross-sectional OCT image of a fresh onion specimen.

The data used as the input for the deconvolution algorithm in Fig. 17a were acquired using an OCT system that, like most OCT systems constructed to date and most other biomedical imaging modalities (excluding ultrasound), records only the magnitude of the image data. A novel approach to signal deconvolution that takes advantage of the complex nature of OCT signals is to perform coherent deconvolution by supplying both the magnitude and phase of the demodulated A-scan data as complex inputs to the deconvolution equation. The advantage of this approach is illustrated in Fig. 18, which illustrates the capability of coherent deconvolution to extract real sample features from what would have been regarded as meaningless speckle in amplitude-only data.

Iterative Restoration Methods

The practical implementation of Fourier domain deconvolution algorithms such as those described by Eq. (20) inevitably leads to a reduction in image dynamic range, as evidence in Fig. 17(b). This is because even small errors in the estimation of the auto- and cross-correlation spectra introduce noise in the resulting impulse response

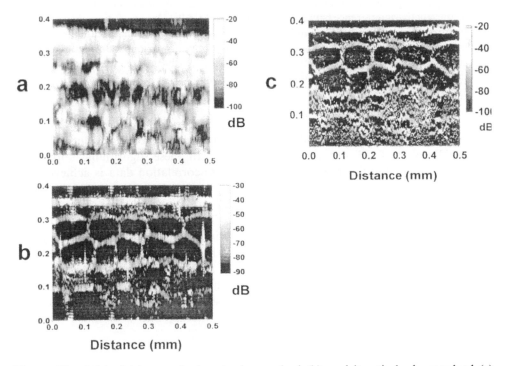

Figure 17 Original (a), magnitude-only deconvolved (b), and iteratively deconvolved (c) cross-sectional OCT images revealing cellular structure in an onion sample. Both deconvolutions resulted in a resolution increase by a factor of ~ 1.5, or $\sim 8\,\mu$m FWHM resolution in the deconvolved images, although the iterative restoration algorithm preserved image dynamic range significantly better. [Images (a) and (c) reproduced from Ref. 48.]

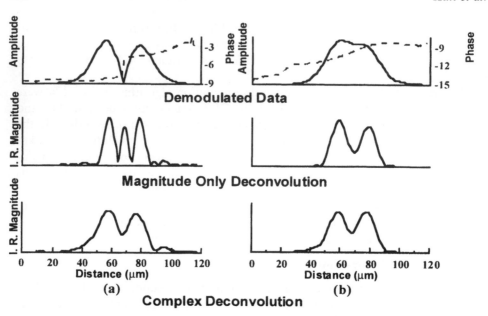

Figure 18 Illustration of coherent OCT deconvolution. Top: Magnitude and phase of demodulated OCT A-scan data obtained from two closely spaced glass/air interfaces with slightly different separations, resulting in (a) destructive (note 180° phase shift at the midpoint) and (b) constructive interference between the reflections. Middle: Deconvolution of the A-scan data performed using only the magnitude of the input data, leading to inaccurate positioning of reflections and spurious reflections in the calculated impulse response. Bottom: Complex deconvolution recovers the true locations of the interfaces in both cases and thus enhances resolution by a factor of ~ 1.5 as well as reducing speckle noise.

image due to the division operation inherent to deconvolution. To alleviate this problem, one study [48] applied advanced constrained iterative deconvolution algorithms [52] to the OCT deconvolution problem. In these algorithms, improved restoration of the impulse response from the cross-correlation data is achieved by using prior knowledge of the properties of the desired impulse response. This use of a prior knowledge provides a consistent extrapolation of spectral components of the transfer function beyond the source bandwidth. The impulse response is then estimated by the method of successive approximations; hence no division operation leading to instabilities and noise is involved. Therefore, the iterative algorithms offer the potential to achieve improvement in OCT resolution with a minimal increase in noise. In a test applying this algorithm to the onion imaging data set displayed in Fig. 17a, resolution enhancement similar to that displayed with the straightforward deconvolution algorithm was achieved, but with much smaller dynamic range loss (~ 2 dB; see Fig. 17c).

CLEAN Algorithm

One report has described promising results in deconvolution of OCT images using the CLEAN algorithm [44]. This algorithm, which is highly nonlinear and can only be described algorithmically, begins with an estimate of a system's impulse response. It then searches a dataset for a peak, subtracts the impulse response from the dataset at the location of the peak, and places a delta function at the location of the peak in the deconvolved dataset. Using a modified version of this algorithm, Schmitt demonstrated somewhat improved resolution and clarity in OCT images of phantoms and skin.

6.4.3 Spectroscopic OCT

Although most OCT systems developed to date have used light exclusively to probe the internal microstructure of sample specimens, the possibility of extracting spectroscopic information from OCT signals is particularly exciting because it may provide access to additional information about the composition and functional state of samples. Relatively little work has been published on this topic, primarily because the number of spectral regions in which sources suitable for OCT is quite limited and because the spectral bandwidths of OCT sources are quite narrow compared to those of light sources used in conventional spectroscopy.

Work in spectroscopic OCT has concentrated in two areas. First, a few reports have appeared concerning spectral ratio imaging of OCT images acquired at two or more spectral bands [53,54]. This approach can be implemented most elegantly by using a wavelength division multiplexer (WDM) to combine light from two or more sources into the source fiber and then electronically distinguishing the resulting signals by their different Doppler shifts resulting from the reference arm scan. Of course, this approach is limited to a choice of wavelengths that can simultaneously be mode-guided in a single-mode fiber. Ratiometric OCT imaging using a pair of sources at 1.3 and 1.5 μm (which are separated by approximately one decade in water absorption coefficient but have similar scattering coefficients in tissues) has been used to probe the water content of samples in three dimensions [53]. Combinations of other wavelength pairs have also been attempted in search of contrast in biological tissues [54].

The second implementation of spectroscopic OCT is that described in the subsection on depth-resolved spectral estimation in Section 6.4.1 in which modifications of the source spectrum caused by the sample can be measured directly from Fourier domain processing of cross-correlation interferometric data. The most successful application of this idea to date has been in Doppler OCT, in which spatially resolved shifts in the sample spectrum due to sample motion are estimated from localized spectral shifts in the cross-correlation data [34,35]. Details of the signal processing techniques used to extract these data and some preliminary applications are described in Chapter 8.

Even if sample motion is absent, however, the techniques described earlier can still be used to extract useful spectral information from samples [25,37]. A simple example of depth-resolved spectroscopy using OCT is provided in Fig. 19. Here, the backscatter spectral characteristics $|H(k)|^2$ of sample arm light reflected from the front and back surfaces (the latter having double-passed the filter) of a commercial interference filter are plotted. These quantities were obtained by applying the Fourier transform of Eq. (19) to an OCT A-scan of the filter, windowed to the vicinity of the glass/air reflection from the front and rear sides of the filter. It is interesting to note that these data illustrate quantitative depth-resolved reflectance spectroscopy demonstrating the equivalent of femtosecond temporal resolution in a simple, inexpensive system suitable for biomedical applications.

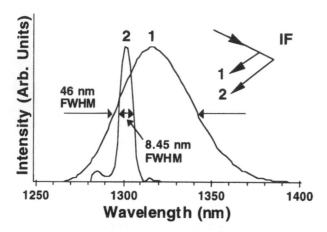

Figure 19 Demonstration of depth-resolved OCT spectroscopy in a discrete optical element. The spectral transfer characteristic $|H(k)|^2$ of the light reflected from (1) the front surface and (2) the rear surface of a commercial interference filter (IF) are plotted. Both spectra were obtained by digital processing of windowed OCT A-scans of the filter. The measured spectral widths correspond well with the manufacturer's specifications (SLD spectral width 47 nm FWHM; filter bandwidth 10 nm FWHM).

6.5 SAFETY IN THE CLINICAL ENVIRONMENT

An important consideration in the implementation of OCT systems for medical diagnostic applications is the issue of operator and patient safety. All hospitals in the United States and most research funding agencies and foundations require Institutional Review Board (IRB) approval of all studies involving human tissues, including excised tissue samples. IRB approval procedures typically include the review of protocols for informed consent of patients who will be used as experimental subjects. Potential hazards to operators of OCT equipment and to patients fall into three categories: biohazards, medical device electrical safety, and optical radiation hazards. Procedures for avoidance of contamination and infection as well as for electrical safety are well established in hospital environments, although they may not be as familiar to researchers with physical science backgrounds. Biohazard avoidance primarily implies utilization of proper procedures for handling potentially infected tissues as well as proper disinfection of probes and other devices that come into contact with patients or tissue samples. Electrical device safety guidelines typically regulate the maximum current that a patient or operator may draw by touching any exposed part of a medical device and are usually followed by including appropriate electrical isolation and shielding into the design of clinical OCT systems (see, for example, Ref. 55).

6.5.1 Optical Radiation Hazards in OCT

A potential operator and (primarily) patient safety concern that is unique to optical biomedical diagnostics devices is the potential for exposure to optical radiation hazards. Although continuous-wave sources used for OCT are typically very weak compared to lasers used in physical science laboratories and even in other medical applications, the tight focusing of OCT probe beams that is required for high spatial image resolution does produce intensities approaching established optical exposure limits. A number of international bodies recommend human exposure limits for optical radiation; in the United States, one well-known set of guidelines for optical radiation hazards are ANSI Z1361, produced by the American National Standards Institute [56]. Unfortunately, these guidelines are specified for laser radiation exposure and are provided only for exposures to the eye and skin. Nonetheless, many analyses of OCT radiation safety have used these standards. The applicable ANSI standards for cw laser exposure to the eye and skin both recommend a maximum permissible exposure (MPE) expressed as a radiant exposure, which is a function of the exposure duration, and tabulated spectral correction factors.

ACKNOWLEDGMENTS

We acknowledge research support from the National Science Foundation (BES-9624617), the Whitaker Foundation, an Olympus Graduate Research Fellowship (A.M.R.), and a National Institutes of Health Research Traineeship (S.Y.).

REFERENCES

1. Sorin WV, Baney DM. A simple intensity noise reduction technique for optical low-coherence reflectometry. IEEE Photonics Technol Lett 4(12):1404–1406, 1992.
2. Rollins AM, Izatt JA. Optical interferometer designs for optical coherence tomography. Opt Lett 24:1484-1486, 1999.
3. Bouma BE, Tearney GJ. Power-efficient nonreciprocal interferometer and linear-scanning fiber-optic catheter for optical coherence tomography. Opt Lett 24(8):531–533, 1999.
4. Abbas GL, Chan VWS, Yee TK. Local-oscillator excess-noise suppression for homodyne and heterodyne detection. Opt Lett 8(8):419–421, 1983.
5. Agrawal GP. Fiber-Optic Communication Systems. Wiley Ser Microwave Opt Eng (K Chang, ed.) New York: Wiley, 1992.
6. Takada K. Noise in optical low-coherence reflectometry. IEEE J Quantum Electron 34(7):1098–1108, 1998.
7. Hee MR, Izatt JA, Jacobson JM, Swanson EA, Fujimoto JG. Femtosecond transillumination optical coherence tomography. Opt Lett 18:950, 1993.
8. Podoleanu AG, Jackson DA. Noise analysis of a combined optical coherence tomograph and a confocal scanning ophthalmoscope. Appl Opt 38(10):2116–2127, 1999.
9. Rollins AM, Ung-arunyawee R, Chak A, Wong RCK, Kobayashi K, Michael J, Sivak JV, Izatt JA. Real-time in vivo imaging of human gastrointestinal ultrastructure using endoscopic optical coherence tomography with a novel efficient interferometer design. Opt Lett 24:1358–1360, 1999.
10. Rollins AM, Yazdanfar S, Ung-arunyawee R, Izatt JA. Real-time color Doppler optical coherence tomography using an autocorrelation technique. In: Coherence Domain Optical Methods in Biomedical Science and Clinical Applications III. San Jose, CA: Soc Photo-Instrum Eng, 1999.
11. Swanson EA, Huang D, Hee MR, Fujimoto JG, Lin CP, Puliafito CA. High speed optical coherence domain reflectometry. Opt Lett 18:1864, 1993.
12. Swanson EA, Izatt JA, Hee MR, Huang D, Lin CP, Schuman JS, Puliafito CA, Fujimoto JG. In vivo retinal imaging by optical coherence tomography. Opt Lett 18(21):1864–1866, 1993.

13. Izatt JA, Kulkarni MD, Wang H-W, Kobayashi K, Sivak MV. Optical coherence tomography and microscopy in gastrointestinal tissues. IEEE J Selected Topics Quantum Electron 2(4):1017–1028, 1996.

14. Izatt JA, Kulkarni MD, Kobayashi K, Sivak MV, Barton JK, Welch AJ. Optical coherence tomography for biodiagnostics. Opt Photon News 8:41–47, 1997.

15. Tearney GJ, Bouma BE, Boppart SA, Golubovic B, Swanson EA, Fujimoto JG. Rapid acquisition of in vivo biological images by use of optical coherence tomography. Opt Lett 21(17):1408–1410, 1996.

16. Tearney GJ, Bouma BE, Fujimoto JG. High speed phase- and group-delay scanning with a grating-based phase control delay line. Opt Lett 22(23):1811–1813, 1997.

17. Sergeev AM, Gelikonov VM, Gelikonov GV, Feldchtein FI, Kuranov RV, Gladkova ND, Shakhova NM, Snopova LB, Shakhov AV, Kuznetzova IA, Denisenko AN, Pochinko VV, Chumakov YP, Streltzova OS. In vivo endoscopic OCT imaging of precancer and cancer states of human mucosa. Opt Express 1(13):432–440, 1997.

18. Rollins AM, Kulkarni MD, Yazdanfar S, Ung-arunyawee R, Izatt JA. In vivo video rate optical coherence tomography. Opt Express 3(6):129–229, 1998.

19. Huang D, Swanson EA, Lin CP, Schuman JS, Stinson WG, Chang W, Hee MR, Flotte T, Gregory K, Puliafito CA, Fujimoto JG. Optical coherence tomography. Science 254:1178–1181, 1991.

20. Izatt JA, Hee MR, Swanson EA, Lin CP, Huang D, Schuman JS, Puliafito CA, Fujimoto JG. Micrometer-scale resolution imaging of the anterior eye in vivo with optical coherence tomography. Arch Ophthalmol 112:1584–1589, 1994.

21. Chinn SR, Swanson EA, Fujimoto JG. Optical coherence tomography using a frequency-tunable optical source. Opt Lett 22(5):340–342, 1997.

22. Windecker R, Fleischer M, Franze B, Tiziani HJ. Two methods for fast coherence tomography and topometry. J Mod Opt 44(5):967–977, 1997.

23. Szydlo J, Delachenal N, Gianotti R, Walti R, Bleuler H, Salathe RP. Air-turbine driven optical low-coherence reflectometry at 28.6-kHz scan repetition rate. Opt Commun 154:1–4, 1998.

24. Kulkarni MD, Izatt JA. Digital signal processing in optical coherence tomography. In: Coherence Domain Optical Methods in Biomedical Science and Clinical Applications. San Jose, CA: Soc Photo-Instrum Eng, 1997.

25. Kulkarni MD, Izatt JA. Spectroscopic optical coherence tomography. In: Conference on Lasers and Electro-Optics. Washington, DC: Opt Soc Am, 1996.

26. Podoleanu AG, Seeger M, Dobre GM, Webb DJ, Jackson DA, Fitzke FW. Transversal and longitudinal images form the retina of the living eye using low coherence reflectometry. J Biomed Opt 3(1):12–20, 1998.

27. Podoleanu AG, Dobre GM, Jackson DA. En-face coherence imaging using galvanometer scanner modulation Opt Lett 23(3):147–149, 1998.

28. Izatt JA, Hee MR, Owen GA, Swanson EA, Fujimoto JG. Optical coherence microscopy in scattering media. Opt Lett 19:590–592, 1994.

29. Bashkansky M, Duncan MD, Kahn DL III, Reintjes J. Subsurface defect detection in ceramics by high-speed high-resolution optical coherent tomography. Opt Express 22(1):61–63, 1997.

30. Fercher AF, Hitzenberger CK, Drexler W, Kamp G, Sattmann H. In vivo optical coherence tomography. Am J Ophthalmol 116(1):113–114, 1993.

31. Schmitt JM, Yadlowsky MJ, Bonner RF. Subsurface imaging of living skin with optical coherence microscopy. Dermatology 191:93–98, 1995.

32. Fujimoto JG, Brezinsky ME, Tearney GJ, Boppart SA, Bouma B, Hee MR, Southern JF, Swanson EA. Optical biopsy and imaging using optical coherence tomography. Nature Med 1:970–972, 1995.

33. Tearney GJ, Brezinski ME, Bouma BE, Boppart SA, Pitris C, Southern JF, Fujimoto JG. In vivo endoscopic optical biopsy with optical coherence tomography. Science 276:2037–2039, 1997.

34. Chen Z, Milner TE, Srinivas S, Wang X, Malekafzali A, van Gemert MJC, Nelson JS. Noninvasive imaging of in vivo blood flow velocity using optical Doppler tomography. Opt Lett 22:1119–1121, 1997.

35. Izatt JA, Kulkarni MD, Yazdanfar S, Barton JK, Welch AJ. In vivo bidirectional color Doppler flow imaging of picoliter blood volumes using optical coherence tomography. Opt Lett 22(18):1439–1441, 1997.

36. de Boer JF, Milner TE, van Gemert MJC, Nelson JS. Two-dimensional birefringence imaging in biological tissue by polarization-sensitive optical coherence tomography. Opt Lett 22:934–936, 1997.

37. Morgner U. Spectroscopic optical coherence tomography. In: Conference on Lasers and Electro-Optics. Baltimore, MD: Opt Soc Am, 1999.

38. Gonzalez RC, Woods RE. Digital Image Processing. Reading, MA: Addison-Wesley, 1992.

39. Wolberg G. Digital Image Warping. Los Alamitos, CA: IEEE Computer Soc Press, 1994.

40. Tearney GJ, Boppart SA, Bouma BE, Brezinsky ME, Weissman NJ, Southern JF, Fujimoto JG. Scanning single-mode fiber optic catheter-endoscope for optical coherence tomography. Opt Lett 21:543–545, 1996.

41. Hee MR, Izatt JA, Swanson EA, Huang D, Schuman JS, Lin CP, Puliafito CA, Fujimoto JG. Optical coherence tomography for micron-resolution ophthalmic imaging. IEEE Eng Med Biol Mag 1995:67–76.

42. Yazdanfar S, Rollins AM, Izatt JA. In vivo imaging of blood flow in human retinal vessels using color Doppler optical coherence tomography. In: Coherence Domain Methods in Biomedical Science and Clinical Applications III. San Jose, CA: Soc Photo-Instrum Eng, 1999.

43. Pan Y, Birngruber R, Rosperich J, Engelhardt R. Low-coherence optical tomography in turbid tissue: Theoretical analysis. Appl Opt 34:6564–6574, 1995.

44. Schmitt JM. Restoration of optical coherence images of living tissue using the CLEAN algorithm. J Biomed Opt 3(1):66–75, 1998.

45. Kulkarni MD. Coherent signal processing in optical coherence tomography. Ph.D. Thesis, Cleveland, OH: Case Western Reserve Univ, 1999.

46. Papoulis A. Systems and Transforms with Applications in Optics. New York: McGraw-Hill, 1968.

47. Mendel JM. Maximum-Likelihood Deconvolution: A Journey into Model-Based Signal Processing. New York: Springer-Verlag, 1990.

48. Kulkarni MD, Thomas CW, Izatt JA. Image enhancement in optical coherence tomography using deconvolution. Electron Lett 33(16):1365–1367, 1997.

49. Cohen L. Time-Frequency Analysis. Prentice-Hall Signal Processing Series. AV Oppenheim, ed. Englewood Cliffs, NJ: Prentice-Hall, 1995.

50. Nawab SH, Quatieri TF. Short-time Fourier Transform. In: Advanced Topics in Signal Processing. AV Oppenheim, ed. Englewood Cliffs, NJ: Prentice-Hall, 1989:289–327.

51. Mallat SG. A theory for multiresolution signal decomposition: The wavelet representation. IEEE Trans Pattern Anal Mach Intel 11(7):674–693, 1989.

52. Schafer RW, Mersereau RM, Richards MA. Constrained iterative restoration algorithms. Proc IEEE 69:432, 1981.

53. Schmitt JM, Xiang SH, Yung KM. Differential absorption imaging with optical coherence tomography. J Opt Soc Am A 15:2288–2296, 1998.

54. Pan Y, Farkas DL. Noninvasive imaging of living human skin with dual-wavelength optical coherence tomography in two and three dimensions. J Biomed Opt 3:446–455, 1998.

55. Olson WH. Electrical safety. In: Medical Instrumentation. JG Webster, ed. New York, NY: Wiley, 1995:751–792.
56. ANSI. American National Standard for Safe Use of Lasers. New York, NY: American National Standards Institute, 1993:37–43.
57. Hee MR, Izatt JA, Swanson EA, Huang D, Schuman JS, Lin CP, Puliafito CA, Fujimoto JG. Optical coherence tomography of the human retina. Arch Ophthalmol 113:325–332, 1995.

7

Speckle Reduction Techniques[*]

J. M. SCHMITT, S. H. XIANG, and K. M. YUNG

Hong Kong University of Science and Technology, Hong Kong, People's Republic of China

7.1 INTRODUCTION

The word "coherence" in optical coherence tomography (OCT) conveys both a primary strength and a primary weakness of this new imaging technology. On the one hand, the measurement technique on which OCT is based, interferometry, relies inherently on the spatial and temporal coherence of the optical waves backscattered from a tissue. On the other hand, this same coherence gives rise to speckle, an insidious form of noise that degrades the quality of OCT images. Speckle arises as a natural consequence of the limited spatial-frequency bandwidth of the interference signals measured in optical coherence tomography (OCT). In images of highly scattering biological tissues, speckle has a dual role as a source of noise and as a carrier of information about tissue microstructure.

This chapter gives an overview of speckle in OCT and attempts to clarify some of the issues that makes its origins and consequences difficult to understand. The first section addresses a central question: Is speckle a source of noise in OCT or is it the signal itself? The concepts of *signal-carrying* and *signal-degrading* speckle are defined in terms of the phase and amplitude disturbances of the sample beam. Four speckle noise-reduction methods—polarization diversity, spatial compounding, frequency

[*] The first three sections of this chapter are an edited version of a paper published in the *Journal of Biomedical Optics* 4:95–105, 1999.

compounding, and digital signal processing—are discussed, and the potential effectiveness of each method is analyzed briefly. The final sections of the chapter are devoted to examples of speckle-reduction techniques that rely on digital signal processing: a modified zero-adjustment procedure (ZAP) and an optimal nonlinear wavelet threshold (ONWT) technique.

7.2 CHARACTERISTICS OF SPECKLE IN OCT

Speckle came to the forefront soon after it was discovered that the reflection of a laser beam from a rough surface has a distinctive granular or mottled appearance [1]. Having no obvious relationship with the texture of the surface, the dark and bright spots formed by the reflected beam change their pattern whenever the surface moves slightly. This phenomenon, known as laser speckle, was found by early researchers to result from random interference between reflected waves that are mutually coherent. It has taken several decades, however, for researchers to realize the full significance of speckle as a fundamental property of signals and images acquired by all types of narrowband detection systems, which include radar, ultrasound, and radio astronomy. In addition to the optical properties and motion of the target object, speckle is influenced by the size and temporal coherence of the light source, multiple scattering and phase aberrations of the propagating beam, and the aperture of the detector. All of these variables contribute to the observed characteristics of speckle in optical coherence tomography of living tissue. A thorough analysis of each of these variables alone and in combination is not possible within the narrow confines of this chapter. We ask the reader to settle instead for a barebones analysis of a small subset of these variables whose effects have been studied at this early stage of development of OCT. Many of the missing elements in the analysis presented in this section can be pieced together from the theoretical analyses given in Ref. 2. Other elements are truly missing, and an analysis of their influence on OCT awaits further research.

7.2.1 Origin

In optical coherence tomography the sample is placed in one of the arms of an interferometer at the focus of a converging lens. As the optical path in the other arm of the interferometer varies during the scanning operation, an ac current is generated by a photodetector at the output of the interferometer. This photocurrent is proportional to the real part of the cross-correlation product of the reference optical field U_r and the optical field U_s backscattered from the sample,

$$i_d \sim \text{Re}\langle U_r U_s^* \rangle \tag{1}$$

where the brackets $\langle \rangle$ denote an average over time and space. When the light source satisfies the quasi-monochromatic condition (i.e., its center frequency, ν_0, greatly exceeds its bandwidth $\Delta\nu$) and the sample field backscatters from a single scattering center, the photocurrent can be expressed in terms of the optical path difference, $\Delta\tau$, between the two arms,

$$i_d(\Delta\tau) = K|g(\Delta\tau)| \cos[2\pi\nu_0\Delta\tau + \phi(\Delta\tau)] \tag{2}$$

where K is a constant of proportionality that relates the optical and electronic variables and $|g(\Delta\tau)|$ and $\phi(\Delta\tau)$ are, respectively, the argument and phase of the cross-correlation in Eq. (1). The function $|g(\Delta\tau)|$ represents the envelope of the temporal coherence function, given by $g(\Delta\tau) = \langle U_s(t)U_s^*(t+\Delta\tau)\rangle$. We see from Eq. (2) that $i_d(\Delta\tau)$ responds to both the phase and the amplitude of the cross-correlation of the scattered and reference optical fields. It is the sensitivity of the photocurrent to the phase that makes OCT susceptible to the effects of speckle. For the ideal case of a perfectly flat reflector placed at the focus of the lens in the sample arm, the complex autocorrelation function of the source determines the magnitude of the phase term $\phi(\Delta\tau)$ in Eq. (2). However, when the sample is a tissue containing densely packed scatterers, both $g(\Delta\tau)|$ and $\phi(\Delta\tau)$ can no longer be treated as deterministic variables because waves from multiple scattering centers combine randomly to form the interference signal [3].

Consider the changes that a focused wave incident on the tissue undergoes as it propagates through the tissue to the sample volume, scatters back, and then propagates once again through the tissue back to the lens (Fig. 1). Two main processes influence the spatial coherence of the returning wave: (1) multiple backscattering of the beam inside and outside of the desired sample value and (2) random delays of the forward-propagating and returning beam caused by multiple forward scattering. Although the first of these is the primary source of speckle in rough-surface imaging, the second must also be considered in coherent imaging systems, like OCT, that utilize penetrating waves. The common feature of the two processes is that they alter the shape of the wave front of the returning beam and create localized regions of constructive and destructive interference that appear as speckle in OCT images [4].

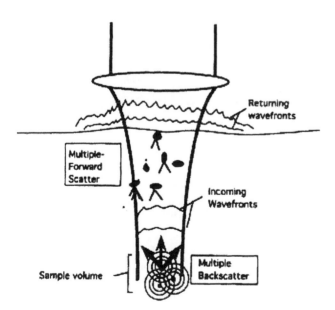

Figure 1 Propagation of a focused beam in tissue. The two main processes that distort the wave front of the returning wave—multiple forward scatter and multiple backscatter—are depicted here.

Multiple backscattering can occur in spite of the short coherence time of the sources used in OCT (usually less than 100 fs). For speckle to form, all that is required is that two or more scatterers in the sample volume backscatter waves that reach some point on the detector out of phase within an interval of time less than the coherence time of the source. Waves backscattered from any pair of point scatterers separated by an optical distance close to an odd multiple of one-half of the wavelength can generate speckle, provided that the optical distance does not exceed the coherence length of the source in the medium. Waves backscattered from different facets of a single large particle can generate speckle in a similar manner. Recent studies suggest that closely packed subwavelength-diameter particles contribute a large fraction of the total optical cross section of the tissue [5–7]. Therefore, the likelihood of finding a pair of scatters or clusters of scatterers within the sample volume that satisfy the conditions for speckle generation is high.

The simulation results in Fig. 2 illustrate how interference noise caused by multiple backscattering can distort the envelope of an OCT signal generated as the sample beam scans along a single line (an OCT A-line). The coherent A-line

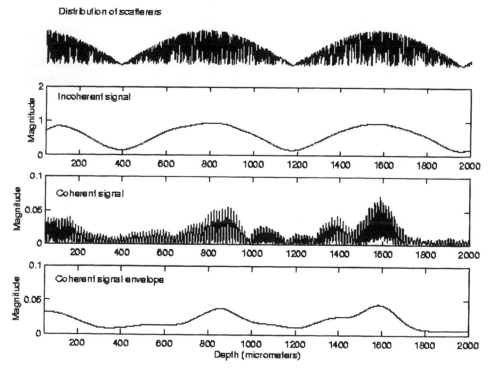

Figure 2 Simulation of the distortion of an OCT A-line caused by the coherent detection process. The uppermost plot shows the ideal backscatter profile generated by a dense random distribution of point particles with cross sections modulated by a cosinusoidal function. Below this plot is the incoherent signal that was formed by convolving the backscatter profile with the Gaussian envelope of the simulated OCT point spread function (15 μm FWHM). The coherent signal was found in a similar way by convolving the backscatter profile with the coherent PSF containing the optical carrier frequency. The lowermost plot is a low-pass-filtered version of the coherent signal.

shown in this figure was computed by convolving a random sequence of scatterers (top line of the figure) with the theoretical coherent point spread function (PSF) of an OCT scanner; the incoherent A-line was computed by convolution with the envelope of the PSF. Details of the simulation method are described in Ref. 8. Note that, unlike those of the incoherent A-line, the variations in the magnitude of the coherent A-line track the density of scatterers poorly. In two-dimensional OCT images formed from a series of A-lines, this type of distortion manifests itself as speckle.

7.2.2 Statistical Properties

Figure 3 is an example of an OCT image that shows high-contrast speckle in regions of strong backscatter below the surface of skin. Note that the appearance of the speckle noise has no obvious dependence on depth, which suggests that the statistical properties of the speckle are dominated by the effects of multiple backscatter rather than by phase aberrations incurred during propagation through overlying tissue. Decorrelation of the incident and returning beams undoubtedly also occurs, but its effects are difficult to discern because the phase aberrations caused by the multiple forward scattering and multiple backscattering process surperimpose. When a large number of polarized quasi-monochromatic waves with random phase combine, a fully developed speckle pattern is formed in which the probability of measuring an intensity I at a given point is described by the negative exponential density function [9],

$$p(I) = \frac{1}{\langle I \rangle} \exp\left[-\frac{1}{\langle I \rangle}\right] \tag{3}$$

where $\langle I \rangle$ is the mean intensity. The image of a speckle pattern that obeys negative exponential statistics has a signal-to-noise ratio (SNR) equal to 1, where the SNR is defined as the ratio of the mean and standard deviation of the intensity,

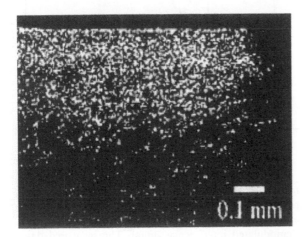

Figure 3 Example of an OCT image (dorsal aspect of a finger) containing high-contrast speckle. The interference signals from which the image was formed were sampled at $1.2\,\mu$m intervals in both dimensions, and the overall size of the image is approximately 1 mm × 1 mm.

$SNR = \langle I \rangle / \sigma_I$. Because intensities close to zero are probable, fully developed speckle patterns are riddled with dark spots.

Although the ac photocurrent, i_d, measured by OCT scanners is proportional to the complex cross-correlation $\langle U_r U_s^* \rangle$, not the intensity $I = \langle U_s U_s^* \rangle = \langle |U_s|^2 \rangle$ in Eq. (3), its squared magnitude $M = i_d^2$ can nevertheless be treated as an analog of the intensity for characterization of the statistical properties of speckle in OCT images. To study these properties, we employed a quadrature-demodulation technique to record the instantaneous phase and amplitude of the ac photocurrent from an OCT scanner [11]. Figure 4 presents the results of a typical set of measurements. Histograms of the intensities and phases of the OCT signals acquired from a highly scattering region of the skin are shown in the right half of the figure. As expected from the random nature of the signals, the phase was found to be almost uniformly distributed between $-\pi$ and π (Fig. 4c). The lack of correlation between the real and

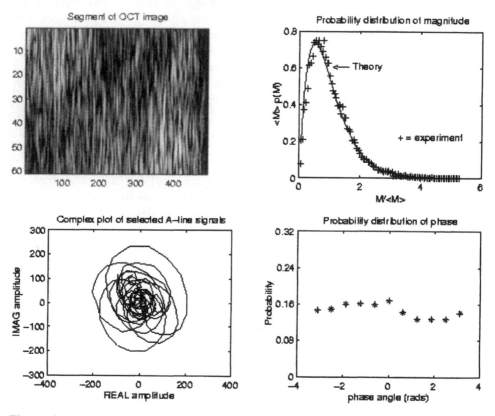

Figure 4 Statistics of the amplitude and phase variations of the OCT interference signal derived from a highly scattering region of living skin tissue. (a) OCT image of the region of the tissue from which the signals were extracted. (b) Histogram of the signal magnitude $M = \sqrt{A_s^2 + A_c^2}$, where A_s and A_c are the amplitudes of the real (cosine) and imaginary (sine) components of the quadrature-demodulated interference signal. The measured data are fit by the solid-line curve, which is a plot of Eq. (4). (c) Histogram of the measured phase, defined as $\tan^{-1}(A_s/A_r)$. (d) Plot of the real and imaginary components of three A-line signals plotted together in the complex plane.

imaginary components of complex amplitudes of the measured OCT signals gives further evidence of the randomness of the phase. Plotted as a curve in the complex plane, the trajectory of the complex amplitude of the signals recorded along a given A-line was found to execute a random walk within a circular area centered on the origin (Fig. 4d). We found a close fit between the histograms of M and the density function expected for speckle generated by reflection of unpolarized light from a rough surface,

$$p(M) = \frac{4M}{\langle M \rangle^2} \exp\left[-2\frac{M}{\langle M \rangle}\right] \tag{4}$$

A close relative of the Rayleigh distribution, this density function describes the random variations in the sum of two oppositely polarized intensities in a speckle field, each of which obeys negative exponential statistics [12]. The SNR of the unpolarized intensity in an unpolarized speckle field is 1.4, a value higher than that of the negative exponential density function (SNR = 1) but lower than that of the Rayleigh density function (SNR = 1.9). Insofar as the open-air interferometer with which the measurements were made is designed to respond equally well to light backscattered in either polarization state, the theoretical conditions underlying the derivation of Eq. (4) are consistent with the experimental conditions. However, it would be presumptuous to claim that Eq. (4) is a universal description of the first-order statistics of the OCT signal magnitude, because the effects of the bandwidth of the source, the aperture of the collection optics, and other instrumental variables are not yet known. Previous studies in other fields indicate, however, that these variables do not alter the first-order statistics of the speckle, except when the number of scatterers in the sample volume is small or the distribution of scatterers is periodic [15]. Preliminary measurements suggest that the SNRs of OCT images of biological tissue lie between 0.5 and 2.0 [10,11,13,14], a range that encompasses the SNRs of polarized and unpolarized speckle patterns.

7.2.3 Classification

The results of the experiments and simulations discussed thus far underscore the importance of multiple backscatter in the formation of speckle in OCT. This type of speckle can be classified as noise because it reduces the correspondence between the local density of scatterers and the intensity variations in OCT images. If somehow all of the waves backscattered from the sample volume could be forced to interfere constructively, the noise would vanish and the contrast of features in the OCT image would be markedly improved. The speckle reduction techniques discussed in the next section (Section 7.3) aim toward this ideal.

A fundamental problem arises, however, when the objective of removing speckle is extended to the extreme of removing speckle entirely. It is here that the types of speckle that we call *signal-carrying* speckle and *signal-degrading* speckle need to be introduced.

The richest source of information in optical coherence tomography is the single-backscattered component of the scattered optical field, because its spatial frequency content extends to the diffraction limit of the imaging optics. Unfortunately, for single backscattering to occur, the incident beam must pass through the overlying tissue without scattering, reflect from one (and only one) particle in the focal plane, and then return to the detector, again without scattering within the overlying tissue. When an optically dense tissue is probed, the probability that only this type of scattering occurs within the temporal coherence interval is diminishingly small. In practice, the returning optical field is corrupted by speckles with correlation spot sizes ranging from less than a wavelength (generated by near-simultaneous backscattering from widely separated particles illuminated by multiply scattered light) to several hundred micrometers (generated by narrow-angle forward scattering and multiple backscattering by large particles) o more than the diameter of the lens (generated by the single-backscattered light). In OCT, the signal-carrying speckle originates from the sample volume in the focal zone of the imaging optics and projects the largest average spot size. The signal-degrading speckle field consists of small speckle spots created by the out-of-focus light that scatters multiple times and happens to return within the delay time set by the difference between the optical paths in the two arms of the interferometer.

Fortunately, the ability to discriminate between signal-carrying and signal-degrading speckle is an inherent characteristic of a scanning interferometer that can be controlled to some extent by the numerical aperture (NA) of the imaging optics. The component of the optical field corrupted by many small speckle spots generates, on average, an interference signal of nearly zero amplitude that fluctuates little as the optical path difference between the arms of the interferometer is scanned. For this reason, the speckle produced by wide-angle multiply scattered light is relatively easy to suppress in OCT. The rms amplitude of the fluctuations produced during scanning by the large speckles in the field is comparatively high. Unfortunately, because of the unfavorable nature of the statistical properties of speckle, a few large speckles or many small speckles are almost equally likely to produce signal amplitudes close to zero for a given sample of the speckle field, and only the second-order statistics (i.e., spatial distribution) of the signal-carrying and signal-degrading speckle differ significantly.

The question posed in the Introduction regarding whether speckle is the signal or the noise in OCT can now be answered succinctly: It is both. To differentiate signal from noise, a well-designed scanner accentuates the interference signals generated by the component of the measured optical field that contains the largest, fastest-moving speckles and suppresses the others.

7.2.4 The Missing Frequency Problem

The earlier subsections discuss speckle from the classical perspective as an interference phenomenon. There is an equivalent, yet much broader, interpretation of speckle to which Fercher [16] and Hellmuth [17] alluded in earlier papers that has important implications for OCT imaging. This interpretation relates to the missing frequency problem [18], which is best understood in the context of information processing. Suppose we regard the desired signal in OCT as a three-dimensional distribution of refractive index variations characterized by a certain spatial frequency spectrum $S(v)$, as illustrated in Fig. 5. $S(v)$ extends from $1/R_0$ to $1/r_0$, where R_0 is the dimension of the largest continuous structure in a given volume of tissue (e.g., a blood vessel) that gives a measurable backscatter signal and r_0 is the smallest (e.g., a protein macromolecule). Owing to the nature of the coherent detection method on which it is based, an OCT scanner can detect only those objects

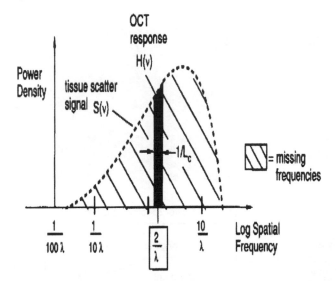

Figure 5 Illustration of the disparity between the broad spatial frequency spectrum of the refractive index variations in tissue, $S(\nu)$, and the narrow spatial frequency response of an OCT scanner, $H(\nu)$. Given by the magnitude of the Fourier transform of the coherent point spread function, $H(\nu)$ is centered on the peak wavelength of emission of the source, λ, and has a width equal to the reciprocal of the coherence length l_c.

whose spatial frequency spectra overlap the band of spatial frequencies between $2/\lambda - 1/l_c$ and $2/\lambda + 1/l_c$, where l_c is the coherence length of the source [17]. A consequence of this bandpass characteristic is that the interior of structures with smoothly varying refractive index profiles is absent from OCT images. Figure 6 illustrates this effect. The simulated OCT image in Fig. 6b was made by convolving the image of a stained tissue section of skin (Fig. 6a) with the theoretical coherent PSF of an OCT scanner ($l_c = 15\,\mu$m; lateral focal spot diameter $= 10\,\mu$m) given in Ref. 8. Notice the severe distortion of the simulated OCT in comparison with the incoherent image, which was computed by convolving the image of the tissue section with the envelope of the PSF (Fig. 6c). The power spectral density curves in Fig. 6d show the distortion of the spatial frequency spectrum of the original image caused by the bandpass filtering property of the coherent detection process. Interestingly, in this example the loss of *low* spatial frequencies appears to have degraded the image quality most. Although blurred noticeably by the attenuation of high spatial frequencies above $1/l_c = 67\,\text{mm}^{-1}$, the incoherent image in this example retains most of the structural detail of the unprocessed tissue section.

This example demonstrates that OCT images suffer from a type of speckle whose effects can be appreciated without directly invoking the concepts of random interference and multiple scattering. By calling this type of noise "speckle," we risk stretching the definition of an already overstretched term. It would perhaps be better to classify this manifestation of speckle and classical speckle together simply as narrowband noise to emphasize their common origin. In fact, the simulation results in Fig. 6 do not accurately represent scattering from real tissue, which contains particles much smaller than the pixels in the original image of the tissue section. Because such particles exist in abundance, truly continuous structures that extend

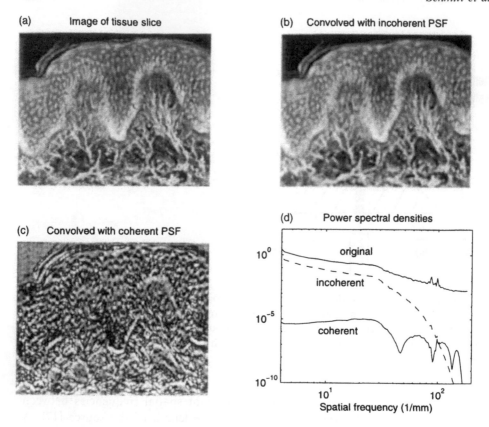

(a) Image of tissue slice

(b) Convolved with incoherent PSF

(c) Convolved with coherent PSF

(d) Power spectral densities

Figure 6 Simulation of the effect of the bandpass filtering property of the coherent detection process in OCT on image quality. (a) Image of a stained tissue section of skin (approximately 1 mm × 1 mm). (b) Image after convolution with the envelope of the simulated point spread function (PSF) of an OCT scanner. (c) Image after convolution with the simulated coherent PSF of an OCT scanner. (d) One-dimensional power-spectral densities of the three images.

over more than a few micrometers are rare; instead, large structures in tissue are assembled from smaller structures, each of which contributes to the total backscatter cross section. For this reason, the edge enhancement that results from the bandpass property of the coherent detection process is not as apparent in OCT images of dense tissue. The small particles, in effect, outline the boundaries of the larger structures; as a result, the high- and low-frequency components of the spatial frequency spectrum of tissue tend to correlate [5]. This fortuitous situation makes OCT images look better than one would expect given the limitations of the coherent detection process.

7.3 SPECKLE REDUCTION

In the context of optical coherence tomography, the objective of speckle reduction is to suppress signal-degrading speckle and accentuate signal-carrying speckle. According to the definitions in Section 7.2.3, these two types of speckle are distinguished by their correlation spot sizes and by the frequencies of the signals they generate during scanning.

Speckle reduction techniques fall into four main categories: polarization diversity, spatial compounding, frequency compounding, and digital signal processing. This section examines the applicability of each of these techniques to OCT imaging and outlines the results of the few studies that have been carried out to date. As the undiminished zeal of researchers with respect to the development of new speckle-reduction methods for medical ultrasound, astronomy, and other fields attest, none of these techniques has proved to be entirely satisfactory. One should not expect, therefore, that a ready solution exists for the speckle problem in OCT. Nonetheless, substantial improvements in image quality should be achievable through the skilful adaptation of available techniques. The preliminary results highlighted later in this section give evidence of the effectiveness of this approach.

7.3.1 Polarization Diversity

Polarization diversity in OCT can be achieved simply by illuminating the sample with unpolarized light and interfering the backscattered light with an unpolarized reference beam. Most OCT scanners based on interferometers built with non-polarization-preserving single-mode fibers automatically implement a form of polarization diversity. However, because most fiber-optic couplers are not completely polarization-independent, equal mixing of light in opposite polarization states cannot be assumed. Configurations of polarization-independent interferometers have been reported for fiber-optic reflectometry that should work equally well for optical coherence tomography of biological tissue [19]. A limitation of polarization diversity i that it increases the SNR of a fully developed speckle pattern by a factor of $\sqrt{2}$ at most. The actual increase in SNR that can be realized in OCT may be considerably less, however, because the polarization signal–carrying component of the speckle may maintain its polarization better than the signal-degrading component generated by multiple wide-angle scattering.

7.3.2 Spatial Compounding

In spatial compounding, the absolute magnitudes of signals derived from the same sample volume or slightly displaced sample volumes are averaged to form a new signal with reduced speckle noise. It is essential that the signals add on a magnitude basis because addition of the amplitudes of signals derived from the different speckle patterns does not improve the SNR [9]. The effectiveness of this approach depends on the number of signals averaged and their mutual coherence. The incoherent average of N uncorrelated signals, each with the same signal-to-noise ratio $\mathrm{SNR} = S_R$, yields a combined signal with an SNR equal to $S_R\sqrt{N}$. Any correlation among the signals reduces the SNR gain. Because the total field of view or angular aperture of the detector must be split to perform the averaging, spatial compounding always results in some loss of resolution.

Figure 7 illustrates one realization of spatial compounding, called angular compounding, that has been applied recently to OCT [13]. An array of detectors located in the back Fourier plane of the objective lens receives light backscattered from the sample volume at different angles. The absolute magnitudes of the demodulated photocurrents from each of the detectors are added to obtained a combined signal with reduced speckle variance. An advantage of this approach is that the number of detectors can be tailored for optimal separation of the signal-carrying

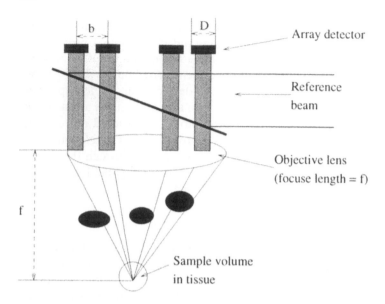

Figure 7 Principle of angular compounding.

speckle from the signal-degrading speckle. For best performance, the NA of the lens should be made as large as possible to increase the light collection angle of each detector while still providing the working distance required to achieve the desired probing depth.

Optical coherence tomographic images of living skin acquired with and without angular compounding are compared in Fig. 8. The uncompounded image (Fig. 8a) was formed from the magnitude of the signal from a single detector in a quadrant array, and the compound image (Fig. 8b) was formed from the sum of the signals from all four detectors. The increase in the number of discernible gray-scale levels of the compounded image is a consequence of the enlarged numerical aperture of the combined detector and the reduced speckle contrast (increased SNR) of the averaged signal [13]. Assuming that the array fills the entire back focal plane of the lens, the extent to which the SNR can be improved at a given resolution using angular compounding is limited by the NA of the lens. As the NA increases, however, the spherical aberration caused by the refractive index mismatch at the surface of the tissue becomes increasingly severe. At the same time, the sensitivity of the interference signal to phase and amplitude aberrations caused by dispersion of the sample beam within inhomogeneous tissue overlying the sample also increases. Unless corrected adaptively, these aberrations can reduce the resolving power to the extent that further increase in the NA above a certain limiting value would be fruitless. The numerical aperture above which aberrations dominate at a given probing depth depends on the optical properties of the tissue and other variables whose effects are still unknown.

Spatial compounding can be done with a single detector by scanning the reference beam back and forth across the detector plane within an interval much shorter than the time constant of the demodulator. This approach has been demonstrated in lidar (light detection and ranging) using an acousto-optical technique [21], but its

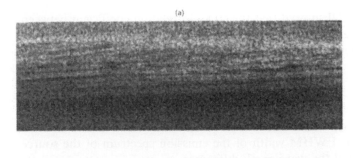

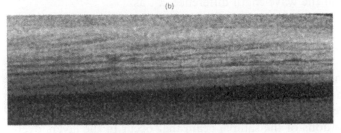

Figure 8 Optical coherence tomographic images before and after angle compounding. The uncompounded image in (a) was formed from the summed amplitudes of the signals generated by the elements of a quadrant detector located in the back focal plane of the objective lens. To form the compounded image in (b), the square root of the magnitudes (sum of the squares) of the interference signals from all four detectors was calculated for each pixel.

application in OCT is complicated by the wide bandwidth of the light source, which necessitates correction for optical dispersion in the acousto-optical scanner. A simple and inexpensive spatial compounding technique for fiber-optic OCT imaging systems has not yet been reported.

7.3.3 Frequency Compounding

Frequency compounding takes advantage of the reduced correlation between speckled images recorded within different optical frequency bands. To ensure sufficient decorrelation for effective averaging of the images, the overlaps of the bands should be as small as possible. Suppose, for example, that the bandwidth, $\Delta\lambda$, of the light source of an OCT scanner with a peak emission wavelength of $\lambda = 1.3\,\mu$m is split into N equal, nonoverlapping bands. Since the phases of the fully developed speckle recorded with nonoverlapping sources are uncorrelated, incoherent addition of the images would reduce the speckle contrast by a factor of $\sqrt{N}$. However, the axial resolution, which is determined by the temporal coherence length of the source, would degrade at the same time by a factor of N. In OCT, this loss of resolution is a steep price to pay. A typical superluminescent diode with a peak emission wavelength of $\lambda = 1.3\,\mu$m and a full-width-at-half-maximum (FWHM) bandwidth of 30 nm has a coherence length in tissue (assuming a mean refractive index of 1.38) of approximately 18 μm. Therefore, applying nonoverlapping frequency compounding to halve the speckle contrast with a typical source would degrade the axial resolution from 18 μm to approximately 72 μm. For most biomedical applications of OCT, such poor axial resolution would be unacceptable.

Melton and Magnin [22] showed that the cross-correlation coefficient between fully developed speckle patterns formed in two equal-width Gaussian frequency bands with center frequencies separated by f_s is approximately

$$\rho_{xy} = \exp\left[-\frac{f_s^2}{2B^2}\right] \tag{5}$$

where B is the width of each band. This correlation coefficient can be written equivalently in terms of the FWHM width of the emission spectrum of the source in wavelength units, $\Delta\lambda$, and the wavelength difference, λ_s, as

$$\rho_{xy} = \exp\left[-\frac{\lambda_s^2}{2\,\Delta\lambda^2}\right] \tag{6}$$

According to this equation, the cross-correlation coefficient remains high even for relatively large wavelength differences. For example, for $\lambda_s = \Delta\lambda/2$, which corresponds to an overlap between the bands of about 50% $\rho_{xy} = 0.88$. But in OCT the phase and amplitude aberrations of the sample beam that occur in the layers overlying the sample volume may cause more rapid decorrelation of the speckle with wavelength than Eq. (6) predicts. The wavelength dependence of the correlation depends on the mean scatter angle and the number of scattering events—the same factors that affect the speckle spot size. Thus, frequency compounding may provide a means of distinguishing the signal-carrying and signal-degrading speckle defined in Section 7.2.3. Reduction of speckle noise could be done adaptively by varying the compounding bandwidths according to the second-order statistics of the recorded image.

The preceding discussion points to the conclusion that a wideband source is prerequisite for effective application of frequency compounding in OCT. A simple way to synthesize a source with a wider spectrum is to combine multiple LED sources [20]. Unfortunately, LED sources generally emit less than $100\,\mu$W in a single spatial mode, and sources with peak emission wavelengths that differ by a few tens of nanometers are not readily available. If these problems can be solved, source synthesis may permit suppression of speckle by frequency compounding without unacceptable loss of resolution. Widening the source bandwidth has the additional benefit of filling in some of the missing spatial frequencies in the tissue spectrum lost in the coherent detection process (see Section 7.2.4).

7.3.4 Digital Signal Processing

Numerous methods have been developed—and continue to be developed—for reducing speckle noise in coherent imaging systems. Most are applied after an image is formed and are commonly referred to as image postprocessing methods. The remaining methods are applied directly to the complex interference signal before the image is recorded and are referred to in this section as complex-domain processing methods.

Among the most popular image postprocessing methods for speckle reduction are median filtering [23], homomorphic Weiner filtering [25], multiresolution wavelet analysis [14,24,31], and adaptive smoothing [26]. All of these methods incorporate either an explicit or implicit statistical model of the spatial frequency spectra of the target features and background. The optimum shape of the passband of a conventional frequency domain- or wavelet-based filter can be derived from the ensemble-averaged spatial frequency spectra of a group of histological tissue specimens with the same microstructure as the tissue being probed. However, insofar as the power spectral densities of signal-carrying and signal-degrading speckle overlap, some loss of useful information is inevitable. By adjusting the passband according to the local mean or standard deviation measured within a window centered on the region of interest, the blurring across the boundaries of heavily speckled regions that results from loss of high-frequency information can be reduced. An optimal nonlinear wavelet threshold (ONWT) technique will be discussed as an example of spatial frequency filtering in Section 7.5.

Digital signal processing can be performed either before or after the absolute magnitude of the OCT interference signal has been calculated for display via demodulation and rectification. Analysis of the interference signal prior to demodulation and rectification has the advantage that changes in the phase as well as the amplitude of the signals can be used to distinguish signal-carrying from single-degrading speckle. One type of speckle reduction method that operates in the complex domain, called the zero-amplitude procedure (ZAP), was first applied by Healey et al. [27] in medical ultrasound. It has been applied recently to optical coherence tomography by Yung and Schmitt [11]. ZAP relies on the location of the zeros of the interference signal in the complex plane to find gaps in the signal caused by destructive interference. One implementation of ZAP is discussed in the following section.

Digital signal processing in the complex domain can also be used to implement a form of adaptive frequency compounding, as suggested in Section 7.3.3. Other complex-domain processing methods that have been applied in OCT include iterative point deconvolution (CLEAN [28,29]) and constrained iterative deconvolution [30]. Although not speckle reduction methods per se, they share a similar aim of reducing the degrading effects of the side lobes of the coherent PSF. Deconvolution of OCT signals performs best, in general, when the scattering targets are separated by the wider of the envelope of the PSF or more; as the number of scatterers in the sample volume increases, the deconvolution becomes increasingly sensitive to noise and performance degrades steeply. This failure is related to the difficulty of interpolating between the gaps in the spatial frequency spectrum that arise from the coherent detection process [18].

7.4 THE ZERO-ADJUSTMENT PROCEDURE (ZAP)*

Tissue is composed of a large number of scatterers that backscatter the light from which OCT images are formed. Each A-line of an OCT image, denoted by $y(n)$, can be modeled as a convolution of the scatterer sequence $x(n)$ and the PSF of the OCT system $h(n)$:

$$y(n) = h(n) \otimes x(n) \tag{7}$$

The PSF, in turn, can be expressed as the product of a Gaussian sequence $g(n)$ and a complex sinusoidal function with a period equal to the wavelength of the light source λ,

---

* This section authored by K. M. Yung.

$$h(n) = g(n)e^{j2\pi n/\lambda} \tag{8}$$

Combining these expressions, we write the A-line signal as

$$y(n) = \left[g(n)e^{j2\pi n/\lambda}\right] \otimes x(n) \tag{9}$$

or

$$y(n) = \left\{g(n) \otimes \left[x(n)e^{-j2\pi n/\lambda}\right]\right\}e^{j2\pi n/\lambda} \tag{10}$$

Now consider the simplest case of destructive interference in which $x(n)$ represents two positive points a and b separated by odd integer multiples of $\lambda/2$,

$$x(n) = \begin{cases} a, & n = 0 \\ b, & n = (N \pm 1/2)\lambda \\ 0, & \text{otherwise} \end{cases} \tag{11}$$

For any integers N and $(N \pm 1/2)\lambda$, the backscatter signal is then

$$y(n) = \left\{ag(n) - bg[n - (N \pm 1/2)\lambda]\right\}e^{j2\pi n/\lambda} \tag{12}$$

In the zero-adjustment procedure (ZAP), the complex backscatter signal is z-transformed and its zeros are found. These zeros are processed in two steps: zero detection and signal correction [11]. The detection process involves locating zeros that lie close to the angular carrier frequency of the signal. Those zeros (called ZAP zeros) that appear inside the sector in the complex plane bounded by the angular carrier frequency plus or minus a fixed fraction of the signal angular bandwidth are assumed to cause speckles. For $y(n)$ given by Eq. (12), only one ZAP zero exists, which is located at

$$z_{\text{ZAP}} = \left(\frac{b}{a}\right)^{2/(2N \pm 1)\lambda} e^{j2\pi/\lambda}$$

After each ZAP zero is found, it is rotated away from the carrier frequency of the signal. The corrected A-line is then obtained by inverse z-transforming the polynomial with roots given by the zeros. For a given angle of rotation of δ, the ZAP-corrected A-line is given by

$$y_{\text{ZAP}}(n) = \left\{ag(n) + a(1 - e^{j\delta}) \sum_{k=1}^{(N \pm 1/2)\lambda - 1} g(n - k) \right. \\ \left. + [a(1 - e^{j\delta}) - b]g\left[n - \left(N \pm \frac{1}{2}\right)\lambda\right]\right\}e^{j2\pi n/\lambda} \tag{13}$$

This procedure, in effect, adds a series of complex numbers with the sample amplitude $a(1 - e^{j\delta})$ in the space between the two original scatters, thereby filling in energy in the region where speckle occurs. To implement ZAP on a signal generated by a sequence of scatterers, the A-line is broken into overlapping segments with lengths close to the axial width of the system PSF. The magnitudes of ZAP-corrected segments are then multiplied with Hanning windows to reduce edge effects and reconstructed to form the corrected A-line.

Column (a) of Fig. 9 consists of simulation results that show the effect of applying the traditional ZAP to demodulated complex backscatter signals formed

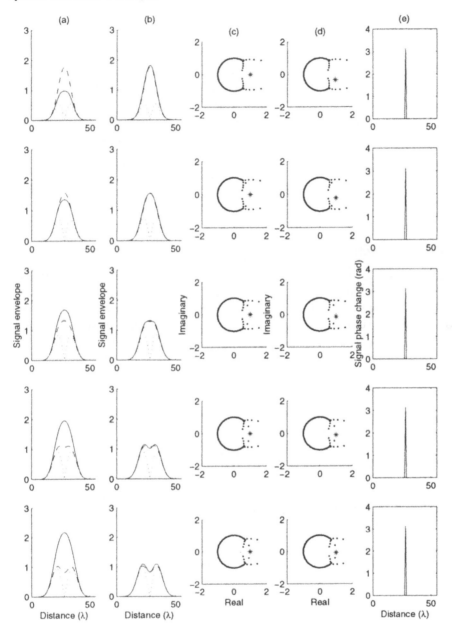

Figure 9 Simulated envelopes, zeros, and phases of the complex OCT backscatter signals after demodulation. The results shown were obtained for pairs of scatterers of unit amplitudes separated by 4.5λ, 6.5λ, 8.5λ, 10.5λ, and 12.5λ (top to bottom). (a) Coherent backscatter envelope (dotted line), ideal incoherent envelope (broken line), and original ZAP-corrected envelope (solid line). (b) ZAP-corrected envelope (solid line) by optimal rotation of ZAP zero. The ZAP-corrected envelope resembles the ideal envelope (broken line). (c) Zeros of z-transformed backscatter signal with ZAP zero plotted as an asterisk. (d) Zeros after optimal rotation of the ZAP zero. (e) Absolute value of the instantaneous phase change. (From Ref. 32.)

with scatter separations of increasing odd integer multiples of $\lambda/2$. The simulated results show that the original ZAP helps to correct the speckled backscatter signal. However, the method is unable to fill in the right amount of energy for different degrees of destructive interference. One can see that the filling-in procedure is too weak in some cases but too strong in others. Figure 9b presents the ZAP-corrected envelope (solid line) by optimal rotation of ZAP zero. The broken line shows the profile of the ideal envelope. Figure 9c illustrates the zeros of the z-transformed demodulated A-lines before ZAP is applied. The asterisks show the locations of the ZAP zeros. Figure 9d gives the ZAP zeros after optimal rotation. Figure 9e shows the absolute value of the instantaneous phase change, which indicates that for backscatter signals formed with pairs of scatterers spaced at 0.5 fractional multiples of wavelength, there must be a phase change of π where destructive interference occurs.

7.4.1 Speckle Detection

In Eq. (12), the complex signal $y(n)$ is represented as a convolution of the scatterer function $x(n)$ with the PSF $h(n)$ centered on a carrier with a period λ. The zeros of $Y(z)$ are the collection of the zeros of $H(z)$ and $X(z)$. The signals from scatterers of amplitudes α and β suffer from destructive interference when the scatterers are separated by an integer distance of $d = (N \pm 1/2)\lambda$ for any integer N. For this case, the scatterer function is given by Eq. (11), which after z-transformation, yields

$$X(z) = \alpha + \beta z^{-d} \tag{14}$$

A speckle-corrupted A-line represented by

$$y_{\text{SPK}}(n) = \left\{ \alpha g(n) - \beta g\left[n - \left(N \pm \frac{1}{2} \right)\lambda \right] \right\} e^{j2\pi n/\lambda} \tag{15}$$

results from destructive interference of the signals generated by two scatterers α and β separated by $(N \pm 1/2)\lambda$. We consider the zeros of $x(n)$ first, which, from Eq. (14) are located in the z-domain at

$$z = \left(\frac{\beta}{\alpha} \right)^{1/d} \exp\left[\frac{j(2n - 1)\pi}{d} \right], \qquad n = 0, 1, 2, \dots, d - 1 \tag{16}$$

$$Z = \left(\frac{\beta}{\alpha} \right)^{1/d} \exp\left[\frac{j2(2n - 1)\pi}{(2N \pm 1)\lambda} \right], \qquad n = 0, 1, 2, \dots, \left(N \pm \frac{1}{2} \right)\lambda - 1 \tag{17}$$

There must exist an $n = (N + 1/2) \pm 1/2$ such that

$$z = z_{\text{ZAP}} = \left(\frac{\beta}{\alpha} \right)^{1/d} e^{j2\pi/\lambda} \tag{18}$$

The angular frequency of $y(n)$ is $\omega = 2\pi/\lambda$, which is the same as the frequency of the zero given by Eq. (18). This derivation shows that destructive interference must produce (ZAP zero) at the signal angular frequency ω. As zeros of the PSF do not lie close to its angular carrier frequency, zeros near ω must be from the scatterer sequence. Therefore, the presence of a zero at or near ω indicates the presence of speckle.

Optimization of the ZAP-Zero Rotation Angle

To correct the distortion caused by destructive interference of signals generated by pairs of scatterers, energy must be added back to the signal within the proper time interval to replace the lost signal energy. One way to accomplish this is to rotate the angle of the ZAP zeros. The closer the separation of the scatterers to 0.5 fractional multiples of the wavelength, the more rotation of the ZAP zeros is required. Rotation of the zeros by a constant angle according to the algorithm of the original ZAP does not properly correct destructive interference of A-lines of different integer and fractional wavelength multiples.

We carried out an extensive simulation of ZAP correction for various pairs of scatterer separations to find an optimal ZAP-zero rotation angle for each case. The ZAP zeros were rotated by an adjustable angle until the ZAP-corrected envelope matched the ideal incoherent envelope as closely as possible.

For the scatterer sequence of Eq. (11), the zeros are located at

$$z = \left(\frac{b}{a}\right)^{2/(2N\pm1)\lambda} \exp\left[\frac{j2(2n-1)\pi}{(2N\pm1)\lambda}\right], \qquad n = 0, 1, 2, \ldots, \left(N \pm \frac{1}{2}\right)\lambda - 1 \qquad (19)$$

The phase angle of each zero is related to the separation of scatterers. In the present case, the separation distance is $(N1/2)\lambda$, so the angle between any two adjacent scatterer zeros is $4\pi/(2N \pm 1)\lambda$. In general, the adjacent scatterer zero-angle difference in terms of multiple of wavelength M is given by

$$\phi_\Delta(M) = \frac{2\pi}{M\lambda} \qquad (20)$$

where λ denotes the wavelength of the light source in number of samples. From Eq. (2), the exact scatterer separation of an A-line can be found given prior knowledge of the adjacent scatterer zero-angle separation. After this division, the angles trace out a triangular wave function related to the multiple of wavelength M and written as

$$\phi_z(M) = \begin{cases} 0.5 - M + \lfloor M \rfloor, & 0 \leq M - \lfloor M \rfloor < 0.5 \\ 0.5 - \lceil M \rceil + M, & 0 < \lceil M \rceil - M \leq 0.5 \end{cases} \qquad (21)$$

where the symbols $\lfloor \cdot \rfloor$ and $\lceil \cdot \rceil$ mean that the quantity inside is rounded toward minus infinity and plus infinity, respectively. After normalizing the rotation angles with a best-fit line and taking in the square root, we obtain a normalized rotation function. This function has a simple profile that can be approximated by a triangular wave according to

$$\phi_{opt}(M) = 1 - 2\phi_z(M) \qquad (22)$$

Hence, once the distance between two scatterers is known, we can estimate how much a ZAP zero needs to be rotated to correctly fill in speckles.

Determination of Scatterer Separation

We now have a procedure for correcting speckled A-lines with an optimal amount of energy based on a modified form of ZAP. With the help of the original ZAP-zero angle and the sum of the absolute phase change, we can estimate the spacing between adjacent scatterers. The problem now is that we do not know the exact multiple of the wavelength by which a given pair of scatterers is separated because the adjacent scatterer zero separation is still unknown. However, according to Eq. (20), it is possible for us to extract an exact distance of scatterer separation in terms of multiples of wavelength from adjacent zero angle differences. The difference in angle between adjacent zeros can be calculated directly by finding the difference of the phase angles between that of a ZAP zero and the closest zero of the same magnitude within the angular bandwidth of the A-line. The zeros beside the asterisks at the months of two Y-structures in the bottom three plots of Fig. 9c illustrate such adjacent zeros. One might ask why we still need to calculate the fractional multiple from either the original ZAP-zero phase angle or the sum of phase change when both integer and fractional multiples can be obtained readily from adjacent zero angles. The reason is that the change of the adjacent zero separation angle becomes negligible for the same integer-multiple of separation distance of widely separated scatterers. To avoid error in calculating the exact scatterer separation, we break the procedure down into three steps. First, an estimate of the exact scatterer spacing is found from the adjacent scatterer zero-angle difference by using Eq. (20). For an A-line for which the angle of ZAP zero is α, the angle difference of adjacent scatterer zeros is β and the summation of phase changes is P, the estimate of scatterer separation in terms of the multiple of wavelength can be found by evaluating $\phi_\Delta^{-1}(\beta)$, where $y = f(x)$ and $x = f^{-1}(y)$ are equivalent. Next, two sets of scatterer spacing are found by computing $\phi_s^{-1}(\alpha/\beta)$ and $\phi_{\text{sum}}^{-1}(P)$. Finally, an element is selected from each set of separations that are closest to the estimate in the first step. The two values are averaged to give a more accurate estimate of the scatterer separation than either of them alone.

A problem arises, however, when the scatterer spacing is between 0 and 6 integer multiples. Referring to the top two plots of Fig. 9c, we observe that no adjacent zeros can be found within the signal bandwidth. Adjacent zeros are hidden by PSF zeros. Without this information, it is impossible for us to know the estimated scatterer spacing. Therefore, when this situation arises, we simply approximate the estimated exact scatterer separation by the median of integer multiples with the problem and then go through the three steps above.

Figure 10 shows OCT images of tissue before and after processing with the original and modified ZAP. A weak low-pass filter was applied on all images in the lateral dimension to smooth the transitions between A-lines. The speckle fluctuations in both of the processed images are clearly smaller than in the original image; however, some features in the original ZAP-processed image are blurred. For reference, the image created by angle compounding using a four-element detector [11,13] is shown in Fig. 10d.

Our preliminary investigation of the ZAP suggested its potential to suppress speckle noise. The disadvantage with the traditional ZAP is that its smoothing effect is sometimes excessive. It is caused by the difficulties with ZAP in filling in speckles with the right amount of energy according to the local signal properties. The modified ZAP we presented in this section is more adaptive to speckles and linear in response. However, applied to real OCT signals, the modified ZAP does not perform as well as our theoretical analysis. One likely reason is that noise in weak OCT signals introduces false phase changes. Another problem is the inability of ZAP to cope with the speckle generated by very large numbers of scatterers in the sample volume. This problem also appears to be a major stumbling block in deconvolution and filtering of OCT images. A better phase-noise filtering procedure needs to be developed as an alternative to the thresholding function now used in our OCT

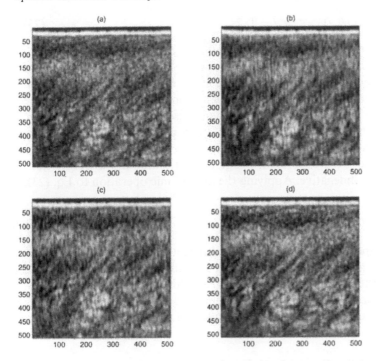

Figure 10 A comparison of the original and modified-ZAP processed OCT images of skin (back side of index finger). (a) Original image. (b) Original ZAP-corrected image. (c) Modified ZAP-corrected image. (d) Image as an ensemble average of four independent channels of an array detector. (From Ref. 32.)

system. Hardware improvements, such as the use of broader band and more powerful sources, may make ZAP more robust.

7.5 OPTIMAL NONLINEAR WAVELET THRESHOLDING*

The method of speckle noise reduction by optimal nonlinear wavelet thresholding (ONWT) was first applied to medical ultrasound imaging [31] and later applied to OCT image processing [14]. Because it is based on optimization of the signal-to-noise (SNR) ratio in the wavelet domain, ONWT can reduce speckle noise while preserving image details. This feature is very important in coherent imaging technologies such as OCT in which weak signal detection is critical. This section gives a brief introduction to the ONWT method. Processed OCT images of living tissues are presented to illustrate the performance of the method.

7.5.1 OCT Speckle Statistics

Speckle noise can be approximated as a type of multiplicative noise that is commonly observed in images generated with highly coherent waves [33]. An OCT image degraded by multiplicative noise, $y'(h, i)$, can be expressed as

---

* This section authored by S. H. Xiang.

$$y'(h, i) = f'(h, i) \times n'(h, i), \qquad h, i = 1, 2, 3, \ldots, N \tag{23}$$

where $f'(h, i)$ denotes the real OCT image pixels that need to be recovered: $n'(h, i)$ denotes independent, identically distributed x^2 random variables with two degrees of freedom; and $y'(h, i)$ represents the observed noisy image data [24]. When the spatial resolution of the imaging system is small in comparison with the details of the imaged object, speckle can be modeled as Gaussian noise provided that the image is sampled coarsely enough that the degradation at any pixel is independent of the degradation at all other pixels [9].

Because $y'(h, i)$ and $f'(h, i)$ represent image intensities and are therefore non-negative, $n'(h, i)$ is also nonnegative. Applying the logarithmic operation to Eq. (23), we obtain

$$y(h, i) = f(h, i) + n(h, i), \qquad h, i = 1, 2, 3, \ldots, N \tag{24}$$

The logarithmic operation transforms the multiplicative noise $n'(h, i)$ into additive noise $n(h, i)$, which is amenable to restoration algorithms based on linear noise models [24]. Because the dynamic range of OCT interference signals is high (80–110 dB), logarithmic compression is generally required before display. For displayed OCT images, the additive white Gaussian noise model is a reasonable approximation for speckle modeling.

7.5.2 Maximization of the Signal-to-Noise Ratio

To deal further with Eq. (24), we now apply the separable dyadic multiresolution analysis developed by Mallat [34]. The basic concept of multiresolution decomposition is to split an image dataset into components of different resolutions. To achieve optimal noise reduction, the localized signal components are reduced if their magnitudes exceed a certain threshold.

Multiresolution analysis is carried out in a series of spaces $V_m \subset \mathbf{L}^2(\mathbf{R})$, $m \in \mathbf{Z}$, such that

$$\cdots \subset V_2 \subset V_1 \subset V_0 \subset V_{-1} \subset V_{-2} \subset \cdots$$

with

$$\overline{\cup_{m \in Z} V_m} = \mathbf{L}^2(\mathbf{R}) \qquad \text{and} \qquad \cap_{m \in Z} = \{0\}$$

which describes a successive approximation sequence to the space $\mathbf{L}^2(\mathbf{R})$ [34]. The symbol $\subset$ means "in"; for example, $V_2 \subset V_1$ means space V_2 in space V_1; $m \in \mathbf{Z}$ means m in the integer space. More precisely, for a given energy-limited OCT image signal $f \in \mathbf{L}^2(\mathbf{R})$, the successive projections $\mathrm{Prov}\, V_m(f)$ on the spaces V_m gives approximations of f with resolution 2^{-m}. If $f(h, i)$ is the signal and $n(h, i)$ is the noise, then by carrying out the discrete wavelet transform (DWT), we obtain $W_s(j, k, l)$ for the signal coefficients and $W_n(j, k, l)$ for the noise coefficients at different levels.

Applying the soft-thresholding λ nonlinearity [31],

$$\eta(j, k, l, \lambda) = \mathrm{sign}\,[W(j, k, l)][|W(j, k, l)| - \lambda] \tag{25}$$

where

$$\text{sign}(W(j, k, l)) = \begin{cases} +1 & \text{when } W(j, k, l) > 0 \\ 0 & \text{when } W(j, k, l) = 0 \\ -1 & \text{when } W(j, k, l) < 0 \end{cases} \tag{26}$$

we obtain denoised coefficients $\eta_s(j, k, l, \lambda)$ and $\eta_n(j, k, l, \lambda)$ for the signal and noise, respectively.

To reconstruct the image signal $f_o(h, i, \lambda)$, which contains the residual image noise $n_o(h, i, \lambda)$, the inverse wavelet transform (IWT) is applied. By defining the SNR as

$$\text{SNR}(\lambda) = \frac{\sum_{h,i}[f_o(h, i, \lambda)]^2}{\sum_{h,i} E[(n_o(h, i, \lambda))^2]} \tag{27}$$

and simplifying Eq. (27), we find

$$\text{SNR}(\lambda) = \frac{N^2\lambda^2 - 2\lambda N\sqrt{\gamma E_s} + E_s}{N^2\lambda^2 - 2\lambda N\sqrt{E_n} + E_n} \tag{28}$$

where

$$E_s = \sum_{j,k,l} |W_s(j, k, l)|^2 \tag{29}$$

and

$$E_n = \sum_{j,k,l} |W_n(j, k, l)|^2 \tag{30}$$

represent the energy of the signal and the energy of the noise in the wavelet domain, respectively. The steps involved in simplifying Eq. (27) to Eq. (28) are given in Ref. 31. In Eq. (28), $\gamma \subseteq [0, 1]$ is a constant that represents the signal inhomogeneity in the wavelet domain. When the image data are transformed into the wavelet domain, the noise projects into the whole wavelet space in (j, k, l), but the most significant coefficients of the signal, in general, project into a limited subspace (j', k', l'). The constant γ in Eq. (28) is defined as

$$\gamma = \frac{1}{2N^2} \sum_{j,k,l} [\text{sign} (|W_s(j, k, l)| - \beta) + 1] \tag{31}$$

where β is the mean of signal coefficients W_s. Since, according to Eq. (31), γ is proportional to the ratio of the total number of wavelet coefficients whose absolute values lie above the mean of W_s and the dimension of the total wavelet space, a smooth image will give a lower value of γ than a sharp image containing more features of high spatial frequency.

Now to obtain an optimal threshold λ_o, the maximizes the SNR, we let

$$\frac{\partial \text{SNR}(\lambda)}{\partial \lambda} = 0 \tag{32}$$

and find

$$\lambda_o = \frac{E_s - E_n - [(E_s - E_n)^2 + 4(\sqrt{\gamma E_s} - \sqrt{E_n})(E_n\sqrt{\gamma E_s} - E_s\sqrt{E_n})]^{1/2}}{2N(\sqrt{\gamma E_s} - \sqrt{E_n})} \tag{33}$$

for the optimal threshold. Note that λ_o depends on the energy levels of the signal and noise in the wavelet domain. When the signal and noise concentrate in different levels, the optimal threshold given by Eq. (33) can reduce noise without destroying useful information in the original signal.

Figure 11 demonstrates the results of ONWT processing on an OCT image of the nail fold, which was acquired by an OCT system that incorporates array detection [20]. The image was contaminated with speckle because the received A-line signals came from the coherent summation of the multiple scatterers. Figure 11b presents the results of ONWT processing. Each A-line signal of the image was transformed into the wavelet domain, with the Daubechies 4 wavelet used as the mother wavelet. The optimal nonlinear threshold based on the statistics of the signal and noise energy level was first obtained from Eq. (33) and then applied to the wavelet coefficients. The image was reconstructed by the inverse wavelet transform. The most important OCT features, such as junctions between the epidermis and dermis as well as the boundaries of the small blood vessels in the dermis area, were preserved during noise reduction. Figure 11c gives the results of applying a threshold 30% lower than the optimum. Although most of the structural details of OCT images were preserved, some of the speckle noise remains. Figure 11d illus-

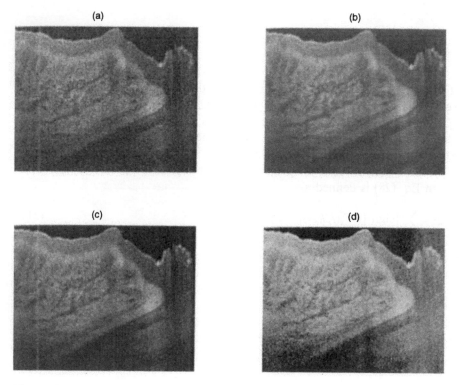

Figure 11 Optical coherence tomographic images of the nail fold region of the index finger of a human subject. Each image covers an area of approximately 1.0 mm (deep)× 2.4 mm (wide). (a) Original OCT image. (b) Processed image after applying optimal threshold. (c) Image reconstructed after applying a threshold 30% below the optimum. (d) Image processed by applying a threshold 2.5 times the optimum.

trates the processing result obtained after applying a threshold 2.5 times the optimum. Although the speckle noise was reduced the most in this case, considerable blurring of the image is evident.

The ONWT technique presented in this section incorporates optimal nonlinear thresholding in multiple spatial frequency bands of OCT interference signals. Using this approach, the SNR is maximized with minimal loss of high spatial frequency information.

7.6 CONCLUSION AND REMAINING PROBLEMS

Speckle is an undesirable consequence of all coherent or partially coherent imaging systems. Any overview of a topic as complex as speckle in OCT inevitably unearths a number of problems for future research. The following is a short list of problems that deserve special attention.

Current understanding of the classes of speckle and their origins is sketchy. More experimental work is needed to understand the relationship between the microscopic scattering properties of tissue and the statistical properties of speckle in OCT images, particularly the second-order properties that specify the distribution of the correlation spot sizes in the projected speckle patterns.

As a fundamental manifestation of coherent noise, speckle is a natural consequence of the limited spatial frequency bandwidth of an interferometric measurement system. To enable effective suppression of speckle effects in OCT, techniques for simultaneously widening the bandwidth of the light source and the light collection aperture must be developed.

Too few studies have focused on ways of adapting spatial- and frequency-compounding methods employed in synthetic aperture radar and medical ultrasound to optical coherence tomography. More work in this area is needed.

The applications of complex-domain processing in OCT merit further investigation, especially those techniques that exploit the phase of the OCT signal.

Topics for further investigation in wavelet-based speckle reduction include methods for optimum selection of mother wavelets and for increasing execution speed.

REFERENCES

1. Rigden JD, Gordon EI. Granularity of scattered optical maser light. Proc IRE 50:6564–6574, 1992.
2. Dainty JC, ed. Laser Speckle and Related Phenomena. New York: Springer-Verlag, 1984.
3. Mandel L, Wolf E. Optical coherence and Quantum Optics. Cambridge, UK: Cambridge Univ Press, 1995, pp 401–414.
4. Wax A, Thomas JE. Measurement of smoothed Wigner phase-space distributions for small-angle scattering in a turbid medium. J Opt Soc Am A 15:1986–1908, 1998.
5. Schmitt JM, Kumar G. Turbulent nature of refractive-index variations in biological tissue. Opt Lett 21:1310–1312, 1996.

6. Dunn A, Richards-Kortum R. Three-dimensional computation of light scattering from cells. IEEE J Selected Topics Quant Electron 2:898–905, 1996.

7. Beuthan J, Minet O, Helfmann J, Herrig M, Müller G. The spatial variation of the refractive index in biological cells. Phys Med Biol 41:369–382, 1996.

8. Schmitt JM, Zhou L. Deconvolution and enhancement of optical coherence tomograms. Proc SPIE 2981:46–57, 1997.

9. Goodman JW. Some fundamental properties of speckle. J Opt Soc Am 66:1145–1150, 1976.

10. Schmitt JM, Knüttel A, Yadlowsky M, Bonner RF. Optical-coherence tomography of a dense tissue: Statistics of attenuation and backscattering. Phys Med Biol 42:1427–1439, 1994.

11. Yung KM, Schmitt JM. Phase-domain processing of optical coherence tomography images. J Biomed Opt 4:125–136, 1999.

12. Goodman JW. Statistical Optics. New York: Wiley 1985:124–127.

13. Schmitt JM. Array detection for speckle reduction in optical coherence microscopy. Phys Med Biol 42:1427–1439, 1997.

14. Xiang SH, Zhou L, Schmitt JM. Speckle noise reduction for optical coherence tomography. Proc SPIE (Euroser) 3196:79–88, 1997.

15. Wagner RF, Insana MF, Brown DG. Statistical properties of radio-frequency and envelope-detected signals with applications to ultrasound. J Opt Soc Am A 4:910–921, 1987.

16. Fercher AF, Drexler W, Hitzenberger CK. Ocular partial coherence tomography. Proc SPIE 2732:229–241, 1996.

17. Hellmuth T. Contrast and resolution in optical coherence tomography. Proc SPIE 2926:228–237, 1997.

18. Fried DL. Analysis of the CLEAN algorithm and implications for superresolution. J Opt Soc Am A 12:853–860, 1995.

19. Kobayashi M, Hanafusa H, Takada K, Noda J. Polarization-independent interferometric optical-time-domain reflectometer. J Lightwave Tech 9:623–628, 1991.

20. Schmitt JM, Lee SL, Yung KM. An optical coherence microscope with enhanced resolving power. Opt Commun 142:203–207, 1997.

21. Strauss CEM. Synthetic-array heterodyne detection: A single-element detector acts as an array. Opt Lett 19:1609–1611, 1994.

22. Melton HE, Magnin PA. A-mode speckle reduction with compound frequencies and compound bandwidths. Ultrasound Imag 6:203–207, 1984.

23. Bernstein R. Adaptive nonlinear filters for simultaneous removal of different kinds of noise in images. IEEE Trans Circuits Syst 34:1275–1291, 1987.

24. Moulin P. A wavelet regularization method for diffuse radar-target imaging and speckle-noise reduction. J Math Imag Vision 3:123–134, 1993.

25. Franceschetti G, Pascazio V, Schirinzi G. Iterative homomorphic technique for speckle reduction in synthetic-aperature radar imaging. J Opt Soc Am A 12:686–694, 1995.

26. Kuan DT, Sawchuk AA, Strand TC, Chavel P. Adaptive noise smoothing for images with signal-dependent noise. IEEE Trans Pattern Anal Mach Intell 7:165–177, 1985.

27. Healey AJ, Leeman S, Forsberg F. Turning off speckle. Acoust Imag 19:433–437, 1992.

28. Högbom JA. Aperture synthesis with non-regular distribution of interferometer baselines. Astron Astrophys Suppl 15:417–426, 1974.

29. Schmitt JM. Restoration of optical coherence images of living tissue using the CLEAN algorithm. J Biomed Opt 3:1998. In press.

30. Kulkarni MD, Thomas CW, Izatt JA. Image enhancement in optical coherence tomography using deconvolution. Electron Lett 33:1365–1367, 1997.

31. Xiang SH, Zhang YT. Sensitivity enhancement using nonlinear optical wavelet thresholding for two-dimensional medical ultrasound transducer. Biomed Eng Appl Basis Commun 9:91–100, 1997.
32. Yung KM, Schmitt JM, Lee SL. Digital processing of noisy OCT signals in phase space. Proc SPIE 3251:2–11, 1998.
33. Wells PNT, Halliwell M. Speckle in ultrasonic imaging. Ultrasonics 19:225–229, 1981.
34. Mallat S. A theory for multiresolution signal decomposition: The wavelet representation. IEEE Trans Pattern Anal Mach Intell 11:675–693, 1989.

8

Doppler Optical Coherence Tomography

THOMAS E. MILNER

University of Texas at Austin, Austin, Texas

SIAVASH YAZDANFAR, ANDREW M. ROLLINS, and JOSEPH A. IZATT

Case Western Reserve University, Cleveland, Ohio

T. LINDMO

Norwegian University of Science and Technology, Trondheim, Norway

ZHONGPING CHEN and J. STUART NELSON

University of California at Irvine, Irvine, California

XIAO-JUN WANG

Georgia Southern University, Statesboro, Georgia

8.1 INTRODUCTION

8.1.1 The Doppler Effect

An effect exhibited in all wave phenomena is the apparent change in frequency (ν_D) due to relative motion between a source and an observer. If the source and observer are approaching each other, the apparent frequency of the wave is greater ($\nu_D > 0$). Conversely, the apparent frequency is lowered ($\nu_D < 0$) if the source and observer are moving away from each other. This effect was first identified and studied in 1842 by the Dutch physicist Johann Christian Doppler, who performed experiments involving the apparent tone of musical instruments played on moving railroad cars. In more recent times, the "Doppler effect" has been used to detect and measure the velocity of moving objects ranging in size from the atomic to galactic scale. Within the last few decades, many biomedical researchers and clinical practitioners have investigated the application of noninvasive Doppler techniques such as ultrasound imaging and laser flowmetry to monitor blood flow.

The use of coherent light sources to measure the velocity of moving particles was first reported shortly after the invention of the laser. In the late 1960s and early 1970s, development of laser Doppler velocimetry proceeded rapidly for a range of applications. The use of laser light to measure blood flow in retinal arteries was first reported by Charles Riva and colleagues. Initially, measurements of blood flow velocity in rabbit retinal vessels were reported [1]. Later, a similar procedure was followed using light from a lower power HeNe laser with a photomultiplier detector and an electronic correlator to measure blood flow in human retinal arteries and veins [2]. Subsequently, a number of investigators developed the methodology further to measure blood flow in a catheter [3] and skin pulsatile flow using a source-and-receiver geometry incorporating optical fibers [4]. One of the earliest reports describing the use of a light source with a broad spectral emission profile or short temporal coherence length for interferometric measurement of fluid flow was given by B. T. Meggitt and colleagues [5]. The power spectrum of light backscattered from a 200 μm measurement volume in a test flow was measured using a Michelson configuration incorporating a low finesse Fabry–Perot recovery interferometer combined with differential detection. Using this technique, the authors measured the power spectrum of interference fringe intensity corresponding to light backscattered from discrete spatial locations in a test flow. More recently, development of high power amplified spontaneous emission (ASE) light sources that provide broad spectral emission profiles in a single transverse spatial mode have allowed high resolution ($\sim 10\,\mu$m) measurement of flow velocity in turbid media [6].

8.1.2 Doppler Ultrasound

In Doppler ultrasound imaging, an acoustic transducer external to the tissue generates ultrasonic waves that are backscattered from moving red blood cells (RBCs) and shifted in frequency (ν_D) by an amount proportional to the velocity. In addition to being noninvasive, the chief advantage of Doppler ultrasound techniques is the ability to record images of the heart and relatively large diameter blood vessels. Although Doppler ultrasound imaging provides a means to resolve blood flow velocities at discrete spatial locations in tissue, the relatively long acoustic wavelengths required for deep tissue penetration limits spatial resolution to approximately 100 μm. Application of Doppler ultrasound to the recording of tomographic images of microvasculature blood flow requires the use of high frequency acoustic waves that are strongly attenuated in tissue.

Differences in the spatial and velocity resolution between Doppler ultrasound and optical coherence tomography (OCT) are due to the large variance between characteristic wavelengths of corresponding optical and acoustic waves in tissue. The spatial resolution of Doppler OCT is an order of magnitude better than what can be achieved with ultrasound tomography [7]. Vessels positioned at depths to 1 mm beneath the tissue surface with diameters as small as 10 μm can be imaged using Doppler OCT. Similarly, the velocity resolution of Doppler OCT is better than in ultrasound because of the difference in respective wavelengths (λ). For ultrasound, $\lambda_{\text{acoustic}}$ depends on the wave frequency and mean velocity of sound through soft tissue (taken to be 1540 m/s). For 10 MHz ultrasound, $\lambda_{\text{acoustic}} = 1540\,(\text{m/s})/10^7\,\text{Hz}$ = 154 μm compared to $\lambda_{\text{optic}} = 0.85\,\mu$m. Assuming equal measurement time (Δt_p) to record a single pixel in acoustic and optical Doppler imaging systems, the ratio of minimum velocity ($V^{\min}$) resolutions is given by

$$\frac{V^{\min}_{\text{acoustic}}}{V^{\min}_{\text{optical}}} = \frac{\lambda_{\text{acoustic}}}{\lambda_{\text{optic}}} = \frac{154}{0.85} = 180$$

The two-order magnitude improvement in $V^{\min}$, together with a tenfold increase in Doppler OCT spatial resolution, allows very high resolution measurement of volumetric blood flow rates on the order of 10–100 pL/s. Notwithstanding the significant disparity in spatial resolution between ultrasound and OCT, the basic physics of the Doppler effect involving acoustic and electromagnetic waves is similar, and many of the signal processing techniques (hardware and software) used to estimate the Doppler shift ν_D are analogous. Moreover, because the evolution of Doppler ultrasound predated OCT by more than a decade, signal processing and data estimation algorithms developed for ultrasound represent a valuable resource for Doppler OCT.

8.1.3 Laser Doppler Flowmetry

In laser Doppler flowmetry (LDF), incident highly coherent light at a single optical frequency (ω) enters the tissue and is multiply scattered by static constituents and moving red blood cells (RBCs). A second fiber collects the backscattered light, a small fraction of which is Doppler shifted by moving RBCs; in comparison, light scattered exclusively by static constituents has little or no frequency change. Detection of the Doppler shift in LDF is founded on the heterodyne beating principle: shifted and nonshifted backscattered light amplitudes mix coherently on the surface of a photoreceiver to produce low frequency ($< 10\,\text{kHz}$) intensity fluctuations. Power spectra of the intensity fluctuations are a function of the RBC velocity distribution and concentration in the microcirculatory network. An LDF blood perfusion signal is given by the first moment of the computed power spectrum of measured intensity fluctuations. Because the LDF signal is due to multiply scattered light with a large variation of optical pathlengths in the tissue, spatial resolution is poor ($> 250\,\mu\text{m}$) and information relevant to bloodflow at discrete positions is lost.

Many investigators have reported experimental and theoretical investigations to improve the LDF spatial resolution and demonstrate application to clinical diagnostic problems. Stern at Johns Hopkins University completed a detailed analysis of Doppler-shifted and multiply scattered light using a Feynman path integral formalism [8]. Obeid et al. [9] reported a two-wavelength LDF system to improve depth discrimination of tissue blood flow. In this technique, two coherent light sources with spectral emission in the visible and infrared are coupled into a multimode optical fiber and incident at a single position on the tissue. Light backscattered from the tissue is collected in a receiving fiber, and the first moment of the power spectrum of measured intensity fluctuations is computed at each wavelength. Because longer wavelength light is scattered less strongly in tissue than the visible wavelengths, penetration is deeper and the near-infrared LDF signal measures RBC velocity over a deeper range of depths. Comparison of visible and near-infrared LDF signals allows coarse depth discrimination of microvascular blood flow. Various investigators have reported application of LDF imaging instruments to clinical diagnostic problems [10]. In LDF imaging instruments, light emitted from a coherent laser source is scanned over a region of interest on the tissue surface. At each beam position on the tissue surface, intensity of backscattered light is measured and the first moment of the power spectrum of intensity fluctuations is computed. A blood perfusion image is produced by displaying the first moment of the power spectrum at each pixel. Because lateral spatial resolution of LDF is limited by the scattering properties of the probed tissue volume, pixel ($250\,\mu\text{m}$) and image ($1–100\,\text{cm}^2$) sizes are relatively large.

8.2 DOPPLER OCT SYSTEM

We present a simple analysis of Doppler OCT by considering a turbid sample positioned in a Michelson interferometer. Spatially coherent light emitted from a source with broad spectral emission $[S_o(\omega)]$ is coupled into the interferometer and split into reference and sample paths. At the interferometer output, interference fringe intensity may be detected using a single-element photoreceiver or an optical spectrum analyzer. In systems that measure interference fringe intensity using a single-element photoreceiver, optical time delay ($\Delta\tau$) between light propagating in reference and sample paths is varied by using a delay line, and scanning of light in the turbid sample may be performed in two manners: (1) continuous scanning in depth followed by an incremental change in lateral position (longitudinal scanning) or (2) continuous scanning of lateral position followed by an incremental change in depth (lateral scanning). In scanning systems, interference fringe intensity is measured over a time delay approximately equal to the coherence time of source light (τ_c) to record position and velocity of static and moving constituents at a single pixel in the turbid sample; information at deeper positions is obtained by measuring fringe amplitude and phase at increased time delays ($\Delta\tau$). A potential practical advantage of measuring fringe intensity in the optical spectral domain is that the requirement for a delay line in the reference path is removed and the optical time delay is scanned electronically by computing the amplitude of various harmonics of corresponding spectral oscillations. Despite the potential advantages in measuring fringe amplitude in the optical spectral domain, fabrication constraints in the detector array readout architectures have hindered practical application of electronic delay line scanning systems.

8.2.1 Doppler OCT Signal

We calculate the Doppler signal current $i_d/(d)$ measured by a single-element photoreceiver (e.g., photodiode) by determining the correlation between light amplitudes in the reference and sample paths of the interferometer. When the sample contains moving constituents (e.g., RBCs), optical time delay ($\Delta\tau$) is due to scanning in the reference path ($\Delta\tau_s$) and possible delays due to Doppler motion of scattering centers parallel to the optical axis in the sample path ($\Delta\tau_D$). The amplitude of light emitted by the source and coupled into the interferometer $[U(t)]$ at time t is written as a harmonic superposition,

$$U(t) = \int_0^\infty \mathcal{U}(\omega)e^{i\omega t}d\omega \tag{1}$$

where $U(t)$ is a complex-valued analytic signal representing the field amplitude emitted by the light source; $\mathcal{U}(\omega)$ is the corresponding spectral amplitude at optical frequency ω. Cross-spectral density of $\mathcal{U}(\omega)$ satisfies

$$\langle \mathcal{U}^*(\omega)\mathcal{U}(\omega')\rangle = S_o(\omega)\delta(\omega - \omega') \tag{2}$$

here, $\langle * \rangle$ is a time average over various realizations of $\mathcal{U}(\omega)$; $S_o(\omega)$ is the optical source power spectral density in watts per hertz (W/Hz); and $\delta(\omega)$ is the Dirac delta function. Light emitted by the source is coupled into the interferometer and split equally into reference and sample spectral amplitudes, each denoted by $\mathcal{U}_o(\omega)$. After splitting, spectral amplitude of light in the reference path propagates forward to the delay line, is reflected, and is coupled back into the interferometer. After return to the 2 × 2 splitter, the reference spectral amplitude is

$$\mathcal{U}_r(\omega) = K_r e^{i\omega\Delta\tau_s}\mathcal{U}_o(\omega) \tag{3}$$

Here, $\Delta\tau_s$ is the variable delay time between light propagating in the sample and reference paths established by the scanning delay line; K_r is the amplitude reflection coefficient of light returning from the delay line. In writing Eq. (3), we have assumed that the delay line is dispersion-free and does not limit the source spectrum. After splitting, spectral amplitude of light in the interferometer sample path propagates forward to the turbid sample, is backscattered, and is coupled back to the splitter. After return to the 2 × 2 splitter, the sample spectral amplitude is

$$\mathcal{U}_s(\omega) = \mathcal{U}_o(\omega)\sum K_s(\Delta\tau_s)e^{i\omega\Delta\tau_D} \tag{4}$$

where the sum is taken over all backscattering centers in the sample. $K_s(\Delta\tau_s)$ is the complex amplitude reflection coefficient of light backscattered from a center position in the sample with time delay $\Delta\tau_s$ established by the delay line in the reference path (for simplicity we assume no spectral modulation of light propagating in the sample); when light backscatters from a moving particle, the phase of light in the sample path varies according to $\omega\Delta\tau_D$, where $\Delta\tau_D$ is the Doppler time delay of light backscattered from moving constituents. Using expressions for the spectral amplitude of light in the reference [Eq. (3)] and sample [Eq. (4)] paths, we derive the temporal coherence function [$\Gamma_{OCT}(\Delta\tau)$] for the interference fringe intensity. Combining harmonic expansions [Eq. (1)] for $\mathcal{U}_s(\omega)$ and $\mathcal{U}_r(\omega)$ and applying Eq. (2) when computing a time average, the temporal coherence function is

$$\Gamma_{OCT}(\Delta\tau = \Delta\tau_s - \Delta\tau_D) = \langle U_r(t + \Delta\tau)U_s^*(t)\rangle$$
$$= K_r\sum\int_0^\infty K_s^*(\Delta\tau_s)S_o(\omega)e^{i\omega(\Delta\tau_s - \Delta\tau_D)}d\omega \tag{5}$$

Because the Doppler signal current is the measured quantity of interest, we write the expression for i_d at time delay $\Delta\tau_s - \Delta\tau_D$ as

$$i_d(\Delta\tau = \Delta\tau_s - \Delta\tau_D) = 2\,\mathrm{Re}\left\{K_r\sum\int_0^\infty K_s^*(\Delta\tau_s)\right.$$
$$\left.\frac{e\eta(\omega)}{h\omega}S_o(\omega)\exp[i\omega(\Delta\tau_s - \Delta\tau_D)]\,d\omega\right\} \tag{6}$$

Here, $\eta(\omega)$ is the quantum efficiency of the detector and h is Planck's constant. When the sample is nondispersive, the source *photon* spectral density is Gaussian with center frequency ω_o and total power P_o, and the quantum efficiency (η) of the detector is constant over the source bandwidth, the Doppler signal is

$$i_d(\Delta\tau_s - \Delta\tau_D) \approx 4\pi K_r\frac{P_o e\eta(\omega_o)}{h\omega_o}$$
$$\sum|K_s(\Delta\tau_s)|\exp\left[-\left(\frac{\Delta\omega(\Delta\tau_s - \Delta\tau_D)}{4\sqrt{\ln 2}}\right)^2\right] \tag{7}$$
$$\cos\left[\frac{2\pi c(\Delta\tau_s - \Delta\tau_D)}{\lambda_o} + \varphi_s\right]$$

Here $\Delta\omega$ is the full width at half-maximum (FWHM) optical bandwidth of the source, and $\lambda_o = 2\pi c/\omega_o$ is the free-space wavelength, ϕ_s is the phase of the complex amplitude K_s. In Doppler OCT systems, the time delay $\Delta\tau_s$ is varied linearly in real time $[\Delta\tau_s = rt]$, and the Doppler delay $(\Delta\tau_D)$ introduced by backscattering from moving constituents is

$$\Delta\tau_D = 2\pi\nu_D t/\omega_o \tag{8}$$

where the Doppler shift ν_D is

$$\nu_D = \frac{1}{2\pi}(k_s - k_i)\cdot V \tag{9}$$

where k_s and k_i are wavevectors of backscattered and incident light, respectively, at the central optical frequency (ω_o) and V is the velocity of the moving constituents. The measured Doppler signal current is approximated by

$$i_d(t) \approx 4\pi K_r \frac{P_o e\eta(\omega_o)}{h\omega_o}$$

$$\times \sum |K_s(\Delta\tau_s)| \exp\left[\left(\frac{\Delta\omega(rt - \Delta\tau_s)}{4\sqrt{\ln 2}}\right)^2\right]\cos\left[\frac{2\pi}{\lambda_o}(cr)t - \nu_D t + \varphi_s(\Delta\tau_s)\right] \tag{10}$$

Because the incident and backscattered light may contain a variety of wavevectors at each optical frequency (ω), the Doppler shift (ν_D) does not have a single value but rather is represented by a distribution. For each backscattering center, uniform variation of time delay in the reference path gives a signal carrier frequency centered at $\nu_o = cr/\lambda_o$. Because the phase (ϕ_s) of the backscattering amplitude K_s is a function of the scanning delay $(\Delta\tau_s)$, speckle effects also influence the power spectrum of the Doppler signal. Effects of probe geometry on the distribution of Doppler shifts (ν_D) are discussed in Section 8.3.1. For a nonzero Doppler shift $(\nu_D \neq 0)$, a requirement is that $k_s - k_i$ must have a nonvanishing component along the velocity (V) of the scattering center. To determine the magnitude of the scattering center velocity $(|V|)$ from i_d, the relative orientation between vectors $k_s - k_i$ and V must be known. In systems that restrict direction of the incident and backscattered light so that $k_s = -k_i$, turbulent motion or spatial variation in the velocity of moving constituents, V, may be detected and creates a distribution of detected Doppler shifts. Doppler OCT of turbulent flow is discussed in Section 8.4.3.

8.2.2 Processing of Doppler OCT Signal

The detected Doppler signal current, $i_d(t)$, is measured by a single-element photo-receiver and input into a coherent detection system to measure the amplitude and phase of the interference fringe intensity. The Doppler shift (ν_D) at each scan position can be determined by computing the time-dependent power spectrum or spectrogram of the recorded interference fringe intensity. A spectrogram [11] is an estimate of the power spectrum of the interference fringe intensity in successive time segments $(t_i, t_i + \Delta t_p)$ and may be represented by a two-dimensional surface in the time–frequency plane containing the time-varying spectral properties of the Doppler signal current. To construct a spectrogram, the Fourier transform is applied to "short-time" (i.e., localized or windowed) segments of the Doppler signal current. Each local Fourier transform provides the spectral information for that particular time segment, and the window is then shifted to a slightly later time to generate another local spectrum. Following this approach, the properties of the signal can be simultaneously analyzed in the temporal and frequency domains. Although a number of algorithmic approaches can be used to estimate the spectrogram of a time-varying signal, a simple approach is to compute the fast Fourier transform (FFT) of the Doppler signal current $i_d(t)$ for each time delay interval. The value of the spectrogram [$S_d(t_i, v_j)$, Eq. (11)] at frequency v_j is given by the squared magnitude of the short-time fast Fourier transform (STFFT) of the Doppler signal current in the ith time-delay interval, $(t_i, t_i + \Delta t_p)$,

$$S_d(t_i, v_j) = \left| \text{STFFT}[i_d(t_i, t_i + \Delta t_p), v_j] \right|^2 \tag{11}$$

The gray-scale value at the ith pixel in a Doppler OCT structural image [$S_{\text{OCT}}(i)$, Eq. (12)] is given by the logarithm of the spectrogram value, $S_d(t_i, v_j)$, at the carrier frequency v_o established by the delay line in the reference path,

$$S_{\text{OCT}}(i) = 10 \log[S_d(t_i, v_o)] \tag{12}$$

The gray-scale value at the ith pixel in a Doppler OCT velocity image [$V_{\text{OCT}}(i)$, Eq. (13)] is given by the Doppler shift (v_D) of the recorded signal

$$V_{\text{OCT}}(i) = \frac{\lambda_o v_D}{2 n_m \cos \theta} = \frac{\lambda_o \left[\sum_j v_j S_d(t_i, v_j) \middle/ \sum_j S_d(t_i, v_j) - v_o \right]}{2 n_m \cos \theta} \tag{13}$$

We have assumed that $k_s = -k_i$ and that θ is the angle between k_i and V and n_m is the mean refractive index of the medium. Velocity resolution is dependent on pixel acquisition time (Δt_p) and the angle (θ) between flow velocity (V) and the incoming and backscattered light directions (k_s and k_i) in the turbid sample; velocity resolution may be improved by reducing the angle (θ) or increasing the pixel acquisition time (Δt_p). The detected velocity is color coded to indicate the magnitude and direction of flow and may be overlaid on the OCT structural image or displayed separately (see subsection on color coding of structure, flow, and variance).

A typical Doppler OCT depth scan (A-scan) is analyzed using a rectangular window (N points) shifted by a decimation factor (d points) along the entire A-scan (L points), resulting in k Doppler spectra, where

$$k = \frac{L - N}{d} \tag{14}$$

For typical parameters ($L = 512$, $N = 32$, and $d = 1$), k corresponds to 480 localized complex fast Fourier transforms per A-scan. Inasmuch as STFFT calculations are computationally intensive (e.g., the processing time for an image with 100 A-scans using a 266 MHz Pentium personal computer is approximately 10 s), real-time acquisition of Doppler OCT images is problematic. Improved algorithms for real-time processing of Doppler signals recorded in vivo are discussed in Sections 8.4.2–8.4.4.

Velocity Resolution and Frame Rate Limitations

The velocity resolution in Doppler OCT, defined as the minimum resolvable velocity, $V_s^{\min}$, is directly proportional to the minimum detectable Doppler shift given by

$v_s^{min} = 1/N\,\Delta t_s$, which is determined by the STFFT window size N and the sampling increment, Δt_s. Substituting v_s^{min} into Eq. (13) [12],

$$V_s^{min} = \frac{\lambda_o}{2n_m\,\cos(\theta)}\left(\frac{1}{N\,\Delta t_s}\right) \tag{15}$$

the velocity resolution can be expressed in terms of the image acquisition or frame rate R_f as [13,14]

$$V_s^{min} = \frac{\lambda_o}{2n_m\,\cos(\theta)}\left(\frac{KLR_f}{N\rho}\right) \tag{16}$$

where ρ is the axial scanning duty cycle and K is the number of A-scans per image with L pixels. For a given set of system parameters, an inverse relationship exists between the desired frame rate (R_f) and the minimum detectable velocity, V_s^{min}. Faster frame rates increase V_s^{min} and reduce Doppler velocity resolution; conversely, increasing precision of the velocity resolution requires a reduced frame rate.

The width of the Doppler spectrum and modulation by speckle in turbid media [ϕ_s in Eq. (10)] also give rise to a trade-off between the velocity estimation precision and frame rate [13,14]. In practice, precision of the estimated Doppler shift is also limited by the Doppler signal bandwidth Δv [14], which is proportional to the optical source spectral width $\Delta\omega$. Thus the practical velocity resolution, V_s^p, is worse than Eq. (16) and is given by the product of V_s^{min} and the number of frequency samples M ($2\,\Delta v\,ND/cL$) spanned by Δv:

$$V_s^p = MV_s^{min} \tag{17}$$

The velocity resolution limits, determined by Eq. (16), for typical design parameters ($\lambda = 1.3\,\mu m$, $n_m = 1.4$, $\theta = 45°$, $K = 100$, $L = 512$, $N = 32$, $\rho = 0.8$) are 0.13 mm/s at a slow image acquisition time of 10 s. High speed imaging (8 fps) results in a theoretical velocity resolution of 10.5 mm/s.

Color Coding of Structure, Flow and Variance

Two color coding formats for Doppler OCT have been reported. One format [14] is consistent with color Doppler ultrasound [15], in which backscatter amplitude is logarithmically assigned a gray-scale value [Eq. (12)], white indicating the highest reflectivity. Flow direction is encoded red or blue, and the flow magnitude is determined by the red or blue saturation. The Doppler velocity image [Eq. (13)] is thresholded to remove velocity noise and superimposed on the amplitude image [Eq. (12)], simultaneously delineating tissue microstructure and blood flow. In the literature, this format is referred to as color Doppler OCT (CD-OCT). A format that uses false color coding has also been used to display Doppler OCT images [16,17]. In this format, backscatter amplitude is displayed with red and green representing high and low backscatter amplitude, respectively. Flow is encoded in a separate image, with black indicating no flow and red indicating saturation proportional to blood flow velocity. In the literature, this format is referred to as optical Doppler tomography (ODT).

Turbulence (or more appropriately, depth-resolved spectral broadening) has been designated [18] (refer to Section 8.4.3) by using green to indicate regions of increased variance, with intensity indicating the extent of spectral broadening. In color Doppler ultrasound, increasing variance adds green to red or blue (producing yellow or cyan, respectively [19]). In work completed, Doppler OCT variance images are presented separately.

8.3 DOPPLER OCT OF IN VITRO SAMPLES

Early demonstration and development of Doppler OCT required testing and experimentation using samples in vitro. These studies and experiments improved our understanding of the effect of instrumentation parameters and optical properties of the media on the measured Doppler OCT signal. In this section we first describe results of a study using a Monte Carlo simulation of the light detection process in an OCT system to identify factors that affect the Doppler signal current, $i_d(t)$. Then we indicate some of the early imaging experiments completed using low speed (100–200 s/image) scanning systems that demonstrated the feasibility of using Doppler OCT to image flow in turbid media with optical properties similar to those of tissue.

8.3.1 Parameters Influencing Doppler Frequency Spectra

Better understanding of how instrumentation parameters and medium properties affect the Doppler signal current [$i_d(t)$] may be gained by Monte Carlo simulation of light propagation in the turbid medium under consideration. The results presented in this section are based on Monte Carlo simulations of an experiment involving an in vitro phantom, where blood flow is confined to a vessel submerged at a fixed depth and oriented parallel to the air/tissue interface in a scattering medium [20]. Simulated photons are launched from the probe in such a way that the numerical aperture is filled with a Gaussian intensity profile. The probe acts as a confocal detector, because the antenna theorem for a heterodyne receiver limits the effective size of an interferometric receiver to twice the diameter of a confocal detector [21,22]. This feature is implemented through the confocality angle δ. Intralipid was chosen as a model medium that could easily be used experimentally to verify predictions resulting from the Monte Carlo study. Both Intralipid and blood were modeled as homogeneous media, each characterized by three optical parameters: the absorption coefficient μ_a, the scattering coefficient μ_s, and the anisotropy parameter g. Based on limited available data at $\lambda = 850$ nm, the following optical parameters were chosen for 1% Intralipid: $\mu_a = 0$, $\mu_s = 2.0 \, \text{mm}^{-1}$, $g = 0.7$; and for blood: $\mu_a = 0.75 \, \text{mm}^{-1}$, $\mu_s = 150 \, \text{mm}^{-1}$, $g = 0.99$.

The geometric model representing the combined emission and detection probe of a fiber-optic Doppler OCT instrument is shown in Fig. 1. The probe is pointed at an incidence angle of α (typically 15°), and we simulate Doppler OCT measurements of blood flow in a vessel immersed at an axial depth of $z_o = 250 \, \mu$m in the scattering medium. The probe is aimed in the direction of point P on the z axis, but owing to refraction at the surface of the medium the focus is shifted to point P' at depth z', where $z' = cz$. The probe has a numerical aperture NA = $\sin \theta$, defined by the focusing lens L and the divergence of the light from the fiber core F. The surfaces S_1 and S_2 define the spherical wave fronts of the beam diverging from the fiber tip and being focused by the lens L to converge toward point P (in air). Photons that are backscattered from the turbid medium meet three criteria for detection: (1) They intersect the surface S_2 defined by the numerical aperture; (2) they deviate from normal

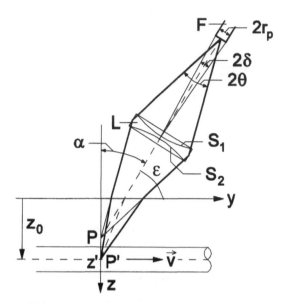

Figure 1 Geometry of Doppler OCT flow phantom for Monte Carlo simulations. A 100 μm diameter wall-less vessel is positioned horizontally in a 2% Intralipid solution at an axial depth of 250 μm. The y axis is taken to be parallel to the vessel axis. The probe is oriented at an incidence angle of α at various focus positions z' on the z axis through the center of the vessel lumen. Blood flow is assumed to have a parabolic velocity profile with on-axis velocity V_o.

incidence on S_2 by less than the confocality angle δ; and (3) they have a total optical path length that deviates by less than the source coherence length L_c from the nominal pathlength for a photon launched from S_2 and scattered from P' back to S_2 in a single backscattering event.

The Monte Carlo simulation consisted of propagating photons into the turbid medium while keeping an account of the accumulated pathlength in medium-equivalent physical distance units. Details of the sampling and phase function used in the simulation have been described [23]. At each scattering interaction with the moving medium in the vessel the resulting Doppler shift (Δ_k) was determined according to Eq. (9), $\Delta_k = \nu_D(k)$. The accumulated Doppler shift from all n_j scattering interactions in the medium was defined as the Doppler frequency, ν_D, of the detected photon:

$$\nu_D \equiv \nu_{Dj} = \sum_{k=1}^{n_j} \Delta_k \tag{18}$$

The average Doppler frequency for photons detected at each position in a longitudinal scan was computed as

$$\bar{\nu}_D \equiv \bar{\nu}_{D_i} = \frac{1}{n_i} \sum_{j=1}^{n_i} \nu_{D_j} \tag{19}$$

where n_i is the number of photons detected for each scan position.

The simulated geometry corresponds to an optical depth from the surface to the top of the vessel of 0.8 mean-free-path (mfp) unit in Intralipid ($g = 0.7$) and an additional optical depth in blood ($g = 0.99$), increasing to 15 mfp units through the full diameter of the vessel. To account for the nonvertical path, these values are multiplied by the factors 1.02 and 1.05 for incidence angles of 10.9° and 18° in the medium, corresponding to incidence angles of 15° and 25°, respectively in air. The final optical pathlengths of detected photons are actually twice the above values due to the round-trip path to the focus position and back to the detector. In the simulations, the number of photons detected was found to be nearly proportional to the source coherence length and the squares of numerical aperture and confocality angle.

Figure 2 shows average Doppler frequencies along a vertical scan through the vessel at its axis. The average Doppler frequency for photons detected from a particular focus position was determined with an accuracy of about 5% deviation from the mathematically expected Doppler frequency as shown by the middle panels in Fig. 2. This result is remarkable considering that the distributions of observed Doppler frequencies were quite broad, with standard deviations typically exceeding 250 Hz (top panels, filled symbols, Fig. 2), compared to the nominal Doppler frequencies of $\nu_D = 1212$ and $\nu_D = 1979$ Hz on the flow axis for $\alpha = 15°$ and 25° incidence angle. Evidently, the averaging of Doppler frequencies over many photons for each focus position represents such a robust estimation procedure that the resulting mean value quite accurately approximates the true frequency. The frequency profiles show the expected increase in maximum value with increasing incidence angle of the probe.

Standard deviations of Doppler frequencies measured within the vessel increase with increasing numerical aperture of the detector (Fig. 2, top panels, filled symbols). This can be explained by simple consideration of the variability in Doppler frequency shifts represented by backscattering events involving marginal rays at minimum and maximum angles with the flow axis, i.e., $(90° - \alpha - \theta)$ and $(90° - \alpha + \theta)$, respectively, giving rise to maximal and minimal Doppler frequencies with differences increasing with NA.

Standard deviations show a maximum around the center of the vessel and diminish away from the flow axis, suggesting a value proportional to the parabolic velocity profile within the vessel. This is evidenced by the precision profiles in the lower panels, which indicate that the coefficients of variance (CVs) are nearly independent of position along the cross section of the vessel. The lower CV for lower NA is apparent, and since the standard deviations show insignificant variation with increasing incidence angle, the CV decreases with increasing incidence angle due to increased mean Doppler frequency (lower right versus lower left panel). The precision of the estimated average Doppler frequency will therefore be considerably improved by using a low NA detection geometry. Results of the Monte Carlo simulations confirm that the precision (i.e., relative standard deviation) of the Doppler frequency on the flow axis will be best for large incidence angles and low numerical aperture.

Closer examination of the individual histories of photons backscattered from the central region of flow reveal that each photon experiences a series of stochastic Doppler shifts on the downward path through the vessel, a large positive Doppler shift upon backscattering, and a series of stochastic Doppler shifts on the upward path through the vessel. Figure 3 shows spectra of Doppler shifts from individual

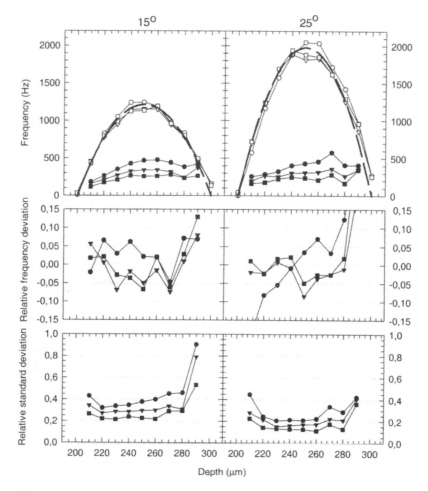

Figure 2 Upper panels, open symbols show Doppler frequency profiles along the z axis obtained from Monte Carlo simulations with the probe at incidence angles of 15° (left) and 25° (right). Data are shown for $L_c = 14\,\mu$m and $\delta = 0.5$°. Different symbols correspond to different numerical apertures: (○,●) NA = 0.4; (▽,▼) NA = 0.2; (□,■) NA = 0.1. The broken line shows the frequency profile determined by the parabolic velocity profile specified as part of the input data for the simulation. Filled symbols show standard deviations of simulated Doppler frequency spectra obtained for incidence angles of 15° (left) and 25° (right). Data are shown for $L_c = 28\,\mu$m and $\delta = 0.5$. Use of $L_c = 14\,\mu$m gave similar results but greater variability due to fewer detected photons. Middle panels show the accuracy of estimated mean Doppler frequencies expressed as relative differences between estimated and theoretical values from upper panels. Symbols indicate detector NA values as noted for upper panels. Lower panels show relative standard deviations (CVs) of estimated Doppler frequencies, i.e., standard deviations divided by mean values from upper panels. Symbols as before.

interactions (open circles) as well as the accumulated Doppler frequencies for detected photons (filled symbols). The bimodal distributions demonstrate the clear distinction between the pronounced Doppler shifts due to backscattering and many small, random Doppler shifts from individual forward-scattering events. The distinc-

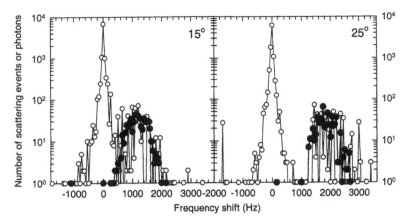

Figure 3 Distributions of Doppler shifts from individual interactions (○) and accumulated Doppler frequencies for photons (●) detected with the probe focus on the flow axis at 250 μm depth. Results are shown for probe incidence angles of 15° (left) and 25° (right). Other detection parameters were NA $= 0.2$, $L_c = 14\,\mu$m, and $\delta = 0.5°$. Detected photons had experienced an average of 18 and 20 scattering interactions for incidence angles of 15° and 25°, respectively.

tion between Doppler noise due to forward scattering in the flow region and the Doppler shift due to backscattering becomes even more pronounced as the probe incidence angle is increased from 15° (left panel) to 25° (right panel). The distributions of accumulated Doppler frequencies (filled symbols) approximate the distributions of backscattering Doppler shifts but show less variability.

8.3.2 Shadowing by Doppler Noise Below Flow Regions

Data from below the vessel (Fig. 4) show similar distributions for the two angles of incidence considered. Both Doppler shifts for individual interactions (open circles) and accumulated Doppler frequencies for detected photons (filled symbols) are distributed around zero, with similar widths for both incidence angles of the probe. The width corresponds to the Doppler noise contribution seen in spectra at positions on the flow axis (Fig. 3). If the individual Doppler shifts are assumed to be stochastically independent, their standard deviations, σ_Δ, can be used to express the standard deviation of accumulated Doppler frequencies, σ_D, as follows:

$$\sigma_D = \sqrt{\bar{m}_j}\sigma_\Delta \tag{20}$$

where $\bar{m}_j$ is the mean number of scattering interactions within the flowing medium for each photon. Estimates of $\bar{m}_j$ obtained by inserting pairs of values σ_Δ and σ_D for photons backscattered from below the vessel were found to be in good agreement with the expected number of interactions:

$$m_j = \int_S \mu_s\, ds = \frac{2\mu_s T}{\cos(\alpha')} \tag{21}$$

Here the integral is taken along the photon path, S, at an incidence angle of α' back and forth through the flowing medium of vertical thickness T.

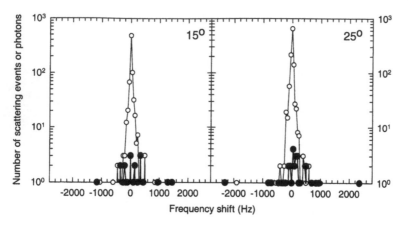

Figure 4 Distributions of Doppler shifts from individual interactions (○) and accumulated Doppler frequencies for photons (●) detected with the probe focus aimed below the vessel at 340 μm depth. Results are shown for probe incidence angles of 15° (left) and 25° (right). Other detection parameters were NA = 0.2, $L_c = 14\,\mu$m, and $\delta = 0.56$°. Detected photons had experienced an average of 34 and 36 scattering interactions for incidence angles of 15° and 25°, respectively.

The influence of some measurement parameters on the Doppler noise generated by multiple forward scattering of photons traversing a flow region can be deduced by a simple analysis based on the geometry in Fig. 5.

The Doppler shift resulting from a single interaction k for photon j when the probe is aimed at focus position i is

$$\Delta_{i,j,k} \equiv \Delta_k = \left(\frac{1}{2}\pi\right)(\boldsymbol{k}_s - \boldsymbol{k}_i) \cdot \boldsymbol{V} = \left(\frac{1}{2}\pi\right) 2kV \cos\alpha \sin\frac{\phi}{2}\cos\zeta,$$
$$k = 1, 2, 3, \ldots, m_j \tag{22}$$

where $\boldsymbol{V}$ is the velocity of the scattering center at the position under consideration and m_j is the number of scattering interactions in the flowing medium for photon j (as opposed to the total number of scattering events for photon j, n_j). The expected value, i.e., mean value, of Δ_k is $\langle\Delta_k\rangle = 0$, because the azimuthal angle ζ varies uniformly between 0 and 2π. The variance of Δ_k is

$$\text{Var}(\Delta_k) \equiv \sigma_\Delta^2 = \overline{[(\Delta_k - \overline{\Delta_k})^2]} = \overline{\Delta_k^2} = (kV\cos\alpha/\pi)^2 \overline{\left(\sin\frac{\phi}{2}\cos\zeta\right)^2}$$

The scattering angle is independent of the azimuthal angle, and the expectation values are therefore obtained as

$$\overline{\left(\sin\frac{\phi}{2}\cos\zeta\right)^2} = \overline{\left(\sin\frac{\phi}{2}\right)^2}\,\overline{(\cos\zeta)^2} = \frac{\overline{1 - \cos\phi}}{2}\left(\frac{1}{2}\right) = \frac{1 - g}{4}$$

Thus

$$\sigma_\Delta = \left(\frac{1}{2}\pi\right)kV(\cos\alpha')\sqrt{1 - g} \tag{23}$$

By combining Eqs. (20), (21), and (23) we obtain

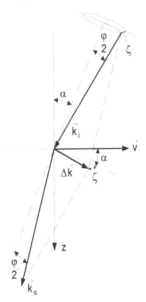

Figure 5   Vector diagram illustrating forward scattering according to Eq. (22).

$$\sigma_D = \left(\frac{1}{2\pi}\right)kV_{\text{ave}}\left[2(1-g)\cos(\alpha')\mu_s T\right]^{1/2} \tag{24}$$

where V_{ave} denotes the flow velocity averaged over the scattering locations along the photon path.

Theoretical values according to Eq. (24) were calculated for various flow conditions and plotted to show the correlation with corresponding Monte Carlo results. The fitted regression line in Fig. 6 indicates a proportionality relationship.[*] Although the data show reasonably good correlation, the proportionality constant (0.43) is quite different from the value of 1.0 that would be expected if Eq. (24) were a correct expression for the standard deviations of Doppler noise spectra for detected photons.

An explanation for systematically smaller observed standard deviations than predicted by Eq. (24) may be that Doppler OCT selectively detects photons that are extremely forward-scattered (apart from the backscattering event). Such selective detection of minimally scattered photons was observed in OCT Monte Carlo simulations [23]. If we define an effective anisotropy parameter $g_{\text{eff}} = \overline{\cos\varphi}$ for detected photons, a value of $g_{\text{eff}} = 0.998$ (as opposed to $g = 0.99$) inserted into Eq. (24) would yield theoretical standard deviations similar to those observed in the Monte Carlo experiments. The fact that values for the 2× diluted blood (filled triangles, Fig. 6) fall below the regression line might indicate that for less optical thickness ($\mu_s T$), forward-scattered photons are even more selectively detected and characterized by an even higher value for g_{eff}.

---

[*] This figure is equivalent to Fig. 11 in Lindmo et al. [20] except that $k' = nk$ was used instead of k in the present analysis, where $k' = 1.37k$

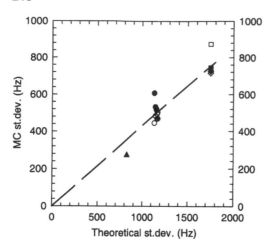

Figure 6 Correlation between theoretical values for standard deviations of Doppler noise from below the vessel according to Eq. (24) and corresponding results from Monte Carlo simulations. Open symbols represent NA = 0.2, filled symbols NA = 0.4. (○,●) Standard flow conditions (parabolic velocity profile with $V_o = 2$ mm/s) at $\alpha = 10–30°$ angles of incidence; (△,▲) standard flow of 2× diluted blood at 15° incidence angle; (◇,◆) 50% increased velocity under otherwise standard conditions ($V_o = 3$ mm/s); (□,■) flat velocity profile ($V_o = 2$ mm/s) using 15° incidence angle. The broken line through the origin is fitted to illustrate a proportionality relationship ($y = 0.43x$).

It is interesting to observe that the correlation between simulated and theoretical values in Fig. 6 is better for NA = 0.2 (open circles) than for NA = 0.4 (filled circles). In fact, in the analysis leading to Eq. (24), the numerical aperture of the probe was assumed to be vanishingly small, corresponding to photon paths close to the optical axis of the probe at incidence angle α. The results in Fig. 6 (filled versus open circles) suggest that there may be an effect on numerical aperture for large incidence angles that is not contained in Eq. (24).

The Monte Carlo simulation results are supported by experimental investigations. Figure 7 shows experimental Doppler signal power spectra representing regions above and below the vessel as well as at the center of the lumen in a geometry corresponding to Fig. 1. Power spectra representing backscattering from static Intralipid are distributed around the carrier frequency (1600 Hz) with mean values in the range 1560–1650 Hz, whereas spectra representing the center of the lumen are shifted to higher frequencies, more so for the larger angle of incidence (Fig. 7, right versus left). Standard deviations of the spectra above the vessel were 310 and 350 Hz for the incidence angles of $\alpha = 15°$ and 25°, respectively (dashed lines), whereas corresponding values for spectra below the vessel were 610 and 650 Hz (thick solid lines).

Standard deviations of experimental Doppler noise spectra recorded at positions below the vessel were thus greater than those of corresponding spectra above the vessel. Although several sources of noise contribute to the width of experimental Doppler signal power spectra, the increased standard deviations of spectra at positions below the vessel are taken to indicate Doppler broadening caused by the blood flow. In agreement with Monte Carlo results, standard deviations of experimental

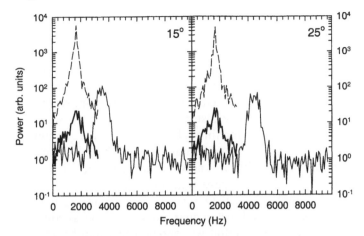

Figure 7 Experimental Doppler power spectra obtained at incidence angles of $\alpha = 15°$ (left) and $\alpha = 25°$ (right). Spectra were averaged over intervals ($\Delta z'$) of $100\,\mu$m (10 pixels) above (dotted lines) and below (thick, solid lines) the vessel, and over $40\,\mu$m at the center of the vessel (thin, solid lines).

Doppler noise spectra revealed no significant differences between values representing different probe incidence angles, despite the significantly higher Doppler frequencies from the flow region at larger incidence angles.

8.3.3 Imaging of in Vitro Samples

To demonstrate the ability of Doppler OCT using a STFFT spectrogram for simultaneous imaging of structure and flow in a scattering medium, images were recorded using in vitro models. In the first model, a polyethylene circular-cross-section conduit (inner diameter $580\,\mu$m) was submerged 1 mm below the surface of a scattering phantom (0.25% Intralipid solution). Polymer microspheres (diameter $2\,\mu$m) suspended in deionized water were used to simulate a biological fluid. A microsphere suspension (3.5×10^8 particles/cm^3) was infused through the conduit at constant velocity by a linear syringe pump.

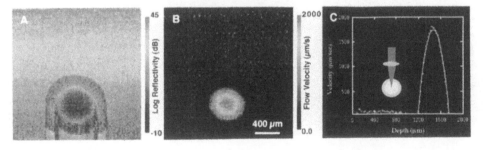

Figure 8 Doppler OCT images of microspheres in a conduit submerged 1 mm below the surface in a turbid sample. (A) Structural image of static microspheres; (B) velocity image of flowing microspheres; (C) velocity profile along a vertical line passing through the center of conduit. (See color plate.)

In Doppler OCT structural images (Fig. 8A, see color plate), backscattered light intensity from the phantom is color coded with red and green representing high and low reflectivity, respectively. The color change from red at the surface to green at the bottom indicates strong attenuation of the probe beam by the phantom. In the Doppler velocity image (Fig. 8B), static regions in the conduit appear dark ($V = 0$), and the presence of beads moving at different velocities is evident. Microspheres near the center of the conduit are observed to move faster than those near the wall. A velocity profile taken from a vertical line passing through the center of the conduit is shown in Fig. 8C, where the open circles are experimental data and the solid line is a theoretical fit assuming laminar flow with a known inner conduit diameter. Agreement between theory and experiment suggests that flow is laminar.

In a second in vitro model, application of Doppler OCT for imaging microstructure and mapping flow profile in a small rectangular cross section glass conduit (lumen size $1000\,\mu m \times 100\,\mu m$). The glass conduit was submerged 1 mm below the surface of a highly scattering 1% Intralipid solution. OCT structural (Fig. 9A) and Doppler velocity (Fig. 9B) images were obtained when a suspension of 1% Intralipid was infused through the conduit at constant velocity by a linear syringe pump (see color plate). Although scattering from 1% Intralipid is high ($\mu_s = 23\,cm^{-1}$) and the conduit was invisible to the unaided eye when viewed from the top surface of the phantom, both the conduit and flowing Intralipid are observed in OCT structural and Doppler velocity images, respectively.

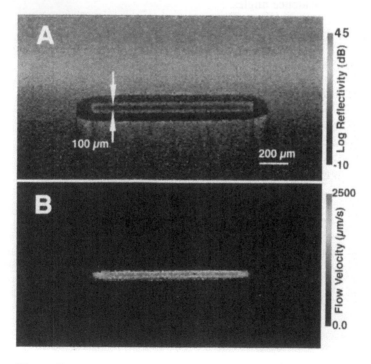

Figure 9 (A) OCT structural and (B) Doppler velocity images of flowing Intralipid in a rectangular glass conduit with inner dimensions of $100\,\mu m \times 2000\,\mu m$ submerged 1 mm below the surface in a turbid sample of Intralipid. The arrows indicate the inner conduit dimension. (See color plate.)

8.4 DOPPLER OCT BIOMEDICAL APPLICATIONS

The noninvasive nature and exceptionally high spatial resolution of Doppler OCT have distinct applications in the clinical management of patients in whom blood flow monitoring is essential. For example, with Doppler OCT it is possible to

> Obtain an in situ three-dimensional tomographic image and velocity profiles of blood perfusion in tissue at discrete spatial locations in either the superficial or deep layers.
>
> Determine burn depth; provide guidance regarding the optimal depth for burn debridement prior to definitive closure.
>
> Determine tissue perfusion and viability immediately after injury, wound closure, replantation, or transposition of either rotational or free skin flaps.
>
> Evaluate the vascular status of a buried muscle flap covered by a split thickness skin graft; perfusion in the superficial and deeper flap components can be monitored separately.
>
> Distinguish between arterial or venous occlusion and determine the presence and/or extent of adjacent posttraumatic arterial or venous vascular injury by providing in situ tomographic image and velocity profile of blood flow.
>
> Monitor the effects of pharmacological intervention on the microcirculation (e.g., effects of vasoactive compounds or inflammatory mediators); determine transcutaneous drug penetration kinetics; evaluate the potency of penetration enhancers, irritation of chemical compounds, patch-test allergens, and ultraviolet radiation; compare the reactivity of the skin microcirculation in different age and ethnic groups.

In human tissue, an important issue is the volume of tissue that may be interrogated and imaged using Doppler OCT. We describe two clinical entities designed to demonstrate how Doppler OCT can assist in the optimal management of patients where imaging blood flow in the skin's most superficial layers (1–2 mm) is important: (1) port wine stain (PWS)—the evaluation of laser therapy efficacy—and (2) superficial basal cell carcinoma—monitoring intratumoral blood flow during photodynamic therapy (PDT).

8.4.1 Port Wine Stain

Port wine stain (PWS) is a congenital, progressive vascular malformation of the dermis; although PWS may occur anywhere on the body, most lesions appear on the face and neck. The pulsed dye laser can selectively coagulate PWS by inducing microthrombus formation within the targeted blood vessels. However, only a small proportion of patients obtain 100% fading of their PWS, even after undergoing multiple laser treatments. Histopathological studies of PWS show an abnormal plexus of layers of dilated blood vessels located 150–750 μm below the skin surface in the upper dermis. These vessels have diameters varying on an individual patient basis and even from site to site on the same patient, over a range of 10–150 μm. Barton et al. [24] reported application of Doppler OCT to investigate the relationship between irreversible photocoagulation of subsurface blood vessels and incident laser dosimetry (dose, pulse duration, and wavelength). Although these studies were completed using an in vivo animal model, application of Doppler OCT to provide a fast semiquantitative evaluation of the efficacy of laser therapy in real time appears feasible.

8.4.2 Superficial Basal Cell Carcinoma—Monitoring Intratumoral Blood Flow During Photodynamic Therapy

Superficial basal cell carcinoma (SBCC) is a malignant tumor arising from the basal cells at the epidermal-dermal junction located 50–500 μm deep in the skin and is by far the most common form of skin cancer; in the United States 400,000–500,000 new cases are diagnosed each year. Existing treatments for these lesions include surgery, curettage with desiccation, and radiation, all of which may leave highly disfiguring scars. In recent years, photodynamic therapy (PDT) has been proposed as a treatment modality that may offer more cosmetically appealing results. Previous basic science studies have attempted to elucidate the mechanism of PDT-induced tumor destruction. Stoppage of tumor blood flow shortly after the initiation of PDT treatment has been demonstrated and also that complete cessation of tumor circulation was required to effect its complete eradication. Noncurative treatments frequently result in resumption of intratumoral blood flow. Taken together, these studies suggest that the vascular compartment represents an important target and that the progress of PDT could potentially be followed by monitoring intratumoral blood flow.

The rationale for using Doppler OCT in the clinical management of SBCC is that the technique offers a means of following the progress of PDT by monitoring intratumoral blood flow in real time. It is expected that blood flow reduction from preirradiation levels as measured by Doppler OCT will be proportional to the total light dosage delivered. At low total light dosage, there are relatively minor effects on the tumor vasculature; after the laser is turned off, reperfusion leads to a return in blood flow to preirradiation levels. Alternatively, high total light dosage effectively destroys the tumor vasculature, leading to complete and permanent reduction in blood flow. In this case, blood flow approaches zero during laser irradiation, and after the laser is turned off there is no return to preirradiation values observed with Doppler OCT. A correlation of tumor necrosis as a function of total light dosage can then be made.

The potential application of Doppler OCT for in vivo blood flow monitoring during photodynamic therapy (PDT) was investigated in the rodent mesentery. Twenty minutes after injection of a 2 mg/kg solution of benzoporphyrin derivative (BPD) through the rodent tail vein, the effect of laser irradiation ($\lambda = 690$ nm, $D = 12$ J/cm^2, and $t_L = 120$ s) on mesenteric blood flow was studied. Doppler OCT images recorded before (Fig. 10A) and 16 min (Fig. 10B) and 71 min (Fig. 10C) after laser irradiation were obtained.

Sixteen minutes following laser irradiation, the diameter of the rodent artery had decreased from 320 μm to 60 μm; 71 min after laser irradiation, the diameter of the artery was 385 μm. As expected and as described by other investigators [25], the artery went into vasospasm after laser exposure. Subsequently, in response to PDT-induced tissue hypoxia, compensatory vasodilation occurs within 1 h of laser irradiation.

Although these results suggest that the application of Doppler OCT to clinical problems of interest is feasible, the processing used to construct these images is based

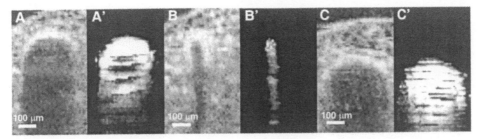

Figure 10 (A) OCT structural and (A′) Doppler velocity images of rodent artery prior to laser irradiation. (B) OCT structural and (B′) Doppler velocity images of rodent artery 16 min after laser irradiation. (C) OCT structural and (C′) Doppler velocity images of rodent artery 71 min after laser irradiation.

on the spectrogram using an STFFT. Because the STFFT is computationally intensive, alternative approaches are required to obtain Doppler OCT imaging in real time.

8.4.3 Alternative Implementations of the Short-Time Fourier Transform

To integrate Doppler OCT with clinical systems, processing must be performed rapidly, generating several flow images per second. Hardware methods for time–frequency analysis are desirable, because these implementations allow faster processing and analysis. This section describes alternative implementations for performing the short-time Fourier transform (STFT), allowing near-real-time acquisition of Doppler OCT images.

Filterbank Approach

As shown schematically in Fig. 11, the STFT can alternatively be implemented as the output of a filterbank [26]. Rather than measuring a spectrum for each window centered at time t_i, the spectrogram can be formed by measuring the temporal response at each frequency v_i. Because the analysis window behaves as a low-pass filter [27], modulating it by $\exp(-j2\pi v_0 n \, \Delta t_s)$ results in a frequency-shifted version, or a bandpass filter (BPF). The summation in the STFFT may be viewed as a convolution summation between the Doppler signal and a BPF centered at frequency v_o:

$$S_d(n \, \Delta t_s, v_o) = i_d(n \, \Delta t_s) \otimes w(n \, \Delta t_s) \exp(-j2\pi v_o n \, \Delta t_s) \tag{25}$$

If several BPFs are employed, then the Doppler frequency at a given time can be taken as the center frequency of the BPF whose output contains the highest energy relative to all other filters [28].

Parallel Demodulation Approach

Alternatively, the filterbank approach to the STFT can be implemented by parallel demodulation [26,28,29] (i.e., demodulating at several frequencies concomitantly). In Eq. (25) grouping the exponential term with the Doppler signal current results in

$$S_d(n \, \Delta t_s, v_o) = [\exp(j2\pi v_o n \, \Delta t_s)][i_d(n \, \Delta t_s) \exp(-j2\pi v_o n \, \Delta t_s) \otimes w(n \, \Delta t_s)] \tag{26}$$

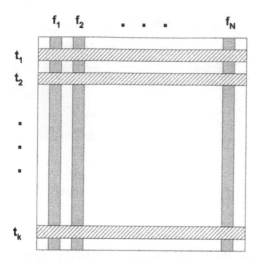

Figure 11 A spectrogram can be implemented vertically or horizontally: by obtaining spectral information at times t_1, t_2, etc. or by arranging temporal information at frequencies f_1, f_2, etc. Currently, a velocity estimate in Doppler OCT is the centroid of the spectrum at some time t_i. Alternatively, the local velocity can be estimated by selecting the filter f_i that has the highest relative energy at that given time (depth).

Here the STFT is a convolution between the modulated detector current and the analysis window, or the operation performed by a quadrature detector at a single frequency. The output is then modulated by $\exp(j2\pi v_o v \Delta t_s)$. For Doppler OCT, this final step can be disregarded, because synthesis (reconstruction of the signal from the STFT) is not necessary and the amplitude is not altered by this omission. Hence, it has been demonstrated that time–frequency analysis in Doppler OCT can be implemented with parallel demodulation electronics. The output of each of the detection channels is nearly instantaneous, allowing real-time implementation of Doppler OCT. Hardware techniques avoid time-consuming computation of fast Fourier transforms used in Doppler processing of images presented above.

Time Domain Autocorrelation Implementation

The Wiener–Khinchin theorem relates the power spectral density of a wide-sense stationary process to its autocorrelation via the Fourier transform:

$$R(\tau) = \int_{-\infty}^{\infty} P(v)e^{i2\pi v\tau}\, dv \tag{27}$$

The center frequency, given by

$$\bar{v} = \frac{\int_{-\infty}^{\infty} v P(v)\, dv}{\int_{-\infty}^{\infty} P(v)\, dv} \tag{28}$$

can thus be directly calculated using the signal autocorrelation

$$\bar{v} = -i\frac{\dot{R}(\tau)}{R(\tau)}\bigg|_{\tau=0} \tag{29}$$

where $\dot{R}(\tau)$ is the derivative of $R(\tau)$ with respect to τ. Because the autocorrelation is typically calculated using a fast Fourier transform algorithm, direct calculation of Eq. (29) may be time-consuming. To simplify the computation, the autocorrelation can be evaluated in terms of the amplitude and phase. Define

$$R(\tau) \equiv A(\tau)e^{i\phi(\tau)} \tag{30}$$

and

$$\dot{R}(\tau) = \left[\dot{A}(\tau) + iA(\tau)\dot{\phi}(\tau)\right]e^{i\phi(\tau)} \tag{31}$$

Equation (29) can now be estimated by taking the derivative of the phase of the autocorrelation [14]:

$$\bar{v} = \dot{\phi}(0) \approx \frac{\phi(T) - \phi(0)}{T} = \frac{\phi(T)}{T} \tag{32}$$

where T is the time delay of the detected signal. Implemented in software, the autocorrelation technique reduces computation time by greater than tenfold.

Experiments to detect flow in an Intralipid phantom in real time using a variation of the autocorrelation technique was recently implemented in hardware [18] as described schematically in Fig. 12. A high dynamic range limiter removes the amplitude dependence of the interferogram, which is then low-pass filtered and split into two paths. One of these paths is electronically delayed with respect to the other by a time τ. A phase detector then measures the difference in phase between the

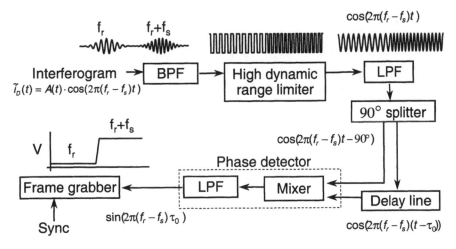

Figure 12 Flow diagram of real-time Doppler OCT using autocorrelation implementation. The interferogram is bandpass filtered (BFP) to reduce noise, then input into a high dynamic range limiter, which removes the envelope, or amplitude dependence, of the Doppler signal. A low-pass filter (LPF) then removes the higher harmonics introduced by the limiter. The signal is split into two paths, one of which is electronically delayed with respect to the other. The two paths are multiplied and low-pass filtered, thus implementing the autocorrelation in hardware. Because the enevolpe has been removed, this process results in a sinusoidal function of the phase of the autocorrelation, which is related to the sample arm Doppler frequency by Eq. (34).

signals from the two paths. The output of the phase detector (i.e., the autocorrelation) is a sinusoidal function of the phase difference between the two paths, given by

$$\tilde{R}(\tau) = \sin[2\pi(v_r + v_s)\tau] \tag{33}$$

which is, equivalently, the autocorrelation of the detector current without the envelope.

By choosing v_r and τ appropriately such that $\tilde{R}(\tau) = 0$ when $v_s = 0$, the autocorrelation reduces to

$$\tilde{R}(\tau) = \sin(2\pi v_s \tau) \tag{34}$$

Therefore, because v_s is related to flow velocity, positive values of the autocorrelation encode flow in one direction, and negative values encode flow in the other direction (Fig. 13). Implemented in hardware, this technique was used to measure flows representative of larger blood vessels at 6 fps [18].

8.4.4 Perfusion and Turbulent Flow Characterization

In Sections 8.3.1 and 8.3.2, multiple scattering of light was observed to broaden the Doppler signal power spectra. When direction of the incident and backscattered light is constrained so that $k_s = -k_i$, turbulent motion or spatial variation in the velocity of moving constituents, V, creates a distribution of detected Doppler frequencies characteristic of the sample under investigation. Turbulent flow, although generally not present in the micrometer-scale vasculature, also leads to Doppler broadening. In this case an estimate of local tissue perfusion or turbulent flow, spectral broad-

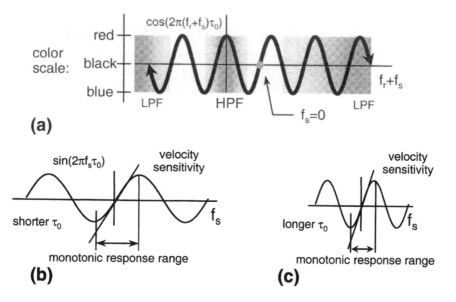

Figure 13 (a) Sinusoidal output of phase detector in Fig. 12, chosen such that zero Doppler shift in the sample corresponds to zero output. Positive and negative Doppler shifts are then represented by red and blue, respectively. (b) Choosing a shorter time delay results in a longer monotonic response range but lower velocity sensitivity. (c) A longer delay improves the sensitivity, but over a smaller response range.

ening can be measured by using the variance of the spectrum. The variance of the local spectrum $S(n\,\Delta t_s, v)$ for an N-point STFT window is given by

$$\sigma^2(n\,\Delta t_s) = \frac{\sum_{i=-N/2}^{i=+N/2}[v_i - \bar{v}(n\,\Delta t_s)]^2 S_d(n\,\Delta t_s, v_i)}{\sum_{i=-N/2}^{i=+N/2} S_d(n\,\Delta t_s, v_i)} \qquad (35)$$

where

$$\bar{v}(n\,\Delta t_s) = \frac{\sum_{i=-N/2}^{i=+N/2} v_i S_d(n\,\Delta t_s, v_i)}{\sum_{i=-N/2}^{i=+N/2} S_d(n\,\Delta t_s, v_i)} \qquad (36)$$

is the corresponding centroid used in the Doppler OCT images.

Spectral broadening was measured [30] in depth-resolved backscattered spectra in the cardiovascular system of a stage 51 [31] *Xenopus laevis* tadpole, shown in Fig. 14 (see color plate). The images were processed using the STFT algorithm described in Section 8.2.2. On the left are velocity images during systole and diastole, and on the right are the corresponding variance images. Note that in the velocity images, motion on the ventricular tissue induced Doppler shifts in the sample arm that were detected using Doppler OCT. This artifactual signal, referred to as clutter [15], is also observed in clinical Doppler ultrasonography. Motion of the ventricle is uniform and thus is not composed of large velocity gradients that lead to spectral broadening. However, blood flow in the ventricle, atrium, and truncus arteriosus contains sufficient velocity gradients to generate uncorrelated random shifts of light backscattered

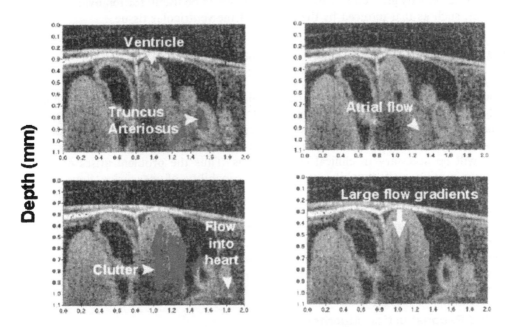

Figure 14 Comparison of velocity (left) and variance (right) images in a stage 51 *Xenopus* tadpole heart [13] during systole (top) and diastole (bottom). Motion of the ventricle induces a uniform Doppler shift that generates cluttered images. Variance images eliminate clutter by identifying regions containing large flow gradients, such as within the ventricle, atrium, and truncus arteriosus. (See color plate.)

from these regions, broadening the Doppler spectrum considerably. Variance within these regions exceeds that induced by the ventricular wall.

In addition to detecting the center Doppler frequency of the signal spectrum, the autocorrelation formulation can be used to approximate the variance of the spectrum as a measure of turbulence in the flow [14]. The variance is given by

$$\sigma^2 = \frac{\int_{-\infty}^{\infty}(v - \bar{v})^2 P(v)\,dv}{\int_{-\infty}^{\infty} P(v)\,dv} = \overline{v^2} - \bar{v}^2 \tag{37}$$

Here, the second derivative of the autocorrelation is also necessary, because

$$\sigma^2 = \left(\frac{\dot{R}(0)}{R(0)}\right)^2 - \frac{\ddot{R}(0)}{R(0)} \tag{38}$$

which can be approximated by

$$\sigma^2 \approx \frac{2}{T^2}\left(1 - \frac{|R(\tau)|}{R(0)}\right) \tag{39}$$

Within the sampling volume of the STFT window, a distribution of scatterers with various velocity vectors (i.e., a velocity gradient within the window) will lead to Doppler broadening of the measured frequency spectrum. Quantification of broadening is particularly useful for estimating tissue perfusion when the dimensions of the vessels are smaller than the dimensions of the STFT window. Depth-resolved spectral broadening was used in Fig. 14 to distinguish regions of the *Xenopus* ventricle with large velocity gradients. This technique may also be useful for removal of image clutter, such as that induced by the motion of the ventricular tissue.

8.4.5 High Precision Velocity Image Reconstruction in Periodic Flows

The minimum resolvable velocity in Doppler OCT is proportional to the image acquisition rate [13,14,17,32]. Images must be acquired relatively slowly ($\gg 1$ s/image) in order to obtain high velocity resolution (< 0.5 mm/s). This prevents imaging of dynamic structures due to motion artifact in living subjects, a task that will be necessary in clinical environments. Thus the problem arises of overcoming motion artifact while retaining the capability of measuring flow in the microcirculation, where velocities approaching the resolution of Doppler OCT may be encountered. In this section, a technique is presented for motion artifact–free reconstruction of flow [13] in a beating *Xenopus* heart. This technique is illustrated with reconstructed Doppler OCT frames displaying the dynamics of the cardiovascular system simultaneously with high velocity resolution Doppler flow mapping. Movies arranged from the reconstructed frames have been published and are available for viewing on-line [13].

Gated Reconstruction Algorithm

With the sample beam incident on the ventral side of each specimen, oblique (45° from sagittal to coronal) sections of the beating heart were acquired with Doppler OCT and analyzed for flow. The heartbeat of the specimen was measured under a microscope, using OCT "optical cardiograms" [33]. Reconstruction of the beating heart was performed by obtaining a 1000 A-scan OCT image that was oversampled in the lateral direction, ensuring that at least five A-scans were acquired per heartbeat while the sample was translated laterally by one focused sample probe beam spot size (14 μm). From this image, separate time-gated cardiac image frames were extracted. Each of the frames was composed of A-scans occurring at the same segment of the cardiac cycle. Therefore, if the number of A-scans per beat was T, sequential frames were composed of $1000/T$ lateral pixels each. Gating of the image data according to the heartbeat was performed by estimating the value of T retrospectively, by selecting that value that completely eliminated motion artifact in the reconstructed frames.

Reconstruction of Cardiac Flow Dynamics

An OCT image through the ventral surface of the specimen is shown in Fig. 15. Although stationary structures are clearly delineated in the OCT image, the motion artifact, indicated by alternating dark and light vertical bands in the center of the image, blurs the image data within the pericardium. The general shape of the heart is apparent, but large structures such as the distinct chambers are not resolvable.

Figure 16 isolates a selected smaller time segment from the OCT image in Fig. 15, demonstrating the repetitive expansion and contraction of the heart that result in motion artifact. This figure illustrates that each heart beat (measured between consecutive and diastolic dimensions) comprised approximately five A-scans. Therefore,

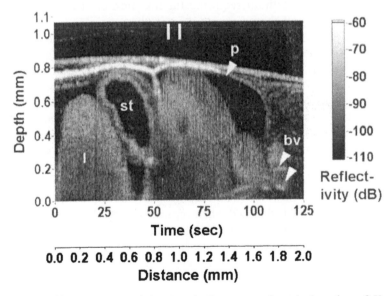

Figure 15 Oblique (45° from sagittal to coronal) optical section of *Xenopus* heart through ventral surface of body. The abscissa is the equivalent time of acquisition for the image. This image is composed of 1000 lateral and 256 axial pixels, spanning 2.0 mm across and 1.07 mm deep (assuming a mean index of refraction of 1.4). Whereas some structures are visible with high resolution, image clarity is drastically reduced in moving structures (i.e., heart and diaphragm). White bars indicate the region magnified in Fig. 14. st, stomach; l, liver; p, pericardium; bv, branched vessels.

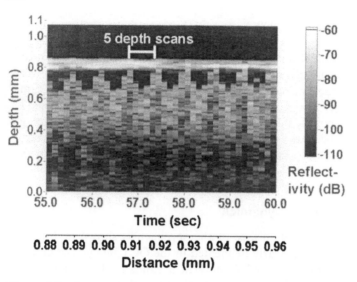

Figure 16 A-scans extracted from Fig. 15 between the vertical white bars within the ventricle. One period of the cardiac cycle required exactly five ($T = 5.00 \pm 0.01$) A-scans.

approximately every fifth A-scan was recorded at the same segment of the cardiac cycle, during which the sample beam was translated laterally 10 μm, less than one focused sample probe beam spot size. This reconstruction method effectively imitates heart beat gated image acquisition without requiring the insertion of electrodes or otherwise independent monitoring of the heart rate.

Figure 17 (see color plate) is a gated Doppler OCT reconstruction of the beating *Xenopus* heart performed using the five sequential time frames extracted from Fig. 15. Using optical cardiograms it was determined that the heart rate was 1.6 beats/s and the number of A-scans per beat $T = 5.00 \pm 0.01$. Color Doppler flow processing was performed solely on the region of interest indicated by the rectangle enclosing the counterpropagating vessels. The appearance of flow in each vessel during the cardiac cycle correlates to its corresponding role in systole or diastole. The contraction of the heart during systole is followed immediately by maximum pulsatile flow in the truncus arteriosus. Also, flow into the heart through the vein occurs preceding and during expansion of the ventricle (diastole). Owing to its pulsatile nature, flow within the truncus arteriosus appears briefly; however, flow through the vein is detected for a longer duration, because blood flow is damped when returning to the heart.

Motion of the vessel walls also results in Doppler shifts in the backscattered light in addition to flow within the truncus arteriosus. In Fig. 17, the upper region of the arterial wall expands during systole, generating negative (blue) Doppler shifts that can be misinterpreted as flow.

This technique requires no additional hardware with current Doppler OCT instrumentation. Because gating assumes that the dynamic process under analysis is periodic throughout acquisition of the image, a potential use for this reconstruction algorithm is for measurement of flow in clinical environments, in which periodic, pulsatile flow is commonly encountered, such as flow in large retinal vessels. Gated reconstruction diminishes motion artifact yet preserves velocity resolution in Doppler OCT.

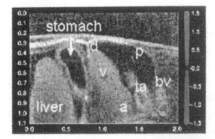 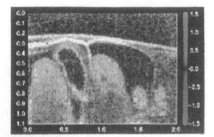

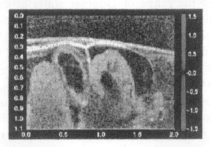

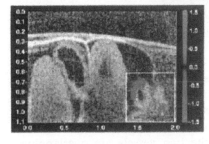 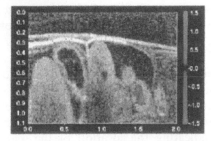

Figure 17 Reconstruction of a beating *Xenopus* heart using the frame gating technique. Doppler processing is restricted to the region indicated by a rectangle. v, ventricle; a, atrium; ta, truncus arteriosus; p, pericardium; bv, branched vessels; d, diaphragm. The highly pulsatile flow of the truncus arteriosus appears only in the frame immediately after ventricular ejection. Meanwhile, flow through the branched vessels is observed in several frames due to its damped nature. (See color plate.)

8.4.6 Applications in Ophthalmology

Evaluation of ocular hemodynamics is a challenging task whose performance has only recently become feasible with the advent of noninvasive and minimally invasive clinical tools. Although the exact effect of ocular disorders on blood flow is unclear, clinicians have noted vascular anomalies that are associated with several pathologies, including diabetic retinopathy, age-related muscular degeneration, glaucoma, and neurogenic optic atrophy [34]. Quantification of blood flow at discrete spatial locations in the retina may lead to a better understanding of the progression and treatment of these disorders.

System Implementation for Retinal Doppler OCT

For retinal imaging, the incident power on the cornea was less than $300\,\mu$W, well within the maximum permissible exposure standards [35]. The sample arm, shown in

Fig. 18, contained a standard slit lamp apparatus modified for viewing of the fundus simultaneously with OCT imaging. A CCD camera sensitive to low intensity and NIR light was used to determine the exact scan location of the fundus during Doppler OCT imaging. Transverse scanning of the OCT beam along the retina was performed using an XY-scanning galvanometric pair, enabling scans in any arbitrary linear or circular direction. The interferometric detector signal was coherently demodulated at the Doppler frequency ν_r induced by the motion of the reference arm (78 kHz). The resulting signal was low-pass filtered at 20 kHz cutoff frequency, encompassing the range of Doppler shifts arising from blood flow in the retinal vessels. Dilation of the pupil was not necessary for these measurements.

To eliminate motion artifact, a registration algorithm [30] was used to align all A-scans. In this algorithm, it was determined at which pixel in the A-scan the backscattered amplitude is above a selected threshold, interactively chosen to isolate the surface of the retina. A profile of the retinal surface is obtained by tracking, as a function of transverse position, the index of the first axial pixel exceeding this threshold. An example of the unregistered profile of the retinal surface is shown in Fig. 17. Assuming that the high frequency components result from motion artifact and the low frequency components represent the topography of the retina, the raw profile was low-pass filtered (5 cycles/image) to indicate the desired profile. Each A-scan is shifted to align with the filtered profile of the retinal surface [36].

Human Retinal Vessels

Retinal imaging of structure and blood flow was performed in the undilated human eye. Figure 19 (see color plate) presents an in vivo Doppler OCT image capable of resolving sub-100 μm diameter vessels within the retina. The conventional amplitude image clearly delineates several layers within the posterior eye. A fundus photograph indicating the location of the scan shows that the two vessels are overlapping. Nevertheless, Doppler OCT can distinguish Doppler shifts arising from the individual vessels.

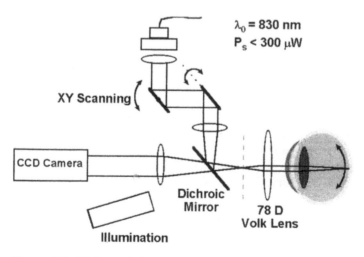

Figure 18 Light path in Doppler OCT sample arm for retinal imaging. P_s, sample arm power; λ_0, source center wavelength.

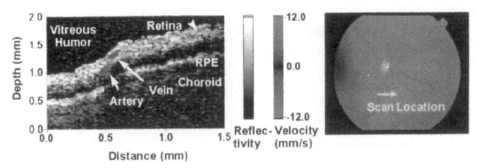

Figure 19 In vivo retinal Doppler OCT image (2048 axial by 100 lateral pixels, acquired in 10 s) of bidirectional flow in the human retina. The axial dimensions indicate the optical depth. Doppler OCT is able to distinguish various layers of tissue as well as quantify blood flow magnitude and direction. A fundus photograph (right) indicates that the linear scan was inferior to the optic nerve head. (See color plate.)

Figure 20 (see color plate) illustrates the effect of motion artifact on retinal imaging of structure and flow. Motion artifact appears in the unprocessed image as oscillations and discontinuities of the retinal surface. For example, the retinal pigmented epithelium (RPE) does not maintain its contiguity throughout the image. These artifactual features are superimposed on the natural retinal curvature, which is a more subtle variation as a function of transverse position. The registered image using the algorithm described earlier eliminates the motion artifact while maintaining the inherent topography of the retina. Figure 21 contains profiles of the retinal

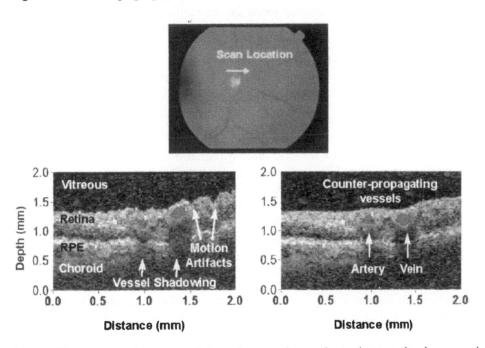

Figure 20 Linear DOCT scan of the retina superior to the optic nerve head, comparing images before (left) and after (right) removal of motion artifact using A-scan registration. Fundus photograph (top) indicates location of image. (See color plate.)

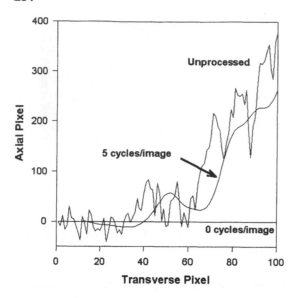

Figure 21 Retinal surface profile before and after correction of motion artifact. Note that if all oscillations are removed (i.e., low-pass cutoff of 0 cycle/image) the processing will flatten the retinal profile.

surface, corresponding to the images in Fig. 20 before and after removal of motion artifact. The unprocessed profile contains low frequency terms attributed to the true topography as well as high frequency terms due to motion artifact. Filtering of the unprocessed profile at 5 cycles/image results in a smooth retinal profile. Another registration algorithm for retinal imaging has also been suggested using a cross-correlation technique [37]. However, this technique fails in regions of the image where the RPE is not visible due to shadowing under vessels. Shadowing beneath the vessels is due to the increased scattering coefficient of blood [36] compared to the surrounding retinal tissue.

Discussion

Doppler OCT was applied for the first time to retinal flow mapping in the human eye. Quantification of retinal flow may have implications for better understanding of ocular hemodynamics and its role in several ocular disorders. Doppler OCT is the first technique to determine, with micrometer-scale resolution, the depth and diameter of vessels within the retina. In addition, this technique is capable of quantifying flow magnitude and direction simultaneously with imaging of the microanatomy of the posterior eye. Unlike fluorescein angiography, Doppler OCT is entirely non-invasive and does not require dilation of the pupil. Furthermore, Doppler OCT operates at longer wavelengths than laser Doppler velocimetry, so light exposure times can be safely increased [32]. In conclusion, Doppler OCT is a viable method for quantification of blood flow within the retina. This imaging technique is able to provide information that is unavailable or uncertain with other methods, such as LDV, fluorescein angiography, or color Doppler ultrasound. Doppler OCT is capable of imaging retinal structure and vasculature beyond the resolution of other techniques, without the need for pupil dilation. Blood flow speeds up to several millimeters per second were identified in sub-100 μm vessels in the retina. Several layers in the posterior eye were clearly delineated, localizing retinal vessels within specific regions of the posterior eye. Accurate knowledge of retinal hemodynamics may prove helpful in understanding several ocular diseases, including diabetic retinopathy, glaucoma, and age-related macular degeneration.

REFERENCES

1. Riva C, Ross B, Benedek G. Laser Doppler measurements of blood flow in capillary tubes and retinal arteries. Invest Ophthalmol 11:936, 1972.
2. Tanaka T, Riva C, Ben-Sira B. Blood velocity measurements in human retinal vessels. Science 186(4166):830–831, 1974.
3. Tanaka T, Benedek GB. Measurement of the velocity of blood flow (in vivo) using a fiber optic catheter and optical mixing spectroscopy. Appl Opt 14:189, 1975.
4. Stern MD. In vivo evaluation of microcirculation by coherent light scattering. Nature (Lond) 254:56, 1975.
5. Meggit BT, Boyle WJO, Grattan KTV, Palmer AW, Ning YN. Fibre optic anemometry using an optical delay cavity technique. Proc SPIE 1314:321–326, 1990.
6. Wang X-J, Milner TE, Nelson JS, Fluid Flow velocity characterization using optical Doppler tomography. Opt. Lett 20:1337–9, 1995.
7. Angelsen BAJ. Waves, Signals and Signal Processing in Medical Ultrasonics, Vols 1 and 2. Trondheim: Norwegian Inst Sci Technol, Dept Physiol Biomed Eng, 1996.
8. Stern MD. Laser Doppler velocimetry in blood and multiply scattering fluids: Theory. Appl Opt 24:1968–1986, 1985.
9. Obeid AN, Bogget DM, Barnett NJ, Dougherty G, Rolfe P. Depth discrimination in laser Doppler skin blood flow measurements using different lasers. Med Biol Eng Comput 26:415–419, 1988.
10. Essex TJH, Byrne PO. A laser Doppler scanner for imaging blood flow in skin. J Biomed Eng 13:190–194, 1991.
11. Hlawatsch H, Boudreaux-Bartels. Linear and quadratic time-frequency signal representations. IEEE Signal Process Mag 9:21–67, 1992.
12. Izatt JA, Kulkarni MD, Yazdanfar S, Barton JK, Welch AJ. In vivo bidirectional color Doppler flow imaging of picoliter blood volumes using optical coherence tomography. Opt Lett 22:1439–1441, 1997.
13. Yazdanfar S, Kulkarni MD, Izatt JA. High resolution imaging of in vivo cardiac dynamics using color Doppler optical coherence tomography. Opt Express 1:424–431, 1997; www.osa.org.
14. Kulkarni MD, v. Leeuwen TG, Yazdanfar S, Izatt JA. Velocity estimation accuracy and frame rate limitations in color Doppler optical coherence tomography. Opt Lett 23:1057–1059, 1998.
15. Kremkaul FW. Principles and pitfalls of real-time color flow imaging. In: Vascular Diagnosis. 4th ed. EF Bernstein, ed. Mosby Year Book, 1993.
16. Chen Z, Milner TE, Dave D, Nelson JS. Optical Doppler tomographic imaging of fluid flow velocity in highly scattering media. Opt Lett 22:64–66, 1997.
17. Chen Z, Milner TE, Srinivas S, Wang X, Malekafzali A, van Gemert MJC, Nelson JS. Noninvasive imaging of in vivo blood flow velocity using optical Doppler tomography. Opt Lett 22:1119–1121, 1997.
18. Rollins AM, Yazdanfar S, Ung-arunyawee R, Izatt JA. Real time color Doppler optical coherence tomography using an autocorrelation technique. Proc SPIE 3598, San Jose, CA, 1999.

19. Kasai C, Namekawa K, Koyano A, Omoto R. Real-time two-dimensional blood flow imaging using an autocorrelation technique. IEEE Trans Sonics Ultrasonics SU-32:458–464, 1985.

20. Lindmo T, Smithies DJ, Chen Z, Nelson JS, Milner TE. Accuracy and noise in optical Doppler tomography studied by Monte Carlo simulation. Phys Med Biol 43:3045–3064, 1998.

21. Siegman AE. The antenna properties of optical heterodyne receivers. Appl Opt 5:1588–1594, 1966.

22. Schmitt JM, Knüttel A, Yadlowsky M. Interferometric versus confocal techniques for imaging microstructures in turbid biological media. SPIE Proc 2135:251–262, 1994.

23. Smithies DJ, Lindmo T, Chen Z, Nelson JS, Milner TE. Signal attenuation and localization in optical coherence tomography studied by Monte Carlo simulation. Phys Med Biol 43:3025–3044, 1998.

24. Barton JK, Welch AJ, Izatt JA. Investigating pulsed dye laser–blood vessel interaction with color Doppler optical coherence tomography. Opt Express 3:251–256, 1998; www.osa.org.

25. Fingar VH, Wieman TJ, Wiehle SA, Cerrito PB. The role of microvascular damage in photodynamic therapy: The effect of treatment on vessel constriction, permeability, and leukocyte adhesion. Cancer Res 52:4914–4921, 1992.

26. Nawab SH, Quatieri TF. Short-time Fourier transform. In: Advanced Topics in Signal Processing. JS Lim, AV Oppenheim, eds. Englewood Cliffs, NJ: Prentice-Hall, 1989, pp 289–327.

27. Oppenheim AV, Schafer RW. Discrete-Time Signal Processing. Englewood Cliffs, NJ: Prentice-Hall, 1989.

28. Yazdanfar S. High resolution in vivo blood flow imaging using color Doppler optical coherence tomography. MS Thesis, Department of Biomedical Engineering, Case Western Reserve Univ, 1998.

29. van Leeuwen TG, Kulkarni MD, Yazdanfar S, Rollins AM, Izatt JA. High flow velocity imaging using color Doppler optical coherence tomography. Adv Opt Imag Photon Migration 21:364–366, 1998.

30. Yazdanfar S, Rollins AM, Izatt JA. In vivo imaging of blood flow in human retinal vessels using color Doppler optical coherence tomography. Proc SPIE 3598, San Jose, 1999.

31. Nieuwkoop PD, Faber J. Normal Table of Xenopus laevis (Daudin). New York: Garland, 1994.

32. Izatt JA, Kulkarni MD, Yazdanfar S, Barton JK, Welch AJ. In vivo bidirectional color Doppler flow imaging of picoliter blood volumes using optical coherence tomography. Opt Lett 22:1439–1441, 1997.

33. Boppart SA, Tearney GJ, Bouma BE, Southern JF, Brezinski ME, Fujimoto JG. Noninvasive assessment of the developing Xenopus cardiovascular system using optical coherence tomography. Proc Natl Acad Sci USA 94:4256–4261, 1997.

34. Alm A. Ocular circulation. In: Adler's Physiology of the Eye: Clinical Application. 9th ed. JWM Hart, ed. St. Louis, MO: Mosby Year Book, Inc, 1992.

35. ANSI. Safe Use of Lasers. ANSIZ136.1. New York: Am Nat Stand Inst, 1993.

36. Roggan A, Friebel M, Dorschel K, Hahn A, Muller G. Optical properties of circulating human blood in the wavelength range 400–2500 nm. J Biomed Opt 4:36–46, 1999.

37. Swanson EA, Izatt JA, Hee MR, Huang D, Lin CP, Schuman JS, Puliafito CA, Fujimoto JG. In vivo retinal imaging by optical coherence tomography. Opt Lett 18:1864–1866, 1993.

9

Polarization-Sensitive Optical Coherence Tomography

JOHANNES F. DE BOER*, **SHYAM M. SRINIVAS, and J. STUART NELSON**

University of California at Irvine, Irvine, California

THOMAS E. MILNER and MATHIEU G. DUCROS

University of Texas at Austin, Austin, Texas

9.1 INTRODUCTION

9.1.1 OCT and Polarization-Sensitive OCT

In the previous chapters, light was treated as a scalar wave. However, light is described by a transverse electromagnetic wave that is markedly different from a longitudinal wave such as sound. The extra degrees of freedom due to the transverse character are described by the polarization state of light. Polarization-sensitive OCT (PS-OCT) uses the information carried by the polarization state to extract extra information from the sample under study. PS-OCT provides high resolution spatial information on the polarization state of light reflected from tissue that is not discernible using existing diagnostic optical methods. This chapter will be devoted to PS-OCT and its application in biomedical imaging.

9.1.2 Optical Properties of Tissue That Influence Polarization

Two mechanisms dominate the changes in the polarization state of light propagating through biological tissue: scattering and birefringence. Scattering changes the polarization of light mainly in a random manner, as will be demonstrated by the following examples. Let us assume circular polarized light incident on an isotropic scatterer (i.e., a spherical particle much smaller than the wavelength). The forward-scattered

---

Current affiliation: Harvard Medical School and Wellman Laboratories of Photomedicine, Massachusetts General Hospital, Boston, Massachusetts

light has the same circular polarization state, but the helicity of the backscattered light is reversed, and light scattered at an angle of 90° from the incident direction is linearly polarized. This example illustrates that a single scattering event can dramatically scramble the incident polarization state. As particle size increases (the scattering becomes more anisotropic), the incident polarization is preserved better [1]. For linearly polarized light, the incident polarization is better preserved by isotropic scattering than by anisotropic scattering [1–3]. For spherical particles and cylinders, exact solutions to the Maxwell equations can be computed by Mie theory [4]. For nonspherical particles, Mishchenko and Hovenier [5] calculated the polarization scrambling, concluding that the difference in polarization scrambling of circularly and linearly polarized light cannot be considered a universal measure of the departure of particle shape from that of a sphere. As the light scatters multiple times, the scrambling effect of single scattering events accumulates, until finally, the polarization state is completely random (i.e., not correlated with the incident polarization state). Assuming a random orientation and arbitrary shape of scattering structures in tissue, the polarization state will be changed in a random manner.

One exception is organized linear structures, such as fibrous tissues, that can exhibit birefringence. Birefringence changes the polarization state of light by a difference (Δn) in the refractive index for light polarized along, and perpendicular to, the optic axis of a material. The difference in refractive index introduces a phase retardation, δ, between orthogonal light components that is proportional to the distance x traveled through the birefringent medium,

$$\delta = \frac{2\pi \, \Delta n \, x}{\lambda} \qquad (1)$$

Birefringence in biological tissues can have two components: Form birefringence results from ordered linear structures surrounded by a ground substance with a different refractive index [6]; intrinsic birefringence results from molecules with different optical retardance arranged in an ordered configuration. Birefringence changes the polarization state in a predictable manner, described by, for instance, the Mueller or Jones matrix of a linear retarder. Many biological tissues, such as tendons, muscle, nerve, bone, cartilage and teeth, exhibit birefringence. The advantage of PS-OCT is the enhanced contrast and specificity in identifying structures in OCT images by detecting induced changes in the polarization state of light reflected from the sample. Moreover, changes in birefringence may, for instance, indicate changes in functionality, structure, or viability of tissues.

9.2 THEORY

9.2.1 Historical Overview

The emphasis in optical coherence tomography (OCT) has been on the reconstruction of two-dimensional maps of changes in tissue reflectivity, and the polarization state of light was of minor importance. However, in 1992, Hee et al. [7] reported the first OCT system able to measure the changes in the polarization state of light reflected from a sample. They demonstrated birefringence-sensitive ranging in a wave plate, an electro-optic modulator, and calf coronary artery. In 1997, the first two-dimensional images of birefringence in bovine tendon were presented, and the effect of laser-induced thermal damage on the birefringence of collagen was demonstrated [8], followed in 1998 by a demonstration of the birefringence in porcine myocardium [9]. To date, polarization-sensitive OCT measurements have attracted active interest from several research groups.

9.2.2 Experimental Configuration

The theory of PS-OCT will be offered based on the experimental configuration first presented by Hee et al. [7]. Figure 1 shows a schematic of this PS-OCT system, which was used for all images presented in this chapter except for Figs 9–12. Light with a short coherence length passes through a polarizer P to select a pure linear horizontal input state and is split into reference and sample arms by a polarization-insensitive beamsplitter (BS). Light in the reference arm passes through a zero-order quarter-wave plate (QWP) oriented at a 22.5° angle to the incident horizontal polarization. Following reflection from a mirror or retroreflector and a return pass through the QWP, light in the reference arm has a linear polarization at a 45° angle with respect to the horizontal. Light in the sample arm passes through a QWP oriented at a 45° angle to the incident horizontal polarization and through focusing optics, producing circularly polarized light incident on the sample. Reflected light from the sample, in an arbitrary (elliptical) polarization state determined by the optical properties of the sample, returns through the focusing optics and the QWP. After recombination in the detection arm, the light is split into its horizontal and vertical components by a polarizing beamsplitter (PBS) and focused on pinholes or single-mode fibers to detect a single polarization state and spatial mode.

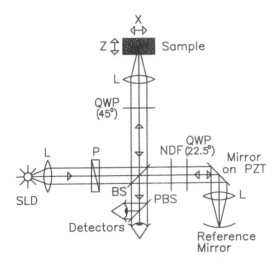

Figure 1 Schematic of the PS-OCT system. SLD: superluminescent diode, 0.8 mW output power, central wavelength $\lambda = 856$ nm, and spectral FWHM $\Delta\lambda = 25$ nm. L, lens; P, polarizer; BS, beamsplitter; QWP, quarter-wave plate; NDF, neutral density filter; PBS, polarizing beamsplitter; PZT, piezoelectric transducer. Two-dimensional images were formed by either axial movement of the sample with constant velocity $v = 1$ mm/s (z direction), repeated after each $10\,\mu$m lateral displacement (x direction), or lateral movement of the sample with constant velocity $v = 1$ mm/s (x direction), repeated after each $10\,\mu$m axial displacement (z direction). The latter allows for focus tracking in the sample.

Two-dimensional images can be formed by lateral or axial movement of the sample at constant velocity v, repeated after each axial or lateral displacement, respectively. The carrier or interference fringe frequency can be generated by axial movement of the sample or the reference mirror, by translating the reference mirror mounted on the piezoelectric transducer over a few wavelengths, or by a combination of both. Transverse and axial image resolutions are determined by, respectively, the beam waist at the focal point and the coherence length of the source.

9.2.3 Jones Matrix Formalism

The polarization state in each arm of the interferometer is computed using the Jones matrix formalism. The intensity detected in each polarization channel can be described by a two-dimensional intensity vector **I**, where the two components describe the horizontal (x) and vertical (y) polarized intensities, respectively. The intensities at the detectors are given by

$$\langle \mathbf{I}(\Delta z) \rangle = \langle \mathbf{I}_r \rangle + \langle \mathbf{I}_s \rangle + \left\langle \begin{matrix} E_{rx}^* E_{sx}(\Delta z) \\ E_{ry}^* E_{sy}(\Delta z) \end{matrix} \right\rangle + \left\langle \begin{matrix} E_{rx} E_{sx}^*(\Delta z) \\ E_{ry} E_{sy}^*(\Delta z) \end{matrix} \right\rangle \tag{2}$$

where E, E^* are the electric field component and its complex conjugate, Δz is the pathlength difference between the two arms of the interferometer, and subscripts r and s denote the reference and sample arms, respectively. The angular brackets denote time averaging. The last two terms of Eq. (2) correspond to the interference between reference and sample arm light. After the polarizer, horizontally polarized source light is described by the Jones vector,

$$\mathbf{E}(z) = E(z) \begin{pmatrix} 1 \\ 0 \end{pmatrix} \tag{3}$$

In our analysis, the electric field amplitude is represented by a complex analytic function $E(z)$ [10], with

$$E(z) = \int \tilde{e}(k) \exp(-ikz)\, dk \tag{4}$$

where $\tilde{e}(k)$ is the field amplitude as a function of free-space wavenumber $k = 2\pi/\lambda$ with

$$\tilde{e}(k) = 0 \qquad \text{if } k < 0 \tag{5}$$

From the Wiener–Khinchin theorem, it follows that

$$\langle \tilde{e}(k)\tilde{e}(k') \rangle = S(k)\delta(k - k') \tag{6}$$

which defines $\tilde{e}(k)$ in terms of the source power spectral density $S(k)$. The beam-splitter splits the light evenly between both arms of the interferometer, and the Jones vector describing the light that enters the sample and reference arm is given by

$$\mathbf{E}_{si}(z) = \mathbf{E}_{ri}(z) = \frac{E(z)}{\sqrt{2}} \begin{pmatrix} 1 \\ 0 \end{pmatrix} \tag{7}$$

First, the polarization state of light reflected from the reference arm is calculated. The Jones matrix for a QWP with fast and slow axes aligned along the horizontal and vertical axes is given by

$$\mathbf{QWP} = \begin{pmatrix} e^{i\pi/4} & 0 \\ 0 & e^{-i\pi/4} \end{pmatrix} \tag{8}$$

A QWP with its fast optic axis at an angle ϕ with the horizontal is found by applying a rotation to the Jones matrix in Eq. (8), $\mathbf{QWP}(\phi) = \mathbf{R}(\phi)\mathbf{QWP}\,\mathbf{R}(-\phi)$, with $\mathbf{R}(\phi)$ given by

$$\mathbf{R}(\phi) = \begin{pmatrix} \cos\phi & -\sin\phi \\ \sin\phi & \cos\phi \end{pmatrix} \tag{9}$$

The polarization state of light reflected from the reference into the detection arm is given by

$$\mathbf{E}_r(z_r) = \mathbf{R}(22.5) \cdot (\mathbf{QWP})^2 \cdot \mathbf{R}(-22.5) \cdot \mathbf{E}_{ri} = \frac{1}{2}E(2z_r)\begin{pmatrix} 1 \\ 1 \end{pmatrix} \tag{10}$$

which describes a linear polarization state at an angle of $45°$ with the horizontal. The horizontal and vertical components of the electric field have equal amplitude and phase. To calculate the polarization state of light reflected from the sample arm, we assume that the optical properties of the sample can be described by a homogeneous linear retarder with a constant orientation of the optic axis. The Jones matrix of the sample, $\mathbf{B}(z, \Delta n, \alpha)$, is written as a product of average phase delay in the sample, rotation matrices, and the Jones matrix of a linear retarder with the fast axis along the horizontal,

$$\mathbf{B}(z, \Delta n, \alpha) = e^{-ikz\bar{n}}\mathbf{R}(\alpha)\begin{pmatrix} e^{ikz\Delta n/2} & 0 \\ 0 & e^{-ikz\Delta n/2} \end{pmatrix}\mathbf{R}(-\alpha) \tag{11}$$

where $kz\bar{n}$ is the average phase delay of a wave propagating to depth z and $\bar{n}$ is the average refractive index along the fast (n_f) and slow (n_s) optic axes, $\bar{n} = (n_f + n_s)/2$. $\Delta n = n_s - n_f$ is the difference in refractive index along the fast and slow axes, and α is the angle of the fast axis with the horizontal. The single-pass retardation δ for the Jones matrix $\mathbf{B}(z, \Delta n, \alpha)$ is $\delta = kz\,\Delta n$. The Jones vector of the light reflected from the sample arm is given by the product of the optical elements in the sample arm and the incident field vector,

$$\mathbf{E}_s(z_s + z) = \mathbf{QWP}(45) \cdot \mathbf{B}(z, \Delta n, \alpha) \cdot \sqrt{R(z)} \cdot \mathbf{B}(z, \Delta n, \alpha) \cdot \mathbf{QWP}(-45) \cdot \mathbf{E}_{si}$$

$$\propto \sqrt{R(z)} \int \tilde{e}(k)\exp[-2ik(z_s + z\bar{n})]\begin{pmatrix} e^{2i\alpha}\sin(kz\,\Delta n) \\ \cos(kz\,\Delta n) \end{pmatrix} dk \tag{12}$$

where $R(z)$ is a scalar that describes the reflectivity at depth z and the attenuation of the coherent beam by scattering, and z_s is the optical pathlength of the arm up to the sample surface. Using the Wiener–Khinchin theorem [Eq. (6)], the interference terms in the horizontally and vertically polarized channels are given by, respectively,

$$A_H(z, \Delta z) = E_{rx}^*E_{sx} + E_{rx}E_{sx}^* \propto \sqrt{R(z)}\int \sin(kz\,\Delta n)\cos(2k\,\Delta z + 2\alpha)S(k)\,dk$$

$$A_V(z, \Delta z) = E_{ry}^*E_{sy} + E_{ry}E_{sy}^* \propto \sqrt{R(z)}\int \cos(kz\,\Delta n)\cos(2k\,\Delta z)S(k)\,dk \tag{13}$$

with z the depth in the tissue and Δz the optical path length difference between sample and reference arms, $\Delta z = z_r - z_s - z\bar{n}$. A Gaussian power spectral density is assumed for the source:

$$S(k) \propto \exp\left[-\left(\frac{k-k_0}{\kappa}\right)^2\right] \tag{14}$$

with the FWHM spectral bandwidth of the source given by $\kappa 2\sqrt{\ln 2}$. The integration over k in Eq. (13) can be performed analytically, and in the approximation that $\kappa z \Delta n \ll 1$, the expressions simplify to

$$A_H(z, \Delta z) \propto \sqrt{R(z)} \sin(k_0 z \Delta n) \cos(2k_0 \Delta z + 2\alpha) \exp\left[-(\Delta z/\Delta l)^2\right]$$

$$A_V(z, \Delta z) \propto \sqrt{R(z)} \cos(k_0 z \Delta n) \cos(2k_0 \Delta z) \exp\left[-(\Delta z/\Delta l)^2\right] \tag{15}$$

with the FWHM of the interference fringes envelope given by $\Delta l 2\sqrt{\ln 2}$, where

$$\Delta l = \frac{1}{\kappa} = \frac{\lambda_0^2 \sqrt{\ln 2}}{\pi \Delta \lambda} \tag{16}$$

and $\Delta \lambda$ is the spectral FWHM of the source in wavelength. The terms in Eqs. (15) for the interference fringe intensities in the horizontal and vertical channels describe the reflected amplitude at depth z, the slow oscillation due to the birefringence $k_0 z \Delta n$, the Doppler shift or carrier frequency generated by the variation of the optical pathlength difference between sample and reference arms, and the interference fringes envelope, respectively. The spatial resolution is determined by the width Δl of the interference fringe envelope. Using Eq. (16), the condition $\kappa z \Delta n \ll 1$ is reformulated as $z \Delta n \ll \Delta l$, which can be interpreted as a condition that the optical pathlength difference between light polarized along the fast and slow optic axes of the sample should be smaller than the coherence length of the source [8]. If the phase retardation $\delta = kz \Delta n$ is assumed independent of the wavelength, i.e., $\delta = k_0 z \Delta n$, the integration in Eq. (13) results directly in Eq. (15) without the condition $z \Delta n \ll \Delta l$ [11]. The angle α of the optic axis of the sample with the horizontal introduces a phase shift between the fringes in the horizontally and vertically polarized channels. In the next sections, this phase shift will be used to extract more information about the exact polarization state of light reflected from the sample.

A_H and A_V are proportional to the light field amplitudes reflected from the sample. Demodulation of the signal eliminates the $\cos(2k_0 \Delta z)$ term in Eqs. (15). After demodulation, the intensity reflected from the sample in the horizontal and vertical polarization channels is proportional to

$$I_H(z) = |A_H(z)|^2 \propto R(z) \sin^2(k_0 z \Delta n)$$

$$I_V(z) = |A_V(z)|^2 \propto R(z) \cos^2(k_0 z \Delta n) \tag{17}$$

The total reflected intensity I_T, as a function of depth is given by

$$I_T(z) = I_H(z) + I_V(z) \propto R(z) \tag{18}$$

and the phase retardation as a function of depth is given by

$$\varphi(z) = \arctan\left[\left(\frac{I_V(z)}{I_H(z)}\right)^{1/2}\right] = k_0 z \,\Delta n \tag{19}$$

Gray-scale-coded OCT and PS-OCT images will be shown side by side, representing the logarithm (base 10) of the total reflected intensity $I_T(z)$ and the phase retardation $\varphi(z)$, respectively. Figure 2 shows OCT and PS-OCT images of mouse muscle. The banded structure in the PS-OCT image clearly demonstrates the presence of birefringence. The limitation of the Jones formalism and the presented detection scheme thus far is the inability to describe or detect the effects of polarization-dependent cross sections (dichroism) or to determine the degree of polarization of the reflected light. In the next sections an analysis based on the Stokes vector formalism is presented that will be able to address these issues.

9.2.4 Stokes Vector and Coherence Matrix Formalism

The Stokes vector is composed of four parameters—I, Q, U, and V (sometimes denoted s_0, s_1, s_2, and s_3)—and provides a complete description of the light polarization state. I, Q, U, and V can be measured with a photodetector and linear and circular polarizers. Let us call I_t the total light irradiance incident on the detector and $I_{0°}$, $I_{90°}$, $I_{+45°}$, and $I_{-45°}$ the irradiances transmitted by a linear polarizer at an angle of, respectively, $0°$, $90°$, $+45°$, and $-45°$ to the horizontal. Let us define also I_{rc} and I_{lc} as the irradiances transmitted by a circular polarizer opaque to, respectively, left and right circularly polarized light. Then the Stokes parameters are defined by

$$I = I_t, \qquad Q = (I_{0°} - I_{90°}), \qquad U = (I_{+45°} - I_{-45°}) \qquad V = (I_{rc} - I_{lc}) \tag{20}$$

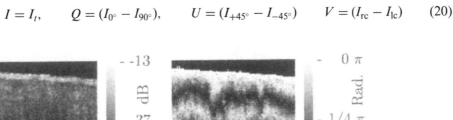

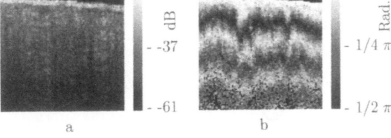

Figure 2 Images of mouse muscle 1 mm wide by 1 mm deep, constructed from the same measurement. (a) Reflection image generated by computing $10\log[I_T(z)]$. The gray scale to the right specifies the signal magnitude. (b) Birefringence image generated by computing the phase retardation φ according to Eq. (19). The gray scale at the right specifies the phase retardation. The banded structure, indicative of birefringence, is clearly visible. Each pixel represents a $10\,\mu m \times 10\,\mu m$ area. (Reprinted from Ref. 12 with permission of the Optical Society of America.)

After normalizing the Stokes parameters on the irradiance I, Q describes the amount of light polarized along the horizontal ($Q = +1$) or vertical ($Q = -1$) axes, U describes the amount of light polarized along the $+45°$ ($U = +1$) or $-45°$ ($U = -1$) directions, and V describes the amount of right ($V = +1$) or left ($V = -1$) circularly polarized light. Figure 3 shows the definition of the normalized Stokes parameters with respect to a right-handed coordinate system, where we have adopted the definition of a right-handed vibration ellipse (positive V parameter) for a clockwise rotation as viewed by an observer who is looking toward the light source. Positive rotation angles are defined as counterclockwise rotations. For practical reasons the Stokes vector is sometimes represented in the Poincaré sphere system [13], where it is defined as the vector between the origin of an x,y,z coordinate system and the point defined by (Q, U, V). The ensemble of normalized Stokes vectors with the same degree of polarization defines a sphere whose radius varies between 0 for natural light and 1 for totally polarized light.

For a well-collimated, uniform, quasi-monochromatic light beam propagating in the z direction with a mean angular frequency ω, we can define the electric field components along the x (horizontal) and y (vertical) axes as follows:

$$E_x(t) = a_1(t)\exp[i(\alpha_1(t) + \omega t)], \qquad E_y(t) = a_2(t)\exp[i(\alpha_2(t) + \omega t)] \tag{21}$$

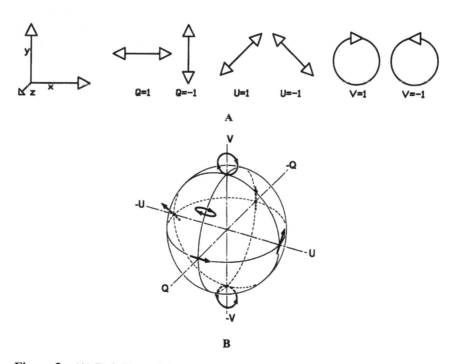

Figure 3 (A) Definition of the Stokes parameters with respect to a right-handed coordinate system. The light is propagated along the positive z axis, i.e., toward the viewer. Q and U describe linear polarizations in frames rotated by $45°$ with respect to each other. The V parameter describes circularly polarized light. (B) Poincaré sphere representation of the Stokes parameters. (Adapted from Ref. 13.)

Then the (non-normalized) Stokes parameters expressed in the variables describing the electric field components can be easily shown to be

$$I = \langle a_1^2 \rangle + \langle a_2^2 \rangle, \qquad Q = \langle a_1^2 \rangle - \langle a_2^2 \rangle$$
$$U = 2\langle a_1 a_2 \cos(\alpha_2(t) - \alpha_1(t)) \rangle, \qquad V = 2\langle a_1 a_2 \sin(\alpha_2(t) - \alpha_1(t)) \rangle \tag{22}$$

Although the Stokes parameters are useful experimentally, the coherence matrix [10] links the polarization state of light more formally to the correlation properties between orthogonal electric field components. The coherence matrix of a well-collimated, uniform, quasi-monochromatic light beam is defined by [10]

$$\mathbf{J} = \begin{bmatrix} \langle E_x^*(t) E_x(t) \rangle & \langle E_x^*(t) E_y(t) \rangle \\ \langle E_y^*(t) E_x(t) \rangle & \langle E_y^*(t) E_y(t) \rangle \end{bmatrix} \tag{23}$$

where $E_x(t)$ and $E_y(t)$ are the components of the complex electric field vector along the x and y axes in the plane perpendicular to the light propagation direction. The diagonal elements are real numbers, and the off-diagonal elements are complex conjugates. The normalized off-diagonal element is defined as

$$j_{xy} = \frac{J_{xy}}{(J_{xx})^{1/2}(J_{yy})^{1/2}}, \qquad 0 \leq |j_{xy}| \leq 1 \tag{24}$$

The normalized off-diagonal element $|j_{xy}|$ is an important parameter, because it measures the degree of correlation between the x and y field components. It is unity for completely polarized light and smaller than 1 for partially polarized light. The elements of the coherence matrix and the Stokes parameters are related by the following formulas:

$$\begin{aligned} I &= J_{xx} + J_{yy} & J_{xx} &= (1/2)(1 + Q) \\ Q &= J_{xx} - J_{yy} & J_{yy} &= (1/2)(1 - Q) \\ U &= J_{xy} + J_{yx} \quad \Leftrightarrow & J_{xy} &= (1/2)(U + iV) \\ V &= i(J_{yx} - J_{xy}) & J_{yx} &= (1/2)(U - iV) \end{aligned} \tag{25}$$

These results will be used in the next section to calculate the Stokes parameters from the coherency matrix.

9.2.5 Calculating the Stokes Parameters of Reflected Light

Combining the principles of interferometric ellipsometry and OCT, the depth-resolved Stokes parameters of reflected light can be determined. As can be seen in Eqs. (13) and (15), the angle α of the sample optic axis with the horizontal gives rise to a phase shift between the interference terms in the horizontal (A_H) and vertical (A_V) polarization channels. The amplitude and relative phase of the interference fringes in each orthogonal polarization channel will be used to derive the depth-resolved Stokes vector of the reflected light. The use of interferometry to characterize the polarization state of light reflected from a sample was first demonstrated by Hazebroek and Holscher [14]. In their work, coherent detection of the interference fringe intensity in orthogonal polarization states formed by HeNe laser light in a Michelson interferometer was used to determine the Stokes parameters of light reflected from a sample. Using a source with short temporal coherence adds pathlength discrimination to the technique, because only light reflected from the sample with an optical pathlength equal to that in the reference arm within the coherence length of the source will produce interference fringes. When using incoherent detection techniques, only two of the four Stokes parameters can be determined simultaneously. In the present analysis, we demonstrate that coherent detection of the interference fringes in two orthogonal polarization states allows determination of all four Stokes parameters simultaneously. Before giving a mathematical description, the principle behind the calculation of the Stokes vector will be discussed. We assume that the polarization state of light reflected from the reference arm is perfectly linear, at an angle of 45° with the horizontal axis. After the polarizing beamsplitter in the detection arm, the horizontal and vertical field components of light in the reference arm will have both equal amplitude and equal phase. Light reflected from the sample will interfere with that from the reference, and the amplitude and relative phase difference of the interference fringes in each polarization channel will be proportional to the amplitude and relative phase difference between horizontal and vertical electric field components of light in the sample arm.

The electric field vector of light reflected from the sample arm can be reconstructed by plotting the interference term of the signals on the horizontal and vertical detectors along the x and y axes, respectively. Figure 4 shows a reconstruction of the electric field vector over a trace of 38 μm. It does not reflect the actual polarization state reflected from the sample, because the light has made a return pass through the quarter-wave plate in the sample arm before being detected. Figure 4 shows the change in polarization state from a linear to an elliptical state as a consequence of tissue birefringence.

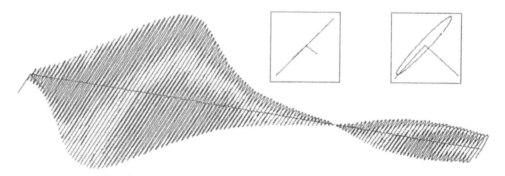

Figure 4 Evolution of the electric component of the electromagnetic wave of the reflected light propagating through birefringent mouse muscle. The electric field is reconstructed from the horizontal A_H and vertical A_V polarized components and relative phase of the interference fringes detected in the experimental scheme shown in Fig. 1. The displayed section is a small part of a longitudinal scan in the middle of the image shown in Fig. 2. The length of the section is 38 μm in a sample with refractive index $n = 1.4$. The beginning of the section shows the reflection from the sample surface modulated by the coherence envelope. The inserts show cross sections of the electric field over a full cycle perpendicular to the propagation direction taken at, respectively, 5.7 μm and 35.7 μm from the beginning of the section. As can be seen from the inserts, the initial polarization state of reflected light is linear along one of the displayed axes, changing to an elliptical polarization state for reflection deeper in the tissue. (Reprinted from Ref. 12 with permission of the Optical Society of America.)

The Stokes parameters can be determined from the signals at the detectors. For instance, if the interference fringes are maximal on one detector and minimal on the other, the polarization state is linear in either the horizontal or vertical plane, which corresponds to the Stokes parameter Q being 1 or -1. If the interference fringes on both detectors are of equal amplitude and exactly in phase, or exactly π out of phase, the polarization state is linear, at $45°$ with the horizontal or vertical, corresponding to the Stokes parameter U being 1 or -1. If the interference fringes on both detectors are of equal amplitude and are exactly $\pi/2$ or $-\pi/2$ out of phase, the polarization state is circular, corresponding to the Stokes parameter V being 1 or -1.

In the mathematical description that follows, the Stokes vector is calculated by Fourier transforming the interference fringes in each channel and computing the relative phase difference and amplitude of the Fourier components at each wavenumber. This will give the Stokes vector for each wavenumber. The Stokes vector of the reflected light is then obtained by summing the Stokes parameters over the spectrum of the source with a weight determined by the power spectral density $S(k)$.

The electric field amplitude of each polarization component is again represented by a complex analytic function, given in Eq. (4), with the conditions given in Eqs. (5) and (6). As derived earlier [Eq. (10)], the light reflected from the reference arm into the detection arm is given by

$$\mathbf{E}_r(z_r) = \frac{1}{2} \int \tilde{e}(k) \exp(-2ikz_r) \begin{pmatrix} 1 \\ 1 \end{pmatrix} dk \tag{26}$$

where z_r is the reference arm length. The electric field amplitude of light reflected from the sample into the detection arm may be written as

$$\mathbf{E}_s(z_s) = \frac{1}{2} \sqrt{R(z_s)} \int \mathbf{a}(k, z_s) \tilde{e}(k) \exp(-2ikz_s) dk \tag{27}$$

where $R(z_s)$ is a real number representing the reflectivity at depth z_s and the attenuation of the coherent beam by scattering, and $\mathbf{a}(k, z_s)$ is a complex-valued Jones vector that characterizes the amplitude and phase of each light field component with wavenumber k that was reflected from depth z_s, with

$$\mathbf{a}^*(k, z_s) \cdot \mathbf{a}(k, z_s) = 1 \quad \text{and} \quad \mathbf{a}(k, z_s) = 0 \quad \text{if } k < 0 \tag{28}$$

Equation (27) is a generic expression describing reflected light without assumption about the cause of the polarization state changes in the sample. Following the notation in Mandel and Wolf [10], the Stokes parameters $s_0 = I$, $s_1 = Q$, $s_2 = U$, and $s_3 = V$ of the electric field amplitude $\mathbf{E}_s(z_s)$ are given by

$$s_j(z_s) = tr[\boldsymbol{\sigma}_j \cdot \mathbf{J}] = \frac{1}{4} R(z_s) \int [\mathbf{a}^*(k, z_s) \cdot \sigma_j \cdot \mathbf{a}(k, z_s)] S(k) dk \tag{29}$$

where the definition of the 2×2 coherence matrix $\mathbf{J}$ [Eq. (23)] and the relation between the coherence matrix elements and the Stokes parameters [Eq. (25)] were used. σ_0 is the 2×2 identity matrix, and σ_1, σ_2, and σ_3 are the Pauli spin matrices, which we take to be[*]

---

[*] This definition of the Pauli spin matrices differs from the widely accepted definition,

$$\sigma_1 = \begin{pmatrix} 0 & 1 \\ 1 & 0 \end{pmatrix}, \quad \sigma_2 = \begin{pmatrix} 0 & -i \\ i & 0 \end{pmatrix}, \quad \sigma_3 = \begin{pmatrix} 1 & 0 \\ 0 & -1 \end{pmatrix}$$

$$\sigma_1 = \begin{pmatrix} 1 & 0 \\ 0 & -1 \end{pmatrix}, \qquad \sigma_2 = \begin{pmatrix} 0 & 1 \\ 1 & 0 \end{pmatrix}, \qquad \sigma_3 \begin{pmatrix} 0 & i \\ -i & 0 \end{pmatrix} \tag{30}$$

From Eqs. (6), (26), and (27), the interference fringe intensity between light in the sample and reference paths measured by the two detectors is given by

$$\mathbf{I}(z_s, \Delta z) = 2\mathrm{Re}\begin{pmatrix} \langle E_{rx}^*(z_r)E_{sx}(z_s) \rangle \\ \langle E_{ry}^*(z_r)E_{sy}(z_s) \rangle \end{pmatrix}$$
$$= \frac{1}{4}\sqrt{R(z_s)} \int 2\,\mathrm{Re}[\mathbf{a}(k, z_s)\exp(-2ik\Delta z)]S(k)\,dk \tag{31}$$

with $\Delta z = z_r - z_s$. The Fourier transform of $\mathbf{I}(z_s, \Delta z)$ with respect to Δz is for notational convenience defined as

$$\tilde{\mathbf{I}}(z_s, 2k) = \frac{1}{2\pi}\int \mathbf{I}(z_s, \Delta z)\exp(2ik\Delta z)\,d\Delta z \tag{32}$$

Retaining only the components for positive k of the Fourier transform $\tilde{\mathbf{I}}(z_s, 2k)$ gives the complex cross-spectral density function for each polarization component,

$$\tilde{\mathbf{I}}(z_s, 2k) = \frac{1}{8\pi}\sqrt{R(z_s)}\mathbf{a}(k, z_s)S(k) \qquad \text{for } k > 0 \tag{33}$$

Using Eq. (33), the Stokes parameters in Eq. (29) can be expressed in terms of $\tilde{\mathbf{I}}(z_s, 2k)$,

$$s_j(z_s) = (8\pi)^2 \int \frac{\tilde{\mathbf{I}}^*(z_s, 2k) \cdot \sigma_j \cdot \tilde{\mathbf{I}}(z_s, 2k)}{S(k)}\,dk \tag{34}$$

The Stokes parameters for each pixel in an image can be calculated according to Eq. (34), with the Fourier components $\tilde{\mathbf{I}}(z_s, 2k)$ determined by the Fourier transform of $I(z_s, \Delta z)$ over Δz intervals on the order of the coherence length of the source light. The power spectral density $S(k)$ in Eq. (34) is given by

$$S(k) = P_0 \frac{\left|\tilde{\mathbf{I}}(z_s, 2k)\right|}{\int \left|\tilde{\mathbf{I}}(z_s, 2k)\right|\,dk} \tag{35}$$

with P_0 the source power. Substituting Eq. (35) into Eq. (34), the Stokes parameters are completely determined by the source power and the Fourier transform of the interference fringes in each polarization channel over an interval Δz around z_s,

$$s_j(z_s) = \frac{(8\pi)^2 \int |\tilde{\mathbf{I}}(z_s, 2k)|\,dk}{P_0} \int \frac{\tilde{\mathbf{I}}(z_s, 2k) \cdot \sigma_j \cdot \tilde{\mathbf{I}}(z_s, 2k)}{\left|\tilde{\mathbf{I}}(z_s, 2k)\right|}\,dk \tag{36}$$

Equation (36) gives the Stokes parameters as measured at the detectors. To determine the polarization state of light reflected from the sample (i.e., before the return pass through the QWP), the Stokes vector computed from Eq. (36) needs to be multiplied by the inverse of the Mueller matrix associated with the QWP in the sample arm, $s_0 \rightarrow s_0$, $s_1 \rightarrow s_3$, $s_2 \rightarrow s_2$, and $s_3 \rightarrow -s_1$. PS-OCT images of the Stokes parameters are formed by gray-scale coding $10\log s_0(z)$ and the polarization state parameters s_1, s_2, and s_3 normalized on the intensity s_0 from 1 to -1. With the incoherent detection technique described in Section 9.2.3, only two of the four Stokes parameters could be determined from a single measurement, s_0 and s_3.

9.2.6 The Degree of Polarization

The complete characterization of the polarization state of reflected light by means of the Stokes parameters permits the calculation of the degree of polarization P, defined as

$$P = \frac{\sqrt{Q^2 + U^2 + V^2}}{I} \tag{37}$$

For purely polarized light the degree of polarization is unity, and the Stokes parameters obey the equality $I^2 = Q^2 + U^2 + V^2$, whereas for partially polarized light the degree of polarization is smaller than unity, leading to $I^2 > Q^2 + U^2 + V^2$. Natural light, characterized by its incoherency has (by definition) a degree of polarization of zero. An interferometric gating technique such as OCT measures only the light reflected from the sample arm that does interfere with the reference arm light. On first inspection, this suggests that the degree of polarization will always be unity, because only the coherent part of the reflected light is detected. We will demonstrate, however, that the degree of polarization can be smaller than unity and that it is a function of the interval Δz over which the degree of polarization is calculated.

An input beam with $P < 1$ can be decomposed into purely polarized beams ($P = 1$), and after propagation through an optical system the Stokes parameters of the purely polarized beam components are added to give the Stokes parameters for the original input beam. In Bohren and Huffman's words [15],

> If two or more quasi-monochromatic beams propagating in the same direction are superposed *incoherently*, that is to say there is no fixed relationship between the phases of the separate beams, the total irradiance is merely the sum of individual beam irradiances. Because the definition of the Stokes parameters involves only irradiances, it follows that the Stokes parameters of a collection of incoherent sources are additive.

Key to our analysis is that a broadband OCT source may be viewed as an incoherent superposition of beams with different wavenumbers.

The degree of polarization can be analyzed in terms of the off-diagonal element of the coherency matrix. From the expression for the electric field amplitude of light reflected from the sample [Eq. (27)], we may write an expression for the normalized off-diagonal element of the coherence matrix as

$$j_{xy} = \frac{\int a_x^*(k, z_s) a_y(k, z_s) S(k)\, dk}{\left[\int |a_x(k, z_s)|^2 S(k)\, dk \right]^{1/2} \left[\int |a_y(k, z_s)|^2 S(k)\, dk \right]^{1/2}} \tag{38}$$

When the polarization state of reflected light is constant over the source spectrum, then $\mathbf{a}(k, z_s) = \mathbf{a}_0$ is constant and $|j_{xy}| = 1$, so the degree of polarization is unity ($P = 1$). When the relative magnitude or phase of the complex numbers $a_x(k, z_s)$ and $a_y(k, z_s)$ change over the source spectrum (i.e., the polarization state of reflected light varies over the source spectrum), we may have $|j_{xy}| < 1$ and the degree of polarization is less than unity ($P < 1$).

A closer look at Eq. (34) or Eq. (36) reveals that the Stokes parameters of each spectral component of the source are determined with a spectral resolution inversely proportional to the Δz interval over which the Fourier transform was taken. The integration over the wavenumber k sums the Stokes parameters of each spectral component with a weight proportional to the power spectral density, $S(k)$. The larger the Δz interval, the higher the resolution in k-space, and the more Stokes parameters of incoherently superposed beams are summed. Using the Poincaré sphere representation, one can visualize that the magnitude of a sum of Stokes vectors will be greatest if the directions of all components are parallel. When the Stokes parameters do not vary over the source spectrum (the polarization state does not vary), then the Stokes vectors add uniformly in one direction and the degree of polarization is unity (note that in our experimental configuration this holds for the input and reference arm beams). When the Stokes parameters vary over spectral components, the polarization state of the various spectral components may be viewed as being distributed over the Poincaré sphere. Because not all components are parallel, when the sum of Stokes parameters over the spectrum is formed, the distribution necessarily results in a sum with P less than unity ($P < 1$).

An alternative argument will lead to the same conclusion. The reconstruction of the electric field vector in Fig. 4 shows that the Stokes parameters can be determined over a single cycle of the field, where at each cycle the degree of polarization will be (very close to) unity. The Stokes parameters over an interval Δz are the sum of the Stokes parameters of single cycles of the electric field vector within the interval. The degree of polarization P of the depth-resolved Stokes vector will be a function of the length of the interval Δz, because Stokes parameters can vary from cycle to cycle.

The reduction of the degree of polarization with increasing depth that is demonstrated in Figs 5 and 7 can be attributed to several causes, such as spectral components that have traveled over different paths with the same length through the sample, spectral dependence of the Stokes parameters of light scattered by (irregularly shaped) particles, the presence of multiply scattered light and speckle in OCT signals, and a decrease in the signal-to-noise ratio. Note that elastic (multiple) scattering does not destroy the coherence of the light in the sense of its ability to interfere with the source light (or the reference arm light). However, spectral phase variations may reduce the coherence envelope similar to the effect of dispersion. Inelastic interactions, such as Raman scattering or fluorescence, do destroy the coherence and the interference with the source light.

9.2.7 Determination of the Optic Axis

From the Stokes parameters, the optic axis of the sample can be determined, assuming that the orientation is constant with depth. The values of Q and U depend on the choice of reference frame (i.e., the orientation of the polarizing beamsplitter in the detection arm). The reference frame, or laboratory frame, is determined by the orientation of orthogonal polarization and vertical axes. If the basis vectors of the reference frame are rotated through an angle β, the transformation from (I, Q, U, V) to Stokes parameters (I', Q', U', V') relative to the new basis vectors is given by

$$\begin{pmatrix} I' \\ Q' \\ U' \\ V' \end{pmatrix} = \begin{pmatrix} 1 & 0 & 0 & 0 \\ 0 & \cos 2\beta & \sin 2\beta & 0 \\ 0 & -\sin 2\beta & \cos 2\beta & 0 \\ 0 & 0 & 0 & 1 \end{pmatrix} \begin{pmatrix} I \\ Q \\ U \\ V \end{pmatrix} \tag{39}$$

The Stokes vector measured in the laboratory frame can be transformed to a new frame, which we will call the sample frame, according to the matrix in Eq. (39). The Mueller matrix for an ideal retarder is given by

$$
\begin{pmatrix}
1 & 0 & 0 & 0 \\
0 & C^2 + S^2\cos\delta & SC(1-\cos\delta) & -S\sin\delta \\
0 & SC(1-\cos\delta) & S^2 + C^2\cos\delta & C\sin\delta \\
0 & S\sin\delta & -C\sin\delta & \cos\delta
\end{pmatrix}
\tag{40}
$$

where $C = \cos 2\alpha$, $S = \sin 2\alpha$, with α the angle of the optic axis with the horizontal and δ the retardance. Equation (40) is the Mueller matrix representation of the linear retarder described by the Jones matrix in Eq. (11), with $\delta = k_0 z\,\Delta n$. Upon specular reflection inside the sample, the Stokes parameters U and V change sign. After the return pass through the retarder, the Mueller matrix is given by

$$
\begin{pmatrix}
1 & 0 & 0 & 0 \\
0 & C^2 + S^2\cos\delta & SC(1-\cos\delta) & -S\sin\delta \\
0 & SC(1-\cos\delta) & -S^2 - C^2\cos\delta & -C\sin\delta \\
0 & -S\sin\delta & -C\sin\delta & -\cos\delta
\end{pmatrix}
\tag{41}
$$

with $\delta = 2k_0 z\,\Delta n$. For example, when right circularly polarized light is incident on a sample with linear retardance, the reflected light polarization state can be defined by the product of the Stokes vector (1,0,0,1) and the matrix of Eq. (41). The reflected light Stokes vector is

$$
\begin{pmatrix} I \\ Q \\ U \\ V \end{pmatrix}
=
\begin{pmatrix}
1 \\
-\sin 2\alpha \sin 2k_0 z\,\Delta n \\
-\cos 2\alpha \sin 2k_0 z\,\Delta n \\
-\cos 2k_0 z\,\Delta n
\end{pmatrix}
\tag{42}
$$

Using Eq. (39) to transform the reflected light Stokes vector into a rotated reference frame, we can show that the Q' parameter equals 0 if the rotation angle β equals $-\alpha$. Therefore, the angle of the optic axis is found by determining the angle of rotation of the reference frame that minimizes the amplitude of oscillations with depth in the Q parameter. This angle defines a rotation of the laboratory frame to a sample frame whose basis vectors are aligned with the optic axes of the sample.

9.2.8 Depth-Resolved Imaging of Stokes Parameters

Rodent muscle was mounted in a chamber filled with saline solution and covered with a thin glass slip to avoid dehydration during measurements. Figure 5 shows images of the four Stokes parameters in the sample frame for right circularly polarized incident light. Several periods of normalized U and V, cycling back and forth between 1 and -1, are observed in muscle, indicating that the sample is birefringent, further demonstrated by the averages of the Stokes parameters over all depth profiles in Fig. 6a. To verify experimentally the orientation of the optic axis computed by rotating the reference frame so as to minimize the amplitude of oscillation in Q, three measurements were performed by replacing the QWP in the sample arm by a half-wave retarder. Light incident on the sample was prepared in three linear polarization

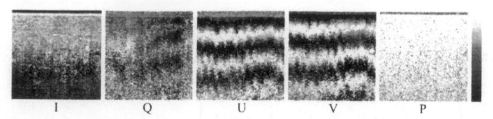

Figure 5 PS-OCT images of ex vivo rodent muscle, 1 mm × 1 mm, pixel size 10 μm × 10 μm. From left to right, the Stokes parameter I, normalized parameters Q, U, and V in the sample frame for right circularly polarized incident light, and the degree of polarization P. The gray scale to the right gives the magnitude of signals, 35 dB range for I, from 1 (white) to −1 (black) for Q, U, and V and from 1 (white) to 0 (black) for P. (Reprinted from Ref. 16 with permission of the Optical Society of America.)

states with electric fields parallel, perpendicular, and at an angle of 45° to the experimentally determined optic axis of the birefringent muscle. Figure 6b shows the average of the normalized Stokes parameter Q over all depth profiles at the same sample location. The negligible amplitude of oscillation in Q for light polarized parallel and perpendicular to the optic axis verified the experimentally determined orientation. When light is incident at an angle of 45° to the optic axis of the sample, Q oscillates with increasing sample depth as expected for a birefringent sample. The similarity of the reflected intensity for circular, parallel, and perpendicular light

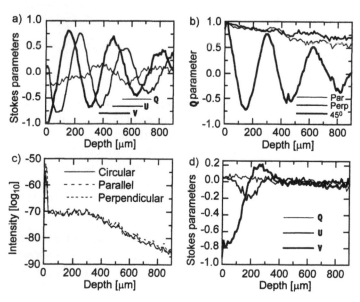

Figure 6 Averages of Stokes parameter I and normalized parameters Q, U, and V in the sample frame over all depth profiles of, respectively, (a) rodent muscle, right circular incident polarization; (b) rodent muscle, linear incident polarization, parallel, perpendicular, and at 45° with the optical axis; (c) rodent muscle, right circular, parallel, and perpendicular incident polarization; and (d) in vivo rodent skin, right circular incident polarization. (Reprinted from Ref. 16 with permission of the Optical Society of America.)

(shown in Fig. 6c) indicates that the polarization state changes are not due to dichroism of the muscle fibers. The birefringence Δn was determined by measuring the distance of a full V period, which corresponds to a phase retardation of $\pi = k_0 z \, \Delta n$, giving $\Delta n = 1.4 \times 10^{-3}$. The similarity between PS-OCT images coding for the phase retardation $\varphi(z)$ and the Stokes parameter V (e.g., Fig. 2b and Fig. 5V) is due to the close algebraic relation between the two.

$$\varphi(z) = \arctan\left[\left(\frac{I_V(z)}{I_H(z)}\right)^{1/2}\right], \qquad V(z) = \cos(2\varphi(z)) \tag{43}$$

Note that $\varphi(z)$ gives the single-pass phase retardation, $\varphi(z) = k \, \Delta n \, z$, whereas $V(z)$ is determined by the double-pass phase retardation, $V(z) = \cos(2k \, \Delta n \, z)$. Figure 7 shows PS-OCT images of the four Stokes parameters in the laboratory frame for right circularly polarized light incident on in vivo rodent skin. Averages of the normalized stokes parameters Q, U, and V over all depth profiles (Fig. 6d, after minimizing the oscillations in Q), indicate oscillations typical of sample birefringence in the first 400 μm. Observed birefringence is attributed to the presence of collagen in skin. Although no preferred orientation of the optical axis is expected in rodent skin, a predominant direction was found at shallow depths. At deeper depths, Q, U, and V approach zero, which is attributed to scrambling of the polarization by scattering and the randomly oriented and changing optic axis.

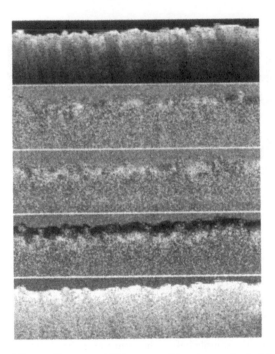

Figure 7 PS-OCT images of in vivo rodent skin, 5 mm × 1 mm, pixel size 10 μm × 10 μm. From top to bottom, the Stokes parameter I; normalized parameters Q, U, and V in the laboratory frame for right circularly polarized incident light; and the degree of polarization P. The magnitude of signals ranged over 40 dB for I; from 1 (white) to -1 (black) for Q, U, and V; and from 1 (white) to 0 (black) for P. (Reprinted from Ref. 16 with permission of the Optical Society of America.)

9.2.9 Polarization Diversity Detection and Speckle Averaging

Figure 8 shows six images reconstructed from a single scan of rodent skin, 3 weeks after exposure to a 100°C brass rod for 20 s. The six images display, respectively, in the left column from top to bottom, the sum of the reflected intensity detected by the detectors, the vertically polarized reflected intensity (detector 1), and the horizontally polarized reflected intensity (detector 2), and in the right column from top to bottom, the normalized Stokes parameters Q, U, and V. The Stokes parameters were calculated as described previously and give the polarization state of light reflected from the sample before the return pass through the QWP. Images display the Stokes parameters normalized on the intensity and gray-scale-coded from 1 to −1. Contour lines indicating 1/3 and −1/3 values were calculated after low-pass filtering by convolving the images with a Gaussian filter of 4 × 4 pixels and overlaid with the original image. The scan was made from normal skin (left) into thermally damaged skin with scar formation (right).

   Two interesting observations can be made. First, the images recorded by a single detector show dark areas indicating low tissue reflectivity that are completely absent from the summed image. These features are solely due to polarization changes in the tissue and are not correlated with tissue reflectivity. Images of the Stokes parameters show the polarization state changing from circular to linear and back as a function of increasing depth.

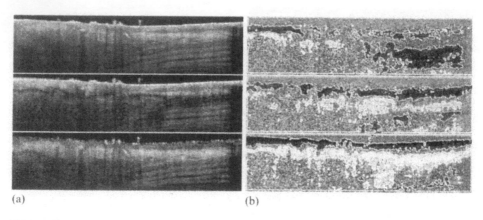

(a)   (b)

Figure 8 (a) OCT and (b) PS-OCT images generated from a single scan of rodent skin, 3 weeks postexposure to a 100°C brass rod for 20 s. Image size is 4 mm × 1 mm. The six images display, respectively, in the left column from top to bottom the sum of the detected reflected intensity, the vertically polarized reflected intensity (detector 1), and the horizontally polarized reflected intensity (detector 2) gray-scale coded on a logarithmic scale, and, in the right column from top to bottom, the normalized Stokes parameters Q, U, and V gray-scale coded from 1 to −1. Incident light was right circularly polarized ($V = 1$). The Stokes parameters Q, U, and V represent the polarization state reflected from the sample before the return pass through the quarter-wave plate. White lines are contours at 1/3 (white to gray transition) and −1/3 (gray to black transition) values. The scan was made from normal (left) into thermally damaged skin with scar formation (right). Punch biopsy and histological evaluation of the imaged location indicate that the banded structure in the lower right half of the summed intensity image is muscle tissue. (Reprinted from Ref. 17 with permission of the Institute of Electrical and Electronics Engineers, Inc.)

Second, the summed image has a smoother appearance, which suggests that speckle noise is averaged. Presently, speckle-averaging algorithms in OCT use four detectors recording light that has traveled over a slightly different path through the sample to the focal point and back [18]. Wave front distortions by tissue inhomogeneities create a different speckle pattern at each detector. However, implementation of this approach in a single-mode fiber is difficult. Because light has two degrees of freedom, at each spatial location two (partially) independent speckle patterns are present, one in each polarization channel. Summing the images recorded in orthogonal polarization channels provides an alternative approach to speckle averaging that is simple to implement in a single-mode fiber. The number of images with (partially) independent speckle patterns can be further increased by modulating the polarization incident on the sample over orthogonal states. Two additional images can be recorded, giving four interference signals available for speckle averaging, which would increase the signal-to-noise ratio (SNR) by a   factor of 2. However, the actual increase in SNR that can be realized may be considerably less, because the speckle patterns in orthogonally polarized channels need not be completely independent due to the low-order scattering of OCT signals [19]. To summarize, PS-OCT is important not only for measuring birefringence but also for accurate interpretation of OCT images. Most fibrous structures in tissue (e.g., muscle, nerve fibers) are birefringent owing to their anisotropy. Single-detector OCT systems can generate images that show structural properties by a reduction in tissue reflectivity, solely due to polarization effects. In addition, polarization diversity detection and polarization modulation in the sample arm could be interesting approaches to speckle averaging in OCT systems based on single-mode fibers.

So far, the source light was assumed to be polarized. The presented analysis is easily extended to include unpolarized sources. An unpolarized source can be described by the addition of two orthogonally polarized sources that are mutually incoherent. The interference fringes at the detector(s) need to be analyzed separately for the two pure polarized states, and the total interference fringe pattern is given by the sum of the fringe patterns of the individual polarized states. An OCT system with an unpolarized source and a single detector does not imply polarization diversity detection. On the contrary, this system is even more sensitive to polarization effects than a system with a polarized source. Consider polarized source light incident on a birefringent sample acting as a linear retarder with its optic axis at 45° with respect to the incident light polarization axis. The polarization state of reflected light that has undergone a π phase retardation is orthogonal to the incident polarization state. Because orthogonally polarized states cannot interfere, light from the sample and reference arms does not produce interference fringes. The same holds for each of the orthogonally polarized states in the decomposition of an unpolarized source into linear states at 45° and −45° to the optic axis. Therefore, for the unpolarized source no interference fringes will be detected either. Suppose now that the decomposition of the unpolarized source is chosen differently for the above-mentioned birefringent sample, such that the two orthogonal linearly polarized mutually incoherent states are along and perpendicular to the optic axis. Both orthogonal polarization states reflected from the sample are unaltered by the birefringence and will produce interference fringes with the reference arm light. However, the interference fringes for orthogonal polarization states are exactly π out of phase and cancel after summation, and no interference fringe pattern is present at the detector. Thus, in this example, the unpolarized source will not produce interference fringes regardless of the orientation of the optic axis (as is expected from symmetry arguments). In contrast, a polarized source would produce interference fringes if the polarization state is (partially) along the optic axis.

9.2.10 Accuracy and Noise: Birefringence, Dichroism, and Scattering

Everett et al. [9] presented an analysis of the systematic error in the phase retardation due to background noise for the incoherent PS-OCT detection scheme described in Section 9.2.3. They showed that for phase retardations close to $0°$ or $90°$ the background noise on the detectors introduces a significant and systematic error of, e.g., $15°$ at a signal-to-noise ratio of 10 dB. The coherent detection scheme described in Section 9.2.5, which calculates the Stokes parameters, has better immunity to this systematic error. A closer look at Eqs. (25), (34), or (36) reveals that in the calculation of the Q parameter (also denoted by s_1) the spectral density in one polarization channel is subtracted from the spectral density in the orthogonal polarization channel, thus eliminating constant background noise terms, and the U (s_2) and V (s_3) parameters are calculated from the cross-correlation between fringes in orthogonally polarized channels, eliminating autocorrelation noise. Noise will decrease the degree of polarization P, because it will be present as autocorrelation noise in the Stokes parameter I. The better noise immunity can be illustrated with the help of Fig. 6a, which shows the Stokes parameters for rodent muscle. In the incoherent detection scheme only V (s_3 in the figure) is measured, and the error in the phase retardation is introduced by the decrease of the amplitude of oscillations with increasing depth. In the coherent detection scheme, the Stokes parameters Q, U, and V can be renormalized on P, restoring the amplitude of the oscillations and thus eliminating the systematic error.

Schoenenberger et al. [11] went further and also analyzed system errors introduced by the extinction ratio of polarizing optics and chromatic dependence of wave retarders, and errors due to dichroism, i.e., the differences in the absorption and scattering coefficients for polarized light in tissue. System errors can be kept small by careful design of the system with achromatic elements but can never be completely eliminated. Dichroism can possess a more serious problem when the results are interpreted as solely due to birefringence. However, Mueller matrix ellipsometric measurements have shown that the error due to dichroism in the eye is relatively small [20,21], and Fig. 6c shows that dichroism is of minor importance in rodent muscle. More research is necessary to determine the importance of dichroism in other types of tissue.

We believe that the dominant noise sources are related to multiple scattering and speckle. As argued earlier, multiple scattering will scramble the polarization mainly in a random manner. This offers some means to distinguish it from birefringence. Reported birefringence values for cornea, tendon, and muscle are on the order of $\Delta n = 10^{-3}$ [8,22–24] which will give a $90°$ phase retardation at a depth on the order of several hundreds of micrometers. Thus, birefringence-induced changes are relatively slow, and the Stokes parameters change according to the Mueller matrix of a linear retarder. However, an optic axis that varies with depth will give changes in the polarization state that will be difficult to distinguish from the randomness of multiple scattering. Measurement of the full Mueller matrix of the sample by varying the incident light over four different polarization states, as recently demonstrated by Yao and Wang [25], will provide additional information that could aid the analysis of PS-OCT signals. More research is necessary on this complex problem.

Speckle introduces noise on the Stokes parameters by the large fluctuations in the interference fringes that could be uncorrelated in the orthogonal detection channels. Speckle-averaging techniques demonstrated by Schmitt et al. [18] will reduce this noise, as will averaging the Stokes parameters over distances greater than the coherence length. Averaging images with different input polarization states will reduce speckle noise also. Speckle noise remains one of the main problems that need to be addressed in OCT.

9.3 IMAGING OF THERMAL DAMAGE WITH PS-OCT

9.3.1 Introduction

Collagen is the dominant structure in human skin. Its birefringence has two components. Form birefringence results from ordered proteins surrounded by a ground substance with a different refractive index; intrinsic birefringence results from chemical groups arranged in an ordered configuration with anisotropic optical retardance. Thermal damage, which starts to take place between 56°C and 65°C, reduces both the form and intrinsic birefringence by changing the collagen from a rodlike to a random coil structure. The reduction of collagen birefringence can be used to determine burn injury, because partial loss of birefringence is known to be an indication of tissue thermal damage [26].

9.3.2 Laser-Irradiated Bovine Tendon

To demonstrate an application of PS-OCT, we present 1 mm and 1.5 mm wide by 700 μm deep images of bovine tendon birefringence before and after pulsed laser irradiation. For comparison, reflection OCT images are shown that were formed by the sum of detected signals in orthogonal polarization channels. A detailed description of the experimental configuration used to obtain Figs. 9–12 is given in de Boer et al. [8]. Measurements on 1 cm × 2 cm samples at least 1 cm thick were done within 48 h of bovine death. In Fig. 9 conventional and birefringence images of fresh bovine tendon are shown. The banded structure in Fig. 9b, indicative of birefringence, is clearly visible up to a physical depth of 700 μm, whereas this structure is completely absent from the conventional reflection image in Fig. 9a. This shows that the banded structure in the birefringence image is not an anatomical artifact in the tendon but is due solely to its birefringence. By measuring the optical versus physical thickness of a thin slice [28], we found the average refractive index of the tendon to be $\bar{n} = 1.42 \pm 0.03$. We determined the birefringence by the average distance between the first and second dark bands from the top of Fig. 9b over the full width (100 lateral scans). The average distance $\bar{z} = 116 \pm 13 \, \mu$m corresponded to a polarization rotation $\varphi = k_0 \bar{z} \delta = \pi$ in Eq. (19). The experimentally determined birefringence $\delta = (3.7 \pm 0.4) \times 10^{-3}$ of bovine tendon (predominantly type I collagen) is in agreement with reported values of $(3.0 \pm 0.6) \times 10^{-3}$ [24] and $(2.8–3.0) \times 10^{-3}$ [22,23] for type I collagen. Fitting $e^{-2z/\gamma}$ at $z = 150$–600 μm depth to the total backscattered intensity I_T [Eq. (18)] in the sample, averaged over the image in Fig. 9a (100 lateral scans) gave

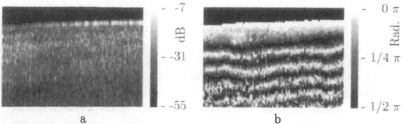

a   b

Figure 9 Images of fresh bovine tendon 1 mm wide by 700 μm deep, constructed from the same measurement. (a) Conventional reflection image generated by computing $10 \log[I_T]$. The gray scale to the right gives the magnitude of the signals. (b) Birefringence image generated by computing the phase retardation φ in Eq. (19). The gray scale at the right gives the angle φ. The banded structure, indicative of the birefringence, is clearly visible. Each pixel represents a 10 μm × 10 μm area. The dynamic range within the image was 48 dB. (Reprinted from Ref. 27 with permission of the Society of Photo-Optical Instrumentation Engineers.)

$\gamma \approx 0.2$ mm. Decay of total backscattered light intensity with depth depends on several factors, among them attenuation of the coherent beam by scattering and the geometry of the collection optics. In Fig. 10 conventional OCT and birefringence images of laser-irradiated bovine tendon are presented. A decrease in the birefringence at the center of the irradiation zone, extending into the tendon over the full depth of the image (700 μm), is clearly seen. Furthermore, the direction of incoming laser light (from the upper left corner, at an angle of 35° with the normal to the surface) is observed. The surface temperature of the tendon was monitored during laser irradiation by infrared radiometry. For comparison, Fig. 10a shows an OCT image of the total backscattered intensity I_T. Although less backscattered light from

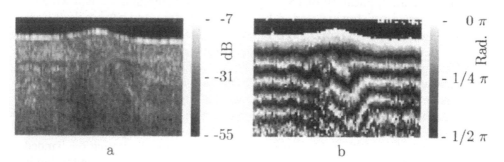

a   b

Figure 10 Images of fresh bovine tendon 1 mm wide by 700 μm deep, constructed from the same measurement. (a) Conventional reflection image generated by computing $10 \log[I_T]$. The gray scale to the right gives the magnitude of the signals. (b) Birefringence image generated by computing the phase retardation φ in Eq. (19). The gray scale at the right gives the angle φ. The bovine tendon was exposed to three consecutive 1 J, 150 μs laser pulses ($\lambda = 1.32$ μm) spaced by 10 ms, incident from the upper left at an angle of 35° with respect to the surface normal. The beam diameter was 2 mm. Initial surface temperature after laser irradiation was 77°C, dropping to 61°C after 0.25 s. The displacement of the banded structure in the image indicates the loss of birefringence due to the thermal damage in the irradiated zone. Each pixel represents a 10 μm × 10 μm area. (Reprinted from Ref. 27 with permission of the Society of Photo-Optical Instrumentation Engineers.)

the irradiated area can be observed, the polarization-sensitive image (Fig. 10b) reveals important structural information not evident in Fig. 10a. In Figs. 11 and 12, conventional and birefringence images 1.5 mm wide by 700 μm deep of laser-irradiated tendon with and without surface cooling are presented. Because loss of birefringence is attributed to thermal damage, comparison of the two figures show the effect of surface cooling on laser-mediated thermal damage. Application of cooling clearly reduces the birefringence loss near the surface in Fig. 12 compared to Fig. 11.

9.3.3 Slowly Heated Porcine Tendon

To investigate the effect of temperature on collagen birefringence, porcine tendon was mounted in a Rose chamber filled with 5% saline solution. A thermocouple monitored the temperature inside the chamber. A heating device was mounted outside the chamber that could increase the temperature inside to 77°C. Lateral scan velocity v (x direction) was 100 μm/s, axial number of scans was 200 at 2 μm increments, giving an image size of 200μm $\times$ 400 μm and a pixel size of 1 μm $\times$ 2 μm. Figure 13 shows the OCT and PS-OCT images of slowly heated tendon at 25, 45, 55, 60, 70, and 77°C, respectively. Image acquisition was started after the Rose chamber had reached the target temperature (15–30 min between consecutive scans). The last scan was taken after the sample was heated for 5 h at 77°C.

The images at 25°C, 45°C, and 55°C (Figs. 13a, 13b, and 13c, respectively) showed no change in the birefringence. The more closely spaced the banded structure, the greater the birefringence, because the accumulated phase retardation is the product of depth z and birefringence Δn. At 60°C (Fig. 13d), a reduction in the birefringence can be observed. The tendon shrank considerably along the axis of the fibers during the scan, which contributed to motion artifacts in the image. At 70°C (Fig. 13e) the birefringence was reduced further, and after 5 h at 77°C (Fig. 13f) the

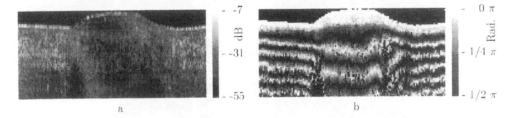

Figure 11 Images of fresh bovine tendon 1.5 mm wide by 700 μm deep, constructed from the same measurement. (a) Conventional reflection image generated by computing $10 \log[I_T]$. The gray scale to the right gives the magnitude of the signals. (b) Birefringence image generated by computing the phase retardation φ in Eq. (19). The gray scale at the right gives the angle φ. The bovine tendon was exposed to three consecutive 1.4 J, 150 μs laser pulses ($\lambda = 1.32 \mu$m) spaced by 10 ms, incident from the upper left at an angle of 35° with respect to the surface normal. The beam diameter was 2 mm. Initial surface temperature after laser irradiation was 88°C, dropping to 70°C after 0.25 s. The displacement of the banded structure in the image indicates the loss of birefringence due to thermal damage in the irradiated zone. Each pixel represents a 10 μm $\times$ 10 μm area. (Reprinted from Ref. 27 with permission of the Society of Photo-Optical Instrumentation Engineers.)

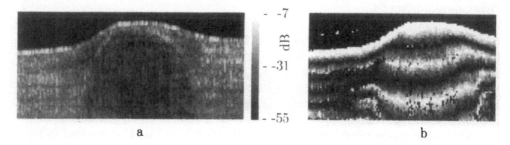

Figure 12 Images of fresh bovine tendon 1.5 mm wide by 700 μm deep, constructed from the same measurement. (a) Conventional reflection image generated by computing 10 log[I_T]. The gray scale to the right gives the magnitude of the signals. (b) Birefringence image generated by computing the phase retardation φ [Eq. (19)]. The gray scale at the right gives the angle φ. The bovine tendon was exposed to three consecutive 1.5 J, 150 μs laser pulses ($\lambda = 1.32$ μm) spaced by 10 ms, incident from the upper left at an angle of 35° with respect to the surface normal. The beam diameter was 2 mm. Prior to exposure to the laser irradiation the surface was cooled to −5°C in 40 ms. Maximum surface temperature of 68°C was reached 330 ms after laser irradiation. The displacement of the banded structure in the image indicates the loss of birefringence due to thermal damage in the irradiated zone. Compared to Fig. 11, the loss of birefringence at the surface is smaller, attributed to the diminished thermal damage due to surface cooling. Each pixel represents a 10 μm × 10 μm area. (Reprinted from Ref. 27 with permission of the Society of Photo-Optical Instrumentation Engineers.)

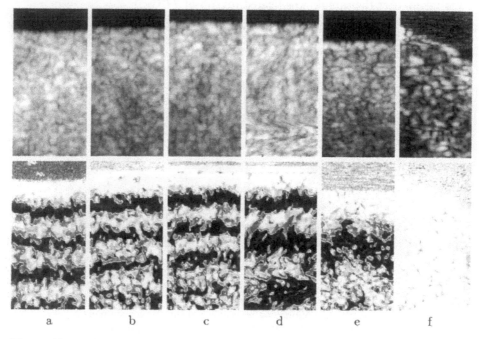

Figure 13 OCT and PS-OCT images of porcine tendon slowly heated in a Rose chamber. Image size: 200 μm × 400 μm, pixel size 1 μm × 2 μm. Upper panels: OCT images; lower panels: PS-OCT images. Temperature and dynamic range: (a) 25°C, 47 dB; (b) 45°C, 46 dB; (c) 55°C, 46 dB; (d) 60°C, 43 dB; (e) 70°C, 36 dB; (f) 77°C, 25 dB. White lines in PS-OCT images are contours at $\varphi = 30$° (white to gray transition) and $\varphi = 60$° (gray to black transition) phase retardation levels, respectively. (Reprinted from Ref. 37 with permission of the Optical Society of America.)

birefringence was completely gone, due to excessive thermal damage. Since Maitland et al. [24] showed that the reduction of birefringence in rat tail tendon is a function of both temperature and time, no quantitative conclusions can be drawn on the reduction of birefringence as a function of temperature alone. However, the presented images demonstrate the capability of PS-OCT to measure the birefringence reduction in collagen due to thermal damage.

9.4 IN VIVO BURN DEPTH IMAGING

In this section, PS-OCT cross-sectional images obtained in normal and thermally injured rat skin will be presented alongside histology of the imaged region. A qualitative relationship between the loss of birefrigence and the depth of burn injuries determined by histology will be demonstrated. This research was conducted by MD/ Ph.D. student S. Srinivas and Ph.D. student B. H. Park [29].

9.4.1 Introduction

Traditionally, thermal burns have been differentiated into first, second, or third degree injuries. This classification is in many respects retrospective. First degree burns show thermal damage limited to the epidermis and are not considered a clinical problem, because skin will regenerate damaged epithelial cells. A second degree or partial thickness burn shows thermal damage extending into the dermis; however, the skin can still heal by re-epithelialization. A third degree burn shows full thickness damage of the epidermis and dermis and fails to heal by regeneration of epithelium from within the wound margins.

The treatment for full thickness burns is skin grafting, either autologous or transplanted. However, a partial thickness burn, which shows destruction of the epidermis and a portion of the underlying dermis, may require a more complex treatment plan depending on the depth of dermal injury. Currently, if a patient has a suspected superficial partial thickness burn, the surgeon will often wait 2–3 weeks to determine if the wound will heal spontaneously from surviving epithelial appendages. If the burn has not healed within this time period, skin grafting is indicated. Conversely, if a deep partial thickness burn is encountered, then skin grafting should be considered as soon as possible, because there is a lower incidence of infection with early eschar removal [30].

A number of methods have been developed to determine the depth of burn injury, including the use of indocyanine green dye fluorescence [31], vital dyes, fluorescein fluorometry, laser Doppler flowmetry (LDF), thermography, ultrasound, nuclear magnetic resonance imaging, and spectral analysis of light reflectance [32]. Clinical estimation by visual and tactile assessment of the wound remains the gold standard for burn depth determination [32]. However, determining whether a deep burn will heal spontaneously is difficult even for an experienced clinician [31,33].

Skin has an abundance of weekly birefringent collagen molecules in the dermis, and ensuing thermal injury will denature this collagen, resulting in a reduction of birefringence. By comparing changes in normal and burned tissues of Sprague-Dawley rats, we will show a qualitative link between the depth of thermal damage and the measurable loss of skin birefringence.

9.4.2 Experiment

Figures 14–17 show typical PS-OCT scans and corresponding histology for normal skin and for burned rat skin produced by a preheated 75°C brass rod for 5, 15, or 30 s exposure time, respectively. Details of the experiment are described in Srinivas et al. [29]. The PS-OCT images were formed by gray-scale coding the single-pass bire-fringence-induced phase retardation from 0° (black) to 180° (white). A white contour line indicating a 90° phase retardation level—90° in the figure labels—in the PS-OCT image was plotted and overlaid with the original image. Scans were always 4 mm long by 1 mm deep cross sections. The start and end points of the scan were marked with India ink by tattooing the skin to identify the scanned region in histology. To determine the relationship between the loss of birefringence in skin and actual depth of thermal damage, the PS-OCT scans are shown side by side with the histological sections that were taken from the biopsied tissue.

9.4.3 Results

Figure 14a shows a control PS-OCT scan, and Fig. 14b displays the abundance of intact hair follicles found in normal rat skin histology. Figure 15a shows an increased depth of the white 90° phase retardation line, and Fig. 15b shows a corresponding purple region near the surface, indicating damage to the dermis, which would be classified as a superficial partial thickness or second degree burn. Figure 16a has an even deeper white 90° phase retardation line, and the purple region indicating damage to the dermis has increased as well (Fig. 16b). Hair follicle damage can be seen, and the burn in Fig. 16b would be classified as a deep partial thickness or, again, a second degree burn. Figure 17a shows the deepest white 90° phase retarda-tion line, and the regressive H & E stain shows damage over the entire dermis (Fig. 17b). Extensive coagulation can be seen in the dermis with a complete absence of hair follicles, classifying the damage in Fig. 17b as a full thickness or third degree burn.

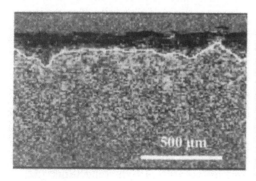
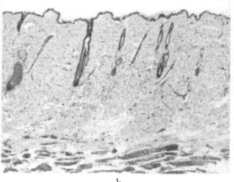

a   b

Figure 14 Typical PS-OCT scan (a) and corresponding histology (b) of normal rat skin. (a) The PS-OCT scan has been gray-scale coded so that black represents 0° phase retardation (the incident polarization) and white is 180° phase retardation. The white contour line in the scan demarcates the depth at which 90° phase retardation has been reached with respect to the incident polarization. (b) The stain used is regressive H & E (mag 157.5×). Note the abundance of intact hair follicles. (Reprinted from Ref. 29.)

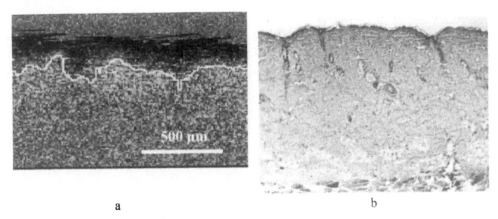

a   b

Figure 15 PS-OCT scan (a) and corresponding histology (b) of rat skin burned by contact with a 75°C brass rod for 5 s. (a) The PS-OCT scan has been gray-scale coded so that black represents 0° phase retardation (the incident polarization) and white is 180° phase retardation. Also note the increased depth of the white 90° phase retardation line in the scan. (b) The regressive H & E stain (mag 157.5×) shows a purple region near the surface, indicating damage to the dermis. This would be classified as a superficial partial thickness burn. (Reprinted from Ref. 29.)

As can be observed in Figs. 14–17, all PS-OCT scans consistently show that the incident circular polarization on the sample (corresponding to 0° of phase retardation and coded as black) is preserved through deeper depths as thermal damage increases. The depths of the 90° phase retardation contour line increase as the duration of the thermal injury exposure increases. This correlation demonstrates that PS-OCT can provide quantitative information for burn depth determination.

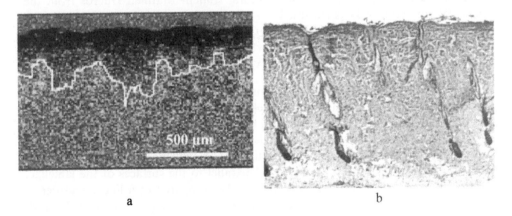

a   b

Figure 16 PS-OCT scan (a) and corresponding histology (b) of rat skin burned by contact with a 75°C brass rod for 15 s. (a) The PS-OCT scan has been gray-scale coded so that black represent 0° phase retardation (the incident polarization) and white is 180° phase retardation. Note the increased depth of the white 90° phase retardation line in the scan. (b) The stain used is regressive H & E (mag 157.5×). The purple region indicating damage to the dermis has increased in depth. Hair follicle damage can also be seen. This would be classified as a deep partial thickness burn. (Reprinted from Ref. 29.)

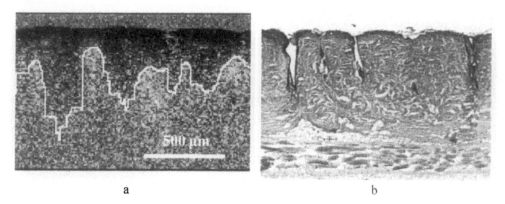

a   b

Figure 17 PS-OCT scan (a) and corresponding histology (b) of rat skin burned by contact with a 75°C brass rod for 30 s. (a) The PS-OCT scan has been gray-scale coded so that black represents 0° phase retardation (the incident polarization) and white is 180° phase retardation. Again note the increased depth of the white 90° phase retardation line in the scan. (b) Here the regressive H & E stain (mag 157.5×) shows damage over the entire dermis. Extensive coagulation can be seen in the dermis with a complete absence of hair follicles. This would be classified as a full thickness burn. (Reprinted from Ref. 29.)

9.5 POLARIZATION-SENSITIVE OPTICAL COHERENCE TOMOGRAPHY OF THE RABBIT EYE

In this section, PS-OCT cross-sectional images obtained in the cornea and retina of enucleated rabbit eyes will be presented. Four polarization images corresponding to the four Stokes parameters of light reflected from any position in the tissue will be used to analyze birefringent structures in the eye.

This research was performed by doctoral student Mathieu Ducros from the Biomedical Engineering Department, University of Texas, Austin, during a visit to the Beckman Laser Institute and Medical Clinic [34].

9.5.1 Introduction

In the eye, the corneal stroma and the retinal nerve fiber layer (NFL) are birefringent. The crystalline lens is also most likely birefringent but will not be discussed here. The corneal stroma is the central and thickest layer of the cornea. It consists of a large number of stacked lamellae. Each lamella has the form of a thin (a few micrometers thick) ribbon. Principal constituents are collagen fibrils, glycosaminoglycans, and water. The fibrils are oriented parallel to the surfaces of the lamellae. Due to this particular structure, a lamella can be compared to a linear retarder in which the slow and fast axes lie respectively parallel and perpendicular to the fibril direction. Each lamella induces a small phase retardation in incoming polarized light. PS-OCT can be used to investigate the corneal stroma structure. Furthermore, depth-resolved polarization images in the cornea may be useful to observe in vivo thermal damage that could occur during treatments such as photorefractive keratectomy (PRK) and laser in situ keratomileusis (LASIK).

The NFL is the most anterior layer of the retina and consists of glial cells and axons of ganglion cells. The axons converge radially to the optic nerve, where they exit the ocular globe. The NFL can be up to $400\,\mu$m thick at the edge of the optic nerve [35]. The NFL birefringence is due to the dense parallel arrangement of axon membranes and microtubules inside the axons [6,36]. Glaucoma is the second leading cause of blindness worldwide and affects the NFL. In glaucoma, the retinal ganglion cells are destroyed and the axons in the NFL disappear. This process is irreversible. An instrument providing a precise and reliable measurement of the NFL thickness and structural integrity could greatly improve glaucoma detection and aid in follow-up examinations.

9.5.2 Phase Retardation Determination

Gray-scale images of the Stokes parameters (I, Q, U, and V) of the cornea, crystal-line lens and retina are presented later in Figs. 19 and 21, respectively. In the I image, pixel brightness is proportional to the local value of I in decibels. In images of Q, U, and V, pixel brightness varies between white for $+1$ and black for -1. For each pixel the phase parameter Φ was calculated as

$$\Phi = \arctan\left[\frac{\sqrt{Q^2 + U^2}}{-V}\right] \qquad (44)$$

In the Poincaré sphere representation [13], Φ is the angle between the Stokes vectors of light reflected from the surface of the cornea ($Q = 0$, $U = 0$, $V = -1$) and that reflected from a given tissue position. According to the known structure of the corneal stroma and retinal NFL, these tissues can be viewed as linear retarders with fast and slow optic axes perpendicular to the light propagation direction (the illumination beam being perpendicular to the corneal surface). In these conditions, Φ represents the phase retardation between two orthogonal polarization components of light reflected from a given tissue element relative to the phase retardation between two orthogonal components of light incident on the eye. Φ equals $0°$ for left circularly polarized light, $90°$ for linearly polarized light, and $180°$ for right circularly polarized light. When the reflected light is unpolarized, or when the intensity is lower than the system noise level, Φ varies randomly.

9.5.3 Methods

Experiments were performed on the enucleated eye of a New Zealand White rabbit. Images were acquired less than 6 h post mortem. The sample holder is diagrammed in Fig. 18. The entry window of the eye holder consisted of a flat glass slide that was gently pressed against the cornea to reduce the refractive power. For imaging the cornea, the beam focus was placed approximately a few hundred micrometers anterior to the apex of the cornea. For imaging the retina, the beam focus was placed anterior to the vitreous/retina interface on the superior and/or inferior region of the optic nerve head where the NFL is the thickest. A red aiming beam, aligned with the broadband infrared SLD beam, was used to determine the imaging position on the retina. The red light was partially transmitted through the choroid and sclera and was visible on the back side of the eye. A blank ink dot was placed on the back of the eye at the lateral edges of the imaged region to identify the corresponding area for histology. After PS-OCT measurements, the eye was fixed in formalin and histology performed.

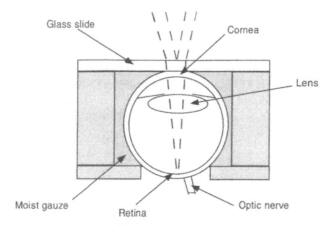

Figure 18   Eye holder. The sample was surrounded by moist gauze. A flat glass slide was placed on the cornea to allow good visualization of the eye fundus. For imaging the cornea, the beam focus was placed a few hundred micrometers above the glass slide at the beginning of the scan. For imaging the retina, the eye was oriented to place the optic nerve in the field of view and the beam focus was positioned above the vitreous/retinal interface. (Reprinted from Ref. 34 with permission of the Institute of Electrical and Electronics Engineers, Inc.)

9.5.4   PS-OCT Imaging in the Cornea

Stokes Parameter Images

Figure 19 presents the Stokes parameter images (from left to right I, Q, U, and V) acquired from the cornea of an enucleated rabbit eye. Each image is 1-mm wide by 3.5-mm deep. The letters to the left of the I image refer to the beginning of the scan (a), the air/glass interface (b), the glass/cornea interface (c), the cornea/aqueous interface (d), the aqueous/crystalline lens interface (e), and the end of the scan (f). As expected, the glass slide (b–c) is transparent (I minimum) and does not induce any change in the light polarization. Q, U, and V appear gray. Their average value is 0, and variations are due only to noise. The reflection from the front and back surfaces of the glass appear bright in the I image, black in the V image, and gray in the Q and U images, meaning that the reflected light polarization is left circular. The helicity of the incident light is reversed as expected for specular reflection. In the cornea (about 0.6 mm thick from c to d), I is relatively low and uniform. No anatomical layers can be clearly differentiated. In contrast, Q, U, and V images of the cornea are nonuniform: the polarization state of reflected light varies as a function of depth and lateral position. Variations of Q, U, and V values in depth in the corneal stroma are due to the cumulative polarization effect of all lamellae, with each lamella acting as a linear retarder. A prominent feature indicating an increase in the V value (from black to white) is observed in the right half of the cornea on the V image, meaning that polarization of reflected light changes from left circular to approximately right circular. Therefore, in this region, the whole corneal stroma acts as a quarter-wave retarder in single pass (half-wave retarder in double pass). A different feature is observed in the left half of the V image. There, backscattered light polarization state changes from left circular at the glass/cornea interface (point c) to approximately linear at

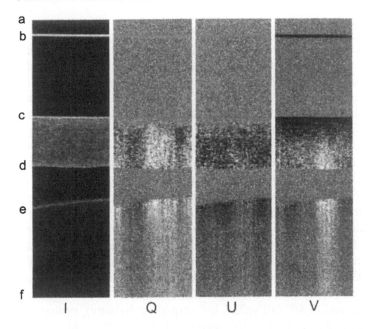

Figure 19 From left to right: Stokes parameters I and normalized parameters Q, U, and V in the rabbit cornea. Each image is 1 mm wide by 3.5 mm deep. The pixel size is $10\,\mu$m × $10\,\mu$m. The letters a and f correspond to the beginning and end of the scan, and b, c, d, and e indicate the air/glass, glass/cornea, cornea/aqueous, and aqueous/crystalline lens interfaces. Five zones can be seen from top to bottom: air (a–b), glass slide (b–c), cornea (c–d), anterior chamber (d–e), and part of the crystalline lens (e–f). In the cornea, the I image is relatively uniform, but the Q, U, and V images show regions where the reflected light has different polarization states indicating structural differences in the corneal stroma. (Reprinted from Ref. 34 with permission of the Institute of Electrical and Electronics Engineers, Inc.)

$-45°$ ($U \sim -1$) at the cornea/aqueous interface (point d). Therefore, the corneal birefringence varies between the left and right sides of the imaged region. In the cornea, we also observe that the Q parameter value decreases (from gray to dark pixels) and increases (from gray to bright pixels) at different lateral positions. This can be explained only by variations in the local optic axis direction as a function of lateral position. Indeed, if the optic axis direction was constant over the imaged region, the Q parameter would vary monotonically as a function of depth but could not increase and decrease.

Our results are consistent with the observations of Chang et al. [23], who used small-angle light scattering. They found that the local birefringence and optic axis of the rabbit cornea depend on lateral position. The glass slide modified the anatomical structure of the cornea and may have induced stress birefringence. However, we expect that the effect was small, inasmuch as we observed similar local variations in the polarization state of backscattered light from corneas that were unstressed. In the Q, U, and V images we see that the polarization state of light is not modified by the anterior chamber fluid and remains approximately constant in the anterior lens. Therefore the aqueous fluid and lens do not appear birefringent.

A-Scan Averages of the Cornea

The amplitude of the Stokes parameters as a function of depth, i.e., in A-scan mode, has a significant noise component due to speckle effects, detector shot noise, and electronic amplification noise. To decrease this noise, we averaged laterally adjacent pixel values (after reregistering A-scan depth positions to align laterally on the glass slide surface). Figure 20 shows an example of an average of 25 adjacent A-scans for the intensity I and phase retardation Φ calculated according to Eq. (44). The left y axis corresponds to I in decibels (solid line) and the right y axis refers to Φ in degrees (dashed line). The letters above the x axis refer to the depth positions described in Fig. 19. In the air (*a–b*), glass slide (*b–c*), and aqueous (*d–e*), the intensity I is minimum. Peak values of I are observed at the air/glass (*b*), glass/cornea (*c*), cornea/aqueous (*d*), and aqueous/crystalline lens (*e*) interfaces. In the cornea (*c–d*), I varies between −70 dB and −80 dB, and in the anterior part of the crystalline lens it decreases slowly down to the noise level (−92 dB). In air (*a–b*), glass slide (*b–c*), and aqueous (*d–e*), the reflected light intensity is below the noise level of the PS-OCT system. In these regions, the value of Φ is not related to the polarization state of the reflected light but varies randomly between 0° and 180° on individual A-scans. Φ averages 65° in Fig. 20, instead of 90° (all values have equal probability), probably because of an imbalance in the detector noise figures. At the air/glass (*b*), glass/cornea (*c*), and aqueous/crystalline lens (*e*) interfaces, we observed that when the

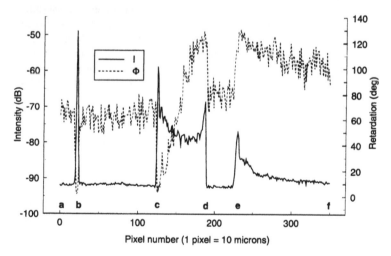

Figure 20   Plots of I and Φ parameters versus depth. The letters *a, b, c, d, e,* and *f* indicate the depth positions introduced on Fig. 19. Plots were calculated by averaging 25 adjacent A-scans of the I and Φ parameter images. Φ was calculated according to Eq. (44). At all interfaces a peak of intensity (I) can be observed. In the air, glass, and aqueous, no light is reflected; and I is about −92 dB and $\Phi = 65°$. In the cornea, I varies between −70 dB and −80 dB, and in the crystalline lens it slowly drops down to the noise level. At the front and back glass slide surfaces, Φ drops to almost 0°; in the cornea (*c–d*) it increases from 0° to 120°. It is still 120° at the aqueous/lens interface, showing that the aqueous did not affect the Φ parameter value. In the anterior part of the crystalline lens it decreases from 120° to 100°. (Reprinted from Ref. 34 with permission of the Institute of Electrical and Electronics Engineers, Inc.)

intensity increases by 6 dB above the noise level, Φ varied by more than 70% of its initial value. Therefore, we decided to consider that Φ was representative of the polarization state of the reflected light when the intensity I is 6 dB or more above the noise level (-86 dB in Fig. 20).

In the cornea, Φ increases from $0°$ to about $120°$, indicating that the polarization state of the reflected light varies from left circular to some right elliptical state between the anterior and posterior surfaces of the cornea. The aqueous does not modify the phase retardation, because Φ equals $120°$ at the posterior cornea and anterior crystalline lens. Within the crystalline lens Φ decreases. The value of Φ computed from pixels 250–350 is unreliable because the intensity is lower than -86 dB.

9.5.5 PS-OCT Imaging in the Retina

Stokes Parameter Images

The Stokes parameter images I, Q, U, and V acquired in the retina of an enucleated rabbit eye, as well as the phase retardation Φ calculated with Eq. (44), are presented in Fig. 21. To reduce speckle noise, each pixel value in the Q, U, and V images was multiplied by the I image pixel value, a low-pass filter was applied to the resulting image, and each pixel was divided by the local average intensity. Each image represents a 3 mm wide by 2 mm deep section. The left edge corresponds approximately to the center of the optic never. Above the optic nerve the posterior hyaloid phase scatters some light and shows up as bright and dark "clouds" in the I and U images, respectively. The dark and light bands following the contour of the retina in the U and V images, respectively, mean that the light reflected from this region is in an elliptical polarization state between right circular and linear at $-45°$. In the Φ image we notice a region on top of the retina (right half) and in the optic nerve (left third) that changes approximately from gray to white as a function of depth, corresponding to an increase approximately from gray to white as a function of depth, corresponding to an increase in phase retardation. In the region where the retina curves into the optic nerve head, this increase is not as pronounced. At these positions, the axons are oriented downward and the optic axis of the tissue is nearly parallel to the incident light propagation direction.

A-Scan Averages of the Retina

Plots of I and Φ as a function of depth in the retina were obtained by averaging 50 laterally adjacent A-scans. An example is presented in Fig. 22. The intensity increases from -104 dB to -81 dB at the vitreous/retina interface, is maintained at -81 dB over approximately $100\,\mu m$, then decreases exponentially to -102 dB in 1 mm. Between pixels 31 and 90 the intensity is greater than 6 dB above the noise level (-102 dB). In this region, Φ describes reliably the polarization state of the reflected light. At the vitreous/retina interface the intensity I increase sharply and Φ drops to about $60°$. Although noise is observed in the Φ plot, the increase after the vitreous/retina interface is significantly higher than the noise amplitude. The distance between the minimum and maximum of the phase retardation was measured on a smoothed Φ plot (a low-pass or median filter can be used). For example, in Fig. 22, Φ increased over a depth of $90\,\mu m$ (pixels 35–44). Since the NFL is

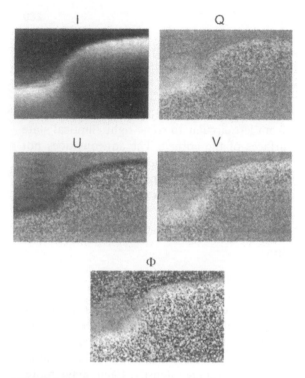

Figure 21 Stokes parameters I, normalized parameters Q, U, and V, and phase retardation Φ images in the rabbit retina. The left edge of each image is at approximately the center of the optic nerve. A significant change in phase retardation can be observed in the Φ image at the position of the NFL. (Reprinted from Ref. 34 with permission of the Institute of Electrical and Electronics Engineers, Inc.)

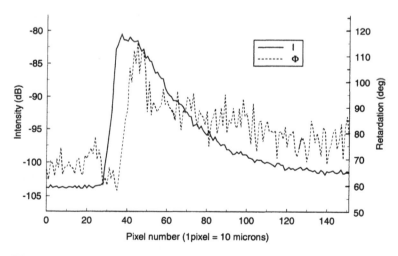

Figure 22 The values of I in decibels (solid line) and Φ in degrees (dashed line) are plotted as a function of depth in the rabbit retina. Each plot is an average of 50 depth scans, corresponding to a lateral scanning distance of $500\,\mu$m. The intensity I, i.e., the conventional OCT signal, increases from $-104\,$dB to $-81\,$dB at the vitreous/retina interface. The retardation Φ, calculated with Eq. (44), increases from about $60°$ to $115°$ over a depth of $90\,\mu$m. (Reprinted from Ref. 34 with permission of the Institute of Electrical and Electronics Engineers, Inc.)

the only known birefringent layer in the retina, we believe that the region representing a significant change in phase retardation corresponds to the NFL. The shape of the Φ versus depth plot depends on the birefringence and optic axis orientation of the tissue as well as on the polarization state of light incident on the retina. In the worst case, light incident on the retina is linearly polarized parallel to the optic axis of the NFL and no change in any of the Stokes parameters is observed. Although the chances of this happening appear remote, the problem could be resolved by probing the eye with more than one incident polarization state.

Comparison with Histology

The thickness of the retinal nerve fiber layer (NFL) was measured on histology slides every $500\,\mu$m between the black ink dots indicating the boundaries of the PS OCT-imaged region. The depth-resolved phase retardation and intensity plots were calculated at the corresponding positions by averaging 50 adjacent A-scans ($500\,\mu$m). The thickness of the region presenting a significant change in phase retardation was measured by the method described in the previous section. Figure 23 shows the NFL thickness as determined by histology and PS-OCT as a function of lateral position. Six points positioned $500\,\mu$m apart were considered. Point 1 corresponds approximately to the center of the optic nerve. The optic nerve diameter was approximately 2 mm. The optic nerve margin was near point 3. Good correlation is observed between NFL thickness measured by both methods except for points 3 and possibly 4. At point 3, the NFL curves into the optic nerve and the measurement on the histology section contains an artifact due to the position and orientation of the section. A birefringent layer was observed for points 1 and 2 that are inside the optic nerve head. This is consistent with the histology results and can be explained by the fact that the imaged section does not pass through the center of the optic nerve where the birefringence should be zero,

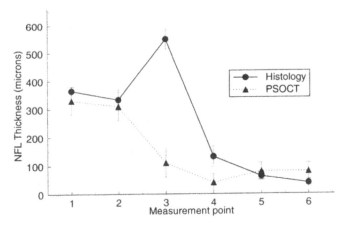

Figure 23 Comparison of NFL thickness measurement in histology section with PS-OCT. The distance between successive measurement points is $500\,\mu$m. Point 1 is approximately at the center of the optic nerve. (Reprinted from Ref. 34 with permission of the Institute of Electrical and Electronics Engineers, Inc.)

because all fibers (and thus the tissue optic axis) are parallel to the incident light propagation direction.

9.5.6 Conclusions

Depth-resolved Stokes parameter images of the corneas and retinas of New Zealand White rabbit eyes were acquired with PS-OCT. We demonstrated that the cornea is birefringent and that the birefringence as well as the optic axis of the stroma vary as a function of lateral position. PS-OCT could be used to study the corneal stroma structure more extensively.

We also imaged the retina and observed a birefringent layer at the vitre-ous/retina interface. The local thickness of the birefringent layer determined using PS-OCT correspond closely to the thickness of the NFL measured from histology slides in four out of six predetermined points. With SLP and OCT, NFL thickness is typically measured in a cylindrical ring around the optic nerve with a diameter of 1.5–1.75 optic discs, corresponding to the location of points 5 and 6 in our experiment. At these points, NFL thickness measured by PS-OCT is in close agreement with the histological results. Furthermore, the magnitude of the birefringence is related to the axon density, and a quantitative analysis of the phase retardation could provide information on axon density within the NFL.

9.6   FUTURE DIRECTIONS IN PS-OCT

The potential biological and medical applications of PS-OCT are just beginning to be explored. Much work remains for further development of PS-OCT. We anticipate that progress will procced in three major areas: instrumentation, biological and medical applications, and data interpretation and image processing. Many clinical applications of PS-OCT will require the development of a fiber-based instrument that can record images at frame rates comparable to those of current OCT systems ($\sim$ 5 fps). Because many components in biological materials contain intrinsic and/or form birefringence, PS-OCT is an attractive technique for providing an additional contrast mechanism that can be used to image and/or identify structural components. Moreover, because functional information in some biological systems is associated with transient changes in birefringence, the possibility of functional PS-OCT imaging should be explored. PS-OCT may hold considerable potential for monitoring, in real time, laser surgical procedures involving birefringent biological materials. Because many laser surgical procedures rely on a photothermal injury mechanism, birefringence changes in subsurface tissue components measured using PS-OCT may be used as a feedback signal to control dosimetry in real time. Finally, many features of PS-OCT interference fringe data require additional interpretation and study. Because polarization changes in light propagating in the sample may be used as an additional contrast mechanism, the relative contribution of light scattering and birefringence-induced changes requires further study and clarification. In principle, one would like to distinguish polarization changes due to scattering and birefringence at each position in the sample and use each as a potential contrast mechanism. In conclusion, we anticipate that PS-OCT will continue to advance rapidly and be applied to novel problems in clinical medicine and biological research.

ACKNOWLEDGMENTS

Research grants from the Institute of Arthritis, Musculoskeletal and Skin Diseases and Heart, Lung and Blood, and the National Center for Research Resources at the National Institutes of Health, U.S. Department of Energy, Office of Naval Research, the Whitaker Foundation, and the Beckman Laser Institute Endowment are gratefully acknowledged.

REFERENCES

1. Schmitt JM, Gandjbakhche AH, Bonner RR. Use of polarised light to discriminate short-path photons in a multiply scattering medium. Appl Opt 31:6535–6546, 1992.
2. MacKintosh FC, Zhu JX, Pine DJ, Weitz DA. Polarization memory of multiple scattered light. Phys Rev B 40:9342–9345, 1989.
3. Bicout D, Brosseau C, Martinez AS, Schmitt JM. Depolarization of multiply scattered waves by spherical diffusers: Influence of the size parameter. Phys. Rev. E 49:1767–1770, 1994.
4. Mie G. Beitrage zur Optik trüber Medien speziell kolloidaler Metallösungen. Ann Phys 25:377, 1908.
5. Mishchenko MI, Hovenier JW. Depolarization of light backscattered by randomly oriented nonspherical particles. Opt Lett 20:1356–1358, 1995.
6. Hemenger RP. Birefringence of a medium of tenuous parallel cylinders. Appl Opt 28:4030–4034, 1989.
7. Hee MR, Huang D, Swanson EA, Fujimoto JG. Polarization-sensitive low-coherence reflectometer for birefringence characterization and ranging. J Opt Soc Am B 9:903–908, 1992.
8. de Boer JF, Milner TE, van Gemert MJC, Nelson JS. Two-dimensional birefringence imaging in biological tissue by polarization-sensitive optical coherence tomography. Opt Lett 22:934–936,1997
9. Everett MJ, Schoenenberger K, Colston BW Jr, Da Silva LB. Birefringence characterization of biological tissue by use of optical coherence tomography. Opt Lett 23:228–230, 1998.
10. Mandel L, Wolf E. Optical Coherence and Quantum Optics. Cambridge, England: Cambridge Univ Press, 1995.
11. Schoenenberger K, Colston BW Jr, Maitland DJ, Da Silva LB, Everett MJ. Mapping of birefringence and thermal damage in tissue by use of polarization-sensitive optical coherence tomography. Appl Opt 37:6026–6036, 1998.
12. de Boer JF, Milner TE, Nelson JS. Two dimensional birefringence imaging in biological tissue using phase and polarization sensitive optical coherence tomography. Trends Opt Photonics (TOPS) 21:321–324, 1998.
13. Shurcliff WA, Ballard SS. Polarized Light. New York: Van Nostrand, 1964.
14. Hazebroek HF, Holscher AA. Interferometric ellipsometry. J Phys E: Sci Instrum 6:822–826, 1973.
15. Bohren CF, Huffman DR. Absorption and Scattering of Light by Small Particles. New York: Wiley, 1983.
16. de Boer JF, Milner TE, Nelson JS. Determination of the depth resolved Stokes parameters of light backscattered from turbid media using polarization sensitive optical coherence tomography. Opt Let 24:300–302, 1999.
17. de Boer JF, Srinivas SM, Park BH, Pham TH, Chen Z, Milner TE, Nelson JS. Polarization effects in optical coherence tomography of various biological tissues. IEEE J Selected Topics Quant Electron, 5:1200–1204, 1999.

18. Schmitt JM. Array detection for speckle reduction in optical coherence microscopy. Phys Med Biol 42:1427–1439, 1997.
19. Schmitt JM, Xiang SH, Yung KM. Speckle in optical coherence tomography. J Biomed Opt 4:95–105, 1999.
20. van Blokland GJ. Ellipsometry of the human retina in vivo: Preservation of polarization. J Opt Soc Am A 2:72–75, 1985.
21. Klein Brink HB, van Blokland GJ. Birefringence of the human foveal area assessed in vivo with Mueller-matrix ellipsometry. J Opt Soc Am A 5:49–57, 1988.
22. Naylor EJ. The structure of the cornea as revealed by polarized light. Quart J Microsc Sci 94:83–88, 1953.
23. Chang EP, Keedy DA, Chien CW. Ultrastructures of rabbit corneal stroma: Mapping of optical and morphological anisotropies. Biochim Biophys Acta 343:615–626, 1974.
24. Maitland DJ, Walsh JT. Quantitative measurements of linear birefringence during heating of native collagen. Lasers Surg Med 20:310–318, 1997.
25. Yao G, Wang L. Two-dimensional depth-resolved Mueller matrix characterization of biological tissue by optical coherence tomography. Opt Lett 24:537–539, 1999.
26. Thomsen S. Pathologic analysis of photothermal and photomechanical effects of laser–tissue interactions. Photochem Photobiol 53:825–835, 1995.
27. de Boer JF, Milner TE, van Gemert MJC, Nelson JS. Two-dimensional birefringence imaging in biological tissue using polarization-sensitive optical coherence tomography. Proc Soc Photo-Opt Instrum Eng 3196:32, 1998.
28. Tearney GJ, Brezinski ME, Southern JF, Bouma BE, Hee MR, Fujimoto JG. Determination of the refractive index of highly scattering human tissue by optical coherence tomography. Opt Lett 20:2258–2260, 1995.
29. Srinivas SM, de Boer JF, Park BH, Malekafzali A, Keikhanzadeh K, Huang L, Chen Z, Nelson JS. In vivo burn depth assessment using polarization-sensitive optical coherence tomography. Proc. Soc Photo-Opt Instrum Eng 3598:70–78, 1999.
30. Park DH, Hwang JW, Jang KS, Han DG, Ahn KY, Baik BS. Use of laser Doppler flowmetry for estimation of the depth of burns. Plast Reconstr Surg 101:1516–1523, 1998.
31. Sheridan RL, Schomaker KT, Lucchina LC, et al. Burn depth estimation by use of indocyanine green fluorescence: Initial human trial. J Burn Care Rehabil 16:602–604, 1995.
32. Heimbach D, Engrav L, Grube B, Marvin J. Burn depth: A review. World J Surg 16:10–15, 1992.
33. Waxman K, Lefcourt N, Achauer B. Heated laser Doppler flow measurements to determine depth of burn injury. Am J Surg 157:541–543, 1989.
34. Ducros MG, de Boer JF, Huang H, Chao L, Chen Z, Nelson JS, Milner TE, Rylander HG. Polarization sensitive optical coherence tomography of the rabbit eye. IEEE J Selected Topics Quant Electron, 5:1159–1167, 1999.
35. Varma R, Skaf M, Barron E. Retinal nerve fiber layer thickness in normal human eyes. Ophthalmology 103: 2114–2119:1996.
36. Zhou Q, Knighton RW. Light scattering and form birefringence of parallel cylindrical arrays that represent cellular organelles of the retinal nerve fiber layer. Appl Opt 36: 2273–2285, 1997.
37. de Boer JF, Srinivas SM, Malekafzali A, Chen Z, Nelson JS. Imaging thermally damaged tissue by polarization sensitive optical coherence tomography. Opt Express 3:212–218, 1998.
38. Chandrasekhar C. Radiative Transfer. New York: Dover, 1960.
39. MacKintosh FC, John S. Diffusing-wave spectroscopy and multiple scattering of light in correlated random media. Phys Rev B 40: 2383–2406, 1989.

10

Optical Coherence Microscopy

HSING-WEN WANG and JOSEPH A. IZATT

Case Western Reserve University, Cleveland, Ohio

MANISH D. KULKARNI

Zeiss Humphrey Systems, Dublin, California

10.1 INTRODUCTION

In this chapter, approaches for increasing the spatial resolution of OCT to enable noninvasive imaging of tissues at the cellular level are discussed. In particular, the dual nature of OCT both as an optical time-of-flight gating instrument and as a confocal microscope are described, and the implications of increasing the numerical aperture of OCT until the width of the axial point spread function of the confocal microscope approaches the width of the axial point spread function of the range gate are analyzed. It is found that the high numerical aperture mode of operation of OCT (here referred to as optical coherence microscopy, or OCM) offers significant advantages for high resolution imaging deep in highly scattering tissues compared to confocal microscopy. However, these advantages come at the price of requiring higher quality optics and sample arm stability compared to conventional OCT.

10.2 RESOLUTION IMPROVEMENT IN OCT

Optical coherence tomography (OCT) has met wide success in initial clinical applications because it offers spatial resolution superior to that of other noninvasive medical imaging techniques such as computed tomography, magnetic resonance imaging, and ultrasound. The 10–15 μm axial and lateral resolution of most OCT systems used to date is sufficient to visualize normal morphology at the tissue level as well as disruptions of normal morphology due to disease processes. However, the resolution of current OCT systems is at least one order of magnitude less than that required to visualize most types of living cells; thus the goal of a true "optical biopsy" capable of conclusive diagnosis of pathologies at the cellular level (such as cancer) remains unrealized.

A number of approaches have been conceived to extend the spatial resolution of OCT. The most straightforward approach makes use of the well-known relation of the full width at half-maximum (FWHM) coherence length l_c of a light source to its center wavelength λ and FWHM spectral bandwidth $\Delta\lambda$ (under the assumption of a Gaussian source frequency spectrum) [1]:

$$l_c = \ln(2)\frac{2\lambda^2}{\pi\,\Delta\lambda} \tag{1}$$

By using shorter wavelength or broader bandwidth light sources for OCT, the coherence length of the source is thus reduced and the axial resolution is increased. Typical parameters for current clinical implementations of OCT include $\lambda = 840\,\text{nm}$, $\Delta\lambda \sim 30$ nm, $\Delta z \sim 10.4\,\mu\text{m}$ for ophthalmic OCT using superluminescent diode sources [2], and $\lambda = 1300$ nm, $\Delta\lambda \sim 70$ nm, $l_c \sim 10.7\,\mu\text{m}$ for endoscopic OCT using semiconductor optical amplifier sources [3,4]. OCT systems using broader bandwidth sources including LEDs, broadband fluorescent sources, and mode-locked lasers have also been reported featuring coherence lengths ranging as short as $2\,\mu\text{m}$ [5–7].

Optical coherence tomographic systems based on ultrabroad bandwidth sources have illustrated dramatic improvements in image quality, including a recent demonstration of cellular resolution imaging in *Xenopus* with $\sim 1.5\,\mu\text{m} \times 3\,\mu\text{m}$ (longitudinal × transverse) resolution imaging using a novel sub-two optical cycle mode-locked Ti : sapphire laser [8]. However, significant signal losses and increased system complexity accompany the use of such sources, including the reduced heterodyne efficiency for shorter coherence length, difficulties in obtaining ultrabroadband fiber couplers, greatly increased difficulties of dispersion matching in the interferometer arms, and (in the case of femtosecond lasers) the dramatically increased complexity of the source itself. In addition, it is noteworthy that decreasing the source coherence length increases the resolution only in the axial dimension. Although the near-surface structures of many biological tissues accessible to OCT demonstrate a layered structure in which axial resolution is more critical than lateral resolution, most biological cell types do not exhibit this structure. Thus, a method for OCT imaging that increases resolution in all three spatial dimensions remains desirable.

A second approach for increasing the resolution of OCT springs from the observation that an OCT scanner is inherently a single spatial mode confocal microscope as well as a range-gating instrument [9,10]. Fundamentally, confocality of the light incident on and returning from the sample is ensured by the heterodyne mixing process, which selects out only the light returning from the sample that occupies the same spatial mode as the local oscillator (the reference light). In fact, OCT systems implemented in single-mode fiber optics are redundantly confocal, because the sample arm fiber also acts as a single-mode aperture for illumination and collection of light from the sample. In contrast to bright-field microscopy, in which the received power in the reflection geometry does not depend on the scatter depth, in a confocal system the reflected power is a function of the scatterer location in all three dimensions [11]. Thus, in addition to the depth resolution that OCT derives from low coherence interferometry (hereafter referred to as the "coherence gate"), any OCT system is also characterized by a depth and lateral response that is purely a function of the sample arm optics (hereafter referred to as the "confocal gate").

Abbé's rule for the lateral resolution Δx of a coherent microscope is given by [12]

$$\Delta x = 1.22 \frac{\lambda}{[NA]_{objective} + [NA]_{condenser}} \tag{2}$$

where the denominator reduces to twice the numerical aperture (NA) of the objective in a confocal microscope operating in the retroreflection configuration (see Fig. 1). Increasing the NA can thus increase the lateral resolution, but it also decreases the confocal parameter (or depth of focus b, given by $b = 2z_R = 2\pi\omega_0^2/\lambda$. Here z_R is the "Rayleigh range," and ω_0 is the minimum beam waist of a Gaussian beam [13]. In conventional OCT, a relatively low numerical aperture objective (NA < 0.2) is typically used in the sample arm for two reasons. First, even a relatively low numerical aperture objective still delivers a lateral resolution Δx of $\sim 10\text{--}20\,\mu m$, thus giving more or less square pixels when the depth resolution is set by the coherence length of a typical OCT light source. Second, the low numerical aperture objective also generates a long depth of focus (b greater than several hundred micrometers), within which the coherence gate may be axially scanned without much loss of light recoupling back into the confocal gate. This latter reason is particularly germane in the design of clinical diagnostic

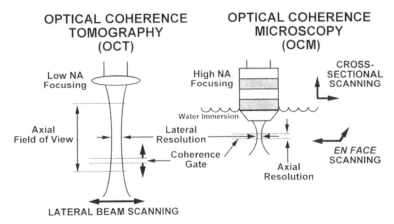

Figure 1 Schematic illustration of sample arm focusing in optical coherence tomography (OCT) and optical coherence microscopy (OCM). In OCT, low numerical aperture focusing is employed to provide a long depth of focus to enable cross-sectional imaging using axial coherence gate scanning. In OCM, sample arm light is focused with a high numerical aperture objective to create a minimal focal volume in the sample. The low coherence interferometric coherence gate is overlapped with the focal volume to provide enhanced scatter rejection of out-of-focus light, while the sample is scanned in either the *xy* or *xz* planes to create *en face* or cross-sectional images, respectively. (From Ref. 53.)

devices, which must be used with living (and moving) patients. For example, an endoscopic OCT probe exiting the distal end of a several-meters-long endoscope deep inside the gastrointestinal tract of a patient cannot be positioned with much greater than millimeter accuracy in position next to the tissue to be imaged (at least without a dramatic redesign of the endoscope). In this case, a long depth of focus in the OCT sample arm optics enables reasonable tissue images to be obtained even if the physician has relatively poor control over the position of the sample arm optics themselves.

Increasing the numerical aperture of the sample arm optics increases both the lateral and axial resolutions of the confocal microscope and is thus an alternative method to increase the resolution in OCT. As shown in the following sections, overlapping the coherence gate of OCT at the same depth as the confocal gate of the confocal microscope increases the depth to which high resolution confocal images can be acquired in highly scattering media. In this book, we define optical coherence microscopy (OCM) as the implementation of OCT with high numerical aperture optics in the sample arm, accompanied by some means to coordinate the coherence gate position to the confocal gate position (Fig. 1). Optical coherence microscopes have been demonstrated using both single and array detection techniques; the former will be discussed in the present chapter, and the latter in Chapter 11.

10.3 CONFOCAL MICROSCOPY IN SCATTERING MEDIA

In this section, we review the principles of confocal microscopy including fiber-optic implementations and imaging performance in scattering media. Confocal microscopy has been successful in imaging up to very high resolution ($< 1\,\mu$m) in relatively weakly scattering biological media and a few scattering depths into highly scattering media [12,14–17]. Combining focused illumination with spatially filtered detection, the confocal microscope collects signal from a diffraction-limited focal volume and rejects background that originates outside that focal volume. In an ideal case using single-point detection, the image intensity of the microscope is given by [12]

$$I(u, v) = \left|(h_{\text{ill}}(u, v)h_{\text{det}}(u, v)) \otimes R(u, v)\right| = \left|h_{\text{confocal}}(u, v) \otimes R(u, v)\right| \quad (3)$$

where

$$u = \left(\frac{8\pi}{\lambda}\right)z \sin^2\left(\frac{\text{NA}}{2}\right), \qquad v = \left(\frac{2\pi}{\lambda}\right)r \sin(\text{NA})$$

where h_{ill} and h_{det} are the illumination and detection point spread functions (PSFs), respectively (given by the Fourier transforms of the condenser and objective pupil functions), u and v are axial and lateral optical units, respectively (in terms of the actual axial and lateral distances z and x), and R is the power reflectivity of the sample object. The quantity $h_{\text{confocal}}(u, v)$ is the product of the illumination and detection PSFs and represents the overall PSF of the confocal imaging system. In the reflection mode of a confocal microscope, the same objective is used for sample illumination and light collection, and thus $h_{\text{ill}} = h_{\text{det}}$. For an ideal point object, the power reflectivity in Eq. (3) simplifies to a three-dimensional delta function, and the axial and lateral components of the response function separate, given by

$$I_{point}(u) = h_{confocal,point}(u) = \left[\frac{\sin(u/4)}{u/4}\right]^4 \tag{4a}$$

$$I_{point}(v) = h_{confocal,point}(v) = \left(\frac{2J_1(v)}{v}\right)^4 \tag{4b}$$

The widths of the functions $I(u)$ and $I(v)$ versus u (or z) and v (or r), respectively, decrease as NA increases. Thus, the axial and lateral resolutions of a confocal microscope are improved at high numerical aperture.

The axial response of a confocal microscope is easier to measure experimentally by measuring the PSF of a uniform planar object such as a mirror by scanning the mirror axially through the focus. In this case, the reflectivity $R(u, v)$ in Eq. (3) is equal to 1 at $u = 0$ for all v. The axial component of the image intensity is then modified to

$$I_{mirror}(u) = h_{confocal,planar}(u) = \left(\frac{\sin(u/2)}{u/2}\right)^2 \tag{5}$$

For an objective with NA = 0.4, the FWHM of the effective PSF, or the FWHM of the measured image intensity of an ideal mirror as a function of the depth, is approximately 8 μm. For NA = 0.3, this FWHM increases to ~ 35 μm.

Considering a finite-sized detector (or equivalently a finite-sized confocal pinhole) $D(v)$, Eqs. (4) and (5) are modified to

$$I_{int}(u) = \int I(u, v)D(v)v \, dv \tag{6}$$

where the signal intensity is integrated over the detection aperture. The axial discrimination or "confocality" is dependent on the size of the confocal pinhole. It has been shown that the confocality, using a pinhole radius v_p in optical units of less than 2.5, is the same as that using an ideal point detector [12]. The optical unit is then defined in Eq. (3) as $(\pi d/\lambda)\sin(NA)$, where d is the diameter of the confocal pinhole. The actual pinhole size is obtained by dividing v_p by the system magnification M between the objective and the detector and should be less than $2.5M\lambda/[\pi \sin(NA)]$ in an ideal point detection case.

The penetration depth of a confocal microscope is limited by the ratio of signal S to background B (S/B). The background noise originates from outside the focal volume if the pinhole is not infinitesimally small (neglecting multiple scattering; see below). The background noise can be greatly attenuated by decreasing the size of the confocal pinhole [14–17]. Assuming a uniform background, Webb et al. [15] and Sheppard et al. [16] demonstrated independently that the background rejection improves the signal-to-noise ratio. The ability of optical sectioning and image contrast is thus improved such that the signal-to-noise ratio rather than the signal-to-background ratio limit the information capacity of an image [14–17]. The penetration depth can be expressed in terms of mean free path (MFP), which is the product of the depth and the extinction coefficient $\mu_t = \mu_s + \mu_a$ of the sample medium. In biological samples, the absorption coefficient μ_a is usually negligible in the near-infrared spectral region; thus the extinction coefficient is dominated by the scattering coefficient μ_s. The penetration depth limit of a conventional confocal microscope has been estimated to be dependent on the numerical aperture and to be 5–9 MFP using single backscatter theory (discussed in the next section) [9,18,19]. However, the penetration depth limit is degraded to 3–4 MFP if multiple scattering is considered [20]. The penetration depth also depends upon the reflectivity of the sample; a highly reflective grating has been resolved through 6 MFP of scattering media by using a confocal pinhole with diameter equal to 1.3 optical units [21].

The single-mode fiber-optic confocal microscope is a relatively new implementation of the confocal scanning microscope. The introduction of optical fibers makes the system more compact with numerous potential remote imaging applications, but it also changes the nature of the imaging point spread function. Because the light source in a fiber confocal microscope is the spatial mode profile of the light exiting the fiber tip (which also defines the confocal pinhole), image formation in this system is different from that of a conventional confocal microscope. In this case, the axial effective point spread function of a planar reflective sample from Eqs. (4) is modified to [22]

$$h_{\text{confocal,planar}}^{\text{fiber}}(u) = \left| \frac{A\{1 - \exp[-(A - iu)]\}}{[1 - \exp(-A)](A - iu)} \right|^2 \tag{7}$$

where

$$A = \left(\frac{2\pi a_0 r_0}{\lambda d} \right)^2$$

Here, the system magnification is assumed to be 1. The dimensionless parameter A denotes the normalized fiber spot size, where a_0 is the pupil radius of the objective, r_0 is the radius of the core of a single-mode fiber, and d is the distance from the fiber tip to the collimating lens. Parameter A plays a role analogous to that of the normalized pinhole radius v_p in a hard-aperture confocal microscope. For an objective with a fixed NA, the width of the PSF becomes broader as A increases. Thus, the strength of the optical sectioning effect (or degree of confocality) decreases with increasing A. Similar to a confocal point, $\sqrt{A}$ is measured relative to the object plane and the actual value of $\sqrt{A}$ must be multiplied by the system magnification M between the object and the detector. For a 20× objective with NA 0.4, assuming $\lambda = 1.31 \, \mu$m, $d = 4.5$ mm, $a_0 \sim$ mm, and $r_0 = 4.5$ um, A is less than 0.5. Since $h_{\text{confocal,planar}}^{\text{fiber}}(u)$ for $A = 0$ and $A = 1$ are nearly identical, the degree of confocality for $A < 1$ is close to the case of an ideal single-point detection in a confocal microscope. For the case of a point reflector and in the limit $A = 0$, the axial PSF of the single-mode fiber confocal microscope simplifies to be the same as the axial component of Eqs. (4) [22].

Unlike in a conventional confocal microscope, however, the received intensity in a fiber-optic confocal microscope is limited by the nonadjustable fiber core size. In the conventional microscope, the confocal pinhole can be opened up to $2.5v_p$ to have image quality equivalent to using an ideal point detector but with higher signal intensity. This flexibility is not available in the optical fiber implementation.

Although fiber-optic confocal microscopes have strong potential for use in in vivo medical diagnostics, most confocal microscopes available commercially for general-purpose applications are table-top systems using bulk optics. This implementation provides the advantages of flexibility in the choice of light sources, scan parameters, and pinhole size. The greatest impediment to the widespread use of fiber-optic confocal microscopes in remote imaging applications such as endoscopy is the difficulty of implementing a lateral scanning mechanism within the restricted volume available at the working end of the probe. A novel solution to this problem that has recently been proposed uses a miniaturized diffraction grating–lens combination with no moving parts [23]. This system encodes the reflectivity of the sample as a function of lateral extent into the spectral content of the detected signal light, using a broadband optical source.

10.4 COHERENCE-GATED CONFOCAL MICROSCOPY

Although confocal microscopy has been used successfully for imaging through relatively thin layers of living biological tissues [24], the mechanism of image formation in the axial dimension immediately gives rise to two important limitations to confocal imaging in a turbid media. First, because turbid media are exponentially scattering (i.e., their reflectivity varies exponentially as a function of depth), an imaging system that aims to image deeply into turbid media should preferably feature an axial PSF, which is a stronger function of distance from the object plane than an exponential. The envelope of the sinc functions in Eqs. (4a) and (5) do not satisfy this criterion. Second, confocal microscopy features no intrinsic mechanism for rejection of multiply scattered light, which inevitably leads to image clouding at sufficient depth [20].

Both of these concerns are alleviated by the addition of coherence grating to confocal microscopy. As will be shown below, the effective axial PSF of an optical coherence microscope approaches a Gaussian function of distance from the object plane (in the ideal case of a source with a Gaussian spectrum), which is a stronger function of distance than an exponential and thus achieves stronger theoretical spatial discrimination than a confocal gate alone. Second, the addition of the coherence gate to the confocal gate provides an additional barrier for increased rejection of non-image-bearing multiply scattered light.

To extend the quantitative analysis of the previous section to the case of coherence-gated confocal microscopy (i.e., OCM), we must first expand the theoretical description of OCT derived in previous chapters to include the axial PSF of the confocal gate, which is always present (but rarely considered because it is usually broad) in OCT. The lateral PSF of an OCM system is not affected by the coherence gate and is given by Eq. (4b) for a hard-edged (i.e., bulk-optic system) confocal aperture. The axial response of OCM depends upon both confocal and coherence gates. The detector current in an OCT/OCM system is in general given by [25]

$$\tilde{i}_d(l_r) \propto \int_0^\infty \sqrt{R_s(l_s)h_s(l_s)}\,\tilde{R}_{ii}(l_r - l_s)\,dl_s \tag{8}$$

where l_r is the reference arm length, l_s is the sample arm length, $R_s(l_s)$ represents the depth-dependent reflectivity of the sample, $h_s(l_s)$ is the axial PSF of the sample arm confocal optics [given by Eqs. (4)–(7) depending upon the normalized aperture of the pinhole or fiber and the nature of the object], and $\tilde{R}_{ii}(l_r - l_s)$ is the source autocorrelation function, which can be thought of as the axial PSF of the coherence gate. The tildes above the detector current and autocorrelation functions denote that these quantities are undemodulated; typically the detector current is demodulated at the carrier frequency of the autocorrelation function (usually given by the Doppler shift of the reference arm light) before being digitized and displayed [26]. The square root sign denotes that in OCM/OCT the detector current is proportional to the electric field amplitude returning from the sample arm rather than its power. The salient feature of Eq. (8) is that the confocal PSF $h_s(l_s)$ *multiplies* with the depth-dependent reflection coefficient profile $R_s(l_s)$, whereas the low coherence interferometric PSF $\tilde{R}_{ii}$ $(l_r - l_s)$ *convolves* with the reflection coefficient profile [27,28].

The Weiner–Khinchin theorem states that the autocorrelation function of a signal is given by the inverse Fourier transform of that signal's power spectral density [29]. Although many sources used in OCT are not ideal, many sources approach the ideal case of having a Gaussian power spectral density (PSD) represented by

$$S_{ii}(k) \propto \frac{2\sqrt{\ln 2}}{\Delta k \sqrt{\pi}} \exp\left\{ -\left[\frac{(k - k_0)^2}{\Delta k/2\sqrt{\ln 2}} \right] \right\} \tag{9}$$

where k_0 is the center wavenumber and Δk the FWHM spectral bandwidth. In this case, the detector current reduces to

$$\tilde{i}_d(l_r) \propto \int_0^\infty \sqrt{R_s(l_s)h_s(l_s)} \exp\left[-\left(\frac{l_r - l_s}{l_c/\sqrt{\ln 2}} \right)^2 \right] \exp[j2\pi k_0(l_r - l_s)] \, dl_s \tag{10}$$

Thus the low coherence interferometric PSF that convolves with the product of the sample reflectivity and confocal gate PSF is a Gaussian function.

The interaction of the confocal and coherence PSFs is illustrated by considering the case of a single planar reflector at depth l_{s0} in the sample arm. In this limit, Eq. (8) simplifies to

$$\tilde{i}_d(l_r) \propto \sqrt{R_s(l_{s0})h_s(l_{s0})} R_{ii}(l_r - l_{s0}) \tag{11}$$

The objective location and reference arm position thus provide independent control over the positions of the peaks of the confocal and coherence gates, respectively. Maximum signal acquisition occurs for $l_r = l_{s0}$, when both functions are overlapped at the desired detection depth. Maintaining perfect overlap of these two functions can be a challenging experimental concern in random media such as biological tissues (see below).

One mode of imaging in OCM is to overlap the confocal and coherence gates and then raster scan in the x–y direction, i.e., at fixed sample arm depth l_{s0} [9,25,30–32]. Another mode is to perform dynamic focusing wherein the focus position is scanned within the tissue in synchrony with reference mirror scanning [33–35]. In this case, Eq. (8) takes the form

$$\tilde{i}_d(l_r) \propto \int_0^\infty \sqrt{R_s(l_s)h_s(l_r - l_s)} R_{ii}(l_r - l_s) \, dl_s \tag{12}$$

In this case, both the coherence and confocal PSFs convolve with the depth-dependent sample reflectivity.

In either scanning mode, however, the Gaussian shaped autocorrelation function falls off more rapidly than the axial response of the confocal microscope; thus the overlap of both functions in OCM provides enhanced scatter rejection of out-of-focus light compared to confocal microscopy alone. As an example, experimental plots of the confocal axial response (for a planar mirror sample) and source auto-correlation function of a laboratory OCM system are illustrated in Fig. 2. The

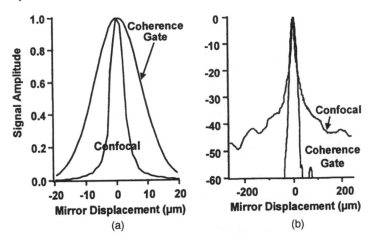

Figure 2 (a) Linear and (b) logarithmic plots of the confocal axial response of an OCM using a 40×, 0.65 NA objective and the source autocorrelation function under conditions of exact spatial overlap. The plots were obtained by translating a mirror through the focal region with the reference arm blocked (confocal only) and unblocked (autocorrelation function). (From Ref. 25.)

confocal axial response was obtained by scanning a mirror through the focus of the objective with the reference arm blocked. The source autocorrelation function was obtained by scanning a mirror through the focal region of the OCM with weak sample arm focusing and is close to a Gaussian function as expected for a semiconductor superluminescent diode source [36]. It is apparent from the plots that near the focus the combined axial response of the OCM is dominated by the axial response of the confocal microscope. However, far from the focus (better seen on the logarithmic plot) the sharper autocorrelation function shape acts to reject scattered light, which is incompletely eliminated by the aberrated wings of the confocal-only axial response. In this case where the confocal PSF dominates on a linear scale, one can think of the coherence gate as essentially isolating a region of depth in the sample within which the confocal microscope operates as usual.

The advantage of OCM over confocal microscopy alone for scattered light rejection in turbid media is illustrated in Fig. 3. This figure illustrates *en face* imaging of absorbing structures placed in highly scattering media, which were not visualized using confocal microscopy alone but which were clearly visualized with the addition of coherence gating. The confocal image in this case was obscured by out-of-focus light rather than electronic noise, which the confocal PSF was incapable of penetrating.

10.5 IMAGE FORMATION IN SCATTERING MEDIA

A complete analytical description of image formation using either confocal or coherence gating that is valid in highly scattering media has not yet been developed. A number of Monte Carlo simulations of confocal microscopy, OCT, and OCM have appeared in the literature [20,37,38], but it is difficult to obtain physical insight from these results. A preliminary theoretical description of single and multiple scattering

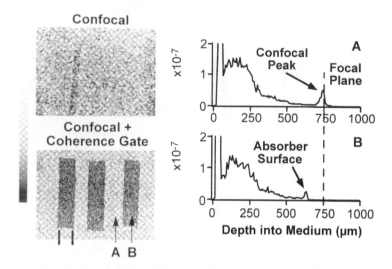

Figure 3 Two-dimensional images of absorbing bars embedded $700\,\mu m$ deep in a scattering medium ($0.3\,\mu m$ diameter polymer microspheres) with scattering coefficient $\mu_s \sim 6\,mm^{-1}$. Top left, confocal image without coherence gating. Bottom left, confocal plus coherence gating reveals the embedded structures. Right, plots of backscatter versus depth at positions both between (A) and over (B) the absorbing bars. (From Ref. 9.)

contributions to OCT has been adapted from atmospheric scattering theory primarily by Schmitt and coworkers [19,38]. Although this model is in no sense complete, it does give considerable physical insight into image formation in scattering media and compares favorably with both experimental and Monte Carlo results published to date.

10.5.1 Single-Backscatter Theory

A single-backscatter model, adapted from atmospheric scattering theory, describes the heterodyne signal from a homogeneous scattering medium under the assumption that only single-backscattering events need to be considered [9,18,19]. Although this model is clearly not valid deep in biological or other turbid media, it does provide experimentally verified accurate results near tissue surfaces and also serves as a starting point for more sophisticated models, which include multiple scattering.

The single-backscatter model depends on the following assumptions [19]:

1. The distance between scatterers is much greater than the wavelength of the light source.
2. The polarization of scattered light is the same as that of the incident beam by the single-backscatter events.
3. The time-averaged return signal from a single scatterer is incoherent with respect to the time-averaged signal from any other scatterer.
4. The scattering phase shifts vary randomly, because the scattering particles are not all identical.

Figure 4 depicts the geometry of three coordinate systems including a transmitter at plane $x'y'$, a scattering plane xy, and a receiver at plane $x''y''$. All have a common z axis, which is the direction of beam propagation. An objective is located at plane $x'y'$, which is overlapped with the $x''y''$ plane. A collimated beam with a Gaussian amplitude distribution (having diameter D at intensity equal to $1/e^2$ of its center intensity) passes through the objective with focal length f and diameter D and is focused at a distance F from the transmitter. The medium between the objective and the sample has refractive index n_1. The surface of the sample, having refractive index n_2 and extinction coefficient μ_t, has a coordinate $(\mathbf{r}, z = 0)$ in the xy plane and is located at a distance a from the transmitter. The time-averaged heterodyne signal power contributed by the scatterers at a distance $L(z) = n_1 a + n_2 z$ from the transmitter can be calculated by summing the scattered power over the scattered plane $\mathbf{r}$ and the axial distance z from the sample surface. Distances a and z are measured in air. F and $L(z)$ are the distances of the focal plane and the scattering plane from the objective expressed in optical pathlengths. After integrating over $\mathbf{r}$ [9,18,19],

$$\langle i_s^2 \rangle = \left[\frac{\eta e}{h\nu}\left(\frac{P_0}{2}\right)\right]^2 \int_0^\infty \frac{\mu_b \pi D^2 \exp(-2\mu_t z)}{4[L(z)]^2\{1 + [\pi D^2/4\lambda L(z)]^2[1 - L(z)/F]^2\}}|\gamma(\tau)|^2\, dz \quad (13)$$

where η is the detector's quantum efficiency, e is the electron charge, $h\nu$ is the photon energy, P_0 is the incident power, and μ_b is the backscattering coefficient. $|\gamma(\tau)|$ is the self-coherence function of a heterodyne detection system, where τ is the optical time delay due to the pathlength difference of two arms. $|\gamma(\tau)|$ is equal to 1 for $\tau = 0$ and diminishes rapidly when the optical pathlength difference exceeds the coherence length l_c of the light source. l_c is defined by $l_c \equiv \int_{-\infty}^\infty |\gamma(\tau)|^2\, d\tau$.

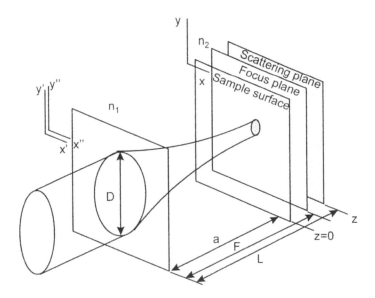

Figure 4   Geometry of the illumination and collection optics used in the single-backscatter model.

Therefore, the time-averaged heterodyne signal current within a coherence length of the center position at $L(z_{AV}) = L$ from the transmitter (or at z_{AV} from the surface of the sample) can be approximated as

$$\langle i_s(z_{AV}) \rangle \approx \frac{\eta e P_0}{2h\nu} \sqrt{R_s(z_{AV})l_c} \tag{14}$$

where

$$R_s(z_{AV}) = \frac{\mu_b \pi D^2 \exp(-2\mu_t z_{AV})}{4L^2[1 + (\pi D^2/4\lambda L)^2(1 - L/F)^2]} \tag{15}$$

$R_s(z)$ is the on-axis reflectance of the sample in the z plane. This expression contains an exponential attenuation term describing light propagation to the scattering site and back and another term describing a local reflectivity peak at the position of the focus, $L = F$.

The focal point of a collimated light beam passing through an objective (focal length f) is extended to nf when the objective is immersed in a medium having refractive index n. In this condition, the optical pathlength of the focal point from the objective, F, and the distance of the scattering plane from the objective, L, are

$$F = n^2 f, \qquad L = n(a + z) \tag{16}$$

When there is an air gap between the objective and the scattering medium, Eqs. (16) are modified to be

$$F = a + n(f - a)\left[n^2\left(\frac{D^2}{4f^2} + 1\right) - \frac{D^2}{4f^2}\right], \qquad L = a + nz \tag{17}$$

Experimental verification of these relationships is provided in Fig. 5. The plots depict experimental profiles of the heterodyne backscatter signal obtained in a polymer microsphere suspension along with the theoretical behavior calculated from Eq. (15). Although the single-backscatter model overestimates the signal magnitude at the focus and near the sample surface, the general behavior of R_s as a decreasing exponential punctuated by a confocal focus is demonstrated.

10.5.2 Comparison of OCM and Confocal Microscopy Under the Single-Scattering Assumption

The single-backscatter model was adapted by Izatt et al. [9] to compare the behavior and calculate the imaging depth limits of OCM and confocal microscopy. Two interesting limits can be readily calculated. First, the imaging depth limit of a confocal microscope was estimated under the condition of coherent detection by assuming that the received signal in a confocal microscope equals the integral of the time-averaged heterodyne current [Eq. (14)] over all depths. When light scattered from other planes exceeds the collected signal from the focal plane, image contrast drops dramatically. This contrast limit to confocal microscopy was estimated by solving Eq. (14) for the depth where the signal from the focal plane equals the signal at the surface. Given in terms of $\mu_t z_1$ or the number of scattering mean free paths, this limit is

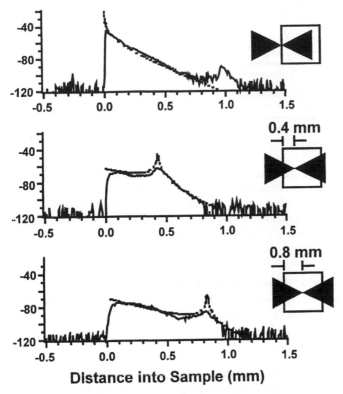

Figure 5 Plots of the heterodyne backscatter signal normalized to the measured reflection coefficient from a mirror versus the imaging depth in a calibrated polymer microsphere suspension ($\mu_s = 6\,\text{mm}^{-1}$). Plots are shown for different focal plane depths of a 20× microscope objective. Dashed curves are predictions of the single-backscatter model. (From Ref. 9.)

$$\mu_t z_1 \leq \frac{1}{2} \ln\left[\frac{\pi^2 D^2}{4\lambda^2}(\text{NA})^2\right] = \frac{1}{2}\ln\left[\frac{\pi^2}{4}M^2\right] \tag{18}$$

where NA is the numerical aperture and M (the lens aperture diameter divided by the focal spot diameter) is the geometrical magnification due to the lens.

A second limit is the depth to which single-backscattered light can be detected given quantum detection and tissue tolerance limits. After Hee et al. [39] and assuming a minimum signal-to-noise ratio of 1, this limit is

$$\mu_t z_2 \leq \frac{1}{2}\ln\left[\frac{E}{2h\upsilon}\mu_b \pi L_c(\text{NA})^2\right] \tag{19}$$

where E is the total energy incident upon the sample for each resolution element. Tissue damage thresholds and reasonable image acquisition times limit the energy that can be delivered to biological samples to a few hundred millijoules per pixel [9,39]. Linear increases in optical power, data acquisition time, and signal averaging affect this limit only logarithmically.

The range in imaging depths between these two limits predicts when OCM outperforms confocal microscopy according to single-scattering theory. Figure 6

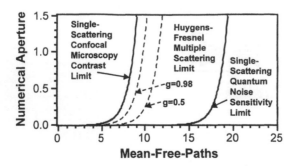

Figure 6 Parametric plot of theoretical limits to OCM in the single and multiple back-scattering models. Solid lines: Predictions of the single-backscatter model. Model parameters: $D = 3.7$ mm, $n_0 = 1.33$, $l_c = 20$ mm, $\lambda = 800$ nm, $\mu_b = 0.3191\mu_s$, $E = 130$ mJ. Dashed lines: Predictions of Huygens–Fresnel multiple scattering theory [38] for maximum single-scattered imaging depth. Model parameters: $n = 1.3$, $f = 5$ mm, $\lambda = 800$ nm.

depicts these limits, assuming typical microscope and tissue scattering parameters. Also plotted on the figure are more realistic predictions from consideration of multiple scattering, which is considered in the following sections.

10.5.3 Role of Multiple Scattering

Multiple scattering becomes important when imaging deeply into dense biological tissues [38,40]. According to the analysis of the previous section, multiple scattering reduces image contrast in confocal microscopy when imaging at a sufficient depth that the probability of multiply scattered light entering the detection pinhole exceeds the extinction of singly scattered light. Analogously, multiple scattering can reduce OCT image contrast (and possibly resolution) when imaging at a sufficient depth that the dual probabilities of multiply scattered light both entering into the detection pinhole and having traveled the correct distance exceed the extinction of singly scattered light. Since OCM is the limiting case of OCT at high numerical aperture, it would be important to understand how multiple scattering affects image formation in this limit. Unfortunately, this is still an open question.

Experimental evidence of multiple scattering in OCT has been presented by several authors. These evidences have included observations of reductions of image contrast and resolution deep in highly scattering media [40–43], the observation of phantom scattered light signals from nonscattering layers in otherwise highly scattering phantoms [40], deviations of A-scans from exponential decay in highly scattering media [40,41,43] (see Fig. 7), and observations of detected electronic power spectrum broadening due to light multiply scattered from particles undergoing Brownian motion [44,45]. In several of these experiments, multiply scattered light was detected in the range of 5–10 scattering mean free paths deep into turbid samples. However, other experimental variables (scattering anisotropy of the sample, numerical aperture of the confocal optics, wavelength and coherence length of the source) varied widely, and to date no comprehensive study of multiple scattering in OCT as a function of these variables has been published.

A few theoretical treatments of multiple scattering in OCT have also appeared [19,38,42,43]. Although largely untested experimentally, the most complete of these

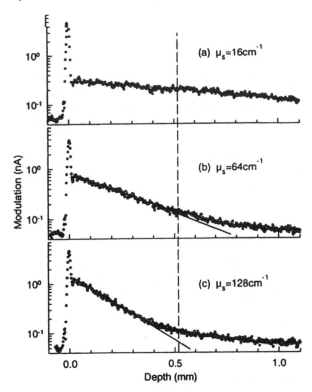

Figure 7 Experimental data illustrating multiple scattering in OCT. Deviations of the detected signal from exponential decay with depth indicate the detection of multiply scattered light for depths greater than ~ 0.5 mm. The samples were various dilutions of Intralipid solution ($g \sim 0.8$, scattering coefficients as indicated), imaged with confocal optics having a numerical aperture of ~ 0.1. (From Ref. 41.)

treatments considers image formation in OCT by adapting the extended Huygens–Fresnel formulation from atmospheric scattering theory [38]. In this formulation, which is more general than the one-dimensional treatment typically applied in OCT, the detector current is described as an integral over the product of the mutual coherence functions (MCFs) of the reference and sample arm beams:

$$i_s^2 = 2\eta^2 q^2 |g(\tau)|^2 \int\int \Gamma_s(\vec{r}_1, \vec{r}_2, z)\Gamma_r(\vec{r}_1, \vec{r}_2, z)\, d\vec{r}_1\, d\vec{r}_2 \tag{20}$$

where $\Gamma_r(\vec{r}_1, \vec{r}_2, z)$ and $\Gamma_s(\vec{r}_1, \vec{r}_2, z)$ are the mutual coherence functions of the reference and sample arm beams, respectively, which describe the spatial correlation of the electric fields of the beams at a given depth z as a function of the lateral position vectors $\vec{r}_1$ and $\vec{r}_2$,

$$\Gamma_r(\vec{r}_1, \vec{r}_2, z) = \langle U_r(\vec{r}_1) U_r^*(\vec{r}_2)\rangle \tag{21}$$

$$\Gamma_s(\vec{r}_1, \vec{r}_2, z) = \langle U_s(\vec{r}_1) U_s^*(\vec{r}_2)\rangle \tag{22}$$

In a turbid medium, the detector current can be expressed as a sum of contributions from single and small-angle multiple scattering events. The single-backscattered component results from a coherent summation over the light field singly backscattered from each of the sample volume scatterers in the vicinity of the beam focus in the sample, as in Eq. (14). Because the phases of signals having experienced pathlength dispersion resulting from multiple scattering are random, the multiply scattered component results from an incoherent sum over the multiply scattered signal powers received.

An interesting limit to OCT and OCM in scattering media suggested by Schmitt occurs at an imaging depth when the magnitudes of the multiply scattered signal overtakes that of the singly scattered signal. This occurs when

$$z_{\max} \approx \frac{1}{2\mu_s} \ln\left(1 + \frac{2R^2}{\rho_0^2}\right) \tag{23}$$

Here μ_s is the scattering coefficient of the sample, R is the $1/e$ radius of the incident probe beam, and ρ_0 is the transverse spatial coherence length of the beam. An approximate relation for ρ_0 valid for small-angle scattering is [46]

$$\rho_0 = \sqrt{\frac{3}{\mu_s z}\left(\frac{2}{k\theta_{\mathrm{rms}}}\right)} = \left[\frac{3}{4\pi^2}\left(\frac{\lambda^2}{\mu_s z(1-g)}\right)\right]^{1/2} \tag{24}$$

Here g is the scattering anisotropy of the specimen, θ_{rms} is the mean scattering angle in the tissue, and the approximate relation $\theta_{\mathrm{rms}}^2 = 2(1-g)$ was used [47].

In expression (23) it is notable that the quantity R^2/ρ_0^2 approximately corresponds to the number of speckle spots resulting from lateral beam incoherence (due to multiple scattering) that are projected onto the detector. This result leads to the surprising conclusion that increasing R (equivalent to increasing the numerical aperture of the sample arm optics for a fixed focal length) *decreases* the sensitivity of the OCM to multiply scattered light. The increase in the coherent (singly scattered) signal amplitude outstrips the increase in uncorrelated (multiply scattered) signal amplitude as a function of numerical aperture. Also, increases in the mean scattering angle (decreases in g) also lead to reduced sensitivity to multiple scattering, because increasing θ_{rms} reduces the lateral coherence length and thus also increases the number of speckle spots projected onto the detector. The dependence of $z_{\max}$ on numerical aperture (NA) and scattering anisotropy g is plotted in Fig. 6 for typical OCM imaging parameters. In rough correlation with experimental results referred to above, the predicted range of $z_{\max}$ is in the range of 5–10 scattering mean free paths for typical imaging parameters. It should be emphasized, however, that the functional dependences of the theoretical predictions have not yet been systematically investigated experimentally.

10.6 EXPERIMENTAL APPROACHES

The challenges encountered in constructing OCM systems include essentially all of the challenges of building confocal microscopes plus the necessity to perform coherence gating with high signal-to-noise ratio. As in conventional confocal microscopy, obtaining high quality objectives is expensive and always involves a trade-off between resolution and working distance. In a high numerical aperture system the confocal parameter may be on the single micrometer scale; thus much more mechanical stability is required for the sample arm optics than in OCT.

As in conventional OCT, two-dimensional OCM images may be acquired in either the xz or xy planes (with reference to Fig. 1) or in some tilted plane in between. When working with a confocal gate of approximately the same dimension as the coherence gate, however, it is a challenging concern to maintain perfect overlap of the two gates while scanning. This is because the axial positions of the confocal and coherence gates have different dependences on the refractive index of the sample. Under the paraxial approximation, when a collimated beam is focused through an objective of focal length f into a medium having refractive index n, axial movement of the objective by a distance Δz results in a movement of the focal point by $n\,\Delta z$. The equivalent optical pathlength is thus moved by $n^2\,\Delta z$. Thus, any axial scan of the OCM objective must be accompanied by a coordinated reference arm scan of n^2 times that amount [9,34]. At sufficiently high numerical aperture that the paraxial approximation cannot be used, this relationship holds true if index-matching fluid is used between the objective and the sample, but it becomes much more complicated if there is an air gap between the objective and the sample [9]. Focus-tracking scan coordination techniques based on deterministic rules may, of course, be achieved using computer-controlled translation stages. However, in samples with unpredictable variations in refractive index such as biological tissue, large variations in the index may decouple the confocal and coherence gates unless alternative means are used for their determination [48].

A second challenge associated with adding coherence gating to confocal microscopy is to implement phase modulation techniques for noise reduction in frequency-selective detection, particularly in *en face* imaging systems in which there is no Doppler shift from a moving reference arm. Several novel approaches have been reported for this purpose.

10.6.1 *En Face* Imaging Systems

The simplest approach to deal with the focus-tracking problem in OCM is to avoid it by acquiring *en face* images in the xy plane after carefully coordinating confocal and coherence gates. This is the approach adopted by Izatt et al. [9,25,52], Podoleanu et al. [30–32,49], and Haskell et al. [50].

Izatt et al. [25] employed a straightforward approach in which a moderate numerical aperture objective in the sample arm (NA = 0.65) was rigidly fixed to an optical table and the sample was raster scanned underneath. Reference arm phase modulations for lock-in detection was achieved by implementing small-amplitude ($< 1\,\mu$m) modulation of the reference mirror position using a PZT stack. This system employed a method suggested by Chinn [51] to eliminate modulation phase instability due to random fiber length changes. For an arm-length-matched OCM system with a PZT-controlled reference mirror, the interferometric component of the detector current may be written in the form

$$i_d = 1 + \cos\left(\pi \frac{V_{\text{in}}}{V_\pi} + \phi\right) \qquad (25)$$

where V_{in} is the piezo modulation voltage, v_{π} is the voltage required to produce a π phase shift in the interferogram, and ϕ is a random phase shift due to fiber length variations. If the PZT voltage is modulated with the waveform $V_{in} = \rho V_{\pi} \sin \Omega t$, then it can be shown that the detector will detect currents modulated at the first and second harmonics of the modulation frequency Ω according to

$$i_{\Omega} = -2J_1(\rho \pi) \sin \varphi \sin \Omega t, \qquad i_{2\Omega} = 2J_1(\rho \pi) \cos \varphi \cos 2\Omega t \qquad (26)$$

The sum of the powers in the first and second harmonics,

$$i_{\Omega}^2 + i_{2\Omega}^2 = J_1^2(\rho \pi) \sin^2 \phi + J_2^2(\rho \pi) \sin^2 \phi \qquad (27)$$

can then clearly be made independent of the random phase ϕ for the proper choice of the modulation amplitude ρ such that $J_1(\rho \pi) = J_2(\rho \pi)$, which occurs when $\rho \pi = 2.6$. Thus, the interferometric fringe amplitude was measured invariantly with respect to random arm length drifts by monitoring the sum of the detector powers demodulated at both harmonics of the PZT driving frequency.

The Izatt system was used to image features of human colon mucosal tissue in vitro. Sample images are reproduced in Fig. 8 and remain among the only images recorded to date using a coherence technique in which individual cells are visualized hundreds of micrometers deep in a highly scattering biological tissue. More recently,

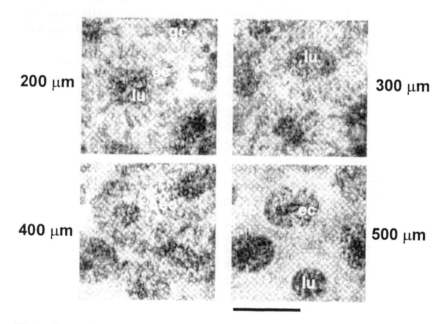

Figure 8 Optical coherence microscopic images corresponding to thin (5 μm FWHM) optical sections obtained parallel to the mucosal surface at the depths indicated in a normal human mucosal specimen in vitro. Mucosal substructure details visualized using OCM include colonic crypt lumens (lu), simple columnar epithelial cells (ec), and lamina propria connective tissue (lp). An individual goblet cell (gc; arrow) is identified as containing a nonscattering spherical mucin droplet. The proportional cross section occupied by connective tissue (lamina propria) versus crypt structures increases near the crypt bases in the deep mucosa. The maximum OCM sectioning depth was 600 mm, limited by the available low coherence power. Bar length = 200 μm. (From Ref. 25.)

the same group reported a rapid raster scan OCM system operating at several frames (4–8) per second [52].

Podoleanu et al. [30–32,49] used a novel sampling function to decode *en face* OCT images of the retina. A schematic diagram of their system is shown in Fig. 9, including two perpendicular galvanometric mirrors to form 2-D raster scans. The centers of both scanners were located on the optical axis of the sample arm optics. When one scanner was fixed, the optical pathlength changed when the other scanner swept the beam from the center of the image plane, O'', to N. The reference arm length was fixed to equal the sample pathlength at position O''. The interferometric signal had maximum intensity when the optical path difference was a multiple of a wavelength. By placing a mirror in plane S and scanning two scanners, nonuniform concentric rings similar to Newton rings were observed. The rings were nonuniform due to nonlinearity of the optical path differences Δ between O'' and N. Since the light source was quasi-monochromatic, the rings appeared within an area $A \sim (\pi/2)l_c r$ assuming the optical path difference Δ was within $l_c/4$. Because the rings contained information about the scanning angles (as a function of time as well as frequency) for each position, the rings were used as a sample function such that the returned signal was modulated in intensity at the frequency f given by

$$f = \frac{8kUx_1\omega}{x_2}\left(\frac{r\alpha}{\lambda}\right) \tag{28}$$

where k is the scanner parameter in degrees per volt, and U and ω are the amplitude and frequency of the driven scanner, respectively.

Using a setup similar to that of Fig 9 but shifting the center of the scanners by δ, the sampling function changed from concentric rings to high density uniform lines [31,32]. Higher spatial frequency of the sampling function corresponds to higher modulation frequency, which reduced the contribution of $1/f$ noise. Using $\omega_x = 300$ Hz, $\omega_y = 0.5$ Hz, and $\delta = 3$ mm, in vivo images of the human retina were obtained. The spatial resolution was $6\,\mu$m. The image acquisition rate was up to several frames per second.

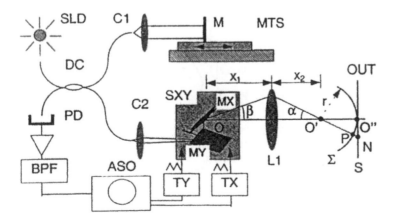

Figure 9 Schematic of OCM using a Newton rings sampling function. (From Ref. 30.)

10.6.2 Focus-Tracking Systems

An ingenious and elegant solution for axial focus tracking at relatively low numerical aperture that depends on the fact that in biological tissue $n^2 \sim 2$ was demonstrated by Schmitt et al. [33,34]. In this implementation (Fig. 10), a retroreflecting prism in the reference arm and the objective lens in the sample arm were both mounted on the same translation stage. When the objective scanned a distance Δz toward the sample, the optical pathlength in the reference arm increased by $2\,\Delta z$ to achieve the pathlength matching. An example of the excellent quality of images obtained in skin using this system is provided in Fig. 11.

Another focus-tracking technique that is suitable for high speed imaging was reported by Lexer et al. [35]. In this technique, a sample beam focus reflected offset from the center of a scanning galvanometer mirror was imaged into the sample. The imaging system translated the angular deviation of the scanner into a depth scan in the sample, and the index of the sample was compensated for by the proper choice of imaging system magnification. This technique was demonstrated for moderate speed (1 image/s) imaging of cellular structure in human corneal samples with an imaging resolution of $14\,\mu\mathrm{m} \times 5\,\mu\mathrm{m}$ (longitudinal × transverse).

10.7 CONCLUSION

Optical coherence microscopy is an extension of optical coherence tomography that capitalizes on the confocal nature of OCT to improve image resolution by imaging with high numerical aperture. From the point of view of practitioners of confocal microscopy, OCM adds the possibility of imaging deeper into highly scattering media at the cost of limiting both the quantity (due to single-mode detection) and nature (coherent scattering processes only, i.e., backscattering, are detected) of the detected light. From the point of view of practitioners of OCT, OCM is the only technique to increase spatial resolution in all three spatial dimensions: however, this comes at the cost of increased overall complexity of the imaging system. Much of the added complexity arises from the need to coordinate sample and reference arm scans

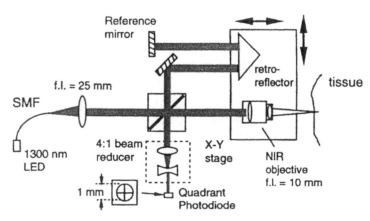

Figure 10   Configuration of optical coherence tomography using a dynamic focusing technique. (From Ref. 33.)

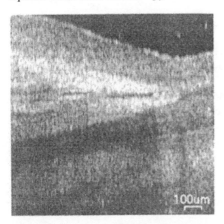

Figure 11 OCM image of living human nail fold region using the dynamic focusing technique. (From Ref. 33.)

in OCM as well as to incorporate high quality optics in the sample arm. Although promising initial results have been obtained, the future of this technique depends upon several unanswered questions. As Fig. 6 illustrates, it is not yet clear over what parameter range OCM enhances confocal microscopy, although some clear improvements have been demonstrated. The potential of OCM in the medical environment rests primarily on the development of microoptical endoscopic systems capable of incorporating confocal-quality scanning optics into an endoscope or other diagnostic probe tip.

ACKNOWLEDGMENTS

We acknowledge research support from the National Science Foundation (BES-9624617), the Whitaker Foundation, and Olympus Graduate Research Fellowship (H-W.W.).

REFERENCES

1. Youngquist RC, Carr S, Davies DEN. Optical coherence domain reflectometry: A new optical evaluation technique. Opt Lett 12:158, 1987.
2. Swanson EA, Izatt JA, Hee MR, Huang D, Lin CP, Schuman JS, Puliafito CA, Fujimoto JG. In vivo retinal imaging by optical coherence tomography. Opt Lett 18(21):1864–1866, 1993.
3. Bouma BE, Tearney GJ. Power-efficient nonreciprocal interferometer and linear-scanning fiber-optic catheter for optical coherence tomography. Opt Lett 24(8):531–533, 1999.
4. Rollins AM, Ung-arunyawee R, Chak A, Wong RCK, Kobayashi K, Sivak MV, Izatt JA. Real-time in vivo imaging of human gastrointestinal ultrastructure using endoscopic optical coherence tomography with a novel efficient interferometer design. Opt Lett 24:1358–1360, 1999.
5. Clivaz X, Marquis-Weible F, Salathe RP. Optical low coherence reflectometry with 1.9 μm spatial resolution. Electron Lett 28:1553–1555, 1992.

6. Schmitt JM, Yadlowsky MJ, Bonner RF. Subsurface imaging of living skin with optical coherence microscopy. Dermatology 191:93–98, 1995.

7. Bouma B, Tearney GJ, Boppart SA, Hee MR. High-resolution optical coherence tomographic imaging using a mode-locked Ti:Al$_2$O$_3$ laser source. Opt Lett 20:1486–1488, 1995.

8. Drexler W, Morgner U, Kartner FX, Pitris C, Boppart SA, Li XD, Ippen EP, Fujimoto JG. In vivo ultrahigh-resolution optical coherence tomography. Opt Lett 24:1221–1223, 1999.

9. Izatt JA, Hee MR, Owen GA, Swanson EA, Fujimoto JG. Optical coherence microscopy in scattering media. Opt Lett 19:590–592, 1994.

10. Kempe M, Rudolph W. Scanning microscopy through thick layers based on linear correlation. Opt Lett 19:1919–1921, 1994.

11. Sheppard CJR, Wilson T. Depth of field in the scanning microscope. Opt Lett 3(3):115–117, 1978.

12. Wilson T. Confocal Microscopy. London: Academic Press, 1990.

13. Siegman AE. Lasers. Mill Valley, CA: 1986.

14. Cox IJ, Sheppard CJR. Information capacity and resolution in an optical system. J Opt Soc Am A 3:1152–1158, 1986.

15. Webb WW, Wells K, Sandison DR, Strickler J. Optical Microscopy for Biology. New York: Wiley-Liss, 1990.

16. Sheppard CJR, Cogswell CJ, Gu M. Signal strength and noise in confocal microscopy: Factors influencing selection of an optimum detector aperture. Scanning 13:233–240, 1991.

17. Sheppard CJR. Stray light and noise in confocal microscopy. Micro Microsc Acta 22:239–243, 1991.

18. Sonnenschein CM, Horrigan FA. Signal-to-noise relationships for coaxial systems that heterodyne backscatter from the atmosphere. Appl Opt 10:1600, 1971.

19. Schmitt JM, Knuttel A, Gandjbakhche A, Bonner RF. Optical characterization of dense tissues using low-coherence interferometry. Proc Soc Photo-Opt Instrum Eng 1989:197, 1993.

20. Schmitt JM, Knuttel A, Yadlowsky M. Confocal microscopy in turbid media. J Opt Soc Am A 11:2226–2235, 1994.

21. Kempe M, Rudolph W, Welsch E. Comparative study of confocal and heterodyne microscopy for imaging through scattering media. J Opt Soc Am A 13:46–52, 1996.

22. Gu M, Sheppard C, Gan X. Image formation in a fiber-optical confocal scanning microscope. J Opt Soc Am B 8:1755–1761, 1991.

23. Tearney GJ, Webb RH, Bouma BE. Spectrally encoded confocal microscopy. Opt Lett 23:1152–1154, 1998.

24. Rajadhyashka M, Anderson RR, Webb RH. Video-rate confocal scanning laser microscope for imaging human tissues in vivo. Appl Opt 38:2105, 1999.

25. Izatt JA, Kulkarni MD, Wang H-W, Kobayashi K, Sivak MV. Optical coherence tomography and microscopy in gastrointestinal tissues. IEEE J Selected Topics Quant Electron 2(4):1017–1028, 1996.

26. Rollins AM, Kulkarni MD, Yazdanfar S, Ung-arunyawee R, Izatt JA. In vivo video rate optical coherence tomography. Opt Express 3(6):219–229, 1998.

27. Pan Y, Birngruber R, Rosperich J, Engelhardt R. Low-coherence optical tomography in turbid tissue: Theoretical analysis. Appl Opt 34:6564–6574, 1995.

28. Kulkarni MD, Izatt JA. High resolution optical coherence tomography using deconvolution. In: Advances in Optical Imaging and Photon Migration. RR Alfano, JG Funjimoto, eds. Orlando, FL: Opt Soc Am, 1996: 227–230.

29. Papoulis A. Systems and Transforms with Application in Optics. New York: McGraw-Hill, 1968.

30. Podoleanu AG, Dobre GM, Webb DJ, Jackson DA. Coherence imaging by use of a Newton rings sampling function. Opt Lett 21(21):1789–1791, 1996.
31. Podoleanu AG, Seeger M, Dobre GM, Webb DJ, Jackson DA, Fitzke FW. Transversal and longitudinal images from the retina of the living eye using low coherence reflectometry. J Biomed Opt 3(1):12–20, 1998.
32. Podoleanu AG, Dobre GM, Jackson DA. En-face coherence imaging using galvanometer scanner modulation. Opt Lett 23(3):147–149, 1998.
33. Schmitt JM. Array detection for speckle reduction in optical coherence microscopy. Phys Med Biol. 42:1427–1439, 1997.
34. Schmitt JM, Lee SL, Yung KM. An optical coherence microscope with enhanced resolving power in thick tissue. Opt Commun. 142:203–207, 1997.
35. Lexen F, Hitzenberger CK, Drexler W, Molebny S, Sattmann H, Sticker M, Fercher AF. Dynamic coherent focus OCT with depth-independent transversal resolution. J Mod Opt 46(3):541–553, 1999.
36. Chinn SR, Swanson EA. Blindness limitations in optical coherence domain reflectometry. Electron Lett 29:2025, 1993.
37. Lindmo T, Smithies DJ, Chen Z, Nelson JS, Milner T. Monte Carlo simulations of optical coherence tomography (OCT) and optical Doppler tomography (ODT). Soc Photo-Instrum Eng 3251:114–125, 1998.
38. Schmitt JM, Knuttel A. Model of optical coherence tomography of heterogenous tissue. J Opt Soc Am A 14:1231–1242, 1997.
39. Hee MR, Izatt JA, Jacobson JM. Swanson EA, Fujimoto JG. Femtosecond transillumination optical coherence tomography. Opt Lett 18:950, 1993.
40. Yadlowski MJ, Schmitt JM, Bonner RF. Multiple scattering in optical coherence microscopy. Appl Opt 34:5699–5707, 1995.
41. Pan Y, Birngruber R, Engelhardt R. Contrast limits of coherence-gated imaging in scattering media. Appl Opt 36:2979–2983, 1997.
42. Kempe M, Thon A, Rudolph W. Resolution limits of microscopy through scattering layers. Opt Commun 110:492–496, 1994.
43. Tearney GJ. Optical characterization of human tissues using low coherence interferometry. Ph.D. Thesis, MIT, Cambridge, MA, 1988.
44. Boas DA, Bizheva KK, Siegel AM. Using dynamic low-coherence interferometry to image Brownian motion within highly scattering media. Opt Lett 23(5):319–321, 1998.
45. Boas DA, Bizheva KK. Imaging in the single-scattering, few-scattering, and light diffusion regimes with low-coherent light. In: Coherence-Domain Optical Methods in Biomedical Science and Clinical Applications III. San Jose, CA: Society of Photo-Instrumentation Engineers, 1999.
46. Lutomirsky RF. Atmospheric degradation of electrooptic system performance. Appl Opt 17:3915–3921, 1978.
47. van de Hulst HC, Kattawar GW. Exact spread function for a pulsed collimated beam in a medium with small-angle scattering. Appl Opt 33:5820–5829, 1994.
48. Tearney GJ, Brezinsky ME, Southern JF, Bouma BE, Hee MR, Fujimoto JG. Determination of the refractive index of highly scattering human tissue by optical coherence tomography. Opt Lett 20:2258–2260, 1995.
49. Podoleanu AG, Dobre GM, Webb DJ, Jackson DA. Simultaneous en-face imaging of two layers in the human retina by low-coherence reflectometry. Opt Lett 22(13):1039–1041, 1997.
50. Haskell RC, Johnson S, Peterson DC, Ungersma S,, Wang R, Williams M, Fraser SE. Optical coherence microscopy in development biology. In: Coherence-Domain Optical Methods in Biomedical Science and Clinical Applications III. San Jose, CA: Soc Photo-Instrum Eng, 1999.
51. Chinn, SR. Personal communication.

52. Wang H-W, Rollins AM, Izatt JA. High-speed full-field optical coherence microscopy. Soc Photo-Instrum Eng 3598:204–212, 1999.
53. Izatt, JA, Kulkarni MD, Kobayashi K, Sivak MV, Barton JK, Welch AJ. Optical coherence tomography for biodiagnostics. Opt Photon News 8:41–47, 1997.

11

Full-Field Optical Coherence Microscopy

H. SAINT-JALMES and M. LEBEC

Université Claude Bernard-Lyon I, Villeurbanne, France

E. BEAUREPAIRE, A. DUBOIS, and A. C. BOCCARA

CNRS, ESPCI, Paris, France

11.1 INTRODUCTION

With the development of new optical technologies and powerful digital image processors, optical microscopy has been moving beyond traditional two-dimensional (2-D) imaging to the reproduction of three-dimensional (3-D) objects. The demonstration in the late 1950s of the confocal scanning principle, with its capacity to reject light from out-of-focus planes, provided a powerful tool for reconstruction of 3-D objects [1]. Confocal laser scanning microscopy, introduced around 1980, is nowadays a well-established tool for biological and biomedical imaging [1–3]. More recently, optical coherence tomography (OCT) [4] was introduced as a novel high resolution noninvasive imaging technique best suited for imaging in scattering media [5]. OCT uses low coherence interferometry to reject scattered light and amplify the single-backscattered component emerging from the sample, and was demonstrated to be an effective technique to produce images with $10–15\,\mu\mathrm{m}$ resolution several hundred micrometers deep inside various biological tissues [6–9]. Optical coherence microscopy (OCM), a variant of OCT that takes advantage of a high numerical aperture (NA) objective lens and produces XY (head-on) rather than XZ images, can provide an order-of-magnitude higher resolution [10–12]. In addition, coherent detection gives access to the optical phase, which can be exploited to image transparent objects, to measure birefringence, or to reconstruct the topography of surfaces.

Full-field optical coherence microscopy [13] is an alternative method developed to retain advantages of scanning OCM systems while enabling simultaneous acquisition of all the pixels of an image. This technique borrows its basic principle from OCT: A low temporal coherence light source is used in a Michelson interference microscope to select single-backscattered photons coming from a given depth in the sample. The main difference is that full-field systems avoid any X-Y scanning by illuminating the whole field of view with a spatially incoherent light source and by taking advantage of a detector array and a parallel coherent detection scheme. A complete slice orthogonal to the Z axis is thus acquired in one shot (Fig. 1). The only mechanical scanning involved in a complete 3-D image acquisition is a relatively slow motion along the Z axis in order to obtain images from different depths in the sample.

Section 11.2 presents the concepts involved in full-field coherent imaging and outlines some advantages of the parallel detection and head-on geometry in the

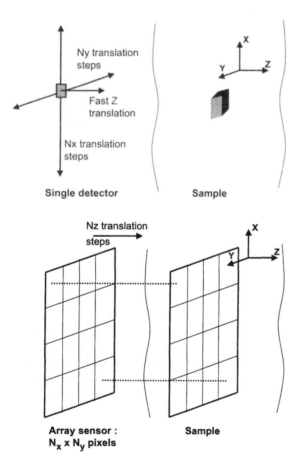

Figure 1 *XY* imaging. In a single-detector experiment, three mechanical movements are required to scan the volume of the sample. With an array of detectors, a plane perpendicular to the Z axis is acquired simultaneously; only a slow Z translation is necessary to acquire the 3-D image of the sample.

context of the optical imaging in scattering media. Section 11.3 describes the layouts that we have been exploring in our laboratory and the associated signal acquisition system. Section 11.4 is devoted to the performance of the full-field optical coherence microscopes in terms of resolution and sensitivity. Section 11.5 presents current applications of these systems.

11.2 FULL-FIELD COHERENT IMAGING

In the development of many techniques, the first milestone has been to establish a point-to-point correspondence between a voxel located in the sample and a single detector. Acquisition of a 2-D or 3-D image data set then required scanning of either the probe or the sample. This was the case, for example, in magnetic resonance imaging (MRI) with a method known as the sensitive point method [14]. Nowadays this method is obsolete, for it has been replaced by direct 2-D or 3-D imaging of the sample [15]. As a matter of fact, if the power of the excitation source is not limited, parallel detection provides a clear improvement in acquisition time over a single-detector method, which we refer to here as the "multichannel advantage." As a positive side effect, the minimization of moving parts also improves the stability and reproducibility of the images. In this section we outline some advantages of the head-on (XY) geometry in the context of OCT, we develop a comparison between single and multiple detectors, and we propose a way to perform a lock-in detection on an array detector.

11.2.1 Head-On (*XY*) Geometry

Most current OCT systems are built around an XZ geometry (Z being the optical axis); they weakly focus the probe beam into the sample and take advantage of a rapid modulation of the reference arm. This geometry imposes a trade-off between lateral (X) resolution and the Z extent of the images [10,16]. Spatial resolution on the order of 10–15 μm is usually achieved in these arrangements. A variant of OCT relying on an *en face* (XY) geometry, which includes the use of higher NA objective lenses and has been dubbed optical coherence microscopy (OCM) [10–12], can provide significantly higher resolution. In the case of systems using a full-field illumination and parallel detection, this geometry is the natural choice; this subsection outlines its specific advantages.

First, as mentioned above, optical coherence microscopy can take advantage of high NA objective lenses and produce images with high diffraction-limited resolution.

Second, in the XY geometry the acquisition time and the excitation power can be chosen according to the depth in the sample to compensate for the exponential attenuation of the excitation intensity with depth [17]. In contrast, a signal-to-noise ratio (SNR) degradation with depth is usually visible in XZ OCT scans, independent of the presence of multiple scattering effects. The use of a strongly focusing objective also allows delivery of a higher optical power to the sample surface when imaging deep within the sample. Indeed, the spread of the excitation beam being wider at the surface, less damage per unit of surface area is done than with an unfocused beam.

Third, the XY geometry makes it possible to naturally combine optical coherence imaging with complementary imaging modalities such as fluorescence [12].

Finally, in the specific case of full-field illumination, advantage can be taken of a spatially incoherent source to perform coherent detection without generating speckle in the whole image.

11.2.2 Serial vs. Parallel Detection

In this section we develop a comparison of the two detection schemes (single/multiple detector) in terms of acquisition time and signal-to-noise ratio (SNR), irrespective to the features common to all OCT arrangements.

In order to compare the two types of experiments (single and multiple detectors), we assume that the detector is not saturated and that the detection is shot noise limited. Coherent detection enables one to amplify the detected signal using a local oscillator (reference arm of the interferometer), and OCT setups usually achieve shot noise limited detection.

The classical expression of the signal-to-noise power ratio $(SNR)_P$ for a single detector is [18]

$$(SNR)_P = \frac{\eta P_S}{h\nu B} \tag{1}$$

where P_S is the optical power received by the detector, ν is the frequency of the light, η is the detector quantum efficiency, h is Planck's constant, and $B \approx 1/2T$ is the measurement bandwidth (with T the acquisition time for one point) (Fig. 1).

Photodiodes and charge-coupled devices (CCDs) have similar light-to-electron conversion properties. For multiple detectors, the signal-to-noise power ratio expression is the same for each element of the $M \times M$ matrix. Assuming that the available power is not limited and that a constant amount of energy can be delivered to every point in the sample, a single-detector instrument requires a total time $T_{total} = M \times M \times T$ to obtain an $M \times M$ image, whereas with a detector array the same image is obtained in time T. In both cases, the voltage signal-to-noise ratio (SNR) can be expressed for each pixel of the image as

$$SNR = \left(\frac{\eta P_s}{h\nu B}\right)^{1/2} \approx \left(\frac{\eta P_s 2T}{h\nu}\right)^{1/2} \tag{2}$$

where T is the observation time for one pixel in the single-detector solution or for the whole $M \times M$ matrix when an array of detectors is used.

We now define an efficiency criterion Γ in order to take into account both SNR and total acquisition time:

$$\Gamma = \frac{SNR}{\sqrt{T_{total}}} \tag{3}$$

The $T^{-1/2}$ factor in the above expression reflects the fact that averaging two acquisitions (thus doubling the acquisition time) improves the SNR by a factor of $\sqrt{2}$.

We see that for a similar acquisition bandwidth and excitation power per pixel, an $M \times M$ detector array provides a gain of M in efficiency over a single detector (Table 1). This illustrates the "multichannel advantage" mentioned above.

Besides the signal-to-noise ratio, other issues must be pointed out.

Table 1 Comparison Between the Single- and Multiple-Detector Solutions[a]

Parameter	Single detector (e.g., photodiode)	Multiple detectors (e.g., CCD array, $M \times M$ pixels)
Signal-to-noise ratio	$\dfrac{S}{N} \approx \left(\dfrac{\eta P_S T}{h\nu}\right)^{1/2}$	$\dfrac{S}{N} \approx \left(\dfrac{\eta P_S T}{h\nu}\right)^{1/2}$
Energy deposition per pixel at the surface of the sample	$E_{\text{pixel}} \propto P_S T$	$E_{\text{pixel}} \propto P_S T$
Total imaging time	$T_{\text{total}} = M^2 T$	$T_{\text{total}} = T$
Efficiency per unit of time	$\Gamma \approx \left(\dfrac{\eta P_S}{h\nu}\right)^{1/2}\left(\dfrac{1}{M}\right)$	$\Gamma \approx \left(\dfrac{\eta P_S}{h\nu}\right)^{1/2}$
Net gain in efficiency	1	**M**

[a] Power deposition, signal-to-noise ratio (SNR) and efficiency comparison between the single- and multiple-detector solutions. An $M \times M$ matrix of detectors provides a net gain of M in efficiency compared to the single-detector scheme.

First, mechanical stability is easily ensured in the parallel detection scheme because there is only one slow mechanical translation, whereas in scanning systems fast movements along two directions may induce artifacts in the image due to vibrations. This may also degrade the reproducibility of the experiments and preclude SNR enhancement by ensemble averaging of several measurements.

Second, simultaneous acquisition of all the pixels of a given slice of the sample in one shot allows one to synchronize the acquisition of a complete image to a physiological event for certain in vivo studies.

In summary, a parallel ($M \times M$) detection scheme is attractive for the following reasons:

1. The mechanical translations and associated vibrations are reduced to a minimum.
2. Acquisition of all the pixels of an image is done simultaneously, yielding a good rejection of motion artifacts (sample motion, breathing, cardiac cycle, etc.) while allowing one to perform a stroboscopic acquisition synchronized on a physiological event (e.g., ECG).
3. The efficiency criterion Γ is improved by a factor M as long as the detection is shot noise limited and the available source power is not limited. As a matter of fact, to fully benefit from the "multichannel advantage," the source should allow delivery of the maximum acceptable amount of power simultaneously to all the pixels of the sample. At the present time, commonly available sources do not fulfil this requirement, especially if one is trying to obtain an *en face* image from deep within the sample, say close to the fundamental limits on OCT probing depth imposed by multiple scattering [19,20]. However, that concern might no

longer be an issue in the near future, conferring a net advantage to parallel detection schemes.

Before going any further, we need to define the principal requirements for an imaging array.

11.2.3 Solid-State Array Detectors

Three types of solid-state array detectors could be used in our application: silicon photodiode arrays (PDAs), CMOS image sensors, and charge-coupled devices (CCDs). The first solution is restricted to line (1-D) imaging because it is constituted of a linear array of photodiodes. CMOS image sensors are based on a bidimensional array of photodiodes. Each pixel also contains transistors to buffer and amplify the collected photocharge. The advantages of this design are the random readout of individual pixels and the use of standard CMOS technology, which enables low-cost volume productions. The main drawbacks are a low filling factor (i.e., the ratio of light-sensitive area to the total size of the pixel) of only 20–30% and also poor linearity of the response. The last family, CCD sensors, have many applications, among which imaging is the most important. The basic light-to-electron conversion mechanism is the same as in photodiodes; the main difference is the collection (or integration) capability of these electrons in a CCD. The electric charges are stored in CMOS capacitors as in wells, and at regular time intervals these wells are emptied and the corresponding charge is transferred serially to the output of the device.

When comparing CCDs and photodiodes, the advantage of having a high number of elements on a CCD (from thousands to millions of pixels) is counterbalanced by the low frame rate of cameras and the limited storage capacity of each well, which limits their dynamic range. This storage capacity is designated as the full well capacity (FWC) of the CCD and is measured in electrons. (In most designs this capacity ranges from $50\,ke^-$ to $400\,ke^-$.) This quantity is of importance, for in a shot noise limited experiment it is a direct measure of the signal-to-noise ratio for a one-shot image: $\text{SNR} = \sqrt{\text{FWC}}$. In the best case, this value of the SNR can be obtained in a time T essentially determined by the maximum pixel readout frequency F_{pix} of the camera: $T = M^2/F_{\text{pix}}$ for an $M \times M$ matrix. If we suppose that the light flux on the matrix is sufficient to reach this FWC in one shot, we can define an efficiency criterion $\Gamma_{\text{CCD}} = \sqrt{\text{FWC}/T} = \sqrt{\text{FWC} \cdot F_{\text{pix}}}/M$, which is directly related to the maximum power that can be measured continuously by the camera given the pixel readout frequency. Again, this supposes that the power limitation comes from the sensor, not from the light source, or from safety issues when irradiating tissues (e.g., maximum permissible exposure). To select a CCD for our application we must then maximize this criterion for a given image size.

Among the other parameters to consider when choosing a CCD camera, most important are the dark current that is generated by thermal activity in the sensor substrate (typical value 0.01 fA/pixel) and the readout noise due to the conditioning electronics (typically 10–20 electrons).

In summary, the selection of the best device is helped by the application of an efficiency criterion, but one must keep in mind that array detectors are slow (less than a few hundred images per second) compared to single detectors.

11.2.4 Parallel Coherent Detection

Optical Path Difference Modulation

In OCM, the useful signal to measure is usually very weak (i.e., interference between the local oscillator and the weak single-backscattered flux returning from the sample) compared to a large detected background due to reference flux and incoherent back-scattered light. A usual remedy for such a situation is to extract the scarce information from the large unwanted signal by modulating the experiment at a given frequency while reading back the signal of interest through a lock-in detector (Fig. 2a). The signal is thus transposed at a frequency f_0 by the modulation, where it can be extracted by multiplication with the reference signal at f_0. This corresponds to a back transposition to a low frequency, where it is easy to minimize the noise by sharp low-pass filtering. This technique has numerous advantages. First, it greatly reduces the sensitivity of the experiment to temporal drifts and allows a precise match of the filter cutoff frequency to the useful bandwidth of the signal. Second, the modulation provides a great way to separate the useful information from the unwanted signal (background, background variations, EMI, etc.).

Applied to OCM, the lock-in detection method consists in modulating the optical pathlength difference between the arms of an interferometer. Thus, only the interference component is modulated in the detected flux, performing an effective discrimination of the coherent backscattered signal. The photoelastic modulator that we have been using to perform this modulation simultaneously in the whole image field is described in Section 11.3.3.

Multiplexed Lock-In Detection

Principle

The theoretical advantage of parallel detection was outlined in Section 11.2.2. We will now consider the main drawback of array detectors. Their low frame rate usually precludes the implementation of lock-in detection, thus canceling most of the potential advantages of parallel detection. As a matter of fact, conventional lock-in detection requires the multiplication of the signal sensor with the modulation reference. But, whereas photodiode bandwidths easily reach hundreds of megahertz (typical lock-in), CCD bandwidths are limited to approximately 1 kHz. Consequently the modulation frequency range allowed for lock-in experiments is reduced, which often precludes the use of lock-in detection with CCD detectors in physical experiments. For instance, our OCM experiments use a 50 kHz optical path difference modulation. At such frequencies, the temporal variations are averaged by the CCD cameras.

However, a way to have the benefit of the lock-in advantage is to modify the typical lock-in detection scheme (Fig. 2). Figure 2a shows the usual diagram, and Fig. 2b outlines the principle of our "multiplexed lock-in detection" method [13,21,22].

The "multiplexed lock-in detection" principle gets rid of the signal multiplication after the sensor (Fig. 2a) by using a secondary modulation. The latter performs the multiplication operation before the light signal reaches the sensor and is subsequently averaged. An example of secondary modulation is light modulation (e.g., light switching). Compared to typical lock-in detection, CCD exposure acts like a low-pass filter, and the integrating time constant is set by the CCD frame rate.

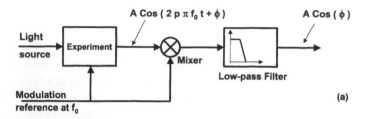

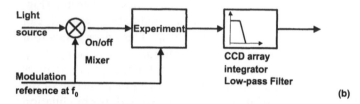

Figure 2 Typical lock-in detection versus multiplexed lock-in detection. The building blocks of the conventional detection scheme (a) are rearranged to get rid of slow array detectors (e.g., CCD) throughput (b).

Analytical Formulation

An analytical formulation of the "multiplexed lock-in" method that applies to any pixel of the CCD matrix is developed below.

Each pixel integrates the incident light flux $\Phi(t)$ during the CCD time exposure T_{FRAME}. We note that S is the signal provided by the CCD camera:

$$S = \int_0^{T_{\text{FRAME}}} \Phi(t)\, dt \tag{4}$$

The incident light flux results from the multiplication of the primary modulation function $x_T(t)$ (reference) by the secondary modulation function $y_T(t)$. Both modulation functions are periodic of period T:

$$\Phi(t) = x_T(t) y_T(t) \tag{5}$$

One modulation can be delayed by a time τ with respect to the other:

$$S(\tau) = \int_0^{T_{\text{FRAME}}} x_T(t) y_T(t + \tau)\, dt \tag{6}$$

Assuming that the CCD exposure time is an integer number K of modulation periods, the signal S detected by the CCD is proportional to the cross-correlation function $\gamma_{xy}^{\circ}(\tau)$ of the $x_T(t)$ and $y_T(t)$ signals.

$$S(\tau) = \int_0^{KT} x_T(t) y_T(t + \tau)\, dt = KT\, \gamma_{xy}^{\circ}(\tau), \qquad \text{with } T_{\text{FRAME}} = KT \tag{7}$$

Since $x_T(t)$ and $y_T(t)$ are real and periodic, cross-correlation $\gamma_{xy}^{\circ}(\tau)$ is also real and periodic. Its Fourier series gives the $x_T(t)$ and $y_T(t)$ cross-power spectrum.

$$SF\{\gamma_{xy}^{\circ}(\tau)\} = \Gamma_{xy}(nF) = X^*(nF) Y(nF), \qquad F = \frac{1}{T}; \ n \text{ an integer} \tag{8}$$

Note that nF signifies that the cross-power spectrum is discrete (periodic signals).

Expression (8) shows that the knowledge of one of the modulation functions permits us to deduce the other:

$$Y(nF) = \frac{X(nF)\Gamma_{xy}(nF)}{|X(nF)|^2}, \qquad |X(nF)| \neq 0 \tag{9}$$

or

$$X(nF) = \frac{Y^*(nF)\Gamma_{xy}(nF)}{|Y(nF)|^2}, \qquad |Y(nF)| \neq 0 \tag{10}$$

Thus, sampling the cross-correlation function permits retrieval of the useful information present in the primary modulation.

In summary, a CCD camera integrates the light flux resulting from an "optical product" of two periodic time functions. The cross-correlation function is sampled by using an electronic device that also introduces delays between the two functions. Thus the acquisition process consists in grabbing several frames, each frame corresponding to a specific delay of the cross-correlation function. A linear combination of the acquired frames then gives access to the useful information about primary modulation. A detailed calculation for a specific example is presented in Section 11.3.4.

11.3 FULL-FIELD OPTICAL COHERENCE MICROSCOPES

11.3.1 Possible Interferometer Geometries

In essence, full-field optical coherence microscopes are based on interference microscopes using low coherence optical sources. In a general manner, interference microscopes can be classified into two categories:

1. Interference microscopes in which the light returning from the object interferes with the light from a reference beam. These interference microscopes, involving two completely separated waves, are based on the Michelson interferometer principle (for observations in reflection) or Mach–Zehnder interferometer (for observations in transmission). These microscopes give the "normal" profile of the object.
2. Interference microscopes in which the image of the object is divided into two identical laterally shifted images that are made to interfere. In the case of small lateral shifts (of the order of the optical wavelength), the differential profile of the object is obtained (first spatial derivative of the "normal" profile). The Nomarski microscope is this kind of system.

In optical coherence microscopy, interference occurs between light backscattered by the object and light reflected by a reference mirror, the light being spatially and temporally incoherent. The analysis of the interference signal provides amplitude images (and possibly phase images) from specific regions in the object, where the interference fringes are localized. Different interferometer geometries can be used: "classical" Michelson [13] (Fig. 3a), Mirau [23] (Fig. 3b), and Linnik [24,25] (Fig. 3c). The drawback in the Michelson and Mirau configurations is that the

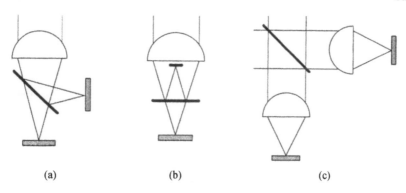

(a)   (b)   (c)

Figure 3   Geometries for Michelson-type optical coherence microscopes. (a) Michelson geometry; (b) Mirau geometry; and (c) Linnik geometry.

beamsplitter can introduce strong aberrations in wide-aperture systems, especially spherical aberration in the axial direction, which increases approximately as the cube of the numerical aperture. Because the reference and object beams share a common path over most of their length, this layout is less sensitive to vibrations than the Linnik configuration. In addition, only one lens is required, although this lens must have a relatively long working distance to accommodate the beamsplitter. The Linnik configuration requires two identical objectives, and because of the long beam paths involved it must be built massively to avoid vibration problems. Nevertheless, the great advantage of this configuration is that objectives with very high numerical apertures can be used (Fig. 3).

11.3.2 Light Sources

The light source used must fulfil several requirements.

1.   Near-infrared wavelengths (typically between 700 and 1300 nm) are used to minimize scattering in tissues and achieve better penetration.
2.   The temporal coherence should be as short as possible in order to avoid degradation of the effective resolution of the instrument when imaging in scattering media. In conventional optical coherence tomography, the axial resolution is principally defined by the coherence length of the source. In contrast, in optical coherence microscopy (OCM), when using a high NA objective lens, axial resolution is predominantly defined by the confocal nature of the signal detection. This is the case in our geometry, as detailed in Section 11.4.1. Nevertheless, the point spread function of the instrument is degraded when imaging deep within scattering media due to the detection of multiply scattered light. Reducing the coherence length of the source is a way to minimize these aberrations.
3.   When full-field illumination is used, the spatial coherence of the source should be as low as possible in order to reduce speckle formation in the image.
4.   Finally, to use the parallel coherent detection technique described in Section 11.2.4, the light source has to be modulated at a frequency of several kilohertz.

In practice, we use light-emitting diodes (LEDs) with typical output power of 40 mW at 840 nm and 20 nm full width at half maximum (FWHM) spectral bandwidth. The emitter size is 240 μm × 240 μm. Light source modulation is achieved by directly modulating its driving voltage. We note that several such sources can be combined using a fiber-optic coupler to increase the spectral bandwidth [26].

11.3.3 Experimental Arrangement

Layout

We have developed in our laboratory optical coherence microscopes based on the Michelson [13] and Linnik [24] interferometer geometries, working with polarized light (Figs 4a and 4b, respectively). An infrared light-emitting diode (LED) is used as a spatially and temporally incoherent light source. Its spectrum is centered at $\lambda = 840$ nm with FWHM ≈ 20 nm, i.e., a coherence length of 20 μm. The spatially incoherent beam produced by the LED is linearly polarized and is separated by a polarizing beam splitter into two orthogonaly polarized beams. A polarizer placed after the LED makes it possible to control the balance of the relative intensities of the two beams. A photoelastic birefringent modulator (see next section) introduces a sinusoidal phase variation of amplitude ψ and frequency $f = \omega/2\pi = 50$ kHz between the two orthogonal components, which are made to interfere by a second polarizer

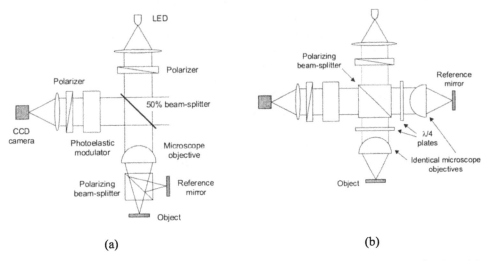

(a)   (b)

Figure 4 Experimental arrangements of polarization coherence microscopes developed in our laboratory In these schematic representations, only one point of the object is imaged on the CCD camera array. Full-field illumination is used to generate parallel cross-sectional images. (a) Michelson geometry. A single objective (0.15 NA) is used to focus the light on the object and on a reference mirror using a polarizing beamsplitter cube. A 50% beamsplitter is used to image the object on the CCD camera array. This configuration is appropriate for low aperture microscope objective lenses. (b) Linnik geometry. Two identical objectives are used. Quarter-wave plates are inserted into the two arms to rotate by $\pi/2$ the linear polarizations after reflection onto the reference mirror and by the object. The light reflected by the object is then totally transmitted by the polarizing beamsplitter whereas the light reflected by the reference mirror is totally reflected. Thus all the useful light is used. High numerical aperture objective lenses can be used.

oriented at 45° from the beam polarizations. The resulting image is finally detected on a two-dimensional CCD detector array.

Photoelastic Modulator

To introduce a stable periodic phase shift between the two orthogonal polarizations, we use a photoelastic birefringence modulator developed in our laboratory [27,28]. The device (Fig. 5) has a rectangular shape and is made of a transparent isotropic material (silica is well adapted for visible applications). A piezoelectric transducer (PZT) ceramic glued on its sides excites the system at its resonance frequency, introducing a periodic longitudinal stress that governs the induced birefringence. The driving voltage is low (a few volts) because we take advantage of the mechanical resonance (quality factor ~ 100). The modulation frequency is given by $f_m = v_{sound}/2L$, where v_{sound} is the speed of sound in the material and L is the modulator length. The PZT is usually glued at $1L/4$ from one of the silica bar's edges (one of the two regions with maximum stress), while the other maximum stress region ($3L/4$ from the same edge) serves as the birefringence modulator. This minimizes residual birefringence induced by the glue.

Issues Raised by the Implementation

At this point, we wish to point out several issues that are raised by the full-field polarization layout described above.

First, we commonly use immersion objectives to reduce the refractive index mismatch between the sample and its surrounding medium. Index mismatch has two consequences that should be avoided. (1) It causes an important specular reflection at the sample surface that limits the amount of light that can be sent to the sample arm without saturating the detector, thereby limiting the effective detector dynamic range. (2) When focusing deep inside the sample, refractive index mismatch introduces an optical path difference between the interferometer arms. In the case of bulk Michelson geometry and nonimmersion objectives, a clever way to compensate for this walk-off has been demonstrated by Schmitt et al. [26]. Because this does not apply here, we try to minimize this effect by using an appropriate medium. In the Linnik geometry, the reference arm length can also be manually modified to compensate for the walk-off and the resulting loss of contrast.

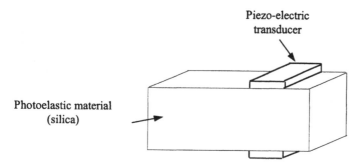

Figure 5 Photoelastic modulator design. A transparent isotropic material is excited on its sides by a PZT ceramic.

Second, because the use of a polarization interferometer is imposed by the modulation method, artifacts may occur when imaging structures having a very strong polarization backscattering dependence, such as collagen or nerve fibers.

Finally, in contrast with scanning OCM systems, full-field illumination precludes the use of a confocal spatial filter to enhance scattered light rejection. Nevertheless, we show in Section 11.4.2 that when using high NA objectives a resolution similar to that of confocal microscopes is achieved.

11.3.4 Signal Acquisition and Processing Instrumentation Principles

When the round-trip optical path difference between the object and reference beams is smaller than the coherence length of the source (see Section 11.4.1), the two beams interfere. The intensity $I(t)$ as a function of time on each pixel of the CCD camera can then be expressed as

$$I(t) = I_0 + A_S^2 + A_R^2 + 2A_S A_R \cos(\phi + \psi \sin(\omega t)) \tag{11}$$

where I_0 is the intensity of the incoherent light (which does not interfere with the light from the reference beam), $A_S \exp(i\phi_S)$ and $A_R \exp(i\phi_R)$ are the complex amplitudes of the mutually coherent waves reflected by the object and by the reference mirror, respectively, and $\phi = \phi_R - \phi_S$. As described earlier, a photoelastic modulator introduces a sinusoidal phase variation of amplitude ψ and frequency $f = \omega/2\pi = 50\,\text{kHz}$ between the object and reference waves. $I(t)$ contains a constant noninterference term and a time-modulated interference term that is proportional to the amplitude A_S. Using the nth Bessel function of the first kind J_n, the intensity $I(t)$ can be expressed as

$$
\begin{aligned}
I(t) = {} & I_0 + A_S^2 + A_R^2 + 2A_S A_R J_0(\psi) \cos\phi \\
& + 4A_S A_R \cos\phi \sum_{n=1}^{+\infty} J_{2n}(\psi) \cos(2n\omega t) \\
& - 4A_S A_R \sin\phi \sum_{n=0}^{+\infty} J_{2n+1}(\psi) \sin((2n+1)\omega t)
\end{aligned}
\tag{12}
$$

The light emitted by the LED is actually also modulated at the resonant modulator's frequency $f = 50$ kHz. Four successive square modulations $M_p(t)$ are applied to the LED supply current (Fig. 6). The square modulations $M_p(t)$ can be written by using Fourier series decomposition as

$$M_{p=0,1,2,3}(t) = \frac{1}{4} + \frac{1}{2} \sum_{n=1}^{+\infty} \frac{\sin(n\pi/4)}{n\pi/4} \cos(n(\omega t + p\pi/2)) \tag{13}$$

The intensity received by each pixel of the CCD camera is then the product $I(t) \times M_p(t)$. Because the camera readout frequency of 200 Hz is much lower than the modulator frequency of 50 kHz, the signal delivered by each pixel of the CCD camera array is proportional to the time average $\langle I(t) \times M_p(t) \rangle$. Four images corresponding to the four time shifts applied to the modulation $M_p(t)$ are successively recorded, the signal delivered by each pixel of these four images being

$M_p(t)$

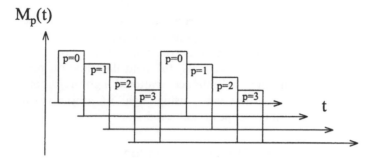

Figure 6 Phase sequencing. Square-wave modulations $M_p(t)$ are applied to the current supply of the light-emitting diode (LED).

$$S_{p=0,1,2,3} \propto \langle I(t) \times M_p(t) \rangle$$

$$= \frac{1}{4}\left[I_0 + A_S^2 + A_R^2 + 2A_S A_R \cos\phi J_0(\psi) \right]$$

$$+ \frac{4}{\pi} A_S A_R \cos\phi \sum_{n=1}^{+\infty}\left[\frac{J_{2n}(\psi)}{2n} \sin\frac{n\pi}{2}\cos np\pi \right] \tag{14}$$

$$+ \frac{4}{\pi} A_S A_R \sin\phi \sum_{n=0}^{+\infty}\left[\frac{J_{2n+1}(\psi)}{2n+1}\sin\frac{(2n+1)\pi}{4}\sin\frac{(2n+1)p\pi}{2} \right]$$

The calculation of the linear combinations Y and Z in Eqs. (15) and (16) give access to the product of the amplitude A_S of the wave backscattered by the object and the constant amplitude A_R of the wave reflected by the reference mirror. The optical phase ϕ can also be obtained [see Eq. (17)].

$$Y = 2(S_3 - S_1) = \frac{16}{\pi} A_S A_R \sin\phi \Sigma_1$$

$$Z = S_0 - S_1 + S_2 - S_3 = \frac{16}{\pi} A_S A_R \cos\phi \Sigma_2 \tag{15}$$

with

$$\Sigma_1 = \sum_{n=0}^{+\infty}(-1)^n\frac{J_{4n+2}(\psi)}{4n+2}$$

$$\Sigma_2 = \sum_{n=0}^{+\infty}(-1)^n\frac{J_{2n+1}(\psi)}{2n+1}\sin\frac{(2n+1)\pi}{4} \tag{16}$$

$$A_S \propto \left(Y^2/\Sigma_1^2 + Z^2/\Sigma_2^2 \right)^{1/2}$$

$$\phi = \arctan\left[\frac{\Sigma_1}{\Sigma_2}\left(\frac{Y}{Z}\right)\right] \tag{17}$$

We point out that interference microscopes detect the amplitude of the optical wave reflected by the object rather than its intensity. Intensity images (as produced by a classical microscope) can, of course, be obtained by calculating the squared amplitude images. An interference microscope can also provide phase images, proportional (modulo $\pi/2$) to the height between the surface of the object and the surface of the reference mirror [23,24]. Unwrapping the phase images gives a 3D representation of the surface.

In practice, our camera is operated at 200 frames per second (fps). Processed images can thus be produced at the rate of 50 per second. Several images are usually averaged to improve the signal-to-noise ratio (see Section 11.4.4).

Architecture Overview

Optical coherence microscopy hardware and software specifications are tabulated below.

Frequency reference	50 kHz
Light source	Switched LED
Primary modulation	Photoelastic (polarization)
Secondary modulation	Light source
Detection technique	Amplitude and phase (four-phase process)
Camera	CA-D1-256S (Dalsa, Waterloo, ON, Canada)

Our design consists of three devices (Fig. 7): an image sensor (camera), a home-made electronic controller ("sequencer"), and a computer equipped with a frame grabber. To perform the signal detection, the camera is synchronized with the reference frequency by the sequencer. The frame grabber transfers the camera frames into the computer main memory. In real time, the computer performs the linear combinations of frames involved in the "multiplexed lock-in detection" and displays the result. Demodulated images are usually averaged to increase their SNR.

"Multiplexed lock-in detection" is a general method used for several physical experiments (see Table 2). Various modulation frequencies, modulation methods, light sources, and cameras are used. Consequently, the system design has to be flexible, and, from this standpoint, several choices are made.

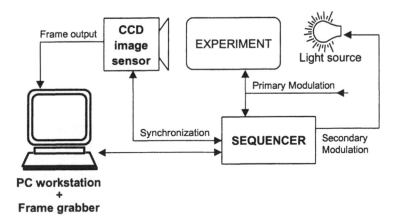

Figure 7 Synchronous imaging kernel architecture. Three devices ⇔ two elemental tasks : grab + processing ⇔ one hardware + software kernel.

Table 2 "Multiplexed Lock-In Detection" Based Experiments

	Biological media speckle imaging [29]	OCM experiments [13, 22, 24]	Photothermal imaging [30]
Frequency reference	2.25 MHz	50 kHz	Variable
Primary modulation	Ultrasound	Photoelastic	Voltage
Secondary modulation	Light source	Light source	Light source
Light source	Switched Laser	Switched LED	Switched LED
Camera	256 × 256 pixels 203 fps	256 × 256 pixels 203 fps	256 × 256 pixels 203 fps
Detection technique	Amplitude and phase (four-image process)	Amplitude and or phase	Amplitude

First, a simple frame grabber is used rather than one with an embedded computing unit such as DSP or programmable logic devices. Obviously, the latter category provides image processing facility and computation power, but these boards have a major drawback: changing the frame grabber model implies the need to entirely rewrite the processing code, because each board holds its specific software architecture (language, function libraries). On the other hand, performing the image processing on the host computer allows the frame grabber to be replaced as easily as the camera without important changes in the software.

Second, we use a conventional PC architecture (Wintel). Since all frame grabber manufacturers provide software drivers for this architecture, we can easily switch between different cameras and acquisition boards. This advantage can be extended to other PC boards necessary in a given experiment (motor controller boards, PIA boards, etc.).

Description of the Acquisition Elements

Both frame grabbing and processing are executed in parallel to achieve the best efficiency allowed by the experimental setups (see Section 11.2.2). This real-time process is the heart of the multiplexed lock-in technique. The frame grabber, the computer, and the sequencer together form hardware and software kernal that we will subsequently refer to as the synchronous image kernel (SIK).

Obviously, the SIK technical part is complex, and it will not be described here. Three relevant technical topics are outlined in the next paragraphs:

1. Camera synchronization: camera operation, exposure time control
2. Sequencer: secondary modulation synthesis, camera synchronization, design
3. Frame grabbing and processing: camera data stream acquisition, memory management, double-buffering algorithm, computation speed optimization

This discussion points out some problems that are generally encountered with any real-time imaging instrument.

Camera (Image Sensor Subset)

At this time, all experimental setups are using a Dalsa (Ontario, Canada) CA-D1-256-S camera, embedding an IA-D1 Dalsa CCD image sensor. Figure 8 shows its spectral response and some specifications.

The frame transfer CCD architecture provides both measurement time optimization and 100% filling factor. Typical frame transfer operation is described below, and CAD1 timings are given.

Reading of the CCD matrix consists of two steps: high speed storage (HSS) and frame transfer (FT). Following an internal trigger, the HSS period starts and the image wells are transferred from the image area to the storage area. This period takes about M cycles of the pixel clock (M^2 is the number of pixels in the CCD matrix). This time corresponds to the parallel shifting of all columns of the image sensor (Fig. 9a). Actual image readout (FT) immediately follows the HSS period. FT takes about $M \times M$ cycles of the pixel clock. This time corresponds to the serial shifting of all the pixels of the CCD matrix (Fig. 9b). Overall, CCD readout takes the sum of the times necessary for HSS and FT.

Without external synchronization the camera operates in "free running mode," meaning that each readout (HSS + FT) is immediately followed by another readout (Fig. 10a). In free running mode, exposure time and FT time are equal. This mode gives the maximum readout frequency of the camera (203 fps for CA-D1-256). To control the exposure time, the readout internal trigger may be replaced by an external synchronization signal (Fig. 10b).

In our system, the exposure time of the CCD array is controlled by an electronic device (sequencer) to match the multiplexed lock-in detection requirements.

Sequencer (Synchronization Subset)

Because square waveforms permit demodulation of a wide range of modulated signals, the sequencer design is essentially digital. It can be separated into two parts: generator and trigger/counter. The generator part synthesizes a TTL-compatible secondary modulation square wave, whereas the trigger/counter block synchronizes the multiplexed lock-in detection operation.

Digital designs provide a simple way to delay square waves. The generator essentially consists of two counters that are shifted relative to one another. Thus the most significant bits (MSBs) of the counters are two TTL signals delayed with respect to each other (Fig. 11). Shifted counts are made thanks to a parallel-load counter (COUNTER 2). In practice, the MSB of COUNTER 1 (MSB 1) is phase-

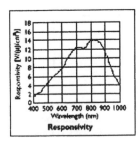

Resolution	256x256
Data bits	8
Full Well Capacity	200 ke⁻
Pixel Clock	15 MHz
Max. frame rate	203 fps

Figure 8 Features of the Dalsa camera. CA-D1-256S.

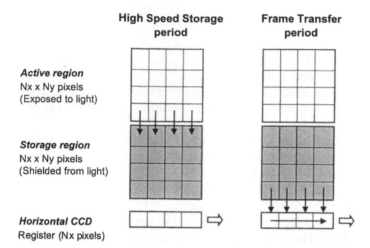

Figure 9 Frame transfer architecture. (a) The active region collects the photoelectrons, then in a very brief time (high speed storage period) the charge is shifted to the storage region. (b) The image region is then ready to accumulate new charges while the pixels from the storage region are read (frame transfer period).

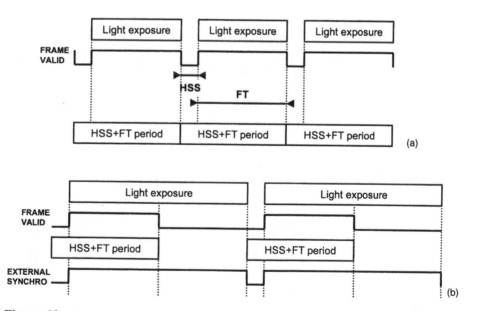

Figure 10 Camera exposure time control. (a) Frame transfer camera operates in "free-running mode." No exposure control signal is needed, and exposure time matches the frame transfer time. During frame transfer, the camera activates a FRAME VALID signal. (b) Thanks to an exposure control signal (EXTERNAL SYNCHRO), exposure time can be controlled by an external electronic device.

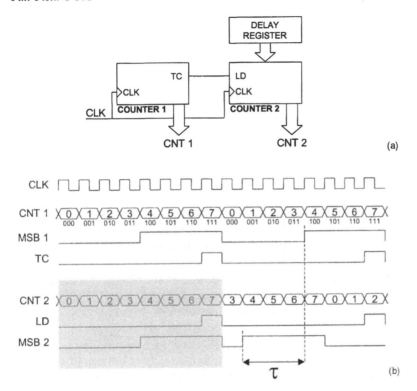

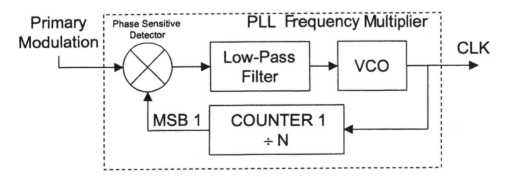

Figure 11 Generator block τ-delayed secondary modulation. (a) Generator block synoptic. (b) Timing diagrams; MSB 2 provides the secondary modulation expected.

locked onto the primary modulation (Fig. 12), and the MSB of COUNTER 2 (MSB 2) provides the τ-delayed secondary modulation.

According to Eq. (7) (Section 11.5.2), correct multiplexed lock-in detection is achieved only if CCD exposure time lasts an integral number of primary modulation periods. With a square wave primary modulation, accurate timings are easily achieved with a programmable binary counter (EXPOSURE COUNTER in Fig. 13) receiving the primary modulation on its clock input. Then, triggering the counter

Figure 12 Generator block or PLL frequency multiplier. To be frequency- and phase-locked on the primary modulation, counter 1 of the secondary modulation generator is included in the feedback loop of a phase-locked loop (PLL).

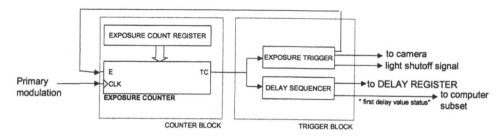

Figure 13 Trigger/counter block—Exposure control.

allows synchronization of the EXPOSURE COUNTER and the camera (HSS + FT periods) (trigger block in Fig. 13). The trigger/counter block also provides a TTL signal used to avoid light flux integration during the HSS period of the camera (i.e., to switch off the light source during HSS).

Finally, the trigger/counter block manages the successive phases of the acquisition process by incrementing the wraparound register (DELAY REGISTER in Fig. 11) each time EXPOSURE COUNTER (Fig. 13) overloads. In addition, it gives a "first delay value" TTL signal that will be checked by the computer subset to synchronize the software part of the SIK design (Section 11.3.4).

As described earlier, the sequencer has to guarantee critical timings of secondary modulation synthesis and camera exposure time. At the same time, the sequencer has to be flexible to match various surrounding devices (Table 2). Flexibility and critical timing are opposite requirements that cannot be easily achieved by a discrete board design. Thus a field programmable gate array (FPGA) programmable logic device has been used in the sequencer design. FPGA integrated circuits realize any kind of digital function (combinatory and/or sequential) according to a program downloaded by the computer through a standard port (e.g., parallel port). Moreover, this reprogrammable architecture offers an easy way to debug.

We designed a motherboard to hold a Xilinx (San Jose, CA) FPGA, a power supply, and several TTL and RS422 buffers. These buffers—connected to the FPGA—allow the sequencer to be easily and quickly upgraded to work with different cameras. A daughter board includes some analog circuits used for primary modulation conditioning and for the PLL multiplier (see generator block discussion) (Fig. 14). Because these subsets belong to a daughter board, the most appropriate technology can be used according to the modulation frequency of the experiment.

Frame Grabbing and Processing (Computer Subset)

Prior to any digital design (hardware and software), data flow rate must be estimated. The CA-D1 maximum frame rate is 203 fps, its frame size is 256 × 256, and its data format is 8 bit, resulting in about 14 Mbytes/s continuous data flow rate. This data stream is stored in the PC main memory by a frame grabber. Current frame grabbers use a PCI bus, whose maximum bandwidth is 132 Mbytes/s (32 bits at 33 MHz). However, this peak value cannot be obtained in sustained data transfer. For a continuous data stream, 100 Mbytes/s data flow rate is a realistic value. Such frame grabbers are said to be "real-time," meaning that frames are stored in PC host memory as fast as they are acquired.

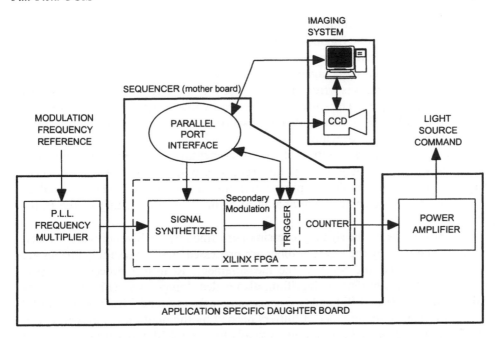

Figure 14 Sequencer design implementation. Mother board: XC4003 Xilinx FPGA running up to 100 MHz provides a hardware programmable kernel to the sequencer. The daughter board brings together all application-specific hardware.

The CA-D1 camera is far from reaching the PCI bus bandwidth limit. The remaining available bandwidth is mainly used for the frame processing. Depending on the data treatment, the bandwidth actually needed by the SIK design can be 2, 3, 4, or more times greater. When software load becomes too important, frames are missed.

The data stream is asynchronous with respect to the operating system and the applications that are running on the computer. Avoiding frame misses during the acquisition can be guaranteed on a 100% basis only on real-time operating systems, which is not the case with Microsoft Windows. In fact, the data transfer is made by a device driver running on the computer. The device driver responds to a hardware event, an interrupt, indicating that the data must be moved. Windows does not have deterministic behavior, especially with respect to hardware interrupts. Nevertheless, thanks to the power of current PCs, quasi-deterministic behavior is achieved. In practice, the time determinism of the operating system behavior depends on its total software load (PCI + CPU).

At this point in the description, each frame grabbed by the computer is anonymous in the multiplexed lock-in detection method. This means that the frames have no relationship to the delay value fixed by the sequencer between the modulation signals. Thus, a "first delay value" synchronization signal is used in the SIK. This signal is provided by the sequencer, and it is checked by a high speed digital port of the computer. This input line can be a generic input/output (I/O) available on the frame grabber or, alternatively, it can be provided by a digital I/O board installed in the computer.

In summary, a continuous grab is performed by the SIK. A time-checking algorithm detects possible frames missed during the concurrent grabbing/processing task. If a frame is missed, the current grab is discarded, the software is synchronized on the first delay value signal again, and the grab is repeated.

The SIK software was written in C because C is the language usually chosen by device driver developers. The software is then easily interlaced to functions libraries driving PC boards. SIK software assumes two basic functions: graphical user interface (GUI) and signal processing.

Briefly, GUI allows control of all experimental parameters and sequencer parameters such as frame grabbing and processing parameters. The latter concern the type of processing (amplitude, phase, etc.), the number of accumulations, and, in the case of an analog camera, the analog-to-digital converter setting of the frame grabber.

We now focus on the signal processing performed by the SIK software. Briefly, the frames acquired by the frame grabber are processed, and the resulting images are averaged to increase the SNR of the measurement. Real-time processing is performed by a double-buffering algorithm, also called "ping-pong" (Fig. 15). It uses a pair of buffers (B1 and B2) and two processing tasks (TA and TB). The B1 and B2 sets of buffers have the number of buffers needed by the multiplexed lock-in detection to retrieve the useful information (typically four in OCM applications). Each set

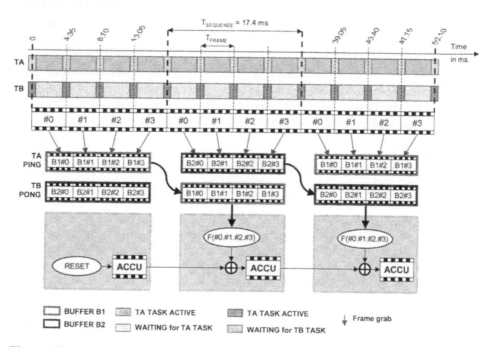

Figure 15 Double-buffer acquisition and processing. At the "reset" pass of the algorithm, and B1 buffers have the "ping" attribute and the B2 buffers have the "pong" attribute. While the TA task fills the "ping" B1 buffers, the TB task computes the "pong" B2 buffers. When both tasks terminate their work, B1 and B2 buffers attributes are switched, and TA/TB tasks are repeated. Again the TA task fills the "ping" buffers, but now these buffers are the B2 ones. In the same way, the TB task processes the "pong" buffers, which are now the B1 buffers.

of buffers owns an attribute whose value can be "ping" or "pong." While the TA task grabs incoming frames in "pong" buffers, the TB task computes the frames previously grabbed. When both tasks terminate their work, the B1 and B2 buffer attributes are switched, and the TA and TB tasks are repeated. Note that each task is working with the complete set of buffers (four buffers in OCM). This process needs an initialization pass that is used efficiently to reset the accumulation buffer.

However, proper operation of this double-buffering algorithm is essential to our application. For this reason we use state-of-the-art programming of this algorithm as much as possible. For example, all these critical tasks are coded in assembly language and take advantage of the internal architecture of the processor (i.e., pipeline, superscalar, and cache-optimized management).

11.4 PERFORMANCE

11.4.1 Axial Resolution

We analyze in this section the ability of our optical coherence microscopes to reject light from out-of-focus planes. The depth response of our microscopes, i.e., their response when the object plane is moved out of the focal plane of the objective lens, depends on both the spectrum width of the source and the numerical aperture of the objective lenses. Without time modulation ($\psi = 0$), the intensity $I(z)$ received by each pixel of the CCD camera as a function of the distance z between the object and the focus plane is [23,31]

$$I(z) = I_0 + A_0^2 + A_S^2 + A_R^2 + 2A_R A_S F_{\text{spect,NA}}(z) \tag{18}$$

where

$$F_{\text{spect,NA}}(z) = \frac{2}{\sin^2 \theta_{\max}} \int S(k) \int_0^{\theta_{\max}} \cos(2kz \cos \theta + \phi) \cos \theta \sin \theta \, d\theta \, dk \tag{19}$$

where $S(k)$ is the spectrum of the light emitted by the optical source and $\theta_{\max}$ is related to the numerical aperture (NA) of the objective lenses by $\text{NA} = n \sin \theta_{\max}$, n being the refractive index of the medium.

Low Numerical Aperture

In the case of objective lenses with low numerical aperture ($\theta_{\max} \approx 0$), $F_{\text{spect,NA}}(z)$ is reduced to

$$F_{\text{spect}}(z) = \int S(k) \cos(2kz + \phi) dk \tag{20}$$

If we assume a Gaussian source line shape,

$$S(k) = \exp\left[-2\left(\frac{k - k_0}{\Delta k} \right)^2 \right] \tag{21}$$

the function $F_{\text{spect}}(z)$ becomes

$$F_{\text{spect}}(z) = \cos(2k_0 z + \phi)\gamma_{\text{spect}}(z) \tag{22}$$

$F_{\text{spect}}(z)$ has a sinusoidal variation of period $\lambda = 2\pi/k_0$, multiplied by an envelope $\gamma_{\text{spect}}(z)$ that also has a Gaussian shape:

$$\gamma_{\text{spect}}(z) = \exp\left[-\Delta k^2 \frac{z^2}{2}\right] \tag{23}$$

The FWHM of $\gamma_{\text{spect}}(z)$ is

$$\text{FWHM}_{\gamma_{\text{spect}}} = \frac{2\sqrt{2\ln 2}}{\Delta k} = \frac{\sqrt{2\ln 2}}{n\pi}\left(\frac{\lambda^2}{\Delta\lambda}\right) \tag{24}$$

which is half the coherence length of the source (n is the refractive index of the medium). Typical infrared LEDs (in air) are characterized by an $\text{FWHM}_{\gamma_{\text{spect}}} \approx 10\,\mu\text{m}$. Lower values could be obtained with a white lamp ($\text{FWHM}_{\gamma_{\text{spect}}} \approx 0.5\,\mu\text{m}$). However, the intensity of a white lamp cannot be modulated at 50 kHz as easily as with an LED.

In conclusion, in the case of narrow-aperture systems, the short coherence length of the optical source determines the resolution in the z direction, which is typically of the order of $10\,\mu\text{m}$.

High Numerical Aperture

In the case of objective lenses with high numerical aperture, the short coherence length of the light may not determine the depth response. If we suppose in the calculation a low-bandwidth optical source ($\Delta k \approx 0$), $F_{\text{spect,NA}}(z)$ is then reduced to

$$
\begin{aligned}
F_{\text{NA}}(z) &= \frac{2}{\sin^2\theta_{\max}} \int_0^{\theta_{\max}} \cos(2kz\cos\theta + \phi)\cos\theta\sin\theta\, d\theta \\
&= \frac{2}{\sin^2\theta_{\max}}\left[\frac{\cos(2kz+\phi) - \cos(2kz\cos\theta_{\max}+\phi)}{4k^2z^2}\right. \\
&\quad \left. + \frac{\sin(2kz+\phi) - \cos\theta_{\max}\sin(2kz\cos\theta_{\max}+\phi)}{2kz}\right]
\end{aligned} \tag{25}
$$

It is worth noting that a more rigorous analysis using Richards and Wolf's vector theory [32] gives the same expression [Eq. (25)] obtained with the scalar approximation [33]. It is interesting to note that this expression is formally identical to the depth response of a confocal microscope [1,23]. The function $F_{\text{NA}}(z)$ exhibits oscillations that decrease with z (Fig. 16). A more explicit expression of the z response can, however, be given under the paraxial assumption ($\cos\theta_{\max} \approx 1$)

$$
\begin{aligned}
F_{\text{NA}}(z) &\approx \frac{2}{\sin^2\theta_{\max}} \int_0^{\theta_{\max}} \cos(2kz\cos\theta + \phi)\sin\theta\, d\theta \\
&= \frac{\sin(2kz+\phi) - \sin(2kz\cos\theta_{\max}+\phi)}{kz\sin^2\theta_{\max}} \\
&= \frac{2}{1+\cos\theta_{\max}}\left(\frac{\sin(kz(1-\cos\theta_{\max}))}{kz(1-\cos\theta_{\max})}\right)\cos(kz(1+\cos\theta_{\max}) + \phi)
\end{aligned} \tag{26}
$$

Finally,

$$F_{\text{NA}}(z) \propto \frac{\sin(kz(1-\cos\theta_{\max}))}{kz(1-\cos\theta_{\max})}\cos(2\alpha kz + \phi), \qquad \alpha = \frac{1+\cos\theta_{\max}}{2} \tag{27}$$

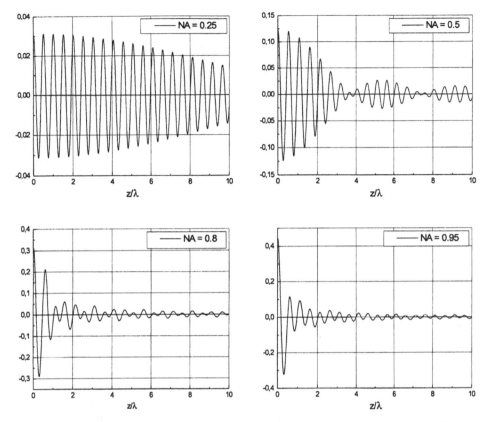

Figure 16 Theoretical calculation of the depth response of an optical coherence microscope [$F_{NA}(z)$] as a function of the numerical aperture (NA) of the objective lenses. The coherence length of the optical source is assumed to be infinite.

From expression (27), we see that $F_{NA}(z)$ has roughly a sinusoidal variation of period modified by the factor α multiplied by an envelope $\gamma_{NA}(z)$ which has a maximum at $z = 0$ and falls off when $|z|$ increases with oscillations like a $(\sin x)\,dx$ function. The FWHM of the envelope $\gamma_{NA}(z)$ is approximately given by

$$\text{FWHM}_{\gamma_{NA}} = \frac{\pi}{k(1 - \cos\theta_{max})} = \frac{\lambda}{2n(1 - \cos\theta_{max})} \qquad (28)$$

The larger the numerical aperture of the objective lenses, the narrower the envelope. In air ($n = 1$), with a numerical aperture $NA = 0.95$ and a wavelength $\lambda = 840\,\text{nm}$, $\text{FWHM}_{\gamma_{NA}} \approx 0.6\,\mu\text{m}$. Thus, the effect of the high numerical aperture of the objectives can yield much better depth resolution than the effect of low coherence length of the optical source.

General Case

In the general case, the depth resolution in OCM depends on both the coherence length of the source and the numerical aperture of the objectives, the range resolution being smaller than its value due to either effect alone. For example, numerical simulations (Fig. 17) show the evolution of the depth resolution (FWHM of the depth

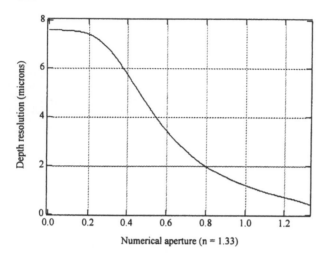

Figure 17   Depth resolution (FWHM of the envelope of the depth response) as a function of the numerical aperture with an 840 nm light source with $20\,\mu$m coherence length in a medium of refractive index $n = 1.33$.

envelope) as a function of the numerical aperture with an 840 nm light source with $20\,\mu$m coherence length in a medium with a refractive index of 1.33. In the Michelson geometry with numerical apertures smaller than 0.2, the depth resolution is imposed by the coherence length of the source ($\approx 7.5\,\mu$m). This situation corresponds to a "pure" optical coherence situation, which is the case in most systems (such as our Michelson-type microscope). In the Linnik configuration, the use of a high numerical aperture objective can improve the depth resolution up to about $0.5\,\mu$m.

Experimental Data

We measured the intensity depth response of our optical coherence microscopes by taking a mirror as the object and measuring the signal intensity $A_S^2(z)$ when the mirror was moved out of the focal plane of the objective. Two numerical apertures were used: NA = 0.15 and NA = 0.95. The measurements are compared with theoretical calculations (Fig. 18). With NA = 0.15, the depth response is determined by the coherence length of the source. The Gaussian shape response, in excellent agreement with theory, has an FWHM of $10\,\mu$m, equal to half the coherence length of the source ($20\,\mu$m). With NA = 0.95, the depth response is then determined by the numerical aperture of the objective lenses. The experimental FWHM is $0.7\,\mu$m, slightly larger than the theoretical value of $0.60\,\mu$m. The difference between theory and experiment is attributed to geometrical optical aberrations at the working wavelength. The depth resolution is thus better than $1\,\mu$m, which means that our microscope is able to reject the light reflected by objects located less than $1\,\mu$m from the focal plane. These experiments were carried out in air. In a medium with refractive index n, the resolution would be improved by a factor equal to n.

11.4.2   Lateral Resolution

If we suppose that the lateral resolution in our microscopes is limited by diffraction, the interference signal I_{int} for an object in the focal plane is of the form

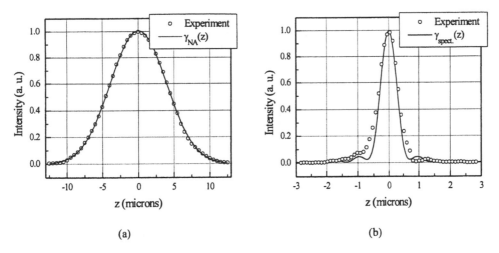

Figure 18 Depth response of our optical coherence microscopes with a $20\,\mu m$ coherence length source at $\lambda = 840\,nm$ and numerical apertures NA = 0.15 (a) and NA = 0.95 (b).

$$I_{\mathrm{int}}(x_0, y_0) = \int\int 2A_R A_S(x, y)\cos(\phi)\big|h(x - x_0, y - y_0)\big|^2 dx\, dy \qquad (29)$$

where $n(x, y)$ is the point spread function of the objectives, which is the Airy function. The amplitude point spread function of our interference microscope is thus given by $|h(x, y)|^2$ and the intensity point spread function by $|h(x, y)|^4$ as it is for the confocal microscope [1]. Because of digitalization by the CCD array, the actual intensity point spread function is the square of the convolution of $|h(x, y)|^2$ with a square distribution of width equal to the pixel dimension in the object plane.

To measure the lateral response of our microscopes, we recorded an intensity profile along a line taken across a cleaved mirror. Two numerical apertures were used: NA = 0.15 and NA = 0.95. The measurements are compared with theoretical calculations (Fig. 19). With NA = 0.15, the experimental 20–80% width of the intensity profile was $1.5\,\mu m$, in good agreement with theory. With NA = 0.95, the experimental 20–80% width of the intensity profile was $0.3\,\mu m$, slightly larger than the theoretical prediction of $0.25\,\mu m$. Again, the difference between theory and experiment is attributed to geometrical optical aberrations. In the calculations, values used for pixel size and wavelength were $0.15\,\mu m$ and 840 nm, respectively.

11.4.3 Sensitivity

We develop an estimate of the sensitivity of our system as usually defined in the OCT context, i.e., the ratio $(K_{\mathrm{min}})^{-1}$ of the power delivered to the sample over the minimum detectable signal.

We first point out that in practice images are accumulated under illumination conditions where the CCD pixels are close to saturation. Let N_0 be the number of polarized photons corresponding to one pixel incident on the objective back aperture during one image acquisition time. Assuming that the initial polarization makes a (small) angle θ with the S axis of the PBS, a fraction $N_0 \sin^2(\theta)$ reaches the reference mirror and $N_0 \cos^2(\theta)$ irradiates the sample. Of the latter, the objective collects a

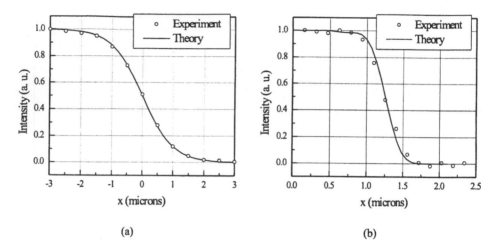

Figure 19 Lateral resolution. Edge response of our optical coherence microscope with a 20 μm coherence length source at λ = 840 nm and numerical apertures Na = 0.15 (a) and NA = 0.95 (b).

fraction $KN_0 \cos^2(\theta)$, which is coherently backscattered from the sample, and an incoherent fraction $K_i N_0 \cos^2(\theta)$. In practice, $\cos^2(\theta) \approx 1$, and the number of photoelectrons on the corresponding CCD pixel of quantum efficiency η is

$$\eta N_\pm \approx \eta \left[\sin^2(\theta) N_0 + KN_0 + \frac{1}{2} K_i N_0 \pm 2 \left(K \sin^2(\theta) N_0^2 \right)^{1/2} \right] \tag{30}$$

The ± sign corresponds to the situation where the backscattered signal and the reference signal are (+) in phase or (−) of opposite phase.

Thus, the modulated signal S that is processed by our parallel lock-in technique and the average flux S_0 can be expressed as

$$S = S_+ - S_- \approx 4\eta N_0 \sqrt{K \sin^2(\theta)}; \qquad S_0 = \eta \left[\sin^2(\theta) + \frac{1}{2} K_i \right] N_0 \tag{31}$$

Assuming that $\sin^2(\theta) \gg K_i$ (the input polarization is oriented so that the noise level is not dominated by the incoherent backscattered light), in the case of shot noise limited signal detection, and if $S_0 \approx \eta \sin^2(\theta) N_0 = S_{sat}$ (where S_{sat} is the saturation level of the CCD pixel), the signal-to-noise ratio for N accumulated image quadruplets can be expressed as

$$\mathrm{SNR}_{4,N} = \frac{S}{\sqrt{4NS}} \approx 2 \left(\frac{N S_{sat} K}{\sin^2 \theta} \right)^{1/2} \tag{32}$$

The minimum detectable signal K_{min} corresponds to the situation where SNR = 1, yielding the following expression for the sensitivity:

$$(K_{min})^{-1} = 4N S_{sat} / \sin^2 \theta \tag{33}$$

In expression (33) the parameter $\sin^2(\theta)$ is in general inversely proportional to the power delivered to the sample. As a matter of fact, it describes the interferometer balance setting that enables one to almost reach the saturation level of the sensor with the signal returning from the reference arm.

Taking $S_{sat} = 2 \times 10^5$ and $\theta = 10°$, a 1 s record of a full image at the maximum speed of the camera (200 images/s) enables one to detect a minimum signal of relative magnitude $K_{min} \approx 7.5^{-10}$, corresponding to a sensitivity of 91 dB. We point out that there is a trade-off between sensitivity and detection bandwidth, so that under the same conditions an 81 dB sensitivity is obtained within 10^{-1} s of recording time.

In the case of single quadrature images, the signal-to-noise ratio for N accumulated image pairs can be expressed as

$$SNR_{2,N} = \sqrt{2}SNR_{4,N} \tag{34}$$

A 1 s record under the conditions specified above would then be characterized by a sensitivity of 97 dB.

We confirmed this estimate by measuring the noise level in featureless images acquired under illumination conditions where the CCD sensor was almost saturated.

Finally, we point out that it is assumed in the above calculation that $\sin^2 \theta \gg K_i$, meaning that the noise does not mainly originate from the incoherent backscattered light. This was typically the case in our experiments with a 0.25 NA objective and a polarizer setting corresponding to $\theta \approx 10°$. However, if an objective lens with higher numerical aperture is used, θ might be increased, depending on the overall backscattering of the sample.

11.4.4 Temporal Resolution and SNR Issues

We saw in the previous section that a sensitivity of ~ 90 dB can be achieved in optimal conditions with an exposure time of about 1 s.

In this derivation we have supposed that the signal backscattered from the structure was stationary on the time scale of our measurement. We can now raise the question of the behavior of such a signal (and of its time average) if the medium under study is quickly changing with time (for example, if the signal originates from scatterers undergoing Brownian or some physiological motion).

In a "classical" OCT system the measurement time per voxel is on the order of a few microseconds and the sample can generally be considered to be static at this time scale. However, line-to-line evolutions (a few milliseconds to a few seconds) usually have to be taken into account in the processing software that reconstructs the final image.

In a full-field approach using a CCD camera, the voxel acquisition time is on the order of a few milliseconds, and, most of the time, averaging over about 1 s is necessary to obtain an acceptable SNR.

If we average *coherently* (with respect to the reference signal) the signals from moving scatterers over 10–100 images, rapid changes in the optical phase of the backscattered wave may wipe out any contrast present in the interference signals. For instance, if the optical phase changes by 2π during the acquisition time, the contrast is zero.

So one may think of first computing the *amplitude* of the interference signal from the four unprocessed images necessary to get the signal, then averaging this value over several acquisitions. Such *incoherent averaging* is obviously valid only if the variance of the noise is smaller than the *signal amplitude* (otherwise noise amplitude rather than signal is averaged). Only in this latter case can signal-to-noise ratio and thus the image quality of the moving sample be improved by averaging.

Thus, a trade-off exists between sensitivity and temporal resolution (or detection bandwidth). Coherent averaging of the images can be performed up to the time scale where the sample is immobile in order to improve the system sensitivity at the expense of temporal resolution. Then, at longer time scales, incoherent averaging increases the SNR in the images without benefit in terms of sensitivity.

Array detectors are usually slower than single detectors, so the temporal resolution is a fundamental feature of parallel coherent systems that may make them suitable or not for a specific application.

11.5   APPLICATIONS

11.5.1   3-D Biological Tissue Imaging

Our optical coherence microscopes can be used to get images through biological materials with a few micrometers depth resolution. Images obtained from onion tissues at various depths using the Michelson and Linnik arrangements are shown in Fig. 20. Structures and tissues organization are clearly revealed. Objective lenses with 0.25 numerical aperture were used. With this objective, the axial resolution is approximately 7 μm (Fig. 17), assuming the average refractive index of the onion is $\sim$ 1.33.

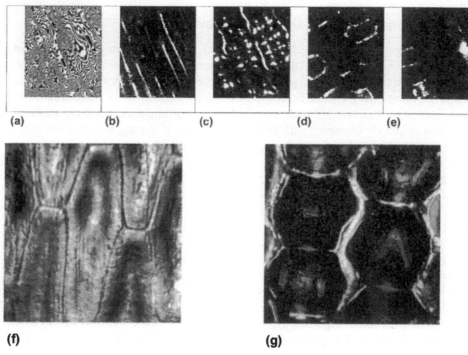

(a)   (b)   (c)   (d)   (e)

(f)   (g)

Figure 20   (a–e) Images from an onion obtained with our Michelson-type low coherence microscope and a 0.25 numerical aperture (NA) objective lens. Field of view 500 μm $\times$ 500 μm. Exposure time 5 s. Optical power incident on the sample 300 mW. (a) Interference fringes obtained from the surface. (b–e) Interference fringes obtained, (b) 15 μm, (c) 60 μm, (d) 140 μm, and (e) 300 μm below the surface. (f–g) Images (onion) obtained at higher resolution using Linnik geometry. The field of view is 260 μm $\times$ 260 μm. Exposure time 1 s. Optical power incident on the sample 500 mW.

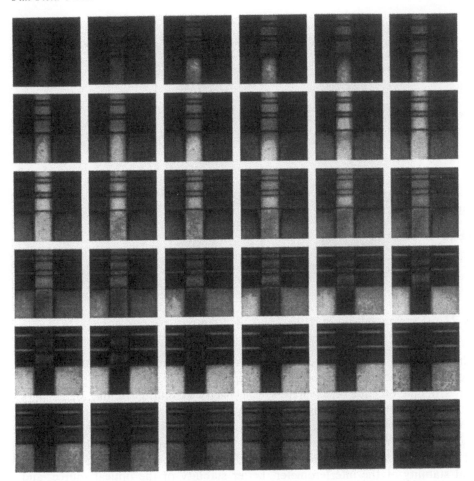

Figure 21 Cross-sectional intensity images at different depths from a multilayer silicon integrated circuit, obtained with our Linnik-type optical coherence microscope. The distance between successive images is $0.1\,\mu$m in the z direction. Each image corresponds to a field of $35\,\mu$m $\times\ 35\,\mu$m. The numerical aperture of the objective lenses was NA $= 0.95$.

11.5.2 Integrated Circuit Inspection

The unceasing advances in optical microlithography and processing technology require more and more powerful optical imaging instruments for characterization and measurement. For this purpose, our high resolution Linnik-type interference microscope is a useful tool. Cross-sectional intensity (A_S^2) images from a multilayer silicon integrated circuit are shown in Fig. 21. Objective lenses with 0.95 numerical aperture were used, which yields $0.7\,\mu$m depth resolution and $0.3\,\mu$m lateral resolution. Two consecutive images are separated by $0.1\,\mu$m in the z direction. Note that off-focus features are suppressed, whereas they are not in classical microscopy (Fig. 22).

11.5.3 Phase Images and Profilometry

As mentioned before, optical coherence microscopes can provide the optical phase, which is proportional (modulo $\pi/2$) to the height between the surface of the object

z = 0   z = 1 μm

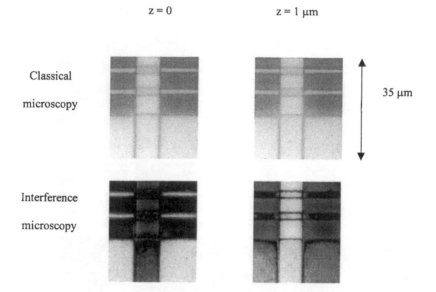

Figure 22   Comparison between classical and interference microscopic images.

and the surface of the reference mirror. Three-dimensional representation of the surface can thus be produced provided the phase is correctly unwrapped. Figure 23 shows details on integrated circuits. The height resolution of the 3-D images produced by our interference microscope depends on how precisely the phase can be measured. The signal-to-noise ratio in the images can be improved by increasing the exposure time. We have measured a height sensitivity better than 0.1 nm with less than 1 s exposure time. This sensitivity could be improved by better mechanical and thermal stability of the interferometer, better stability of the optical source, and

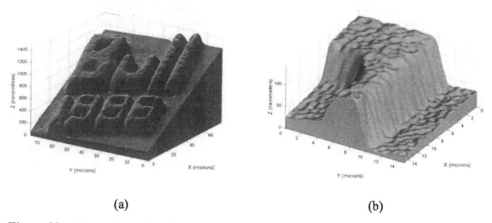

(a)   (b)

Figure 23   Three-dimensional topographic representation of structures from microelectronic devices. (a) Metal inscriptions deposed on a silicon wafer. The field of view is 80 μm × 80 μm. (b) Image of a detail on a pixel of a field emission display device, covered by a 30 μm thick dielectric layer. The image corresponds to an area of 15 μm × 15 μm. The roughness of the structures is clearly revealed (~ 5 nm rms), and the slopes are resolved.

better electronics [34]. With 0.95 NA objective lenses, the lateral resolution, almost limited by diffraction, was about $0.5\,\mu$m. Reducing the optical wavelength to 400 nm using a blue LED would improve the lateral resolution to approximately $0.25\,\mu$m.

11.6 CONCLUSION AND PERSPECTIVES

Full-field illumination and parallel detection have been demonstrated with optical coherence microscopy (OCM). Using high NA objective lenses, the technique allows imaging with micrometer spatial resolution in the three directions and 20 ms temporal resolution.

This approach is attractive for the following reasons:

Head-on (XY) geometry allows high resolution imaging. Three-dimensional submicrometer resolution is achieved using a high-NA objective lens. In contrast with XZ OCT imaging, the resolution is the same everywhere in the full XY image, because the whole field of view is in the plane of focus of the objective lens.

Head-on (XY) geometry allows adjustment of the acquisition time and of the intensity irradiating the sample according to the imaging depth.

If the source power is not limited, parallel detection requires a shorter amount of time than serial detection to achieve a given SNR in the image. In the coming years it is expected that more powerful light sources and faster cameras will make it possible to take full advantage of this approach.

Scanning and associated vibrations are reduced to a minimum.

Simultaneous acquisition allows the acquisition of a complete image to be synchronized to a physiological event.

There are some limitations of this method that may make it unsuitable for certain applications:

The achievable temporal resolution per pixel is limited to one-fourth of the camera frame rate ($\sim$ milliseconds).

Confocal filtering cannot be implemented in a full-field detection as in scanning OCM systems. However, the interference microscope geometry formally plays the same role as a confocal pinhole (see Section 11.4.1).

Artifacts may be present when imaging samples with strong birefringence and backscattering polarization anisotropy with a polarization interferometer. However, the layouts presented here can easily be modified to become polarization-sensitive and then be used to measure sample birefringence.

One of our main motivations was to explore layouts allowing high resolution OCT imaging in the three dimensions. The use of high NA objective lenses in an XY (*en face*) imaging geometry effectively provides 3-D submicrometer resolution, which makes it an alternative approach to XZ imaging with spectrally wide sources [35]. Furthermore, parallel detection in coherence microscopy is a tempting approach, provided that one is not limited by the available power. We are currently investigating the use of white light sources, CCD cameras with higher full well capacities and frame rates, and fast modulators (liquid crystal, ~ 1 MHz) to improve the sensitivity and temporal resolution of these systems.

ACKNOWLEDGMENTS

We thank J. Mertz for many fruitful discussions. This research was supported by the Centre National de la Recherche Scientifique (CNRS) and by the Direction Générale de l'Armement (DGA).

REFERENCES

1. Wilson T, Sheppard CJR. Theory and Practice of Scanning Optical Microscopy. New York: Academic, 1984.
2. Pawley J ed. The Handbook of Confocal Microscopy. 2nd ed. New York: Plenum Press, 1995: 445.
3. Wilson T. Confocal Microscopy. London: Academic, 1990.
4. Huang D, Swanson EA, Lin CP, Schuman JS, Stinson WG, Chang W, Hee MR, Flotte T, Gregory K, Puliafito CA, Fujimoto JG. Optical coherence tomography. Science 254:1178, 1991.
5. Izatt JA, Hee MR, Owen GM, Swanson EA, Fujimoto JG. Optical coherence microscopy in scattering media. Opt Lett 19:590, 1994.
6. Tearney GJ, Bouma BE, Boppart SA, Golubovic B, Swanson EA, Fujimoto JG. Rapid acquisition of in vivo biological images by use of optical coherence tomography. Opt Lett 21:1408, 1996.
7. Tearney GJ, Brezinski ME, Bouma BE, Boppart SA, Pitris C, Southern JF, Fujimoto JG. In vivo endoscopic optical biopsy with optical coherence tomography. Science 276:2037, 1997.
8. Boppart SA, Brezinski MA, Bouma BE, Tearney GJ, Fujimoto JG. Investigation of developing embryonic morphology using optical coherence tomography. Dev Biol 177:54, 1996.
9. Schmitt JB, Yadlowsky MJ, Bonner RF. Subsurface imaging of living skin with optical coherence microscopy. Dermatology 191:93, 1995.
10. Izatt JA, Kulkarni MD, Want H-W, Kobayashi K, Sivak MV Jr. Optical coherence tomography and microscopy in gastrointestinal tissues. IEEE J Selected Topics Quantum Electron 2:1017, 1996..
11. Kempe M, Rudolph W, Welsch E. Comparative study of confocal and heterodyne microscopy for imaging through scattering media. J Opt Soc Am A 13:46, 1996.
12. Beaurepaire E, Moreaux L, Amblard F, Mertz J. Combined scanning optical coherence and two-photon excited fluorescence microscopy. Opt Lett 24:969, 1999.
13. Beaurepaire E, Boccara AC, Lebec M, Blanchot L, Saint-Jalmes H. Full-field optical coherence microscopy. Opt Lett 23:244, 1998.
14. Hinshaw WS. Image formation by NMR: The sensitive-point method. J Appl Phys 47:3709, 1976.
15. Lauterbur PC. NMR Zeugmatographic imaging by true 3D reconstruction. J Comput Assist Tomogr 5:285, 1981.
16. Boppart SA, Bouma BE, Pitris C, Southern JF, Brezinski ME, Fujimoto JG. In vivo optical coherence tomography cellular imaging. Nature Med 4(7):861, 1998.
17. Schmitt JM, Knüttel A, Gandjbakhche A, Bonner RF. Optical characterization of dense tissues using low-coherence interferometry. SPIE Proc 1889:197, 1989.
18. Yariv A. Optical Electronics. 4th ed. Saunders, Philadelphia, 1991.
19. Schmitt JM, Knüttel A. Model of optical coherence tomography of heterogeneous tissue. J Opt Soc Am A 14:1231, 1997.
20. Yadlowsky MJ, Schmitt JM, Bonner RF. Multiple scattering in optical coherence microscopy. Appl Opt 34(25):5699, 1995.

21. Boccara AC, Charbonnier F, Fournier D, Gleyzes P. French Patent FR90.092255 and international extensions (1990).
22. Gleyzes P, Boccara AC, Saint-Jalmes H. Multichannel Nomarski microscope with polarization modulation: Performance and applications. Opt Lett 22(20):1529, 1997.
23. Kino GS, Chim SC. Mirau correlation microscope. Appl Opt 29:3775, 1990.
24. Dubois A, Boccara AC, Lebec M. Real-time reflectivity and topography imagery of depth-resolved microscopic surfaces. Opt Lett 24:309, 1999.
25. Davidson M, Kaufman K, Mazor I, Cohen F. An application of interference microscopy to integrated circuit inspection and metrology. In: KM Monahan, ed. Integrated Circuit Metrology, Inspection, and Process Control. Proc. SPIE 775:233, 1987.
26. Schmitt JM, Hee SL, Yung KM. An optical coherence microscope with enhanced resolving power in thick tissue. Opt Commun 142:203, 1997.
27. Badoz J, Billardon M, Canit JC, Russel MF. Sensitive devices to determine the state and degree of polarization of a light beam using a birefringent modulator. J Opt (Paris) 8:373, 1977.
28. Canit JC, Badoz J. New design for a photoelastic modulator. Appl Opt 22:592, 1983.
29. Lévêque S, Boccara AC, Lebec M, Saint-Jalmes H. Ultrasonic tagging of photons paths in scattering media: Parallel speckle modulation processing. Opt Lett 24:181, 1999.
30. Forget BC, Grauby S, Fournier D, Gleyzes P, Boccara AC. High resolution AC temperature field imaging. Electron Lett 33:1688, 1997.
31. Sheppard CJR, Wilson T. Effects of high angles of convergence on V(z) in the scanning acoustic microscope. Appl Phys Lett 38:858–859, 1981.
32. Richards B, Wolf E. Electromagnetic diffraction in optical systems: II. Structure of the image field in an aplanetic system. Proc Soc Lond Ser A 253:358, 1959.
33. Chang FC, Kino GS. 325-nm interference microscope. Appl Opt 37:3471, 1998.
34. Laeri F, Strand TC. Angstrom resolution optical profilometry for microscopic objects. Appl Opt 26:2245, 1987.
35. Drexler W, Morgner U, Kärtner FX, Pitris C, Boppart SA, Li XD, Ippen EP, Fujimoto JG. In vivo ultrahigh-resolution optical coherence tomography. Opt Lett 24:1221, 1999.

12

Spectral Radar: Optical Coherence Tomography in the Fourier Domain

M. W. LINDNER, P. ANDRETZKY, F. KIESEWETTER, and G. HÄUSLER

University of Erlangen-Nuernberg, Erlangen, Germany

12.1 INTRODUCTION

This chapter will discuss white light interferometry within scattering media. White light interferometry at nonspecular surfaces was discovered only about 10 years ago [1]. The physics of white light interferometry at "rough" surfaces or within scattering objects is rather different from Michelson's white light interferometry. Interferometry on non-smooth objects has to satisfy strong requirements about spatial coherence, temporal coherence, observation aperture, and lateral photodetector resolution.

In white light interferometry on rough or within scattering objects, the subjective speckle pattern in the observation plane is the source of information. Hence we have to take care that the aperture of illumination is smaller than the aperture of observation, in order to create sufficient speckle contrast. Furthermore, the photodetector elements have to be not much larger than the speckles, in order to avoid speckle reduction by averaging. One serious difference from smooth surface interferometry is the achievable accuracy: The interference phase within each speckle is arbitrary and random. The phase variation between different speckles depends on the roughness and may be as great as $10\text{--}20 \times 2\pi$ for ground or milled surfaces. Hence, the achievable measuring uncertainty is limited and is equal to the surface roughness (which is usually much smaller than the coherence length of the source) [2].

Measurements within the bulk of strongly scattering media require conditions similar to those mentioned above. Specifically, the source of information is still the speckle contrast. One major difference from rough surface measurements is that this

335

speckle contrast is usually extremely small if the measured volume is deeper than the coherence length of the source. In those objects, we observe a measuring uncertainty and a depth resolution not much better than the coherence length.

During the last 10 years, our group developed a couple of sensors based on white light interferometry on rough surfaces or within scattering media. The first was "coherence radar" [1,2]. Here the reference is mechanically scanned through the measuring volume. The name "coherence radar" suggests itself because it essentially measures the local time of flight to each object pixel by use of the coherent reference "clock." The sensor can measure the shape of rough surfaces with an accuracy equal to the surface roughness, which is usually in the $1 \mu m$ regime. The objects may be volume scatterers such as ceramics or skin. One exciting feature of coherence radar is that the measuring uncertainty does not depend upon the object distance or the observation aperture: We can measure in deep boreholes without loss of accuracy.

One modification of coherence radar is "dispersion radar" [3]. Here we introduce a dispersive element within the reference arm before we spectrally evaluate the interferometer output. The major advantage of this method is that we can have a large measuring range even with a low cost spectrometer.

The last modification is what we call "spectral radar" [4], which will be discussed in this chapter. We hope that this short introduction has given the reader some idea of the physics of this new type of interferometry and its potential applications.

12.2 BENEFITS AND LIMITATIONS OF LOW COHERENCE INTERFEROMETRY

An important medical aim in dermatology is the early diagnosis of pathological tissue alterations (e.g., skin cancer). High resolution imaging methods are needed that are not harmful to healthy tissue. During recent years noninvasive cross-sectional imaging methods under the heading "optical tomography" have been developed. The sensing methods are manifold but are based on a common feature: The tissue (which is a volume scatterer) is illuminated, and the number of photons scattered back to the detector is measured as a function of the pathlength in the tissue. This principle gives, to a certain extent, access to the scattering amplitude $a(z)$, which is the key to examining the local scattering and absorption behavior in the tissue. The hope is that pathological tissue displays significant scattering properties and can therefore be separated from healthy tissue. The pathlength distribution of the photons can be measured directly by time-of-flight measurements or by using low coherence interferometry.

Optical coherence tomography (OCT) uses a broad bandwidth light source in an interferometric setup. Interference is detected only if the object pathlength equals the reference pathlength. The pathlength of the photons to be detected (backscattered from the tissue) can be adjusted by the reference pathlength. The main advantage of OCT is that the pathlength resolution is roughly given by the coherence length l_C of the light, which can be in the micrometer range.

The major problem in optical tomography is the strong scattering of most types of biological tissue (more in skin than in the retina). As a result of multiple scattering, photons that have traveled the same optical pathlength may have traveled along different individual paths reaching different depths in the scatterer. This affects the depth uncertainty of the measurements. By confocal imaging of back-scattered photons onto a fiber core, photons that have been scattered several times and with low correlation between run time and depth information will no longer hit the fiber.

We again mention one important aspect of the signal formation: Imaging with a finite aperture causes subjective speckle at the entrance of the fiber. Speckle contrast is the actual carrier of information. Because of the strong incoherent background, this speckle contrast is extremely low for strongly scattering media. Sophisticated electronics and data processing are necessary. As a consequence, the requirements for an extremely high dynamic range limit access to the deeper layers of the skin. So consideration of the achievable dynamic range will play an important role in the comparison of competing methods.

12.3 THE FAMILY OF OCT SENSORS

In order to investigate the morphological 3-D data of biological objects, methods based on optical coherence tomography (OCT) have become more and more important during recent years. The OCT methods can be divided into two classes, with sensors based on time domain measuring principles (TDOCT) or on Fourier domain principles (FDOCT).

Both TDOCT and FDOCT use a broad-bandwidth light source in an interferometric setup. For measurement along an axis (z axis) from the surface into the bulk (A-scan) with TDOCT, the reference mirror has to be scanned through the depth. Interference contrast is detected only if the object pathlength equals the reference pathlength. The pathlength of the photons to be detected can be adjusted by the reference pathlength. In TDOCT the scatterers are measured sequentially. Therefore, light that is scattered back from each scatterer contributes to the interference signal only if the distance between the reference pane and the scatterer is less than the coherence length. Only a fraction of the light that is scattered back during the entire measuring time is utilized. Time domain methods have been investigated in a multitude of modifications [5–15].

Fourier domain principles avoid scanning of the reference through the depth range. These OCT sensors acquire depth information by evaluation of the spectrum of the interferogram. The Fourier transformation of the spectrum delivers the depth information. All scatterers are simultaneously measured by FDOCT sensors. Light that is scattered back from each scatterer within the volume contributes to the interference signal over the entire measuring time. For sensors of this type there are several approaches. A broad-bandwidth light source is used for the illumination of the interferometer. The interferometer output is spectrally decomposed, and the whole spectrum is detected by an array of photodiodes. This specific implementation can be adapted for measurements on the (transparent) eye [5–7] as well as for measurements of strongly scattering skin [4,16–19]. In a further modification, the spectrum can be produced by a tunable laser and then be detected by a single photodiode [20,21].

In both classes of OCT sensors the speckle contrast is the actual source of information [22,23].

12.4 SPECTRAL RADAR IN A NUTSHELL

As explained in the Introduction, we called our implementation of FDOCT "spectral radar" because it is one modification of coherence radar. Spectral radar uses an OCT sensor working in the Fourier domain [4,18,19]. The measuring principle is based on spectral interferometry. Spectral radar measures the scattering amplitude $a(z)$ along one A-scan within one detector exposure. No scanning in depth is necessary, so a short measurement time is generally possible. For two-dimensional imaging a transverse scan is necessary (B-scan). The sensor is a Michelson interferometer (Fig. 1) coupled with a spectrometer.

In one specific implementation, the light source is a superluminescent diode (SLD) in the near-infrared range with a short coherence length l_C (central wavelength $\lambda = 840$ nm, FWHM 20 nm, coherence length $l_C = 35 \, \mu$m; output power $P = 1.7$ mW). The SLD is imaged onto the object surface and onto a reference mirror. The signal from the object consists of many elementary waves emanating from different depths z. We neglect the dispersion in the object. The scattering amplitude of the elementary waves versus depth is $a(z)$ [$a(z)$ is assumed to be real here]. The object signal is superimposed with the plane reference wave a_R. At the exit of the interferometer we locally separate the different wavenumbers $k(= 2\pi/\lambda)$ by use of a spectrometer. The interference signal $I(k)$ is in principle [4,18] (a detailed description is given in Section 12.5.1)

$$I(k) = S(k)\left(1 + \int_{-\infty}^{\infty} a(z)\cos(2knz)\,dz + \text{AC terms}\right) \tag{1}$$

where $S(k)$ is the spectral intensity distribution of the light source and n is the refractive index of the scatterer.

It can be seen that $I(k)$ is a sum of three terms. Besides a constant offset the second term encodes the depth information of the object. It is a sum of cosine functions, where the amplitude of each cosine is proportional to the scattering amplitude $a(z)$. The depth z of the scattering event is encoded in the frequency $2nz$ of the cosine function. This term describes the well-known Müller fringes of spectral interferometry [24]. It will be seen that $a(z)$ can be acquired by a Fourier transfor-

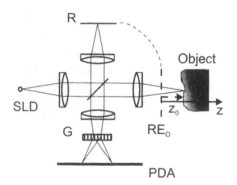

Figure 1 Basic principle of the setup of spectral radar. SLD, superluminescent diode; R, reference; RE$_o$, reference plane in the object arm; G, grating spectrometer; PDA, photodiode array; a(z), scattering amplitude.

mation of the interferogram [25]. The third, autocorrelation term (AC terms), describes the mutual interference of all elementary waves [Eq. (5)].

The main feature of all FDOCT sensors is that the total distribution of the scattering amplitude $a(z)$ along one A-scan is measured at one time. The light that is scattered back from each scatterer in the volume contributes to the interference signal during the entire measuring time. This is the crucial difference between FDOCT sensors and TDOCT sensors. For an A-scan by TDOCT sensors, the reference mirror has to be scanned through the depth. The scatterers are measured sequentially. Therefore, only a fraction of the light that is scattered back during the total measuring time can be considered.

These differences between the two techniques have a strong influence on the dynamic range, which is the ratio of the maximum and minimum measurable power P of the signal emanating from the object. It has been shown that the shot noise of the photons is the main physical limitation of the dynamic range [18,19]. From this fact it can be deduced that the dynamic range is limited only by the number of photons from the object that contribute to the interference signal within the measuring time. The dynamic range of FDOCT sensors is [18,19]

$$ D_{\mathrm{FD}} = 10 \log \left[\frac{4}{\mathrm{SNR}_F^2} \left(\frac{P_O t \eta}{h \nu} \right) \right] \tag{2} $$

where SNR_F is the minimal necessary signal-to-noise-ratio (which will be set to a value of 2 later), P_O is the total power from the object, $h\nu$ is the energy of one photon, and η is the quantum efficiency of the photodiode.

Here the central result has to be emphasized: The more photons from the object contribute to the interference signal, the higher is the dynamic range. Therefore FDOCT sensors have a higher dynamic range than TDOCT sensors, because in FDOCT the light from all scatterers contributes to the signal during the total measuring time, whereas in TDOCT only a fraction of the backscattered light causes interference contrast. The dynamic range of FDOCT can in principle be greater by typically 14 dB. We summarize these and other considerations in Table 1.

The speed of both methods is presently limited by the exposure time needed to integrate sufficient photons or, in other words, by the power of the source. If strong sources eventually become available, the speed of TDOCT might be limited by the mechanics of the depth scan.

One interesting further difference is the requirement for the spectral quality of the source. The correlogram $A(z)$ [see Section 12.5.1 and Eq. (9)], which is the spatial impulse response of both types of sensors, is the Fourier transform of the source spectrum $S(k)$. If $S(k)$ is not a soft function (such as a Gaussian) but is disturbed by some high frequency modulation, then $A(z)$ displays peaks far away from $z = 0$. Because we want to see extremely small signals deep in the skin, even small peaks of $A(z)$ are extremely disturbing, because these artifacts cannot be distinguished from real structure.

Here FDOCT offers a solution: We can compensate for a non-Gaussian spectrum by dividing $I(k)$ by $S(k)$ [see Eq. (9)]. $S(k)$ can be a easily measured in a separate step in our system. This is not possible with TDOCT. It should be mentioned that the unavailability of good sources is the bottleneck of optical tomogra-

Table 1   Fourier Domain OCT vs. Time Domain OCT

Parameter	FD OCT	TD OCT
Dynamic range	$D_{SD} = 10 \log N_0 = D_{TD} + 14\,\text{dB}$	$D_{TD} = 10 \log N_0 - 10 \log(\Delta z / l_C)$
Speed	Limited by source	Limited by source
Source requirements	Low spectral quality	High spectral quality
Vibration sensitivity	Sensitive for $T > 10\,\text{ms}$	Not very sensitive
Technology	Sophisticated	Less sophisticated, mechanical scan

phy. A smooth spectrum $S(k)$ is difficult to generate, because of the high coherence: Longitudinal modes are unavoidable owing to parasitic reflections at the different surfaces of the system.

Finally, we should mention some drawbacks of FDOCT. All waves that are scattered within the volume display interference during the exposure time. Hence, FDOCT is more sensitive to vibration, or moving scatterers, than TDOCT. In TDOCT we measure only a fraction of the volume at the same time; hence our system is less sensitive to motion artifacts by a factor of the ratio of coherence length to measured depth. However, if the total measuring time is less than $10\,\text{ms} - 1\,\text{ms}$, we found that the interference patterns appear stable.

Finally, there is one disadvantage to the use of FDOCT: the considerable technical effort needed for the high resolution spectrometer. This disadvantage comes specifically into play for larger wavelengths (e.g., 1300 nm) that cannot be detected by silicon technology.

12.5   PHYSICS OF SPECTRAL RADAR

12.5.1   Fiber-Optic Setup

For two-dimensional imaging, transverse scanning is necessary (B-scan). In order to perform in vivo measurements at different sites in the human body, spectral radar is implemented as a (single-mode) fiber interferometer [4]. The sensor is a modified Michelson interferometer (Fig. 2). The light source is a near-infrared superluminescent diode (SLD). In order to find the location of the measurement on the skin we use an additional pilot laser in the visible range. The light is coupled into the interferometer by a 50/50 fiber coupler.

In the reference arm we focus the beam onto a reference mirror. In the object arm the same combination of lenses is used to focus the light onto the skin. We use this combination to have two degrees of freedom in the setup. First we need to adjust the optical pathlength in both arms. The reference plane is positioned in a distance z_0 of about $200\,\mu\text{m}$ in front of the object surface, in order to get rid of the source spectrum ("correlogram") and the autocorrelation terms (described below). Second, we can vary the position of the focus of the illumination beam within the skin. The light is focused into the skin at a depth of about $200\,\mu\text{m}$. The diameter of the spot at the surface is about $50\,\mu\text{m}$, and the power in the focus is about $360\,\mu\text{W}$. The light is focused within the skin in order to enhance the interference contrast in deeper

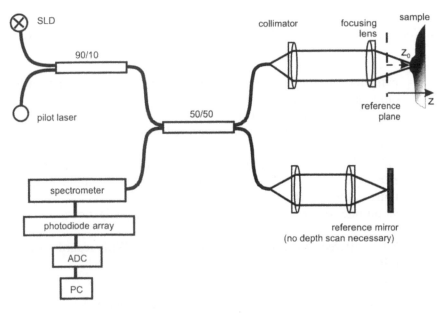

Figure 2 Fiber-optic implementation of spectral radar.

regions of the object [11]. The waves scattered back from different depths of the object are coaxially observed.

Imaging with a finite aperture causes subjective speckle at the entrance of the fiber. The speckle contrast is the actual carrier of the information. With an accepting aperture NA = 0.1 of the fiber core, there is only one speckle on the core. The confocal imaging of the backscattered photons onto the fiber core also has the advantage of spatially separating the photons. For photons that have been scattered several times, there exists hardly any correlation between run time and depth information [22]. Now just these photons will no longer hit the fiber.

The backscattered wave is superimposed with the reference wave. At the interferometer exit we use a grating spectrometer to locally separate the different wavelengths. The resolution of the spectrometer is 0.05 nm. The spectrum is imaged onto an array of 1024 photodiodes, each $2.5\,\text{mm} \times 25\,\mu\text{m}$. Each photodiode can collect 6×10^7 photons to give low photon shot noise and a large dynamic range. The signal is transferred to the host computer by a 14 bit A/D converter. Then the Fourier transformation is performed (which actually limits the dynamic range).

12.5.2 Signal Formation

The measuring principle is based on spectral interferometry. The signal from the object consists of many elementary waves emanating from different depths z. We neglect the dispersion in the object. The scattering amplitude of the elementary waves versus depth is $a(z)$. The object signal is superimposed with the plane reference wave a_R. At the exit of the interferometer a spectrometer locally separates the different wavenumbers $k(= 2\pi/\lambda)$. The interference signal $I(k)$ is

$$I(k) = S(k) \left[a_R e^{i2kr} + \int_0^\infty a(z) \exp\{i2k[r + n(z)z]\} \, dz \right]^2 \tag{3}$$

where

$2r$	= pathlength in the reference arm (Because we care only about path differences we define $r = 0$, arbitrarily.)
$2(r + z)$	= pathlength in the object arm
$2z$	= pathlength in the object arm, measured from the reference plane (Table 1)
z_0	= offset distance between reference plane and object surface (Table 1)
n	= refractive index ($n = 1$ for $z < z_0$ and $n \approx 1.5$ for longitudinal positions in the object $z > z_0$)
a_R	= amplitude of the reference (For further investigations we set $a_R = 1$.)
$a(z)$	= backscattered amplitude of the object signal. With regard to the offset z_0, $a(z)$ is zero for $z < z_0$ (see Fig. 4)
$S(k)$	= spectral intensity distribution of the light source

With these assumptions the interference signal $I(k)$ can be written as

$$I(k) = S(k) \left[1 + \int_0^\infty a(z) e^{i2knz} \, dz \right]^2 \tag{4}$$

or

$$I(k) = S(k) \left(1 + 2 \int_0^\infty a(z) \cos(2knz) \, dz + \int_0^\infty \int_0^\infty a(z) a(z') e^{-i2kn(z - z')} \, dz \, dz' \right) \tag{5}$$

It can be seen that $I(k)$ is a sum of three terms. The first term is a constant offset. The second term encodes the depth information of the object; it is a sum of cosine functions, where the amplitude of each cosine is proportional to the scattering amplitude $a(z)$. The depth z of the scattering event is encoded in the frequency $2nz$ of the cosine function. This term describes the well-known Müller fringes in spectral interferometry [24]. It will be shown that $a(z)$ can be acquired via a Fourier transformation of the interferogram [25]. The third(autocorrelation) term describes the mutual interference of all elementary waves.

We can get $a(z)$ by Fourier transformation of $I(k)$ under the assumption that $a(z)$ is symmetrical with respect to z. Fortunately $a(z) = 0$ for all $z < z_0$. So we can replace $a(z)$ by the symmetrical expansion $\hat{a}(z) = a(z) + a(-z)$. After the Fourier transformation we have to restrict ourselves to $z > z_0$, which gives us the depth information about the object

$$I(k) = S(k) \left(1 + \int_{-\infty}^\infty \hat{a}(z) \cos(2knz) \, dz + \frac{1}{4} \int_{-\infty}^\infty \int_{-\infty}^\infty \hat{a}(z) \hat{a}(z') e^{-i2kn(z - z')} \, dz \, dz' \right) \tag{6}$$

$$I(k) = S(k) \left(1 + \int_{-\infty}^{+\infty} \hat{a}(z) e^{-i2knz} \, dz + \frac{1}{4} \int_{-\infty}^{+\infty} \mathrm{AC}[\hat{a}(z)] e^{-i2knz} \, dz \right) \tag{7}$$

In this notation $\mathrm{AC}[\hat{a}(z)]$ is the autocorrelation.

$$I(k) = S(k)\left(1 + \frac{1}{2}\mathrm{FOU}_z\{\hat{a}(z)\} + \frac{1}{8}\mathrm{FOU}_z\{\mathrm{AC}[\hat{a}(z)]\}\right) \tag{8}$$

Performing the inverse Fourier transformation we get

$$\mathrm{FOU}^{-1}\{I(k)\} = \mathrm{FOU}^{-1}\{S(k)\} \otimes \left([\delta(z)] + \frac{1}{2}\hat{a}(z) + \frac{1}{8}\mathrm{AC}[\hat{a}(z)]\right) \tag{9}$$

$$= A \otimes (B + C + D)$$

where $\otimes$ indicates convolution. From this result the symmetrized scattering amplitude $\hat{a}(z)$ and therefore $a(z)$ can be deduced. In other words, we can see the strength of the scattering versus the depth. The main feature of all FDOCT sensors is that the total distribution of the scattering amplitude $a(z)$ along one A-scan is measured at once. Light that is scattered back from each scatterer in the volume contributes to the interference signal during the whole measuring time.

Figure 3 demonstrates the signal evaluation for a mirror like object. Spectral radar measures the scattering amplitude in the Fourier domain [Eq. (5)], and the evaluation by Fourier transformation delivers the scattering amplitude in the spatial

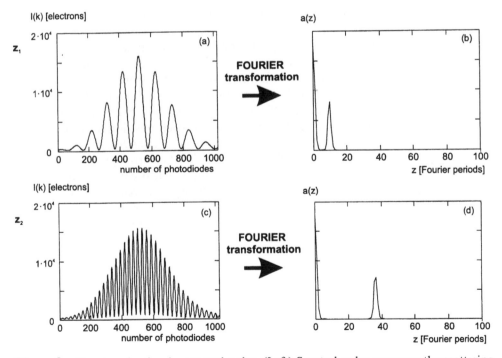

Figure 3 Signal evaluation by spectral radar. (Left) Spectral radar measures the scattering amplitude (a,c for different distances z) in the Fourier domain. (Right) Evaluation by Fourier transformation delivers the scattering amplitude in the spatial domain (b,d). (a) Interference spectrum $I(k)$ versus 1024 photodiodes of the detector array. Intensity is measured as number of electrons of each photodiode. (b) Fourier transformation gives the frequency of the cosine function, measured in Fourier periods FP (1 FP $= 7.2\,\mu$m). (c,d) For a larger distance between the mirror and the reference plane, the cosine function displays a higher frequency.

domain [Eq. (9)]. The interference spectrum $I(k)$ for a mirror at a distance z_1 from the reference plane is shown in Fig. 3a. The signal contains the cosine function $a\cos(2kz_1)$, which is multiplied with $S(k)$. The Fourier transform gives the frequency of the cosine function (Fig. 3b). In the spatial domain the frequency is measured in Fourier periods (FP): 1 FP = 7.2 μm. For a larger distance z_2 between the mirror and the reference plane the cosine function has a higher frequency (Figs 3c, 3d). The finite full width at half-maximum (FWHM) of the frequency peak of about 2 FP is caused by the convolution of the scattering amplitude with the correlogram of the light source [Eq. (9)].

Equation (9) contains the information about the scattering amplitude $a(z)$. However, besides the signal term C there are three further terms A, B, and D. These terms are well known from holography. As in holography we can get rid of them by an offset z_0 of the reference plane with respect to the object surface.

In the first term, $A \otimes B$, we get the Fourier transform of the source spectrum ("correlogram" = A) located around $z = 0$. To separate the correlogram A from the signal C we place the reference 200 μm in front of the surface of the object. A distance of 200 μm is sufficient for the separation, because the correlogram is much shorter (coherence length $\sim 35 \mu$m) if $S(k)$ is a smooth function without ripples.

There is one more disturbing term: $A \otimes D$ denotes the autocorrelation terms, which describe the mutual interference of all scattered elementary waves. In the strongly scattering skin the influence of D can be neglected because the autocorrelation term is much weaker than the signal term, which is weighted by the strong reference amplitude. Moreover, these terms are also located around $z = 0$. Therefore, the center of the autocorrelation term is separated from the object signal $a(z)$ even for a small offset z_0 (Fig. 4). As mentioned earlier, the outer lobes of the AC terms are too weak to disturb us. If the object shows high backscattering from large depths, there is still the possibility to perform at each position a second measurement with no reference signal and subtract that signal from $I(k)$.

Finally, we have a convolution of the signal C with the correlogram of the light source. To achieve high resolution measurements the spectral characteristic of the light source has to be taken into account. Only if the light source has a broad and smooth spectrum without noise or ripple will the convolution peaks be sufficiently narrow. Otherwise we can overcome the influence of the convolution by dividing Eq. (9) by the correlogram of the light source.

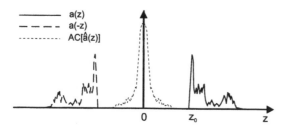

Figure 4 Sketch of the scattering amplitude $a(z)$ and the autocorrelation terms. $a(z)$ is zero up to the object surface that is located at z_0. Due to the reference offset z_0, the object reconstruction is separated from the AC terms, which are located around $z = 0$.

12.5.3 Measuring Range and Measuring Uncertainty

The measuring range Δz of spectral radar is basically limited by the resolution of the spectrometer [17]. A large difference between the object and reference optical paths will cause a high frequency in the spectrum. According to the sampling theorem the sample frequency of the photodiode array has to be twice as large as the highest occurring frequency in the spectrum. For $z = z_{\text{MAX}}$, the period of the cosine fringes is $\delta k = \pi/nz_{\text{MAX}}$. Therefore the spectrometer has to resolve at least $\delta k/2$. With $|\delta k| = 2\pi\delta\lambda/\lambda^2$, we get

$$\Delta z = \frac{1}{4n}\left(\frac{\lambda^2}{\delta\lambda}\right) \tag{10}$$

With the parameters in our setup the measuring range is $\Delta z = 2.4$ mm ($n = 1.5$).

However, if we measure a mirror at variable distance z, we observe a decay of the signal peak with increasing distance. This decay is caused by the finite width of the photodiodes ($1/\delta\lambda$) of the spectrometer, although the reflected amplitude stays the same. To get the real scattering amplitude $a(z)$ we must first compensate for this decay by normalization. Each measurement is normalized by dividing the measured signal by the measured decay.

The achievable spatial resolution depends on the coherence length of the light source and the scattering characteristics of the object. According to our experiments on the behavior of the spatial impulse response during signal propagation in volume scatterers with OCT methods [22], the minimum resolvable distance decreases with decreasing coherence length. However, it is finally limited by the scattering characteristics of the object. To determine the spatial resolution of spectral radar we measured a well-defined multilayer object with scattering coefficients adapted to human skin [26]. It turns out that the achievable spatial resolution within a range of $1000\,\mu$m is about $10\,\mu$m or less.

12.6 EXPERIMENTAL RESULTS

12.6.1 Measurements on Biological Objects

Spectral radar was implemented as a fiber-optic system, and in vivo measurements were performed [4,18,19]. Figure 5 shows the head of the spectral radar including the collimation optics, the devices to adjust the reference plane and the depth of focus, and the lateral scanner.

Figure 6 displays two optograms comparing human skin at the forearm and the hand. We can distinguish the typical layer structure of human skin in both measurements. The scattering amplitudes along two A-scans (lines A and B) are shown at the bottom of the figure. Along each A-scan we see first a high peak obtained from direct reflection at the surface (position $\sim 100\,\mu$m) and the strongly scattering stratum corneum (s.c.). The next layer of the skin is the boundary of the weakly scattering stratum germinativum (s.g.) followed by the strongly scattering stratum papillare (s.p.). In Fig. 6 the difference between different types of skin is evident. The structure in the forearm (e.g., thickness of the s.g.: 70–80 μm) is thinner than the structure at the hand (thickness of the s.g.: 300–350 μm).

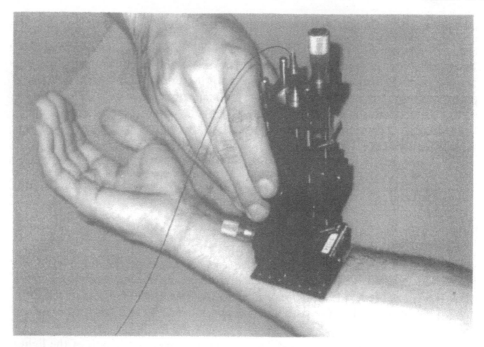

Figure 5 Spectral radar is used to check a patient's arm.

The main aim of OCT is to investigate alterations of the skin. We investigated the influence of increased moisture content on the morphological structure of the skin by OCT. In the result the thickness of the epidermis with increased moisture content leads to an average extension of the epidermis of about 10% [4]. We can demonstrate the difference between healthy skin and a superficial spreading melanoma [4]. Further, we measured the morphological structure of a fingernail and that of the growing nail beneath the skin [19].

In Fig. 7, a malignant melanoma and Bowen's disease, a preliminary stage of skin cancer, are compared. The melanoma causes an accumulation of melanin in the cells of the epidermis and therefore high backscattering. In addition, the layer structure of the healthy skin is destroyed. The epidermis is extended, and the back-scattering caused by the melanin is very strong and homogeneous. The layer structure of the skin has vanished in the malignant melanoma as in the Bowen's disease (Fig. 7). Differently from the melanoma, the scattering amplitude in the Bowen's disease decays exponentially. This picture shows the possible first step of spectral radar to differentiate alterations in the skin. Many further measurements have to be done to confirm the result.

The optogram of Fig. 8 displays a tunnel in the epidermis built by a larva migrane transferred by a midge bite. The tunnel in the epidermis is characterized by an almost vanishing scattering amplitude due to tissue missing from the longitudinal position beneath $150\,\mu$m. The tunnel was too deep for its end to be detected.

Our most recent measurements have been performed with a more powerful SLD (output power in the fiber $P = 10\,$mW; central wavelength $\lambda = 840$ nm; FWHM $= 20\,$nm; coherence length $l_C = 35\,\mu$m). According to our considerations

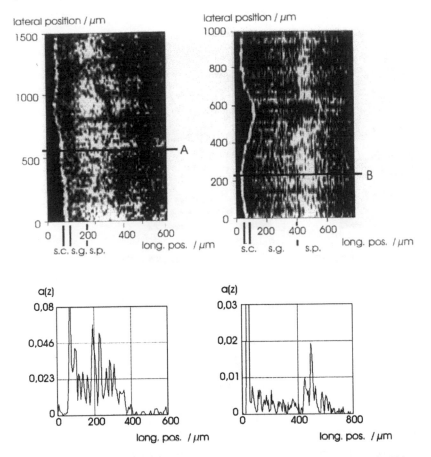

Figure 6 Optograms from two different parts of the human skin. Left: Skin at the forearm. Right: Skin at the hand.

about the dynamic range, the measuring range increases with increasing output power. In measurement with the former SLD (output power $P = 1.7$ mW) we could achieve a depth of only about $600\,\mu$m in the skin of the fingertip (Fig. 6). Now we are able to measure scattering amplitudes up to a depth of more than 1 mm with the new SLD. Figure 9 displays an optogram of human skin at the fingertip obtained with the new SLD. The epidermis (first two layers) has a thickness of about $250\,\mu$m. The third layer with high signal due to backscattering and dark zones below is the stratum papillare. The surface of the skin follows the waves of papillary ridges in the depth. The lateral B-scan is performed over the range of 2 mm. The measuring time for the whole optogram is 21 s. (About half of the time is for scan and control of the spectrometer. The exposure time for one A-scan is 20 ms.)

The lateral boundary between normal skin and a malignant melanoma can be seen in Fig. 10. The melanoma causes an accumulation of melanin in the cells of the epidermis and therefore high backscattering (white areas at the bottom of the image). The epidermis is extended, and the typical layer structure is destroyed. At the top of the image you see healthy human skin with a three-layer structure. The result delivered in Fig. 10 corresponds well to the histology. The melanoma has an average

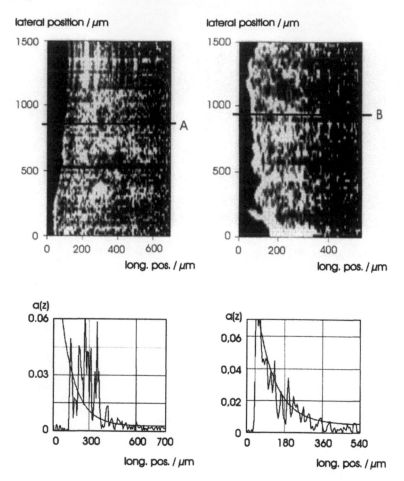

Figure 7 Optograms of malignant melanoma (left) and Bowen's disease (epithelioma) (right). Both skin alterations destroy the layer structure of the healthy skin. The epidermis is extended. The scattering amplitude in the malignant melanoma is strong and homogeneous. The scattering amplitude of the Bowen's disease decays exponentially.

thickness of about 550 μm. This depth was confirmed by further measurements. The measurement was performed with the 10 mW SLD.

12.6.2 Technical Applications

Although spectral radar was developed for the acquisition of 3-D data of biological tissue, it can be used for the examination of technological objects as well [18]. In Fig. 11 we show the structure of a multilayer printed circuit board. The board contains four layers of conducting lines, at depths of about 200, 400, 600, and 700 μm. The first layer is on the surface. The last one is the copper baseplate. The conduction lines are also made of copper. Because the light cannot penetrate copper, no signal can be acquired from underneath the metal. Another application is the measurement of the thickness of paint. Three layers of paint on a car body can be detected and measured.

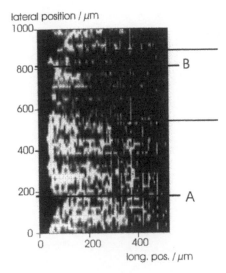

Figure 8 Optogram of a tunnel in the epidermis built by a larva. Tunnel diameter $250\,\mu m$.

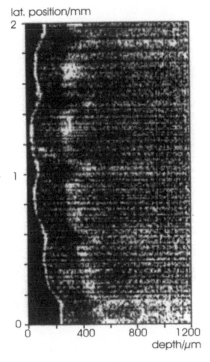

Figure 9 Optogram of human skin at a fingertip. With the new SLD (output power $P = 100\,mW$) the A-scans shows the scattering amplitude in a depth of up to nearly 1 mm.

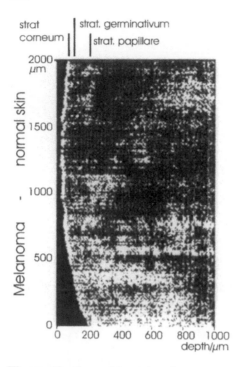

Figure 10 Lateral boundary between normal skin and a malignant melanoma. The measurement was performed with the 10 mW SLD.

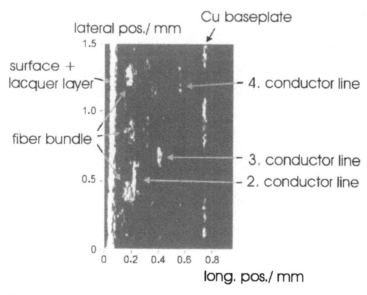

Figure 11 Structure of a multilayer printed circuit board. Fiber bundles and conduction lines in several layers are visible.

12.6.3 Supplementation by Optical Coherence Profilometry

In addition to OCT measurements of the morphological structure of the skin, clinically relevant data about alterations of the skin can be acquired by measurements of the surface skin topology. Alterations in the surface can also be detected by low coherence interferometry. We call this method optical coherence profilometry (OCP) [4] or coherence radar [28]. For in vivo OCP on human skin we use fiber-optic coherence radar [18,27].

The experimental setup for coherence radar uses a Michelson interferometer (Fig. 12). The light source is a light-emitting diode (LED). The reference mirror and the skin are illuminated by a plane wave. Light scattered back from the surface of the skin is imaged onto the CCD camera. Imaging with a finite aperture causes speckle in the image plane. Each speckle has a constant but arbitrary phase. Therefore, the speckles are the actual signal carrier in interferometry on rough surfaces [28].

White light interference displays maximum contrast in a plane, where the object optical pathlength is equal to the reference pathlength. To get the 3-D shape, the reference plane has to be scanned through the object. During the scan, within each pixel of the CCD camera an intensity variation occurs, called a correlogram. Its period is one-half of the average wavelength of the light source. For each pixel the contrast of the correlogram is measured during the scan. The maximum contrast defines the locus of equal optical pathlengths. Outside the center of the correlogram, the interference contrast decays rapidly, dependent on the coherence length of the light source. Special hardware is used to detect this maximum and to save the actual position of the translation stage. This is done for each of the 256,000 pixels in parallel. The speed of depth measurement is $v_s = \lambda/6T$, which is $4\,\mu m/s$ using a standard video camera with a 25 Hz frame rate. By modification of the sensor, the speed can be increased to $70\,\mu m/s$ [29].

The measuring uncertainty δz (standard deviation) of measurements with continuous coherence radar is caused by the statistical phase in the speckle. Therefore δz is mainly limited by the roughness of the object and not by parameters of the sensor (e.g., observation aperture). Industrial surfaces can be measured with $\delta z < 1\,\mu m$ [28].

The algorithm is based on measuring the contrast of the correlogram, not its phase. Therefore movements of the object leading to distortions of the phase will not influence the contrast. This is why in vivo measurements of a slightly moving object such as human skin are possible.

The conventional setup for coherence radar, developed for technical objects, is fixed on a bulky translation stage. The part of the human body to be measured has to be brought to the sensor. This limits the flexibility of the system. Therefore we implemented a fiber-optic version of coherence radar with a translation stage separated from the sensor head [18,27].

For the separation of the translation stage from the sensor head, a fiber has to be used in the reference arm of the interferometer (Fig. 13). To ensure equal optical pathlengths in the object and reference arms, a second fiber has to be placed into the object arm. This is done by inserting an additional beamsplitter (BS1 in Fig. 13), which splits the incoming light up into reference and object beams before the main beamsplitter of the coherence radar (BS2 in Fig. 13) is reached. This setup is equivalent to a combination of a Mach–Zehnder interferometer and a Michelson interferometer. The scan in the z-direction is done in the reference arm of the Mach–

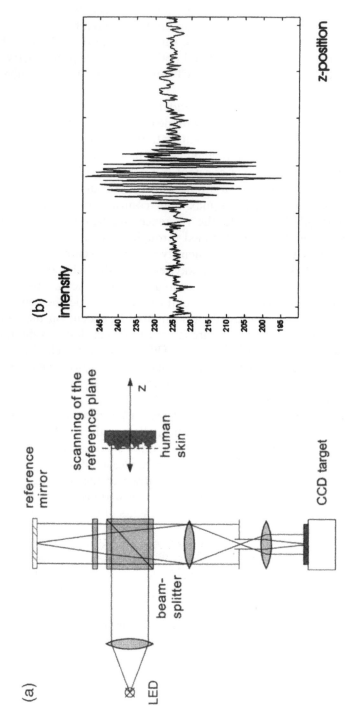

Figure 12 (a) Experimental setup for conventional coherence radar. (b) Correlogram of an in vivo measurement of human skin.

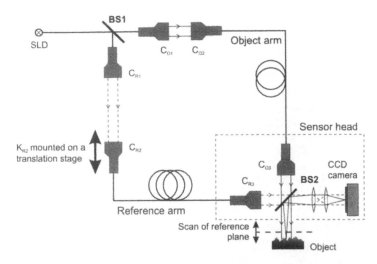

Figure 13   Setup for fiber-optic coherence radar.

Zehnder interferometer by varying the optical pathlength between the two collimators C_{R1} and C_{R2}. Because the sensor head contains no mechanical moving parts, it can be miniaturized and becomes mobile.

Figure 14 illustrates the fiber-optic implementation of coherence radar. The sensor consists of two spatially separated components: the sensor head and a module containing the translation stage. The two parts are connected by single-mode fibers. The light source is an SLD. An additional pilot laser in the visible range is used for aiming.

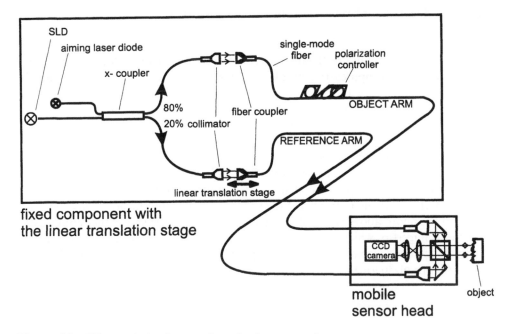

Figure 14   Fiber-optic implementation of coherence radar.

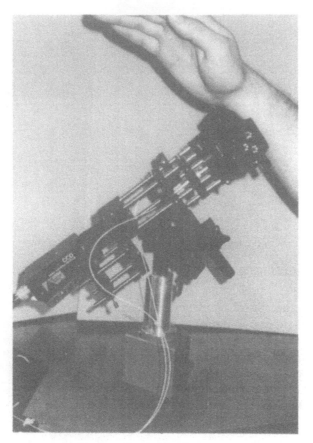

Figure 15 Mobile sensor head of the coherence radar instrument.

The sensor head contains the main part of the coherence radar for in vivo OCP. A beamsplitter superimposes the parallel reference beam with the light scattered back from the surface of the skin (Figs. 14 and 15). The measurable area of the skin surface depends on the output power of the light source and on the reflectivity of the surface. Presently the field of view is 5 mm × 5 mm.

In vivo OCP measurements of several regions of the body—i.e., hand, forearm, nose, belly, etc.—have been performed [27]. Figure 16 displays two gray-level-encoded height maps of measurements. The field of view is 2.5 mm × 2.5 mm. Both measurements were performed without any preparation of the skin and at a z speed of 4 μm/s. At the bottom of Fig. 16 the profile of the surface along the line depicted in the photo above is displayed. The picture to the left shows the wrinkles of the skin of a fingertip, which have a depth of about 80 μm. The measurement of the forearm on the right displays a mesh of deep wrinkles (depth of 80 μm) and shallow wrinkles (depth of 30 μm).

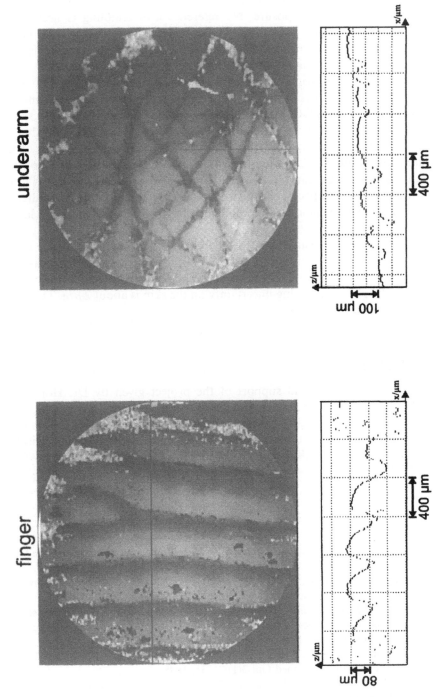

Figure 16 In vivo OCP measurements with the fiber-optic coherence radar.

12.7 CONCLUSION

Spectral radar is an optical sensor for the acquisition of skin morphology. The scattering amplitude $a(z)$ along one vertical axis from the surface into the bulk can be measured within one exposure. No reference arm scanning is necessary. The dynamic range is limited by the maximum power of the object. The more photons from the object contribute to the interference signal, the higher is the dynamic range. The experimental determination of the dynamic range is $D = 79$ dB. The dynamic range is, for the present implementation, limited by the A/D converter. Spectral radar works in the Fourier domain and has the same advantage over standard (time-domain) OCT as Fourier spectroscopy has over standard spectroscopy: the dynamic range of FDOCT is higher than that of TDOCT. In Table 1, FDOCT and TDOCT are compared "in a nutshell." We showed optograms of in vivo measurements of human skin obtained with a fiber-optic implementation of the sensor. The thickness of the skin layers at different locations of the body in vivo is accurately displayed. With spectral radar we can distinguish different skin alterations such as malignant melanoma, Bowen's disease, and skin damage by larva migrane.

In addition to OCT measurements of the morphological structure of the skin, clinically relevant data about alterations of the skin can be acquired by measurements of the surface skin topology. We used fiber-optic coherence radar for in vivo OCP on human skin. The measuring uncertainty on the skin is about $2 \, \mu\text{m}$. The field of view is presently $5 \, \text{mm} \times 5 \, \text{mm}$.

ACKNOWLEDGMENT

We acknowledge suggestions and support of the project given by Dr. Hoppe of Beiersdorf AG and by Prof. Schaefer and Dr. Dauga of l'Oréal Recherche. We further acknowledge in vivo measurements on patients, interpretation of the results, and valuable suggestions and support by Dr. Kiesewetter of the Dermatologische Universitätsklinik und Poliklinik, Erlangen. This chapter was funded by the BMBF, registration 13N7148.

REFERENCES

1. Lee BS, Strand TC. Profilometry with a coherence scanning microscope. Appl Opt 29:3784–3788, 1990.
2. Ettl P, Schmidt B, Schenk M, Laszlo I, Häusler G. Roughness parameters and surface deformation measured by coherence radar. Proc SPIE, 1998.
3. Bail M, Gebhardt B, Herrmann J, Höfer V, Lindner M, Pavliczek P. Optical range sensispatially modulated coherence. Proc Intl Symp on Laser Applications in Precision Measurements, Balatonfüred, Hungary, June 3–5, 1996.
4. Häusler G, Lindner MW. "Coherence radar" and "spectral radar"—New tools for dermatological diagnosis. J Biomed Opt 3(1):21–31, 1998.
5. Fercher AF, Hitzenberger CK, Kamp G, El-Zaiat SY. Measurement of intraocular distances by backscattering spectral interferometry. Opt Commun 117:43–48, 1995.
6. Fercher AF. Optical coherence tomography. J Biomed Opt 1(2):157–173, 1996.

7. Baumgartner A, Möller B, Hitzenberger Ch K, Drexler W, Fercher AF. Measurements of the posterior structures of the human eye in vivo by partial coherence interferometry using diffractive optics. SPIE 2981:85–93, 1997.

8. Lankenau E, Welzel J, Birngruber R, Engelhardt R. In vivo tissue measurements with optical low coherence tomography. SPIE 2981:78–84, 1997.

9. Welzel J, Lankenau E, Birngruber R, Engelhardt R. Optical coherence tomography of the human skin. J Am Acad Dermatol 37(6):958–963, 1997.

10. Clivaz X, Marquis-Weible F, Salathe RP, Nowak RP, Gilgen HH. High-resolution reflectometry in biological tissues. Opt Lett 17(1):4–6, 1992.

11. Izatt JA, Hee MR, Owen GM, Swanson EA, Fujimoto JG. Optical coherence microscopy in scattering media. Opt Lett 19(8):590–592, 1994.

12. Brunner H, Lazar R, Seschek R, Meier T, Steiner R. OCT images of human skin. SPIE 3194, 1997.

13. Lazar R, Brunner H, Steiner R. Optical coherence tomography (OCT) of human skin with a slow-scan CCD-camera. SPIE 2925:143–151, 1996.

14. Knüttel A, Breit M, Böcker D. Tissue characterization with optical coherence tomography (OCT). SPIE 2981:7–18, 1997.

15. Schmitt JM, Knüttel A, Yadlowsky M, Eckhaus MA. Optical coherence tomography of a dense tissue: Statistics of attenuation and backscattering. Phys Med Biol 39:1705–1720, 1994.

16. Häusler G. German Patent DE 41 08 944 (1991).

17. Bail M, Häusler G, Herrmann JM, Lindner MW, Ringler R. Optical coherence tomography with the "spectral radar"—Fast optical analysis in volume scatterers by short coherence interferometry. SPIE 2925:298–303, 1996.

18. Lindner MW. Optische Kohärenz-Profilometrie (OCP) und optische Kohärenz-Tomographie (OCT) in der Dermatologie. Dissertation, Lehrstuhl für Optik, Universität Erlangen-Nürnberg, 1998.

19. Andretzky P, Lindner MW, Herrmann JM, Schutz A, Konzog M, Kiesewetter F, Häusler G. Optical coherence tomography by "spectral radar," dynamic range estimation and in vivo measurements of skin. SPIE 3567, 1998.

20. Haberland U, Jansen P, Blazek V, Schmitt HJ. Optical coherence tomography of scattering media using frequency modulated continuous wave techniques with tunable near-infrared laser. SPIE 2981:20–28, 1997.

21. Chinn SR, Swanson EA, Fujimoto JG. Optical coherence tomography using a frequency-tunable optical source. Opt Lett 22(5):340–342, 1997.

22. Häusler G, Herrmann JM, Kummer R, Lindner MW. Observation of light propagation in volume scatters with 10^{11}-fold slow motion. Opt Lett 21(14):1087–1089, 1996.

23. Tuchin VV. Coherence and polarimetric optical technologies for the analysis of tissue structure. SPIE 2981:120–159, 1997.

24. Müller J. Poggendorfs Ann 69:98, 1846.

25. Wolf E. Three-dimensional structure determination of semi-transparent objects from holographic data. Opt Commun 1:153–156, 1969.

26. Bail M, Eigensee A, Häusler G, Herrmann JM, Lindner MW. 3D imaging of human skin—optical in vivo tomography and topology by short coherence interferometry. SPIE 2981:64–75, 1997.

27. Andretzky P, Lindner MW, Bohn G, Neumann J, Schmidt M, Ammon G, Häusler G. Modifications of the coherence radar for in vivo profilometry in dermatology. SPIE 3567, 1998.

28. Dresel Th, Häusler G, Venzke H. Three-dimensional sensing of rough surfaces by coherence radar. Appl Opt 31:919–925, 1992.

29. Ammon G, Andretzky P, Bohn G, Häusler G, Herrmann JM, Lindner MW. Optical coherence profilometry (OCP) of human skin in vivo. SPIE 3196, 1997.

13

Alternative OCT Techniques

CHRISTOPH K. HITZENBERGER and ADOLF F. FERCHER

University of Vienna, Vienna, Austria

13.1   OPTICAL DIFFRACTION TOMOGRAPHY AND OPTICAL COHERENCE TOMOGRAPHY

In optical tomography, the spatial structure of the illuminated object is reconstructed from scattered light data. Because the wavelength of optical radiation is not appreciably smaller than the structural elements of the object to be resolved, diffraction plays an important role. Hence, high resolution optical tomography must be based on diffraction physics. The diffraction projection theorem yields a solution for the corresponding inversion problem and provides the mathematical frame of optical diffraction tomography (ODT) [1]. It states that some of the three-dimensional spatial Fourier components of the scattering potential can be determined from measurements of amplitudes and phases of the scattered field [2]. This theorem has been used with many types of radiation in addition to optical radiation [3], for example, with X-rays [4,5] and in ultrasonics [6].

"Tomographic" imaging techniques derive two-dimensional data sets from a three-dimensional object to obtain a slice image of the internal structure. In optical coherence tomography (OCT) [7], scattered field data are derived from backscattered light. The depth position of light-remitting sites is detected by a partial coherence interferometric (PCI) depth scan (so-called optical A-scan), whereas lateral positions are determined by scanning the probe beam across the object. Usually, a Michelson interferometer with a short coherence length light source is used to perform the depth scan. The OCT image is synthesized from a series of laterally adjacent PCI depth-scan signals.

The diffraction projection theorem is derived with the assumption of weakly scattering objects. This assumption means that photons are scattered at most once. Hence, the scattered photons carry information about one light-scattering site. In

359

this case the scattered field can be obtained by the first Born approximation as a volume integral extended over the illuminated object volume $V(r')$ [1]. In OCT the object is illuminated by a rather narrow light beam. Therefore, far-field scattering is a reasonable approximation that leads to a simplified version of the diffraction projection theorem [8,9]:

$$E_O(\mathbf{r}, \mathbf{K}, t) \propto \frac{1}{r}\exp\left(i\mathbf{k}^{(S)}\mathbf{r} - i\omega t\right)\int_{V(\mathbf{r}')} F_O(\mathbf{r}')\exp\left(-i\mathbf{K}\mathbf{r}'\right) d^3\mathbf{r}'$$

$$= \hat{F}_O(\mathbf{K})\exp\left(i\mathbf{k}^{(S)}\mathbf{r} - i\omega t\right) \tag{1}$$

$E_O(\mathbf{r}, \mathbf{K}, t)$ is the electric field scattered by the object. $\mathbf{k}^{(i)}$ is the wave vector of the incident wave, $\mathbf{k}^{(S)}$ is the wave vector of the scattered wave, and $\mathbf{K} = \mathbf{k}^{(S)} - \mathbf{k}^{(i)}$ is the scattering vector. $|\mathbf{k}^{(i)}| = |\mathbf{k}^{(S)}| = k = 2\pi/\lambda = \omega/c$ is the wavenumber, λ is the wavelength, ω is the frequency, c is the velocity of light, and $\mathbf{r}$ is the position vector. $F_o(\mathbf{r})$ is the scattering potential of the object (we call it the "object structure"):

$$F_o(\mathbf{r}) = -k^2\left[m(\mathbf{r})^2 - 1\right] \tag{2}$$

where $m(\mathbf{r})$ is the complex refractive index of the object. Equation (1) is basically a Fourier transformation. It can easily be understood in terms of Huygens' principle: The scattered wave (with wave vector $\mathbf{k}^{(S)}$) is composed of elementary waves with amplitudes and phases determined by the Fourier transform $\hat{F}_o(\mathbf{K})$ of the scattering potential of the object [9]. Hence, the three-dimensional scattering potential $F_o(\mathbf{r})$ can be obtained by an inverse Fourier transform of the complex amplitude of the scattered field $E_o(\mathbf{r}, \mathbf{K}, t)$.

However, access to the Fourier data is considerably restricted. That can be seen from the Fourier data geometry in $\mathbf{K}$-space, Fig. 1. For any direction of $\mathbf{k}^{(S)}$ the scattering vector $\mathbf{K}$ points to the surface of the so-called Ewald sphere. As can also been seen from Fig. 1, backscattering with monochromatic light gives access to only one high spatial frequency, i.e., discontinuities of the scattering potential. A wavelength range from λ_1 to λ_2 obtains Fourier components of the scattering potential in the spatial frequency range $[\mathbf{K}_{1Z}, \mathbf{K}_{2Z}]$ and therefore has access to a finite range of

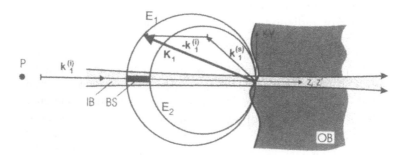

Figure 1 K-space geometry of backscattering (backscattered light is detected at P). $\mathbf{k}_1^{(i)} =$ wave vector of illuminating wave at wavelength λ_1; $\mathbf{k}_1^{(S)} =$ wave vector of scattered wave at λ_{1j} $\mathbf{K}_1 =$ scattering vector corresponding to λ_1; $E_1, E_2 =$ Ewald spheres corresponding to wavelengths λ_1 and λ_2; IB = illuminating beam; BS = Fourier data accessible by backscattering; OB = object.

Fourier components. Nevertheless, again only relatively abrupt changes in the scattering potential, occurring within a few wavelengths, can be seen by backscattering tomography.

In the optical regime, diffraction tomography presents considerable difficulties. Only a few experimental works concerning three-dimensional or even two-dimensional computational reconstruction from measured ODT data can be found in the literature [3]. No lasting biomedical application has been reported so far, though an interesting aspect of ODT is the possibility of quantitative imaging [10].

A straightforward application of ODT is also hindered by the large amount of (three-dimensional) data that would have to be collected in order to provide high resolution (two-dimensional) tomograms. Because the scattered field data belong to the three-dimensional Fourier spectrum, an N^2 pixel (two-dimensional) tomogram would roughly require N^3 three-dimensional Fourier data, which means that a photodetector array with N^3 detector elements would have to be used. Hence, modifications of ODT have been sought [11].

One class of successful modifications are the spectral interferometric techniques. Only one direction of scattering is detected with these techniques, usually the backscattering dirction. A spectrometer is used to disperse different wavelengths on a linear photodetector array. Hence, a two-dimensional version of the Fourier slice theorem [2], following straightforwardly from the Fourier integral, is useful:

$$\iint F_O(x, y, z) \, dx \, dy = \int \hat{F}_O(0, 0, K_z) \exp[iK_z z] \, dK_z = FT^{-1}\left\{\hat{F}_O(K)\right\} \tag{3}$$

where $\hat{F}_o(0, 0, K_z) \equiv \hat{F}_o(K)$ are the wavelength-dependent backscattered field data. This theorem relates the Fourier transform of the object along a line in Fourier space $[\hat{F}(0, 0, K_z)]$ to the Fourier transform of a two-dimensional projection (in the xy plane) of the object. Hence, to maintain transverse resolution the object must be illuminated by a slim light beam (narrow in the xy plane) as is usual in OCT.

Depth resolution is defined by the Fourier uncertainty relation. Using the full width at half-maximum (FWHM) Δz as a measure of the minimal extension of a scattering potential in direct space that can be resolved using a light source with FWHM bandwidth ΔK_z in Fourier space, and assuming a Gaussian shape of the scattering potential and of the source spectrum, we obtain a space–bandwidth product

$$(\Delta z)_{\text{FWHM}} (\Delta K_z)_{\text{FWHM}} = 8 \ln 2 \tag{4}$$

and a minimum resolvable spatial extension of the scattering potential,

$$(\Delta z)_{\text{FWHM}} = \frac{2 \ln 2}{\pi} \left(\frac{\lambda^2}{(\Delta \lambda)_{\text{FWHM}}} \right) \tag{5}$$

This defines OCT depth resolution. It equals the so-called round-trip coherence length of the light, which has been used as a definition of coherence length [12,13]. It should be noted, however, that light in backscattering travels along the same path twice—there and back—through the object. Hence, the corresponding FWHM coherence length l_C is twice as large [14]:

$$l_C = \frac{4 \ln 2}{\pi} \left(\frac{\lambda^2}{\Delta \lambda} \right) \qquad (6)$$

This definition of coherence length will be used later in this chapter.

13.2 SPECTRAL OCT TECHNIQUES

13.2.1 Complex Spectral Interferometric OCT

A direct implementation of this technique is the complex spectral interferometric OCT technique [15]. In this technique the wavelength-dependent amplitudes and phases of $\hat{F}_o(K)$ are obtained with the help of a phase interferometric spectrometer. This is, for example, a Michelson phase interferometer with a spectrometer at the interferometer exit. (In contrast to a fringe interferometer, which displays object phase structures implicitly as fringes, a phase interferometer determines the object wave phases explicitly.) The spectrometer displays the monochromatic field components. In the phase interferometer an additional piezoelectric translator is used in the reference arm to perform a direct phase measurement (see Fig. 2). A series of known phase changes are induced between the object and reference beams in the interferometer, generating a series of spectral intensity data at the spectrometer exit plane. A corresponding number of intensity frames are recorded.

The reference beam phase is changed in a known manner. From changes in the spectral intensity data the wavelength-dependent amplitudes and phases of the scattered field are directly calculated [16] and $\hat{F}_O(K)$ is obtained. According to Eq. (3), an inverse Fourier transform of the complex amplitude of the scattered wave yields the object structure.

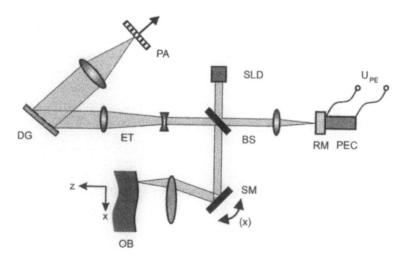

Figure 2 Complex spectral OCT. U_{PE} is the piezoelectric driving voltage to perform a series of known phase changes of the reference beam. BS = beamsplitter; DG = diffraction grating; ET = beam-expanding telescope; OB = object; PA = photodetector array; PEC = piezoelectric crystal; RM = reference mirror; SLD = superluminescent diode; SM = scanning mirror.

This technique gives direct access to absorption properties of the object. In the macroscopic theory of electrodynamics the linear absorption coefficient [17]

$$\alpha = \frac{2\omega\kappa}{c} \tag{7}$$

depends on the extinction coefficient $\kappa(\mathbf{r})$, which is part of the complex refractive index m:

$$m(\mathbf{r}) = \eta(\mathbf{r}) + i\kappa(\mathbf{r}) \tag{8}$$

and can be obtained from the complex scattering potential $F_o(\mathbf{r})$ of the object, for example, by splitting the complex scattering potential into real and imaginary parts. $\eta(\mathbf{r})$ is the phase refractive index. First imaging applications of complex spectral interferometric OCT in dermatology and dentistry have been reported [14,15]. Figure 3 (see color plate) presents a complex interferometric OCT image of an in vivo human finger-nail.

13.2.2 Spectral Interferometry and Spectral Radar

In the spectral interferometric and spectral radar OCT techniques a Michelson interferometer with a spectrometer at the interferometer exit is also used. This technique was described about a decade ago [18,19] and was later mainly used in the dermatological field [20]. There is a basic difference compared to the complex spectral interferometric OCT technique. An inverse Fourier transform of the spectral intensity of the scattered waves does not yield the object structure but yields the autocorrelation function (ACF) of the object structure:

$$FT^{-1}\{I_o(K)\} \propto \int F_o^*(z)F_o(z+Z)\,dz = \mathrm{ACF}_F(Z) \tag{9}$$

However, because autocorrelation is not a useful presentation of the object structure, an additional singular light-reflecting interface (mirror) positioned near the object is used. This yields a reference structure with a fixed phase. Then the inverse Fourier transform yields, among other terms, one term with the object structure (namely, the cross-correlation of the object structure with the delta-like reference structure).

In the spectral techniques the reference wave encodes the object phase in the resulting interferogram term implicitly. It is not used to determine the phase of the

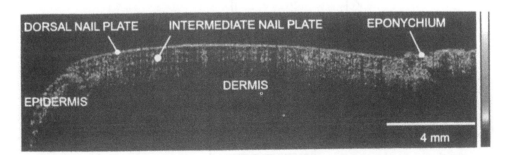

Figure 3 Complex spectral OCT image of a human fingernail. $\lambda = 850$ nm; $\Delta\lambda = 18$ nm. The magnitude of the scattering potential is logarithmically encoded in false colors. Depth dimensions are in terms of optical path length. (See color plate.)

scattered field explicitly. It serves to introduce a carrier frequency in the spectrum in order to separate the various correlation terms in the reconstruction. Hence, these techniques are generalizations of the old channeled spectra interferometric technique [21]. An important advantage of the spectral techniques is that the reference mirror need not be mechanically moved. A disadvantage is the limited wavelength coverage of available photodetector arrays. A further disadvantage is the usually large dc component on the photodetector array, which limits the dynamic range of the detector because a straightforward ac coupling, as with single photodetectors, is not possible with CCD arrays.

13.2.3   Wavelength Tuning (Chirp) OCT

Wavelength tuning OCT (WT-OCT) is related to spectral interferometry. (This technique is sometimes called chirp OCT, a term derived from the corresponding frequency-modulated electronic radar technique.) In this case, however, the wavelength-dependent intensity data are not recorded simultaneously by use of a broadband light source and a spectrometer; instead, they are recorded subsequently by illuminating the interferometer with a tunable narrowband laser and recording the intensity at the interferometer exit by a single photodetector.

Similar to spectral OCT, this technique has been used so far only with backscattered light, i.e., to obtain depth information on the object. Lateral information is obtained by performing several WT interferometric (WTI) scans at adjacent positions.

We explain the measurement of a path difference $2L$ in an interferometer with reference to Fig. 4. If the wavelength λ of the tunable laser diode is kept at a fixed value, the intensity at the photodetector can be calculated as

$$I = I_1 + I_2 + 2\sqrt{I_1 I_2}\cos(2\pi\,\Delta\Phi) \tag{10}$$

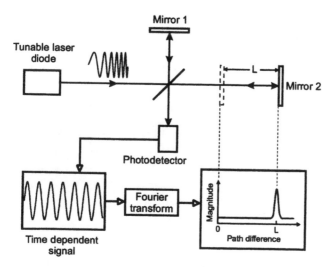

Figure 4   Schematic diagram of the principle of wavelength tuning interferometry. (Adapted from Ref. 28.)

where I_1 and I_2 are the light intensities reflected at mirrors 1 and 2, respectively, and $\Delta\Phi$ is the phase difference of the two beams. This phase difference is given by

$$\Delta\Phi = 2\frac{L}{\lambda} = 2L\frac{k}{2\pi} \tag{11}$$

where k is the wavenumber corresponding to λ. If the wavenumber is changed, the phase difference changes accordingly. This causes the intensity at the photodetector to oscillate with a frequency f:

$$f = \frac{d\Delta\Phi}{dt} = \frac{d\Delta\Phi}{dk}\frac{dk}{dt} = \frac{L}{\pi}\frac{dk}{dt} \tag{12}$$

Hence, the frequency is directly proportional to the tuning rate of the wavenumber dk/dt and to the path difference L. If dk/dt is constant, L can be obtained by a Fourier transform of the time-dependent intensity signal recorded by the photodetector during tuning. If the object contains several reflecting or backscattering surfaces located at different depth positions, each individual path length difference $2L_i$ gives rise to a corresponding frequency f_i. A Fourier transform retains all of the corresponding distances and reflectivities, i.e., the backscattering potential distribution along the z axis. Hence, the Fourier transform of the time domain signal recorded during wavelength tuning retains the same information as an optical A-scan recorded by PCI.

The advantage of this technique compared to standard OCT techniques is again that a fixed reference arm length is used and no moving parts are needed. The use of a single photodetector has the advantage of simple elimination of the unwanted dc intensity terms by high-pass filtering of the photodetector signal. This enhances the usable dynamic range of the detection system considerably.

The drawback of WTI and WT-OCT, which restricted its use to only a few demonstrations [22–28], are the constraints of the available laser sources. The wavelength of the laser must be continuously tunable, without mode hops. The tuning range $\Delta\lambda$ determines the depth resolution according to Eq. (15). The wider the tuning range, the better the resolution. Two different types of compact tunable laser diodes have been used up to now: external cavity laser diodes [22,24–26] and distributed Bragg reflector (DBR) laser diodes [23,27,28]. External cavity laser diodes have a wide tuning range of 10 nm and more. However, their slow tuning speed restricted the use of this large bandwidth to in vitro objects. DBR laser diodes can be tuned within milliseconds, but their tuning range is low and hence the resolution obtained is poor (on the order of $100\,\mu m$). Moreover, their tuning rate is not constant, and they are not mode-hop-free. This situation can be improved, however, by using advanced solid-state laser technology. Recently, the first experiments with a Cr^{4+}:forsterite laser demonstrated scan repetition rates of 2 kHz, yielding WTI with a resolution of $15\,\mu m$ [29].

A first application of the use of a three-section DBR laser diode for measuring intraocular distances in vivo by WTI has recently been reported [28]. The problems of the nonlinear tuning rate and the mode hops were solved by using an auxiliary Michelson interferometer that provided a reference signal for numerically correcting the nonlinearities of dk/dt and for eliminating the signal distortion caused by the mode hops. Figure 5 shows a schematic diagram of the instrument. With a tuning range of 2 nm, a depth resolution of $\sim 150\,\mu m$ was obtained. Figure 6 shows the

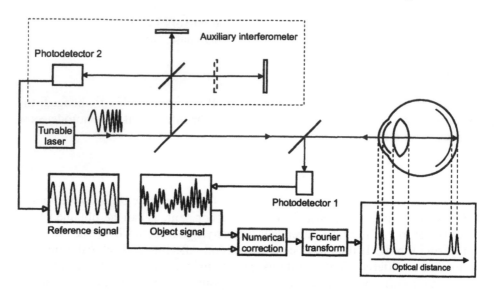

Figure 5 Schematic diagram of wavelength-tuning interferometer used for intraocular ranging. (Adapted from Ref. 28.)

result of a WTI scan carried out parallel to the optic axis of the eye of a healthy volunteer. In this case, the anterior corneal surface was used as the reference surface. Anterior chamber depth, lens thickness, vitreous depth, retinal thickness, and axial eye length were measured; the recording time was 16 ms.

The first two-dimensional WT-OCT tomogram was recorded by Chinn et al. [24]. Using an external cavity laser diode, these authors recorded a section through a stack of microscopy cover glasses (see Fig. 7). The laser had a scan repetition rate of 10 Hz and was tuned over a wavelength range $\Delta\lambda \cong 20$ nm. A depth resolution of

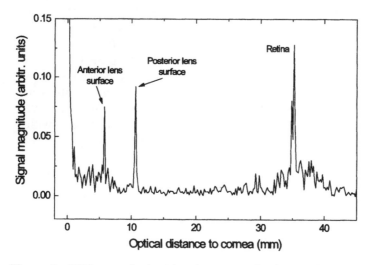

Figure 6 WTI scan obtained in a human eye in vivo. (Adapted from Ref. 28.)

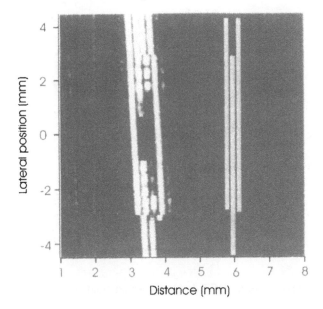

Figure 7 WT-OCT image of a stack of microscopy cover glasses. The figure contains a sketch of the object as an insert. (Courtesy of J. G. Fujimoto, MIT. Reprinted from Ref. 24 by permission of the Optical Society of America.)

38 μm was obtained. The first WT-OCT images of a scattering phantom were reported by Haberland et al. [27]. These authors used a DBR laser diode. They also claim that information on flow velocities can be obtained with this technique.

13.3 DUAL-BEAM OCT

In dual-beam OCT the object is illuminated by both beams exiting from a Michelson interferometer (or another two-beam interferometer) [30]. In the optical scheme of Fig. 8 a superluminescent diode illuminates a Michelson interferometer. The interferometer splits the beam into two subcomponents, generates a path difference, and recombines the two subcomponents. The recombined beams leave the interferometer as a coaxial "dual beam." A beamsplitter at the interferometer exit reflects the dual beam toward the object. A lateral scanning mirror directs the beam to transversely adjacent positions at the object (here the eye's fundus). The reflected beams pass through the interferometer exit beamsplitter and are detected by the photodetector.

The basic principle of the dual-beam technique is to match the path difference generated by the interferometer to path differences between the light-remitting sites in the object. This makes the dual-beam technique insensitive to distance variations between object and interferometer. The optical scheme is explained in more detail with the help of Fig. 9.

The two subcomponents E' and E of the dual beam that leave the interferometer toward the object have a path difference corresponding to twice the interferometer arm length difference, $2z$. A PCI depth scan is performed by shifting one of the interferometer mirrors, subsequently called the "measurement mirror" (MM). This mirror is moved, for example, by a stepper motor with a constant speed v, which

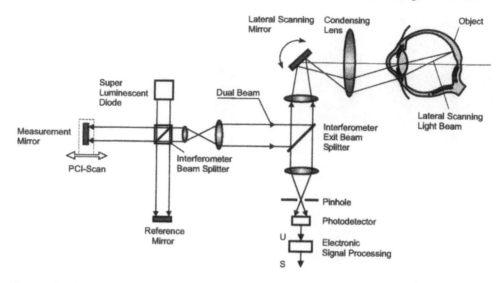

Figure 8 Optical scheme of a bulk optics dual-beam OCT device for ocular fundus imaging.

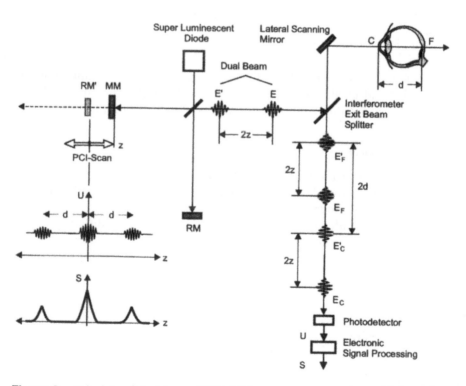

Figure 9 Principle of dual-beam OCT. MM = measurement mirror; RM = reference mirror; RM′ = virtual position of reference mirror in the measurement arm. E' and E are the dual-beam subcomponents. Both subcomponents experience an additional path difference of $2d$ by the object; and d is the optical length. Interference occurs if $2d = 2z \pm l_C$, where l_C is the coherence length of the light. Note the resulting symmetry of the photodetector signal U as well as that of the PCI signal S.

causes a Doppler shift $f_D = 2v/\lambda$ of the light frequency of the corresponding beam. Each subcomponent is reflected at the object interfaces separating regions of different refractive indices. For example, the components E_F' and E_F in Fig. 9 have been reflected at the fundus (F) of the eye, whereas the components E_C' and E_C have been reflected at the anterior corneal surface (C). If $z = d$, the components E_F and E_C' overlap and generate a photodetector signal alternating at a frequency f_D. The photodetector signal is then amplified and filtered by a bandpass filter that transmits only signals with f_D. The envelope of the rectified signal (S in Fig. 9) is the final PCI signal and is recorded as a function of the interferometer's arm-length difference z with a personal computer.

The dual-beam technique is somehow ambiguous. The same signal will appear at the photodetector at an interferometer path difference $z = -d$ (indicated in Fig. 9). In fact, the autocorrelation of the object structure is obtained. This, however, does not create a severe problem. Either one of the object interfaces (in the case of the eye, for example, this is provided by the anterior corneal interface) generates a strong wave, leading to dominating autocorrelation terms, or a corresponding interface may be attached to the object.

The PCI scans or optical A-scans recorded in this way contain signal peaks characteristic of the object interfaces. From the positions of these peaks on the z axis the respective optical distances of the object structure can be determined (typically, as usual in OCT, within the so-called round-trip coherence length, $\pm l_C/2$ [12]). The geometrical distances are obtained by dividing the optical distances by the group index of the respective medium. The dual-beam PCI technique has found important medical applications itself, in particular in the ophthalmological field of intraocular distance measurement [31–35]. Its exceptional stability in an axial direction is rather helpful, in particular if the depth scans go over some millimeters. For example, it has recently been shown that the refractive outcome of cataract surgery can be improved substantially if PCI biometric data are used [36].

In dual-beam OCT, as usual, the image is synthesized from a series of laterally adjacent PCI depth scans [37]. These positions can be addressed by the lateral scanning mirror. The unique depth measurement stability of the dual-beam PCI technique may be used here too and lead to high precision OCT depth and thickness measurement techniques. Investigation of dual-beam OCT has only recently been started [38]. In a first step a simple lateral scanning unit was added to a PCI interferometer. As an example, Fig. 10 shows a horizontal foveal cross-sectional dual-beam tomogram of a patient with macular edema. The low transverse resolution is due to a detection aperture of less than 0.1 and caused by the laboratory-type instrument permitting reproducible transverse steps only on the order of 0.5°.

One drawback of the dual-beam OCT technique in ophthalmological fundus imaging is the poor signal-to-noise ratio due to the wave front mismatch of the two interfering beams reflected at the anterior corneal surface and the retina. If the probing beam is collimated, the light reflected at the retina will be collimated by the optical elements of the eye whereas the beam reflected at the cornea will be divergent. If the probing beam is focused at the cornea, the light reflected at the retina will be divergent. In either case, a concentric ring-shaped interference fringe system is formed. The diameter of the pinhole in front of the photodetector has to be small enough that only a single fringe is transmitted onto the detector

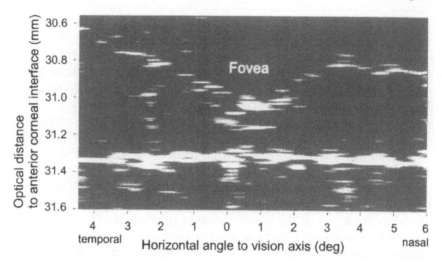

Figure 10   Horizontal foveal cross-sectional dual-beam tomogram of a diabetic retinopathy patient with macular edema [38]. Thickness values are optical; the geometrical values are obtained by dividing the optical distances by the group index (≈ 1.4). SLD with $\lambda = 855$ nm; $\Delta\lambda = 24.6$ nm.

surface. This leads to a pinhole diameter in the $50\,\mu$m range, resulting in a rather low light power at the detector surface and a correspondingly poor signal-to-noise ratio.

To overcome this drawback, a diffractive optical element (DOE) can be used [39]. A Fresnel zone lens can be implemented in front of the eye to focus part of the incident light beam on the vertex of the cornea and transmit part of the beam uninfluenced. The latter part is focused by the optics of the eye onto the retina. The beams reflected by the anterior corneal surface and the retina will thereby both be converted to parallel beams on their way back to the detection unit. A corresponding DOE has been designed to focus 40% of the intensity of the incident light beam on the vertex of the cornea and to let 60% pass through as a collimated beam. This led to an increase of about 20–25 dB in the signal-to-noise ratio for in vivo measurements [40].

We used the dual-beam OCT technique to demonstrate the depth resolution obtainable in retinal tomograms of a human eye in vivo. The closest distance of two layers that can be resolved is usually $\approx l_C/2$, which is inversely proportional to the source bandwidth $\Delta\lambda$. Therefore an increased bandwidth improves the resolution. To increase the bandwidth compared to that of a conventional SLD ($\Delta\lambda \approx 25$ nm), a synthesized light source generated by superimposing two spectrally displaced SLDs (at 830 and 855 nm) was used. The two combined light sources had an effective spectral width of $\Delta\lambda = 50$ nm; the corresponding coherence length is $l_C \approx 15\,\mu$m in air.

However, if measurements are performed through dispersive media, caution has to be taken. Because the measurement beam travels, for example, through the dispersive eye media whereas the reference beam travels through air, the coherence envelope of the optical A-scans broadens and resolution decreases. If the length of a dispersive medium in one of the interferometer arms is L and the group dispersion of the medium is $dn_g/d\lambda$, the width of the coherence envelope, after double passing through the medium, is [41,42]

$$l_{C,m} = \left[l_C^2 + \left(\frac{dn_g}{d\lambda} 2L \, \Delta\lambda \right)^2 \right]^{1/2} \tag{13}$$

With a mean group dispersion of the ocular media of approximately -1.8×10^{-5} nm^{-1} [43] and a mean axial eye length of $L = 24$ mm, a signal width of approximately $21 \,\mu$m is obtained. Hence, use of the larger bandwidth light source does not improve resolution but degrades it. Optimum resolution can be achieved only by placing a dispersion-compensating plane-parallel plate in the longer interferometer arm. This element must fulfill the condition

$$L_{el} \left(\frac{dn_g}{d\lambda} \right)_{el} = L_{ob} \left(\frac{dn_g}{d\lambda} \right)_{ob} \tag{14}$$

where "el" and "ob" refer to the compensation element and the object, respectively [41,42]. For example, in the measurement described here, a plane-parallel BK7 optical glass plate of $L_{el} = 12$ mm and $(dn_g/d\lambda)_{el} \approx 3.46 \times 10^{-5}$ nm^{-1} at $\lambda = 830$ nm was used.

Figure 11 (see color plate) shows a corresponding dual-beam tomogram demonstrating the depth resolution achieved using the synthesized light source and dispersion compensation. As usual in OCT images of the foveal region, the foveal depression and microstructural layers such as the inner limiting membrane and the photoreceptor layer can be seen. However, the posterior side of the retina shows three narrow well-separated highly scattering bands. These bands have not yet been resolved in OCT. They might correlate with the retinal pigment epithelium and

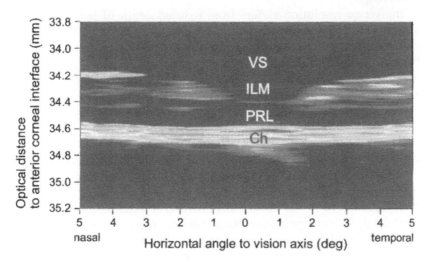

Figure 11 Dual-beam tomographic image of a horizontal section through the fovea centralis, from 5° temporal to 5° nasal. VS = vitreous; ILM = inner limiting membrane; PRL = photoreceptor layer; Ch = choroid. Synthesized light source of two SLDs: $\lambda_1 = 830$ nm, $\lambda_2 = 855$ nm; with an effective wavelength bandwidth of $\Delta\lambda = 50$ nm and dispersion compensation $l_C \cong 8 \,\mu$m in air. (See color plate.)

some of the choroidal layers [44]. An analysis of the corresponding PCI depth-scan signals showed that the use of the synthesized light source in combination with dispersion compensation did reduce the FWHM of these bands by about $7\,\mu$m [39], compared to the case of a single SLD without dispersion compensation.

We point out here that this dual-beam tomographic image was recorded using a simple experimental laboratory setup in which each lateral scanning position had to be adjusted manually. Therefore the total scanning time was several minutes and the lateral resolution is, on the one hand, rather poor ($\cong 150\,\mu$m). On the other hand, this demonstrates the exceptional stability of dual-beam OCT in an axial direction. In spite of the long measuring time, the individual A-scans that were recorded in vivo (!) at different angles with time intervals of tens of seconds were compiled into OCT images without any additional image processing required to correlate the longitudinal positions of the A-scans. This property is useful not only in cases where digital postprocessing of the images could lead to loss of image details, but also in the application of optical contrast enhancement techniques, which, like transverse differentiation of adjacent A-scan signals, might otherwise merely manifest artifacts. In particular, we expect that the dual-beam technique will be of great value in quantitative imaging of histological layers such as the retinal nerve fiber layer.

13.4 DYNAMIC COHERENT FOCUS OCT

Most current medical in vivo imaging technologies offer resolutions ranging from 10 mm to 1 mm. But early-stage tissue abnormalities like those associated with cancer and atherosclerosis require microscopic resolution, i.e., resolution in the 1 μm range. OCT has the micrometer scale resolution potential and therefore can pave the way to in vivo histology.

Improved transverse resolution suffers from reduced depth of field. Usually OCT is used to generate depth scans, and therefore extended depth of field is an important issue in OCT. Dynamic coherent focus (DCF) OCT is a technique that circumvents the depth-of-field problem.

In OCT depth (= longitudinal) and transverse resolution are uncoupled. OCT depth resolution is determined by half the coherence length, $l_C/2$, of the light used [see Eq. (5)]. At present, commercially available single-quantum-well AlGaAs heterostructure SLDs have FWHM spectral bandwidths up to $\Delta\lambda = 77$ nm at $\lambda = 820$ nm, leading to a depth resolution of 3.9 μm, for example.

OCT transverse resolution is limited like transverse resolution in classical imaging optics by the Rayleigh criterion. Two incoherent points are defined as "barely resolved" when the center of the Airy disk generated by one point falls on the first zero of the Airy disk generated by the second. Because two adjacent coherence scans are mutually incoherent, an analogous resolution criterion applies here. Because of the Gaussian intensity distribution we have to replace the "first zero of the Airy disk" by the $1/e^2$ intensity. Hence, the minimum separation of two transversely resolved image points in OCT is determined by the beam waist radius of the scanning object beam [14]:

$$w_0 = \frac{\lambda}{\pi\vartheta} \tag{15}$$

where ϑ is the asymptotic angle of beam divergence.

There is, however, a specific depth-of-focus problem in OCT. Most OCT techniques generate depth tomograms (i.e., sections perpendicular to the object surface). Hence, it is not only the transverse resolution that counts but also the depth of focus. Depth of focus (DOF) is usually defined by twice the confocal beam parameter $DOF = 2z_0$ [14]. There is a rather nonlinear dependence of depth of focus versus the transverse resolution:

$$z_0 = \frac{\pi w_0^2}{\lambda} \tag{16}$$

For example, most OCT devices use a rather large confocal beam parameter z_0 and consequently a correspondingly low transverse resolution, i.e., a large beam waist radius w_0. For example, on the one hand, at a wavelength of $\lambda = 820$ nm a confocal beam parameter of $z_0 = 500\,\mu m$ leads to a beam waist radius of $w_0 = 11.5\,\mu m$; on the other hand, however, a beam waist radius of $w_0 = 1.15\,\mu m$ leads to a confocal beam parameter of only $5\,\mu m$.

Several attempts have been made to obtain high transverse resolution throughout a reasonable object depth. For example, the focusing lens can be shifted synchronously with the reference mirror during the depth scan [45]. This, however, involves the (rapid) movement of at least two optical components. Hence, we have designed the dynamic coherent focus technique, in which only one mirror has to be moved [46]. The optical scheme is shown in Fig. 12. Here we use a reflectometer configuration.

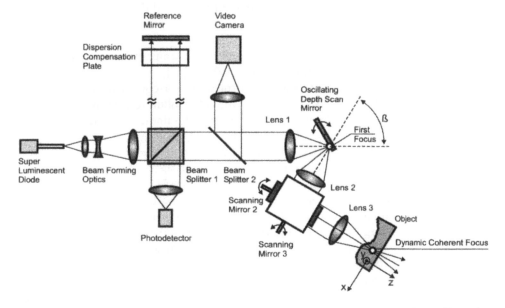

Figure 12 Dynamic coherent focus (DCF) OCT. The reference beam contains a dispersion compensation plate to compensate for the optics in the measurement beam. The measurement beam of the Michelson interferometer is focused at a first focus near the oscillating depth scan mirror and finally at the "dynamic coherent focus" within the object.

The beam of a fiber pigtailed superluminescent diode is collimated by a high numerical aperture microscope lens and expanded by a Galilean telescope in a beam-forming optics ensemble. Nonpolarizing beamsplitter 1 divides the beam into reference and measurement beams. The measurement beam is focused by microscope lens 1 at a first focus near the depth scan mirror. The depth scan mirror oscillates by a tilt angle of approximately $\pm 10°$ and reflects this beam toward lens 2. The periodic tilt of the depth scan mirror performs two tasks: First, it periodically shifts the mirror image of the first focus approximately along the axis of lens 2, and second, it modulates the pathlength of the measurement beam. Besides, a beam deviation of $\beta - \pi$ occurs at this mirror. The beam leaving lens 2 enters the X-Y scanning unit (scanning mirrors 2 and 3) and is focused by lens 3 at the object. This focus is conjugate to the periodically shifting mirror image of the first focus and therefore dynamically scans the object depth. The pathlength modulation is matched to the focus shift by properly choosing the focal lengths of lenses 2 and 3. Hence, the dynamic focus maintains its coherence with the reference beam during the whole depth scan.

The reference beam passes through a dispersion-compensating plate and is reflected at the reference mirror. Both returning beams are focused onto the photodetector. A video camera is used to monitor the object and the position of the dynamic coherent focus.

Focusing the object beam in a medium with a refractive index different from that of air causes an additional pathlength mismatch. First, the focus formed within the object is shifted by refraction at the interface between the air and the object (with phase refractive index n) from z to z'. Second, in OCT the optical pathlength in a medium equals the geometrical pathlength multiplied by the group refractive index n_g. Hence, the dynamic focus is approximately at an optical depth of

$$z'' = n \, n_g \, z \tag{17}$$

Using two Ronchi rulings we recently demonstrated a transverse resolution of the order of $2 \, \mu m$ over a depth of approximately $430 \, \mu m$ [47].

First in vitro measurements were performed with a cornea of a 70-year-old human. The corneal surface was kept moist with Glycerolum to prevent drying and avoid damage to the epithelium. A pigtailed superluminescent diode SLD 371 (Superlum Ltd.) was used. This diode has a center wavelength of approximately $\lambda = 820 \, nm$ and (at nominal driving current) an FWHM spectral bandwidth of $\Delta\lambda = 77 \, nm$. However, at the nominal driving current there are side lobes in the coherence function, decreasing the longitudinal resolution. The optimum longitudinal resolution ($l_C/2 = 4.5 \, \mu m$) was obtained at a driving current of 130 mA, i.e., somewhat below the nominal current. The distance between two adjacent coherence scans was $3 \, \mu m$. The resulting tomogram (Fig. 13, see color plate) consists of 300 pixels in the y direction and 1000 pixels in the z direction. The acquisition time was 1.6 s.

The signal at the anterior surface is very strong due to the high difference in refractive index between air and the (moistened) anterior surface. The weakly scattering layer below the anterior surface is about $75 \, \mu m$ thick and can be associated with the epithelium, although we cannot identify the internal cell structure. Bowman's layer is visible, and there are many bright spots in the stroma, which might point to nuclei of keratocytes. At the posterior surface of the cornea a discrete structure is seen corresponding to the single-cell endothelial layer.

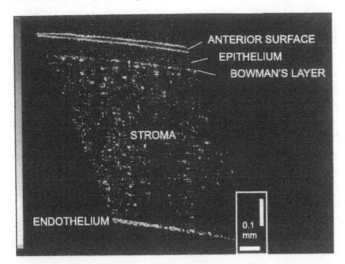

Figure 13 OCT image of a section of a human cornea obtained by the dynamic coherent focus technique. SLD: $\lambda = 820$ nm, $\Delta\lambda = 67$ nm. Transverse resolution is $w_0 = 2\,\mu$m; depth resolution is $l_C/2 = 4.5\,\mu$m in air and $3.2\,\mu$m in tissue. (See color plate.)

This experiment demonstrates resolution at the threshold of cellular structures (with respect to corneal cells). Further increase of the illuminating aperture and of the light wavelength bandwidth seems important to resolve cellular structures.

13.5 TRANSVERSE OCT

In conventional OCT, longitudinal cross sections (i.e., perpendicular to the surface of the sample) are generated by recording several adjacent longitudinal PCI scans (optical A-scans). Three-dimensional information on the distribution of the back-scattering potential in the object can be obtained by recording several adjacent longitudinal cross sections. Once a three-dimensional data set is recorded, sections of arbitrary geometry can be extracted by appropriate data processing algorithms. In this way, transverse cross sections or *en face* images (i.e., images parallel to the object surface) can be obtained by conventional OCT. However, if one is primarily interested in transverse OCT images, a more convenient way is to avoid the detour of three-dimensional data acquisition and record the transverse images directly. Application fields where this technique might be of advantage are OCT microscopy and combinations of OCT with confocal imaging techniques.

Different approaches to transverse OCT have been reported. Their common feature is that the depth of the transverse section is determined by the position of the reference mirror in the partial coherence interferometer. The reference mirror remains in a fixed position during the recording of one transverse image. Subsequent transverse images corresponding to sections at increasing depth locations are generated by shifting the reference mirror in steps between the recording of the individual cross sections.

Whereas in conventional OCT the carrier frequency of the heterodyne signal is provided automatically by the Doppler shift induced in the reference beam by the moving reference mirror, transverse OCT usually requires an additional means for generating the carrier frequency. In an early demonstration of OCT microscopy in scattering media, Izatt et al. [48] used a piezoelectric fiber stretcher for this purpose. A transverse OCT image is recorded by transverse raster scanning of the sample under the illuminating sample beam in x and y directions while the fiber stretcher periodically modulates the phase of the reference arm, thereby generating the carrier frequency. The depth position of the transverse cross section is determined by the position of the reference mirror, and the thickness of the transverse slice corresponds to the coherence length.

Other methods of generating carrier frequencies use electro-optic modulators and acousto-optic frequency shifters. Another method of obtaining transverse cross sections in OCT microscopy does not depend on transverse scanning of the object or the sample beam. Instead, a whole transverse image is recorded in parallel by using a CCD array and a photoelastic modulator for pathlength modulation [49].

Podoleanu et al. [50,51] demonstrated an alternative method of obtaining transverse OCT images by raster scanning the sample beam over the object. This method does not require an additional carrier frequency generator. Instead, the pathlength modulation caused by transverse raster scanning itself was used to generate the heterodyne signal. One of the attractive features of this technique is that it can be combined with a confocal scanning laser ophthalmoscope because both instruments use the same transverse scanning optics [52].

We explain this method with reference to Fig. 14. The instrument uses a fiber-optic Michelson interferometer with an SLD as the light source. In the reference arm, the light beam exiting from the fiber is collimated toward the reference mirror, where it is backreflected and coupled into the fiber again. The reference mirror can be moved to determine the depth position of the transverse cross-sectional plane in the sample. The sample arm consists of a collimation lens, an X-Y scanner block, a lens, and the sample. The backscattered sample beam is coupled into the fiber and superimposed with the reference beam at the directional coupler (DC), and the recombined beam is converted to an electric signal by the photodetector. The

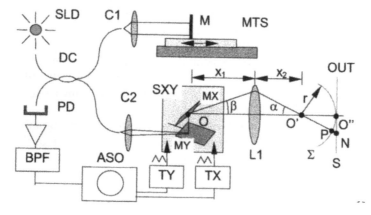

Figure 14 Sketch of transverse OCT instrument using transverse scanning for generation of carrier frequency. (Courtesy of A. G. Podoleanu, University of Kent. Reprinted from Ref. 50 by permission of the Optical Society of America.)

pivot point O on the scanning mirror MX is conjugate to the point O' (for simplicity, the distance between mirrors MX and MY is neglected). Therefore all rays traveling from O to O' have equal pathlength irrespective of the scanning angle β. However, the pathlength from O' to a plane sample surface (OUT) does depend on β, as can be seen in Fig. 14. Therefore, the pathlength of the sample arm is modulated during xy scanning thereby providing a carrier for the heterodyne signal detection. As can be seen in the figure, the pathlength variation is not linear with the scanning angle. For small scanning angles, the pathlength variation is proportional to the square of the scanning angle. This causes a varying heterodyne frequency, requiring a rather large filter bandwidth in the electronic demodulation circuit, which has the drawback of a reduced signal-to-noise ratio.

A detailed analysis shows [50] that this kind of acquisition of transverse OCT images corresponds to a sampling of the object with a sampling function consisting of Newton-ring-like concentric circles. This causes an angle-dependent transverse resolution: Near the center of the image (at about zero scanning angle) the transverse resolution is poor; it improves with distance from the center. This fact is another drawback of the method. Its advantage, however, is its simplicity and the lack of need for an additional carrier frequency generator.

This method has been used to record transverse cross sections of the human retina in vivo [51]. Figure 15 shows a series of such transverse images with increasing depth position generated by increasing the reference arm length between the recordings of the individual images. Compared to confocal scanning laser ophthalmoscopy (SLO), the depth resolution is improved by about an order of magnitude.

Two methods for overcoming the drawback of reduced central resolution have been proposed. One possibility is to use an additional carrier frequency generator for the central part of the image [51]. The obvious drawback is the increased complexity of the instrument. Because the heterodyne frequency still varies with the scanning angle, the problem of increased signal bandwidth and reduced signal-to-noise ratio remains. The other proposed solution is to displace the beam incident on the scanning mirrors away from their rotation axis [53]. This adds a linear term to the above-mentioned quadratic term of the optical path difference on the tilt angle. This causes a change of the Newton-ring-like sampling function to a shape consisting of a grid of approximately equidistant and parallel lines that is superior for imaging purposes. Among the drawbacks of this method are that the sampling function is superimposed on the coherence image in the form of narrow stripes and that no modulation appears if the shape of the sample surface matches the wave front shape. Consequently, some features may be lost. This should be considered with the interpretation of the images.

13.6 SIDE-SCATTERING OCT

At present, practically all OCT techniques use photons backscattered at a single object site. It is rather straightforward to decipher the information about the object structure carried by these photons. Multiply scattered photons collect information about several object sites. To derive the information carried by these photons is substantially more complex. Backscattering at a scattering angle of about π, on the one hand, has also been shown to be far more efficient than other scattering configurations [54]. On the other hand, backscattering is limited to a narrow cone

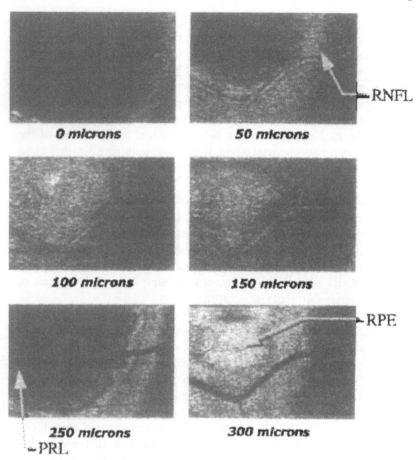

Figure 15 Transverse OCT images obtained from the retina of a human eye in vivo at increasing depth positions (indicated below each image). RNFL, retinal nerve fiber layer; PRL, photoreceptor layer; RPE, retinal pigment epithelium. (Courtesy of A. G. Podoleanu, University of Kent. Reprinted from Ref. 51 by permission of SPIE.)

around the illumination direction and thus limits the photon flux available for the tomographic A-scan. Limited photon flux at the photodetector limits the penetration depth of OCT techniques.

Sufficient penetration depth is of particular importance in such fields as dermatological melanoma diagnosis [55]. For example, it is the growth in depth direction that best correlates with clinical outcomes. But standard OCT techniques are limited to penetration depths in skin (at wavelengths of about 850 nm) of 1 mm or less. Hence, for applications in strongly scattering media like skin, alternative OCT techniques have been developed.

One apparent possibility is the use of all photons reflected from the object surface. This has been the strategy of H. Brunner and colleagues. Because of the limited dynamic range of the photodetector arrays they used, the high intensity light reflected at the so-called illumination spot where the probing beam enters the tissue had to be blocked (this light mainly contains the singly backscattered photons).

Initially, detectors were positioned in a wide area outside of the illumination spot [56]. Later, it was found that detectors placed at greater distance from the illumination spot yield stronger signals from deeper regions at the cost of poorer resolution in the upper layers [57].

Figure 16 depicts the most recent optical scheme [57]. It is a modified Mach–Zehnder interferometer with a superluminescent diode as a light source. A plane glass plate is used as a beamsplitter to separate the reference beam from the measurement beam. The length of the reference beam is adjusted by means of a linear positioner together with a piezo actuator. The measurement beam is focused via a small prism onto the object surface. The beam reflected from the object and the reference beam are combined on a beamsplitter cube positioned at the interferometer exit. Attached to each of the two exit surfaces of the beamsplitter are two groups of complementary photodetectors. Each group comprises three line detectors and is placed on opposite sides of the image of the illumination spot. Hence, two corresponding groups were positioned at each of the exit planes. Because of the complementarity of the two coherent outputs of the Mach–Zehnder interferometer, the difference between the two signals corresponds to the coherent part of the detected light. The incoherent part yields the same intensity distribution on both exit planes and is therefore cancelled.

The linear positioner is used to adjust the reference arm length to select the required optical path length of the photons scattered at the object. Here it becomes clear that a price has to be paid for increased sensitivity. The coherence gate is open

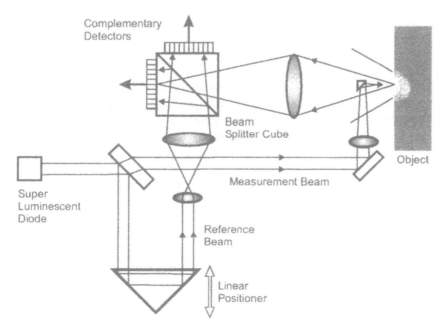

Figure 16 Mach–Zehnder type of interferometric setup for side-scattering OCT. The linear positioner is used to adjust the length of the reference beam. The measurement beam is focused via a small prism onto the subject surface. The beamsplitter cube at the interferometer exit has attached two groups of complementary photodetectors.

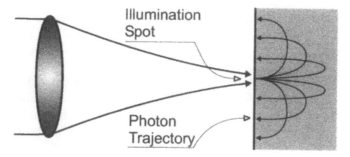

Figure 17 Photon trajectories of equal length through the object.

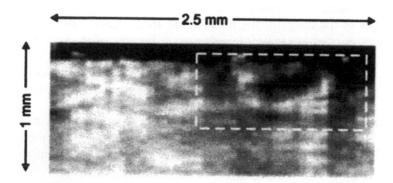

Figure 18 Normal skin (left) and junctional cell nevus (within the dashed rectangle). Note the increased absorption in the cell nevus due to its high melanin content. (Courtesy of H. Brunner, University of Ulm, Germany.)

for all photons that have traveled (within the coherence length) the same optical path irrespective of the detailed course. Some of these trajectories are depicted in Fig. 17. Hence, a substantial averaging over the object structure can occur and reduce the contrast of any image structure. A delicate balance must therefore be found between the need to collect as many photons as possible and the need to reduce averaging of the object structure.

Early measurements showed promising results for imaging human skin structures down to a depth of approximately 2mm [56]. As an example, a tomographic image of a junctional cell nevus is shown in Fig. 18.

ACKNOWLEDGMENTS

Thanks are due to our coworkers at the Institute of Medical Physics. Our own work is based on projects financed by the Austrian Science Foundation (FWF projects P7300-MED, P9781-MED, and P10316-MED).

REFERENCES

1. Wolf E. Three-dimensional structure determination of semi-transparent objects from holographic data. Opt Commun 1(4):153–156, 1969.
2. Kak AC, Slaney M. Principles of Computerized Tomographic Imaging. New York: IEEE Press, 1988.
3. Wolf E. Principles and development of diffraction tomography. In: A Consortini, ed. Trends in Optics, Vol 3. San Diego: Academic Press, 1996:83–110.
4. Harding G, Kosanetzky J. Energy dispersive x-ray diffraction tomography. Phys Med Biol 35(1):33–41, 1990.
5. Brase J, Yorkey T, Trebes J, McNulkty I. Image reconstruction for x-ray holographic microscopy. In: CJ Jacobsen, JE Trebes, eds. Soft X-Ray Microscopy. Bellingham, WA: SPIE, 1993:234–240.
6. Sponheim N, Gelius LJ, Johansen I, Stamnes JJ. Ultrasonic tomography of biological tissue. Ultrason Img 16(1):19–32, 1994.
7. Huang D, Swanson EA, Lin CP, Schuman JS, Stinson WG, Chang W, Hee MR, Flotte T, Gregory K, Puliafito CA, Fujimoto JG. Optical coherence tomography. Science 254:1178–1181, 1991.
8. Fercher AF, Bartelt H, Becker H, Wiltschko E. Image formation by inversion of scattered field data: Experiments and computational simulation. Appl Opt 18(14):2427–2439, 1979.
9. Fercher AF, Hitzenberger CK, Kamp G, El-Zaiat SY. Measurement of intraocular distances by backscattering spectral interferometry. Opt Commun 117:43–48, 1995.
10. Wedberg TC, Stamnes JJ. Quantitative imaging by optical diffraction tomography. Opt Rev 2(1):28–31, 1994.
11. Fercher AF, Drexler W, Hitzenberger CK. OCT techniques. Proc SPIE 2930:164–174, 1996.
12. Swanson EA, Huang D, Hee MR, Fujimoto JG, Lin CP, Puliafito CA. High-speed optical coherence domain reflectometry. Opt Lett 17:151–153, 1992.
13. Bouma B, Tearney GJ, Boppart SA, Hee MR, Brezinski ME, Fujimoto JG. High resolution optical coherence tomographic imaging using a mode-locked Ti:Al$_2$O$_3$ laser source. Opt Lett 20:1486–1488, 1995.
14. Fercher AF, Hitzenbergner CK. Optical coherence tomography in medicine. In: T Asakura, ed. International Trends in Optics and Photonics, Vol ICO 4. New York: Springer-Verlag, 1999:359–389.
15. Fercher AF, Leitgeb R, Hitzenberger CK, Sattmann H, Woitkowski M. Complex spectral interferometry OCT. Proc SPIE 3564:172–178, 1998.
16. Robinson DW, Reid GT. Interferogram Analysis. Philadelphia: Inst Phys Pub, 1993.
17. Loudon R. The Quantum Theory of Light. Oxford: Clarendon Press, 1985.
18. Fercher AF, Hitzenberger C, Juchem M. Measurement of intraocular optical distances using partially coherent laser light. J Mod Opt 38(7):1327–1333, 1991.
19. Fercher AF, Hitzenberger CK, Drexler W, Kamp G, Strasser I, Li HC. In vivo optical coherence tomography in ophthalmology. In: G Müller et al., eds. Medical Optical Tomography: Functional Imaging and Monitoring. Vol. IS 11. SPIE Press, 1993:355–370.
20. Häusler G, Lindner MW. "Coherence RADAR" and "spectral RADAR"—New tools for dermatological diagnosis. J Biomed Opt 3(1):21–31, 1998.
21. Born M, Wolf E. Principles of Optics. New York: Pergamon Press, 1980:265.
22. Lexer F, Hitzenberger CK, Kulhavy M, Fercher AF. Measurement of the axial eye length by wavelength tuning interferometry. Proc SPIE 2930:202–206, 1996.
23. Haberland U, Jansen P, Blazek V, Schmitt H. Optical coherence tomography of scattering media using frequency modulated continuous wave techniques with tunable near-infrared laser. Proc SPIE 2981:20–28, 1997.

24. Chinn SR, Swanson EA, Fujimoto JG. Optical coherence tomography using a frequency-tunable optical source. Opt Lett 22:340–342, 1997.
25. Hitzenberger CK, Drexler W, Baumgartner A, Lexer F, Sattmann H, Esslinger M, Kulhavy M, Fercher AF. Optical measurement of intraocular distances: A comparison of methods. Laser Light Ophthalmol 8:85–95, 1997.
26. Lexer F, Hitzenberger CK, Fercher AF, Kulhavy M. Wavelength tuning interferometry of intraocular distances. Appl Opt 36:6548–6553, 1997.
27. Haberland UHP, Blazek V, Schmitt HJ. Chirp optical coherence tomography of layered scattering media. J Biomed Opt 3:259–266, 1998.
28. Hitzenberger CK, Kulhavy M, Lexer F, Baumgartner A, Fercher AF. In vivo intraocular ranging by wavelength tuning interferometry. Proc SPIE 3251:47–51, 1998.
29. Golubovic B, Bouma BE, Tearney GJ, Fujimoto JG. Optical frequency-domain reflectometry using rapid wavelength tuning of a Cr^{4+}:forsterite laser. Opt Lett 22:1704–1706, 1997.
30. Fercher AF. Optical coherence tomography. J Biomed Opt 1(2):157–173, 1996.
31. Fercher AF, Roth E. Ophthalmic laser interferometry. Proc SPIE 658:48–51, 1986.
32. Hitzenberger CK. Optical measurement of the axial eye length by laser Doppler interferometry. Invest Ophthalmol Vis Sci 32(3):616–624, 1991.
33. Hitzenberger CK, Drexler W, Dolezal C, Skorpik F, Juchem M, Fercher AF, Gnad HD. Measurement of the axial length of cataract eyes by laser Doppler interferometry. Invest Ophthalmol Vis Sci 34(6):1886–1893, 1993.
34. Drexler W, Baumgartner A, Findl O, Hitzenberger CK, Sattmann H, Fercher AF. Submicrometer precision biometry of the anterior segment of the human eye. Invest Ophthalmol Vis Sci 38(7):1304–1313, 1997.
35. Hitzenberger CK, Drexler W, Baumgartner A, Lexer F, Sattmann H, Esslinger M, Kulhavy M, Fercher AF. Optical measurement of intraocular distances: A comparison of methods. Lasers Light Ophthalmol 8(2):85–95, 1997.
36. Drexler W, Findl O, Menapace R, Rainer G, Vass C, Hitzenberger CK, Fercher AF. Partial coherence interferometry: A novel approach to biometry in cataract surgery. Am J Ophthalmol 126(4):524–534, 1998.
37. Fercher AF, Hitzenberger CK, Drexler W, Kamp G, Sattmann H. In vivo optical coherence tomography. Am J Ophthalmol 116(1):113–114, 1993.
38. Drexler W, Findl O, Menapace R, Kruger A, Wedrich A, Rainer G, Baumgartner A, Hitzenberger CK, Fercher AF. Dual beam optical coherence tomography: Signal identification for ophthalmologic diagnosis. J Biomed Opt 3(1):55–65, 1998.
39. Möller B, Rudolph G, Klopffleisch A, Donnerhacke KH, Dorsel A. Application of diffractive optics for axial eye length measurement using partial coherence interferometry. Proc SPIE 2930:175–182, 1996.
40. Baumgartner A, Hitzenberger CK, Sattmann H, Drexler W, Fercher AF. Signal and resolution enhancements in dual beam optical coherence tomography of the human eye. J Biomed Opt 3(1):45–54, 1998.
41. Hitzenberger CK, Drexler W, Baumgartner A, Fercher AF. Dispersion effects in partial coherence interferometry. Proc SPIE 2981:29–36, 1997.
42. Hitzenberger CK, Baumgartner A, Drexler W, Fercher AF. Dispersion effects in partial coherence interferometry: Implications for intraocular ranging. J Biomed Opt 4:144–151, 1999.
43. Drexler W, Hitzenberger CK, Baumgartner A, Findl O, Sattmann H, Fercher AF. Investigation of dispersion effects in ocular media by multiple wavelength partial coherence interferometry. Exp Eye Res 66:25–33, 1998.
44. Richard G. Choroidal Circulation. Stuttgart: G. Thieme, 1992.
45. Schmitt JM, Lee SL, Yung KM. An optical coherence microscope with enhanced resolving power in thick tissue. Opt Commun 142:203–207, 1997.

46. Lexer F, Fercher AF, Sattmann H, Drexler W, Molebny S. Dynamic coherent focus for transversal resolution enhancement of OCT. Proc SPIE 3251:85–90, 1998.
47. Lexer F, Hitzenberger CK, Molebny S, Sattmann H, Sticker M, Fercher AF. Dynamic coherent focus OCT with depth-independent resolution. J Mod Opt 46(3):541–553, 1998.
48. Izatt JA, Hee MR, Owen GM, Swanson EA, Fujimoto JG. Optical coherence microscopy in scattering media. Opt Lett 19:590–592, 1994.
49. Beaurepaire E, Boccara AC, Lebec M, Blanchot L, Saint-Jalmes H. Full-field optical coherence microscopy. Opt Lett 23:244–246, 1998.
50. Podoleanu AG, Dobre GM, Webb DJ, Jackson DA. Coherence imaging by use of a Newton rings sampling function. Opt Lett 21: 1789–1791, 1996.
51. Podoleanu AG, Seeger M, Dobre GM, Webb DJ, Jackson DA, Fitzke FW. Transversal and longitudinal images from the retina of the living eye using low coherence reflectometry. J Biomed Opt 3:12–20, 1998.
52. Podoleanu AG, Rogers JA, Webb DJ, Jackson DA, Fitzke FW, Wade AR. Compatibility of transversal OCT imaging with confocal imaging of the retina in vivo. Proc SPIE 3598:61–67, 1999.
53. Podoleanu AG, Dobre GM, Jackson DA. En-face coherence imaging using galvanometer scanner modulation. Opt Lett 23:147–149, 1998.
54. Yoon G, Roy DNG, Straight RC. Coherent backscattering in biological media: Measurement and estimation of optical properties. Appl Opt 32(4):580–584, 1993.
55. Pan Y, Farkas DL. Noninvasive imaging of living human skin with dual-wavelength optical coherence tomography in two and three dimensions. J Biomed Opt 3(4):446–455, 1998.
56. Brunner H, Lazar R, Seschek R, Meier T, Steiner R. Imaging of skin structures by optical coherence tomography. In: W.U.R. Waidelich, ed. Lasers in Medicine, Springer, 1997:593–596.
57. Lazar R, Brunner H, Seschek R, Meier T, Steiner R. A fast OCT assembly using wide area detection. Proc SPIE 3194:323–327, 1998.

14

Optical Coherence Tomography for High-Density Data Storage

STEPHEN R. CHINN*

Lincoln Laboratory, Massachusetts Institute of Technology, Lexington, Massachusetts

ERIC A. SWANSON[†]

Coherent Diagnostic Technology, Concord, Massachusetts

14.1 INTRODUCTION

High density storage of data and information (including video and audio content) has become an increasingly important part of everyday life. Although magnetic disk storage has been the primary medium for most recent computer systems, there is an ever-increasing demand for high density data storage in optical media, particularly for CD-ROM data and documents and image/movie storage in CD-sized disks [1]. Even with impressive improvements in magnetic storage, that medium is limited by minimum domain sizes that can be created and read on a surface. Optical storage, on the other hand, can use the interior volume of the storage medium, with a theoretical volume limit on the order of a cubic wavelength per bit.

While alternatives such as holographic data storage are being explored to use the full media volume, several strategies have been employed to achieve higher data densities in more conventional types of optical disks. One method has been to decrease the optical wavelength used in reading the disk, because shorter wave-

This work was sponsored by the Department of the Air Force under contract number AF19628-95-C-002. Opinions, interpretations, conclusions, and recommendations are those of the authors and are not necessarily endorsed by the United States Air Force.

Current affiliation: Malachite Technologies, Methuen, Massachusetts

[†]*Current affiliation*: Sycamore Networks, Chelmsford, Massachusetts

lengths can be focused to smaller spot sizes [2], allowing more closely spaced data. Another, more recent and complementary approach to exploit volumetric storage has been to use several layers of data on the same disk [3–5]. The latest commercial advance, digital video disk (DVD), shortens the wavelength slightly to 635–780 nm and offers the option of having two layers per side, on two sides (the disk must be turned to change sides) [6]. The track pitch is reduced from $1.6 \mu m$ (CD) to $0.74 \mu m$, and the minimum pit length is reduced from $0.83 \mu m$ to $0.4 \mu m$ [7]. If the dual layer option is used, an important parameter for later comparison is the layer separation, $35–55 \mu m$ [6,8]. The net improvement in storage capacity is from 650 MB (conventional CD) to a maximum of 17 GB (DVD, two layers on each of two sides) [6].

In this chapter we will discuss a new readout concept [9] using optical coherence domain reflectometry that can extend the capability of reading multilayer disks with a number of layers an order of magnitude greater than previously achieved. Although this is not a quasi-static imaging application, we will refer to the technique as optical coherence tomography (OCT), for consistency with the rest of this volume. Much of the material in this chapter is based upon our previously published work [10,11] with the addition of more detailed analyses and explanations and new experimental data on multilayer disks. Figures 1–9, 11, 12, 14 and 15 are adapted from Refs. 10 and 11.

Optical coherence tomography uses broadband light from a source such as continuous wave (cw) superluminescent light-emitting diode (LED), with interferometric detection [12–15], and is capable of high resolution three-dimensional imaging inside partially transparent media, as has been demonstrated in various biomedical imaging applications described in other works and elsewhere [16] in this volume. This method's high sensitivity with good lateral and depth resolution make it an excellent candidate for reading optical data stored in many closely packed layers. Because diffraction-limited imaging of local regions is used (as opposed to volumetric holography), much of the existing single-layer disk technology can be employed.

Another simpler but related method for improving multilayer readout simply replaces the laser diode in a conventional CD system with the same type of broadband source [11,17], with no other changes to the system except for possibly improving the intensity detection sensitivity. Improvements from the broadband source replacement in this direct-detection (DD) system arise from the reduction of coherent interlayer cross-talk signal fluctuations. Although this method does not have the depth resolution or sensitivity of the OCT system, it does provide improved performance over laser-based systems and provides an interesting comparison to the OCT method. Its main virtue is that required modification of existing system design is reduced.

Section 14.2 contains a more detailed description of the multilayer readout concept using OCT. In Section 14.3 we present analytical descriptions of beam propagation through multilayer media, which has a direct influence on optical signal quality. Similarly, in Section 14.4 we discuss the signal degradation arising from reflective cross-talk among the layers. System sensitivity issues and limits are presented in Section 14.5. Experimental methods and results on imaging one-, two-, and three-layer disks are given in Section 14.6. A summary and conclusions are given in Section 14.7. Throughout this chapter, the emphasis is on readout of multilayer media, which could be most easily produced by mass replication methods adapted from current technology. Other possible media fabrication issues and alternatives will be discussed in Section 14.7.

14.2 DESCRIPTION OF OCT MULTILAYER OPTICAL DISK CONCEPT

A schematic drawing of the essentials of an OCT multilayer optical disk readout system is shown in Fig. 1. Light from a broadband incoherent source, such as a superluminescent LED, a doped-fiber amplified spontaneous emission source, or a short-pulse supercontinuum generator, is divided into two paths. Although the paths are shown in free space with bulk optical components, optical fiber and fiber components can also be used. Light in the signal path is imaged onto and reflected from a target (the desired data layer), and light in the reference path is reflected from a mirror whose optical path distance is the same as the signal's. These two reflected signals are recombined in the interferometer (at the beamsplitter or fiber coupler) onto a detector. The method resembles that of coherence scanning microscopy, except for placement of the focusing objective after the interferometer rather than before it [18]. Since the source has a broad bandwidth, the signal and reference fields will interfere coherently at the detector only when their optical pathlengths are closely matched. As the bandwidth of the source increases, the coherence length decreases and the matching length requirement becomes more stringent, giving better distance resolution. If the optical beam in the reference path is phase-modulated or frequency-shifted, demodulation after the detector provides heterodyne detection of the signal. This path-matching requirement provides depth discrimination for selecting a particular data layer in addition to that provided by the depth of focus of the signal objective lens. Spurious reflections will be generated from other layers of the

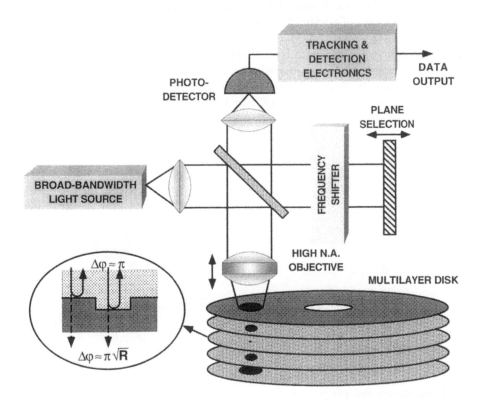

Figure 1 Schematic illustration of an OCT optical disk readout system. [From Ref. 11, Fig. 1.]

disk. Because their optical pathlengths will be different from that of the reference path to the desired layer, the spurious heterodyne signals will be greatly reduced by the combination of smaller coherent interference and increased optical defocusing.

The broadband direct detection (DD) version would be similar to a conventional CD system and would lack the reference path and interferometer used with OCT. The DD system operates functionally in most respects like a conventional laser-based system but would not suffer from unwanted interference effects arising from the narrower laser source linewidth. The differences between OCT and DD occur in the noise fluctuation characteristics, which will be described below for the specific example of a single-spatial-mode receiver.

We describe one particular implementation of information storage, shown in Fig. 2. It resembles that of conventional compact disks and allows relatively straightforward analysis and comparison of the OCT and DD methods. Moreover, as discussed below, the resulting low optical reflectivity and large transmission of each data layer interface are well suited for disks having many layers. Binary signal levels are produced by the absence or presence of data pits or regions, approximately one-quarter wavelength deep, at the interface of two layers having slightly different indices of refraction. We note that this technology is extendible to m-ary storage where the bits have m symbols representing $ln_2 m$ bits by using modified pit depths. As shown in the cross section of the left-hand portion of Fig. 2, light reflected from the top and bottom surfaces of the pit will have π relative phase shift $\Delta\phi_R$. With appropriate optical focus waist and pit size, the reflected beam can be greatly altered in the presence of a pit region. Actual disks may have not only circular data pits but also elongated depressions of varying length. For simplicity of analysis, we limit our model to circular pits, which should give good qualitative insight. Experimental results presented later will show data from actual disks.

In our analyses we will consider both the source and receiver to be near-diffraction-limited, so that (in the ideal case) light at the data layer is in a diffraction-limited focal spot, and the received signal can be found from the overlap of the reflected beam with the diffraction-limited single-receiver mode. For appropriate

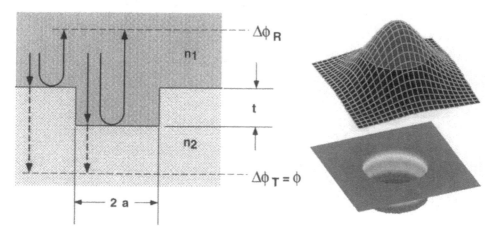

Figure 2 Cross section and perspective view of data layer interface in one example of a multilayer optical disk storage medium. [Adapted from Ref. 11, Fig. 2.]

focus and pit parameters, the beam reflected from a pit can be made nearly spatially orthogonal to the input mode, giving a null in the detected signal when a pit is present. The right-hand portion of Fig. 2 illustrates this case, where the pit size and optical mode waist are such that the integrated optical intensity inside and outside the pit are equal. For simplicity, we assume that the diffraction-limited source and receiver modes are Gaussian beams The lighter shaded top of the Gaussian intensity surface shows the region with π-reflected phase shift. In this example the Gaussian mode waist $w_0 = a\sqrt{2/(\ln 2)}$, where a is the pit radius. Also, in the interest of simplicity, we assume that depolarization effects are negligible. If the disk media significantly depolarize the reflected signal beam, then a polarization diversity receiver could be implemented for the OCT system. Recent work concerning issues of vector diffraction and polarization effects in optical disks is discussed in Refs. 19 and 20.

Because we expect some degree of beam degradation in using many data layers, we first analyze how a Gaussian beam propagates and find the statistics of the received signal under various conditions. This analysis will find the degradation in the received beam quality caused by scattering of light from the intermediate data layers as the signal beam propagates through them to the desired data layer and then reflects back. Then we perform a similar analysis of how spurious cross-talk signals reflected from other data layers interfere with the signal from the desired layer. Our results will show that such interlayer cross-talk plays a dominant role in limiting the receiver eye opening or bit error rate. These two analyses are important factors in determining overall system performance. For practical systems, it is important that the beam quality not be degraded (or the received signal level significantly attenuated) as deeper layers are addressed. In addition to this condition, it is necessary that interlayer cross-talk be low so that reliable bit decisions can be made. Our results will show that OCT is well suited to the requirements imposed by optical disks with many layers.

14.3 PROPAGATION ANALYSIS

The goal of propagation analysis is to obtain as quantitative a model as possible while making it both analytically and numerically tractable. The propagation of a focused beam through multiple data layers and its reflection back through the same layers are simplified as much as possible while retaining the essence of the physical problem. For forward propagation, each data layer interface is idealized as a zero-thickness phase mask, because the quarter-wave thickness of the pits is assumed to be a very small fraction of the separation between different data interfaces and a negligible distance in affecting propagation. To isolate the effects of beam distortion, we do not include the weak Fresnel reflectivity of the interface, which could easily be added as a multiplicative factor. The pit depth is t, so the relative phase difference of beams propagating through pit and planar region is

$$\phi = \Delta\phi_T = \frac{2\pi(n_1 - n_2)t}{\lambda} \tag{1}$$

where λ is the mean free-space wavelength of the source, and n_1 and n_2 are the refractive indices of the adjacent layer media. Because we have chosen the reflective phase shift $\Delta\phi_R$ to be π, the pit depth is

$$t = \frac{\lambda}{4n_1} \tag{2}$$

causing the transmitted phase difference to be

$$\phi = \frac{\pi(n_1 - n_2)}{2n_1} \cong \pm\pi\sqrt{R} \tag{3}$$

where

$$R = \left|\frac{n_1 - n_2}{n_1 + n_2}\right|^2 \tag{4}$$

is the interface's power reflection coefficient (Fresnel reflectivity). Propagation through a pit region is approximated by multiplying the complex optical field in that region by $\exp(j\phi)$. We will use a paraxial approximation for the field propagation, so no angular dependence of the phase factor will be included. For simplicity, we will also use a scalar field approximation that neglects depolarization effects.

Another assumption that one might question is the ability of a pit with fixed depth to provide a π phase shift or reflective null for a broadband source. A simple physical argument shows that this is not a significant problem. Consider a short-pulse coherent source having bandwidth equivalent to a cw incoherent source. The portions of the pulse reflected from the top and bottom of the pit will suffer a relative time delay given by $\lambda/2c$. For a Gaussian temporal pulse, the full width at half-maximum (FWHM) duration is $0.4413\lambda^2/c\Delta\lambda$, so the fractional offset between these portions is $1.133\Delta\lambda/\lambda$. Most practical sources will have fractional bandwidths less than 5%, so the reduction in reflective phase nulling due to bandwidth spread should be negligible. This argument can be quantified and demonstrated by performing the appropriate integrations in the frequency domain.

14.3.1 Analytical Formulation

In the analytical formulation of beam propagation through multiple data layers we try to find an expression for the field transmitted to and reflected from the desired data layer, which is then detected by a single-spatial-mode receiver. This simplifies the problem from one requiring a complete field analysis to an evaluation of the coupling, or overlap, of the receiver field and the receiver spatial mode. Because the fields will be randomly affected by the phase mask patterns of intermediate data layers, we will try to find statistical means and deviations of the received signal levels.

After propagating through each data layer interface, the projection of the transmitted beam onto the ideal receiver Gaussian beam is given by the amplitude coupling coefficient

$$\kappa = \int E^*(r)E(r)Z(r)\,dA \tag{5}$$

where the field $E(r)$ is the complex normalized Gaussian field at the interface and $Z(r)$ is the multiplicative phase function of the data pattern, which is assumed to have values 1 (in regions outside the pits) or $\exp(j\phi)$ (inside the pit regions). Each data layer is described by a grid of square cells, with a circular data pit present or absent (each with probability 1/2) at the center of each cell. The ratio of the circular pit area, C, to the square cell area, A, is ρ. Figure 3 shows a schematic drawing of

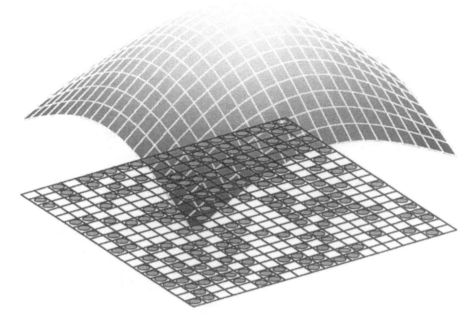

Figure 3 Illustration of analysis formulation of data region shown below an intensity contour of a defocused readout beam. The square grid shows the coordinate system of the data cells and may be displaced by arbitrary fractions of a data cell from the beam coordinate center. [Adapted from Ref. 11, Fig. 3.]

this subdivision, below a typical defocused Gaussian intensity profile. The coupling coefficient is then expressed as the sum

$$\kappa = (1 - \rho) \sum_m I_m A + \rho \sum_m I_m A Z_m \tag{6}$$

where $I_m A$ is the integral of the intensity over the mth square cell, and Z_m is a random variable having values 1 or $\exp(j\phi)$ with probability 1/2. For a fine enough grid, the first (nonrandom) intensity sum over all grid cells is approximately equal to the integral of intensity over the plane, which has been normalized to 1, $\sum_l I_l A = 1$. Each layer will contribute a factor of κ^2 to the overall coupling because the beam traverses the layer twice, in the forward and backward directions. For our purposes, the phase of κ is unimportant, so we evaluate only the magnitude of κ^2, which is given by

$$|\kappa|^2 = (1 - \rho)^2 + \rho(1 - \rho) \sum_m I_m A (Z_m + Z_m^*) + \rho^2 \sum_l \sum_m I_l I_m Z_l^* Z_m A^2 \tag{7}$$

To give an example of the statistical methodology, we show how the mean of Eq. (7) is found. Steps in derivation of the mean of the second term are straightforward. Define

$$\bar{Z}_m = \frac{1}{2}(1) + \frac{1}{2} e^{j\phi}, \qquad \bar{Z}_m^* = \frac{1}{2}(1) + \frac{1}{2} e^{-j\phi}$$

$$V_m \equiv \bar{Z}_m + \bar{Z}_m^* = 1 + \cos \phi, \qquad W_{lm} \equiv \frac{\overline{Z_l Z_m^* + Z_m Z_l^*}}{2} \tag{8}$$

In the third term for $|\bar{\kappa}|^2$,

$$W_{lm} = 1, \qquad\qquad l = m$$

$$= \frac{\overline{Z_l Z_m^*} + \overline{Z_l^* Z_m}}{2}, \qquad\qquad l \neq m \qquad (9)$$

$$= \frac{1}{2}\left\{\left[\frac{1}{2}(1) + \frac{1}{2}e^{j\phi}\right]\left[\frac{1}{2}(1) + \frac{1}{2}e^{-j\phi}\right](2)\right\} = \frac{1 + \cos\phi}{2}, \qquad l \neq m$$

where we have used the independence of different cells for $l \neq m$. The third term of Eq. (7) is rewritten as

$$\rho^2 A^2 \left\{\sum_l I_l^2 W_{ll} + \sum_l \sum_{m \neq l} I_l I_m W_{lm}\right\} = \rho^2 A^2 \left\{\sum_l I_l^2 + \sum_l \sum_{m \neq l} I_l I_m \frac{1 + \cos\phi}{2}\right\}$$

$$= \rho^2 A^2 \left\{\sum_l I_l^2 \left[\frac{1 + \cos\phi}{2} + \frac{1 - \cos\phi}{2}\right]\right.$$

$$\left. + \sum_l \sum_{m \neq l} I_l I_m \frac{1 + \cos\phi}{2}\right\}$$

$$= \rho^2 A^2 \left\{\sum_l I_l^2 \left[\frac{1 - \cos\phi}{2}\right] + \sum_l \sum_m I_l I_m\right.$$

$$\left. \frac{1 + \cos\phi}{2}\right\}$$

$$= \rho^2 \frac{1 - \cos\phi}{2} A \sum_l I_l^2 A + \rho^2 \left(\sum_l I_l A\right)^2$$

$$\frac{1 + \cos\phi}{2}$$

$$= \rho^2 \frac{1 + \cos\phi}{2} + \rho^2 \frac{1 - \cos\phi}{2} A \sum_l I_l^2 A$$

$$(10)$$

The total average of all the terms in Eq. (7) is

$$\mu \equiv \overline{|\kappa|^2} = (1 - \rho)^2 + (1 + \cos\phi)\left[\rho(1 - \rho) + \frac{\rho^2}{2}\right] + \frac{\rho^2}{2}(1 - \cos\phi)A\sum_l I_l^2 A$$

$$(11)$$

Using another integral approximation to the sum, the last summation term in Eq. (11) is $A/\pi w^2$, where w is the Gaussian mode waist at that layer. This approximates the inverse of the number of bit cells, N, in the mode area at a given data layer. Neglecting this last term, assumed to be small for a fine enough grid subdivision or large enough waist, a little algebraic manipulation gives

$$\mu = 1 - (1 - \cos\phi)\rho\left(1 - \frac{\rho}{2}\right) \qquad\qquad (12)$$

and for small values of ϕ, expected for low interface reflectivity,

$$\mu \approx 1 - \phi^2 \frac{\rho}{2}\left(1 - \frac{\rho}{2}\right) \tag{13}$$

This result agrees with the expectation that as the interface phase shift or reflectivity vanishes, there is no beam distortion. Similarly, at the limit of zero fill factor, no differential phase exists, causing no distortion. To find the standard deviation of $|\kappa|^2$, we have to evaluate $|\kappa|^4$. This is done in a manner similar to that of finding the mean, except that products of as many as four sums of random variables occur. Their statistical evaluation requires that these products be separated into terms having sums over the same cells or independent cells. After much algebraic manipulation similar in method to the above derivation, we find that the variance of the coupling coefficient to lowest order in $1/N$ is

$$\sigma^2 \equiv \overline{|\kappa|^4} - \overline{|\kappa|^2}^2 \approx (1 - \cos\phi)^2 \frac{\rho^2(1 - \rho)^2}{N} \tag{14}$$

and for small ϕ, the standard deviation is

$$\sigma \approx \frac{\phi^2 \rho(1 - \rho)}{2\sqrt{N}} \tag{15}$$

The above mean and variance apply to a single layer through which the reading beam propagates back and forth. These terms are the same for all layers except for the value of N, which will vary as the beam propagates through the multilayer medium and the Gaussian mode size changes at each layer. For multiple layers on top of the desired data layer, the total amplitude coupling coefficient is the product of the individual layer coefficients. The individual coefficients are statistically independent of each other because the data pit distributions in different layers are uncorrelated. Therefore, the mean of the total coupling coefficient is the product of the individual layer means:

$$\mu_T = \left[1 - (1 - \cos\phi)\rho\left(1 - \frac{\rho}{2}\right)\right]^M \tag{16}$$

The total random coupling coefficient is

$$|\kappa|_T^2 = |\kappa|_1^2 \, |\kappa|_2^2 \, |\kappa|_3^2 \cdots |\kappa|_M^2 \tag{17}$$

and its total variance is

$$\sigma_T^2 = \overline{|\kappa|_T^4} - \overline{|\kappa|_T^2}^2 = \overline{|\kappa|_1^4} \, \overline{|\kappa|_2^4} \, \overline{|\kappa|_3^4} \cdots \overline{|\kappa|_M^4} - \overline{|\kappa|_1^2}^2 \, \overline{|\kappa|_2^2}^2 \, \overline{|\kappa|_3^2}^2 \cdots \overline{|\kappa|_M^2}^2 \tag{18}$$

or

$$\sigma_T^2 \approx (\sigma_1^2 + \mu^2)(\sigma_2^2 + \mu^2)(\sigma_3^2 + \mu^2) \cdots (\sigma_M^2 + \mu^2) - \mu^{2M} \tag{19}$$

If the ratio of standard deviation to mean for each layer is small, the ratio of the total standard deviation to total mean is approximately

$$\sigma_T^2 \approx \mu^{2M}\left[\left(\frac{\sigma_1^2}{\mu^2} + 1\right)\left(\frac{\sigma_2^2}{\mu^2} + 1\right)\left(\frac{\sigma_3^2}{\mu^2} + 1\right) \cdots \left(\frac{\sigma_M^2}{\mu^2} + 1\right) - 1\right] \tag{20}$$

or

$$\frac{\sigma_T}{\mu_T} \approx \frac{(\sum_{l=1}^{M} \sigma_l^2)^{1/2}}{\mu} \tag{21}$$

If we give the distance of layer l from the reference 0 layers as $L_l = l \times L$, then the number of pits in the defocused Gaussian waist is

$$N_l = \frac{\pi w_0^2}{A}\left[1 + l^2\left(\frac{L}{z_R}\right)^2\right] \approx \frac{\pi w_0^2}{A} l^2 \left(\frac{L}{z_R}\right)^2, \qquad \frac{L}{z_R} \geq 2 \tag{22}$$

where L is the layer separation and z_R is the Rayleigh range (focal depth) of the Gaussian beam, defined by

$$z_R \equiv \frac{\pi w_0^2}{\lambda} \tag{23}$$

with mode waist w_0 (the $1/e$ field radius) at the data layer. A typical value for w_0 is $2\,\mu$m.

Using these results and the relations among the pit radius, cell area, and fill factor, we can find a bound for an infinite sum in Eq. (21),

$$\begin{aligned}
\frac{\sigma_T}{\mu_T} &\leq \frac{0.755(1 - \cos\phi)\sqrt{\rho(1-\rho)}}{(L/z_R)[1 - (1 - \cos\phi)\rho(1 - \rho/2)]} \\
&\approx \frac{3.726R\sqrt{\rho(1-\rho)}}{L/z_R}, \qquad R \ll 0.1
\end{aligned} \tag{24}$$

Equations (16) and (24) give the statistical parameters for the received amplitude coupling coefficient of the beam reflected from a pit-free region (which we will call a 1), because this case will cause an incident Gaussian beam to be reflected on itself. By using the coupling coefficient, we are not concerned with the details of the field scattered out of the receiver mode (a formulation that implicitly neglects multiple scattering back into the mode). If the data at the desired layer were a 0, by design of the pit and focal waist the ideal coupling would be zero. An analytical formation of the exact, nonzero result would have to find the amount of actual reflected field that is scattered back into the receiver mode through scattering processes in both directions of the beam. We have not found a simple analytical technique for this calculation, which is performed only with the numerical method described below. Only the 1's case will provide an analytical comparison with those numerical results.

14.3.2 Numerical Formulation

The numerical analysis of distortion caused by interfering data layers uses a standard fast Fourier transform (FFT) beam propagation method [21]. The basis of this method is an approximate paraxial simplification of Maxwell's equations using a slowly varying envelope approximation. Because we are treating each data layer as a thin phase mask separated by a thick homogeneous region from the next mask, at first glance it would appear that the entire propagation between phase masks could be done in one step in the Fourier domain, because there are no variations in the medium to alter the plane wave decomposition of the beam. In principle this would be correct if boundary condition effects were negligible. The use of the unwindowed FFT imposes implicit constraints that the solutions are periodic over the interval of computation. As long as the fields are negligible at the boundaries this would present no problem. For practical reasons of memory limitations and computation time, however, we have to limit the computation grid to be not much larger than the largest beam waist. To avoid the effects of aliasing (implicit periodic boundary conditions), thin absorbing regions are imposed at the grid boundaries to remove spurious reflected beams. Accurate use of these absorbing layers requires inverse transformation to the spatial domain at several smaller increments through the homogeneous medium between phase masks. Therefore the final technique is the so-called split-step FFT method over several small propagation increments per layers, transforming back and forth from spatial to spatial frequency (wave vector) domains). At each data plane, the spatial domain field is multiplied by the complex exponential phase mask function representing the data pattern.

The phase mask for each layer is generated by using random numbers to determine the presence or absence of a circular data pit in each grid cell. Also, the coordinate center of each intermediate layer's frame of reference with respect to the beam center is offset by a random amount, between $\pm 1/2$ of a cell width in each direction. Both of these randomization steps are used to simulate each layer of a multilayer CD-ROM. Once generated, each random data mask is retained for use in the reverse propagation computation. Each layer has a 19×19 array of data cells in a 256×256 element computation grid. The value of ρ used in the analytical and numerical calculations is 0.503. The calculations are performed with as many as eight data layers through which the beam propagates. At the layer where the beam comes to a focus, we examine the two cases of reflection from a "1" (no phase alteration) or a "0" (π reflected phase shift region centered with respect to the focal point). For both the analytical and numerical cases the coupling coefficients are normalized with respect to the reflectivity from the desired data layer. Also, to isolate the effects of propagation distortion, the Fresnel reflectivity and power loss at each intermediate layer are neglected. For large numbers of layers, there would be such a practical requirement for small reflectivity to avoid excessive beam attenuation. We will discuss this point below in more detail.

A single measurement sample is found by calculating the forward and backward beam propagation through the out-of-focus data layers, with a midpoint reflection from the centered, in-focus data layer (from a "0" or "1"), and then numerically calculating the beam overlap with the receiver mode. The histograms and statistics for the overall coupling coefficients are found from Monte Carlo repetition of this process with different randomly generated data layers. Calculations and data display were performed using Fortran code on a Macintosh 68040 processor computer. Two-dimensional patterns of the field intensity at various depths were saved for example members of the ensemble, to allow visualization of different degrees of beam distortion. Illustrations of such a comparison for different reflectivities are shown in Fig. 4 (see color plate), for propagation back and forth through eight data layers, with a layer thickness equal to the Gaussian beam Rayleigh range. At the top of Fig. 4 are examples of "1" and "0" beam intensity profiles for a Fresnel reflectivity of $R = 0.001$. Intensities are shown on a logarithmic false-color scale, with each gradation of color corresponding to a 2 dB increment. The intensities at the edges of the frames approach zero because of the absorbing boundary conditions. In each frame pair, the left-hand part shows the distorted beam and the right-hand part the undistorted (receiver) beam. At the bottom of the figure is a similar comparison (using the same randomly generated data layers) for the case of

R = 0.001 , Bit = 1   R = 0.001 , Bit = 0

R = 0.04 , Bit = 1   R = 0.04 , Bit = 0

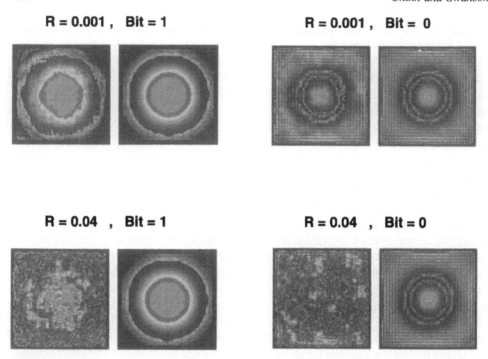

Figure 4 Images of beam intensities after propagation back and forth through eight data interfaces with separation equal to a Rayleigh length. Interface reflectivity R and data at focus are indicated in each pair of profiles (Bit = 1 means no pit; Bit = 0 means pit in focal plane). The left-hand image of each pair is the undistorted intensity with no data in the interfering layers. The images are shown in logarithmic false color scales, with each gradation equal to 2 dB. (See color plate.) [From Ref. 11, Fig. 4.]

$R = 0.04$. As shown previously [Eq. (3)], the transmitted phase shift through a pit region is proportional to the square root of R, and the difference in propagation quality for $\sqrt{R} = 0.033$ and $0.2(R = 0.001$ and $0.04)$ is dramatic. Thus, it is crucial for good beam quality and successful readout from multilayer media that the reflectivity per layer interface be very low. However, low reflectivity can stress the receiver signal-to-noise ratio as discussed later.

14.3.3 Comparison of Analytical and Numerical Formulations

Graphs of the amplitude coupling coefficient for the case of eight data layers are shown in Fig. 5. The graphs illustrated correspond to the beam profile examples of Fig. 4, except that many propagation cases were evaluated to generate the graphs. The vertical bars mark the positions of the mean values of the amplitude coupling coefficient. Note the gaps and scale changes in different positions of the horizontal axes. The data have been normalized to convert them to probability densities, such that the integral of each of the four curves (zeros and ones for two reflectivity values) is unity (the integrals may not appear equal because of the axes' scale changes). The numerical values of the means and standard deviations shown in the figure were found from the ensemble of coupling coefficient results. The analytic comparisons for the "1" data were derived using Eqs. (12), (14), (19), and (22). Given the approx-

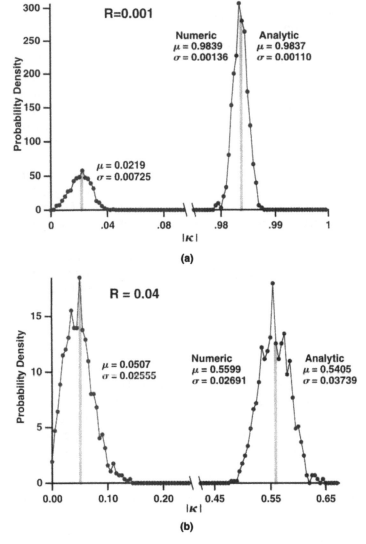

Figure 5 Graphs of amplitude-coupling coefficients after propagating back and forth through eight data layers, each separated by a Rayleigh length. (a) $R = 0.001$; (b) $R = 0.04$. Note the breaks and scale changes in the bottom axes and the difference in scales between (a) and (b). [From Ref. 10, Fig. 2.]

imations involved in these formulas, the agreement is surprisingly good. This agreement gives confidence in the validity of using the analytical results in cases where the numerical modeling would be impractical, as for larger numbers of data layers.

An interesting result of the evaluation of $|\kappa|_T$ for the "1" case is its analytical form for small reflectivity,

$$\overline{|\kappa|_T} = \left[1 - \phi^2 \frac{\rho}{2}\left(1 - \frac{\rho}{2}\right)\right]^M = \left[1 - R\pi^2 \frac{\rho}{2}\left(1 - \frac{\rho}{2}\right)\right]^M \tag{25}$$

showing a signal loss due to scattering that resembles a reflectivity loss.

We discuss the difference between OCT and DD signals in more detail below. For purposes of comparing the propagation results with these two methods, recall that DD will sense the received intensity, which will be proportional to the square of the amplitude coupling coefficient. The OCT signal results from the heterodyne mixing of a constant reference field and varying signal field, the latter of which is linearly proportional to the amplitude coupling coefficient. The beam distortion itself is independent of the means of detection, so the only difference in the OCT and DD analyses is in the choice of evaluating either the received field or intensity of the distorted beam. Note that in finding the average intensity of the received beam using the square of Eq. (25), the average power loss effects of data scattering resemble Fresnel losses but may be even larger. For example, if $\rho = 0.5$, the coefficient of R in Eq. (25) is 1.85. If power loss due to reflectivity alone were considered, the coefficient of R would be 1, corresponding to the usual power attenuation factor $1 - R$ per interface. When both effects are considered, the total effective reflectivity for loss considerations is equivalent to $2.85R$.

The effects of scattering of the light in a multilayer optical storage medium can be severe. It is important that the reflectivity per layer (which is proportional to the scattering coefficient) be kept small so that the average received light level is nearly constant as a function of depth and so the variance around these levels does not cause bit errors.

14.4 CROSS-TALK ANALYSIS

In this section we discuss the effects of signal interference by reflections from layers other than the desired one. We assume that the Fresnel reflectivity from each data layer interface is small, so multiple back-and-forth reflections can be neglected. This approximation is also justified in light of the larger geometrical defocusing factors for multiply reflected beams. We also assume that the signal received from a spurious reflection can be calculated when using beams that are undistorted by propagation through the data layers. This approximation has been validated by the above propagation calculations if the Fresnel reflectivity and data propagation phase shift are small enough, as they need be for good system performance. Because distortion of the spuriously reflected beam would reduce the received cross-talk signal, we are doing a worst-case analysis. The main factors that are included for both OCT and DD are the geometrical defocusing reduction of signals reflected from out-of-focus layers, the effects of random data on this reflection, and the effects of source coherence on the total cross-talk signal.

These points are illustrated schematically in Fig. 6, which shows ray paths of incident (solid) and reflected (dashed) beams from the signal layer (at the beam focus) and one interfering data layer. The phase front curvatures are also indicated by corresponding thinner lines perpendicular to the beams. The arrow diagrams at the right edge of the figure are phasor representations of the relative time dependence of the reflected signal and cross-talk fields. The reflected cross-talk field is shown as an arc of blurred phase (from the temporal decorrelation) whose mean is tipped (from differences in propagation distances) and reduced (from defocusing and data effects) with respect to the reflected signal phasor (vertical arrow). The mean tipping angle has a randomness associated with unknown layer thickness variations relative to an optical wavelength.

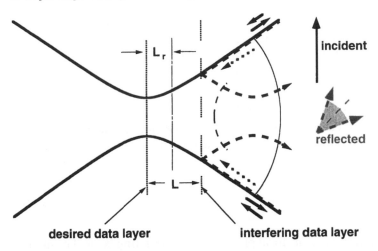

desired data layer   **interfering data layer**

Figure 6 Cross-sectional illustration of beams used in calculation of reflective feedback effects. The heavy solid line is an iso-intensity ray incident and reflected from the signal layer, and the thin solid line is a perpendicular phase front. The heavy dashed line is a ray incident and reflected from one cross-talk layer, and the thin dashed line is its perpendicular phase front. The right-hand arrow diagrams represent temporal phasors for the reflected signal and cross-talk fields, described more fully in the text. [From Ref. 11, Fig. 6.]

Let the amplitude of the field that is incident on the desired data be

$$E_{\text{in}} = E(t)\exp(j\omega_0 t) \tag{26}$$

where $E(t)$ is the slowly varying envelope of a carrier at radian frequency ω_0. The temporal behavior of $E(t)$ will depend on its coherence properties. The field quantities are defined as amplitudes of the receiver spatial mode, whose spatial dependence is not shown. The reflected field detected at the receiver is

$$E_R = \sqrt{R}\left\{ d_i E(t)\exp[j\omega_0 t] + \sum_{l\neq 0} \kappa_l E(t - t_l)\exp[j\omega_0(t - t_l)] \right\} \tag{27}$$

In Eq. (27) a constant shift of time arguments with respect to the incident field is unimportant and is omitted. The signal variable d_i has values 1 or 0, depending on whether a data pit is absent (giving unity normalized signal) or present (giving zero coupling into the receiver mode). The cross-talk summation is over reflections from all layers except the desired data layer, including those above and below it. The quantities κ_l are reflective amplitude coupling coefficients similar to those defined in the propagation analysis. They will be described in more detail below. The temporal arguments of the cross-talk fields are shifted because of their different propagation distances with respect to the signal layer.

The reflective coupling coefficient from layer l is

$$\kappa_l = \int E_f(r)E_b^*(r)Z(r)\,dA \tag{28}$$

where subscripts f and b denote forward and backward (reflected) fields. The normalized fields have Gaussian spatial dependence, with mode waist w and radius of curvature R_c. The complex field product in the integral is

$$E_f(r)E_b^*(r) = \frac{2}{\pi w^2} \exp\left[-\frac{2r^2}{w^2}\left(1 + \frac{jkw^2}{R_c}\right)\right] \qquad (29)$$

Because the radius of curvature changes sign on reflection, an imaginary component of the exponent is present that represents defocusing ($j = \sqrt{-1}$). Using the properties of Gaussian beams, the imaginary component can be simplified as

$$j\frac{kw^2}{R_c} = j\frac{z}{z_R} \equiv j\xi, \qquad w^2 = w_0^2\left(1 + \frac{z^2}{z_R^2}\right) \qquad (30)$$

The variable z is the separation of the focal plane and the interfering layer. The mode waist w is an increasing function of separation, with minimum value w_0 at the desired data layer. The function $Z(r)$ is the reflective phase function of the data pattern, with values 1 in regions outside the data pits and -1 inside the data pits. If $Z(r)$ were uniformly 1, then κ_l would have value $1/(1 + j\xi)$ due to geometric defocusing.

Statistical distributions of $|\kappa_l|$ were calculated using numerical techniques similar to those described in Section 14.3.2, with randomly generated data patterns. Three different numerical approaches were used: (1) direct integration (numerical summation over 256×256 points) in the spatial plane of each layer, (2) integration in the far field of the reflected and reference beams (using Fourier transform), and (3) analytical conversion of Eq. (28) to a sum of one-dimensional integrals, performed by numerical integration. All three approaches gave identical results and were checked with special data patterns that allowed $|\kappa_l|$ to be evaluated analytically. Histograms of $|\kappa_l|^2$ are shown in Fig. 7 for five adjacent data layers, with layer separation equal to one Rayleigh range. The data have been normalized to make them unit-integral probability densities.

14.4.1 OCT

In optical coherence tomography, the received signal is found from the sum of a broadband incoherent reference field and the reflection of this field from the medium being probed. To eliminate the effects of uncontrolled environmental phase drifts between these fields and to avoid problems associated with base-band detection, generally some form of phase or frequency modulation is imposed on one of fields. In this section, we analyze the OCT cross-talk using one common form of modulation that shifts the frequency of the reference field and uses heterodyne detection of the beat frequency. The complex reference field is written as

$$E_{\text{ref}} = E(t)\exp[j(\omega_0 + \Omega)t] \qquad (31)$$

where Ω is the radian frequency shift. The reflected field is

$$E_R = \sqrt{R}\left(d_i E(t)\exp[j\omega_0 t] + \sum_{l \neq 0} \kappa_l E(t - t_l)\exp[j\omega_0(t - t_l)]\right) \qquad (32)$$

The received intensity is the square of the sum of these fields,

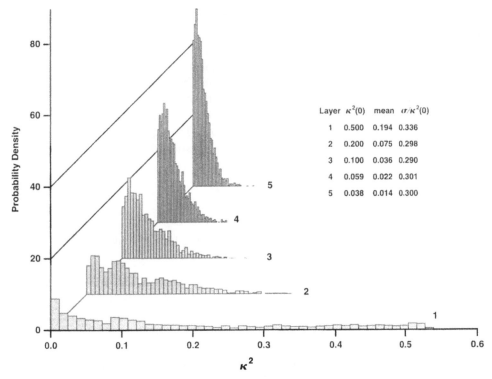

Layer	$\kappa^2(0)$	mean	$\sigma/\kappa^2(0)$
1	0.500	0.194	0.336
2	0.200	0.075	0.298
3	0.100	0.036	0.290
4	0.059	0.022	0.301
5	0.038	0.014	0.300

Figure 7 Histograms of reflective coupling coefficients with data present in defocused, interfering layers. Diagrams 1–5 show results for layers separated from the focal layer by 1–5 Rayleigh lengths. All the histograms have been normalized to have unit area. [Adapted from Ref. 11, Fig. 7.]

$$I = \left| E_{\text{ref}} + E_R \right|^2 = \left| E_{\text{ref}} \right|^2 + \left| E_R \right|^2 + E_{\text{ref}} E_R^* + E_{\text{ref}}^* E_R \tag{33}$$

Only the last two terms have components at the beat frequency,

$$I_\Omega = \exp[-j(\omega_0 + \Omega)t]\sqrt{R}\left(d_i E(t) E^*(t) \exp[j\omega_0 t] \right.$$
$$\left. + \sum_{l \neq 0} \kappa_l E(t - t_l) E^*(t) \exp[j\omega_0(t - t_l)] \right) + \text{c.c.} \tag{34}$$

giving the time-average heterodyne signal

$$\langle I_\Omega \rangle = \sqrt{R}\left\langle \left| E(t) \right|^2 \right\rangle \left(d_i + \sum_{l \neq 0} \kappa_l A(t_l) \exp[-j\omega_0 t_l] \right) \exp(-j\Omega t) + \text{c.c.} \tag{35}$$

In Eq. (35) we use the normalized coherence function, defined as

$$A(\tau) = \frac{\langle E(t) E^*(t - \tau) \rangle}{\left\langle \left| E(t) \right|^2 \right\rangle} \tag{36}$$

which is real and symmetrical in delay τ, with $A(0) = 1$. With an incoherent source, the value of the coherence function decreases for larger temporal displacements, corresponding to larger separations of the reflecting layers. All time averages are with respect to the field envelope function and have nothing to do with averaging over data. Because the exact optical phases of the reflections from each layer are presumed not to be known (i.e., each data layer location is not known to a fraction of a wavelength), we absorb these phase uncertainties into the phase of κ_l and treat κ_l as a real quality with magnitude $|\kappa_l|$ and uncertain phase ϕ_l.

For later comparison of OCT with DD, we take the square of this signal (finding the power at Ω, and dropping 2Ω terms). The squaring process is of no consequence in evaluating the signal-to-noise degradation due to cross-talk.

$$\frac{\langle I_\Omega \rangle^2}{2} = R\langle |E(t)|^2 \rangle^2 \left\{ d_i^2 + 2d_i \sum_{i \neq 0} A(t_l)\kappa_l \cos \phi_l \right.$$

$$\left. + \sum_{l \neq 0} \kappa_l^2 A^2(t_l) + 2 \sum_{l \neq 0} \sum_{m=l+1 \neq 0} \kappa_l \kappa_m A(t_l) A(t_m) \cos(\phi_l - \phi_m) \right\} \tag{37}$$

Within the braces of Eq. (37), the first term represents signal × signal, the second, signal × cross-talk, and the last two terms, cross-talk × cross-talk. Of the latter, the first comes from summation terms with $l = m$ and the second comes from summation terms with $l \neq m$. Both terms decrease with layer separation, as the coherence function becomes smaller.

To obtain the statistical behavior of this OCT signal (and later for DD), we first numerically generate ensembles for the reflection coefficients as described in the introduction to Section 14.4, with histograms (proportional to the probability density functions) shown in Fig. 7 for several values of layer separations. Note that because of symmetry, the five layers shown in Fig. 7 are sufficient to simulate cross-talk from a total of 10 layers, with five on either side of the data layer.

Once we have generated large ensembles of coupling coefficients (one ensemble for each layer separation), we pick a set of random phase angles, one for each cross-talk layer. The summations of Eq. (37) are then performed, using for the coupling parameters randomly selected members of the large ensembles of coupling coefficients. Using random selection from the ensembles is an alternative to creating and using approximations for the probability density functions. This procedure is repeated many times in a Monte Carlo simulation with $d_i = 0$ and 1 to generate an ensemble of values of the received signal for "0" and "1" data given by Eq. (37).

14.4.2 Direct Detection

The normalized signal received in a direct detection (DD) system is the intensity (magnitude squared of the field), giving

$$|E_R(t)|^2 = R\left\{ d_i^2 |E(t)|^2 + d_i \sum_{i \neq 0} [\kappa_l^* E(t) E^*(t - t_l) \exp(j\omega_0 t_l) + \kappa_l E^*(t) E(t - t_l) \right.$$

$$\left. \exp(-j\omega_0 t_l)] + \sum_{l \neq 0} \sum_{m \neq 0} \kappa_l^* \kappa_m E^*(t - t_l) E(t - t_m) \exp[j\omega_0(t_l - t_m)] \right\} \tag{38}$$

Taking the time average of this quantity gives

$$\left\langle |E_R(t)|^2 \right\rangle = R\left\langle |E(t)|^2 \right\rangle \left\{ d_i^2 + d_i \sum_{l \neq 0} A(t_l)[\kappa_l^* \exp(j\omega_0 t_l) + \kappa_l \exp(-j\omega_0 t_l)] \right.$$

$$\left. + \sum_{l \neq 0} \sum_{m \neq 0} \kappa_l^* \kappa_m A(t_l - t_m) \exp[j\omega_0(t_l - t_m)] \right\} \tag{39}$$

Equation (39) then becomes

$$\left\langle |E_R(t)|^2 \right\rangle = R\left\langle |E(t)|^2 \right\rangle \left\{ d_i^2 + 2d_i \sum_{l \neq 0} A(t_l)\kappa_l \cos\phi_l \right.$$

$$\left. + \sum_{l \neq 0} \kappa_l^2 + 2 \sum_{l \neq 0} \sum_{m=l+1 \neq 0} \kappa_l \kappa_m A(t_l - t_m) \cos(\phi_l - \phi_m) \right\} \tag{40}$$

In the cross-talk × cross-talk double-sum decomposition, the first sum with $l = m$ represents the sum of cross-talk powers from other layers. There is no coherence function reduction of this term, as in the OCT case. The second sum represents power from the coherent addition of the interlayer cross-talk fields and can be greatly reduced by using broadband sources. However, the coherence function appears only linearly, rather than quadratically as in OCT. The previous arguments about making the coupling coefficients real and using undetermined phase factors have been applied. The statistics of this signal are evaluated in the same way as in the OCT case. Note that there is a one-to-one correspondence of the terms within the braces for OCT and DD, but with significant differences between the details of the summation terms in the two cases.

14.4.3 Comparison of OCT and DD Cross-Talk

We now present a quantitative comparison of the evaluation of Eqs. (37) and (40). In the numerical evaluation of the signal distributions for OCT and DD we assume a Gaussian coherence function and use a modified spatial argument instead of a temporal argument, because propagation distance difference is proportional to time delay difference:

$$A(z) = \exp\left[-\left(\frac{z}{L_e}\right)^2\right] \tag{41}$$

The argument z is the distance from the data plane at the beam waist to any cross-talk layer. In this definition, the parameter L_e is the $1/e$ half-width of the scan coherence function. The spatial coherence function used here is the normalized envelope function of the interferometric photocurrent signal produced by scanning a reference mirror with respect to a fixed mirror. Its spatial argument is the scanning mirror displacement, which is half the round-trip difference between the signal and reference paths. By using the mirror displacement argument instead of the round-trip path difference, the depth of reflections from inside the signal medium are shown directly as arguments in the measured autocorrelation function (except for scaling from differences in index of refraction), and the spatial resolution of reflection sources is determined from Eq. (41). In these normalized numerical calculations, we do not include refractive index scaling, and we set $n = 1$ in both signal and reference paths. From definition (41), L_e can be related to the other standard definition of the coherence length used elsewhere in this volume. If the broadband source has a Gaussian frequency spectrum, the coherence function (with time argument) is the Fourier transform of the spectrum. After converting from time difference to path-length difference and using wavelength instead of frequency, the full width at half-maximum coherence length is inversely proportional to the spectral width:

$$L_C = \frac{(4 \ln 2)\lambda^2}{\pi \Delta\lambda} \tag{42}$$

where λ is the center wavelength and $\Delta\lambda$ is the spectral full width at half-maximum. Our $1/e$ scan parameter can be related to the coherence length [recalling that the z argument of Eq. (41) is twice the path difference] by $L_e = L_C/\sqrt{\ln 2} = 1.201 L_C$. The numerical evaluations are parameterized by dimensionless ratios of the layer thickness to Rayleigh range (L/L_r, where L_r is the same as the previously defined z_R), and layer thickness to $1/e$ scan parameter (L/L_e).

In Fig. 8 we compare the "0" and "1" signal distributions having cross-talk from five layers below and five above the desired data layer, with ratio $L/L_r = 1$ for different L/L_e coherence length ratios. The relative signal distributions are plotted as a function of normalized signal level, with the cross-talk free "0" signal having value 0 and "1" level having value 1. For OCT all cross-talk terms become small for sufficiently small coherence length, and we see significant "eye-opening" for $L/L_e \geq 1.5$ or $L/L_C \geq 1.8$. Since DD always has a residual cross-talk power term independent of coherence length, this particular example shows that no DD "eye-opening" between normalized "0" and "1" levels ever exists for layers so densely packed.

In a second example, shown in Fig. 9, the layer separation has been increased to $L/L_r = 2$, and the sum is over two interfering layers on either side of the data layer. Now the OCT method has good threshold discrimination for $L/L_e \geq 1$ or $L/L_C \geq 1.2$; that is, the correlation length can be slightly longer if the layer defocusing is increased. The DD method now also has an "eye-opening" at $L/L_e \geq 1$ ($L/L_C \geq 1.2$), but not as large as in the OCT case. What is significant for the DD case is that its performance can be improved by decreasing the coherence length such that $L_e < L/2$.

The analytical forms for the OCT and DD interlayer cross-talk [Eqs. (37) and (40)] show great similarity. The first two terms are identical, but the last two terms differ in their dependence of the coherence function. In the limit of very broad bandwidth sources, the coherence function approaches a delta function. In this limit, all the cross-talk terms of the OCT system vanish, and perfect bit decisions can be made. For the DD case, the residual randomly fluctuating powers detected from the interfering layers remain. If the layers are closely spaced with respect to a Rayleigh range, then the resulting cross-talk will be significant and cause bit errors. If the layers are more widely spaced (yielding poorer volume data density), then the geometric defocusing factors (included in the reflective coupling coefficients) will minimize the detected power from interfering (but out-of-focus) data layers, allowing reliable bit decisions. In general, shorter coherence lengths will allow DD systems to have significantly higher volume densities (closer layer spacing) up to a point where the layer spacing becomes comparable to a Rayleigh range (one or more interfering

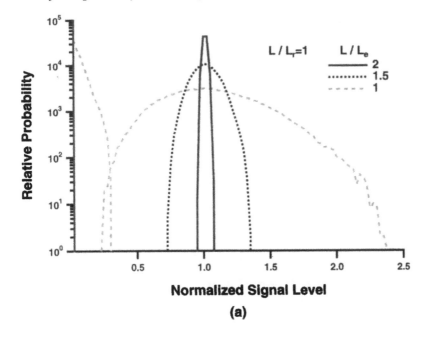

(a)

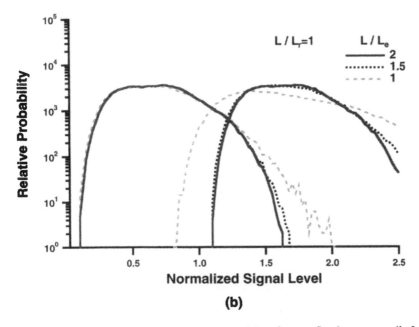

(b)

Figure 8 Relative probability densities arising from reflective cross-talk for "1" and "0" signal levels with five interfering data layers (thickness = one Rayleigh length) on either side of the focal layer. Results are shown for different ratios of layer separation to coherence length. (a) Results using OCT detection; (b) results using direct detection. Note that the "0" level OCT functions for $L/L_e = 1.5$ and 2 appear as delta functions overlapping the left-hand vertical axis in graph (a). [From Ref. 11, Fig. 8.]

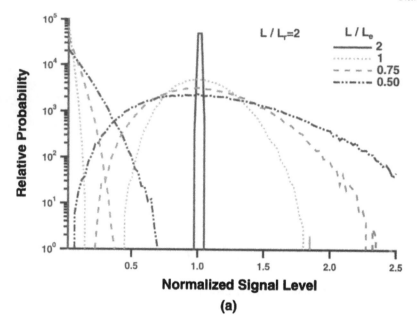

(a)

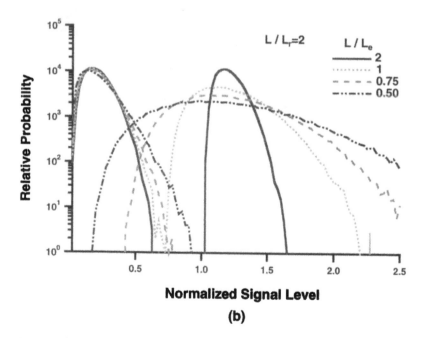

(b)

Figure 9   Relative probability densities arising from reflective cross-talk for "1" and "0" signal levels with two interfering data layers (thickness = two Rayleigh lengths) on either side of the focal layer. Results are shown for different ratios of layer separation to coherence length. (a) Results using OCT detection; (b) results using direct detection. Note that the "0" level OCT function for $L/L_e = 2$ appears as a delta function overlapping the left-hand vertical axis in (a). [From Ref. 11, Fig. 9.]

layers are within the focus). At that point, OCT systems can be used to achieve even higher volume density. OCT systems have the additional advantage of greater system receiver sensitivity, discussed below.

14.5 SYSTEM SENSITIVITY ISSUES

Signals from different layers will have some intrinsic differences in strength because of attenuation and distortion. In this section, we discuss these differences and their relation to system performance. We will compare parameters for an OCT system, a low power broadband DD system, and a more conventional higher power DD system. Typical parameters that will be used for the example calculations are a wavelength of 780 nm (photon energy $h\nu = 2.55 \times 10^{-19}$ J), track radius $r = 30$ mm, bit separation $\Delta l = 0.001$ mm ($1 \,\mu$m), and rotation speed $\Omega = 1800$ rpm. These factors combine to give a data rate

$$f_D = \frac{2\pi r}{\Delta l}\left(\frac{\Omega}{60}\right) = 5.7 \times 10^6 \,\text{bits/s}$$

The first case we consider is an OCT system with a broadband source having 1 mW total power equally divided between signal and reference beams. A heterodyne detection sensitivity of 100 photons/bit can be achieved for an uncorrected bit error rate (BER) of 10^{-9}. At the above data rate, this sensitivity corresponds to a minimum detectable power of $P_{\min} = 100 f_D h\nu = 1.45 \times 10^{-10}$ W. To allow for practical implementation losses and the diversion of some signal power for tracking considerations, $P_{\min}$ is derated by a factor of 10, giving a minimum detectable power of 1.45×10^{-9} W. This means that the smallest allowable reflectivity from a data layer is bounded by the ratio of the minimum detectable power to the input signal power, or $R_{\min} = (1.45 \times 10^{-9}\,\text{W})/(0.5 \times 10^{-3}\,\text{W}) = 2.9 \times 10^{-6}$. This corresponds to a minimum refractive index difference between layers of $\Delta n_{\min} \approx 2\bar{n}\sqrt{R_{\min}} \approx 5.3 \times 10^{-3}$ (at an average index of 1.57).

The optical power in the diffraction-limited mode of the signal beam will be attenuated by scattering and reflection as it passes through data layers. To limit signal strength variation with data layer depth, we impose a constraint that the nominal read signal not drop below 90% of its initial value from the first or top data layer. This ensures a nearly constant receiver eye-opening as different data layers are addressed, and reduces any need for automatic gain control. From the previous propagation analysis, we found that scattering introduces a loss factor of 1.85 times the Fresnel reflectivity. If we include this in a total effective reflectivity, then $R_{\text{eff}} = 2.85R$. The normalized read-field *amplitude* (appropriate for heterodyne detection, and not the intensity) after going back and forth through N data layers (traversing each of N layers twice) is $(1 - R_{\text{eff}})^N$, which we require to be greater than 0.9. In the limit of small R, this is equivalent to $NR_{\text{eff}} \leq -\ln(0.9) = 0.105$. Using the smallest allowable value of R from the detection limit, $R_{\min,\text{eff}} = 2.85 \times 2.9 \times 10^{-6} = 8.3 \times 10^{-6}$, which gives a maximum value for $N = 1.3 \times 10^4$. This bound establishes a limit on the number of layers in an OCT system solely from signal sensitivity and attenuation factors. Material uniformity problems may require the refractive index difference to be larger than the limit from detection sensitivity. Also, other practical engineering problems such as excessive total thickness and focusing aberration provide a much smaller limit.

As an example of a practical aberration problem, we have examined focal depth issues for a typical aspheric focusing lens of the type used in standard CD systems, with a numerical aperture of 0.55, at a wavelength of 780 nm, optical disk thickness of 1.2 mm, and polycarbonate disk refractive index of 1.57. The phase function at the lens pupil is calculated from the optical path difference as a function of ray angle from the focal spot at the design depth in the medium, 1.2 mm. This phase function is assumed to be flattened by the aspheric lens as it collimates the beam originating from the focus at the data layer. Conversely, the same phase function is imposed on the incident flat-phase collimated beam, to focus it at the required depth. Then with the surface of the medium translated with respect to the lens, a second phase function at the lens is recalculated from the rays originating at a new focal spot at a different depth in the medium. Because the focal depth is no longer at the optimal point in the medium for which the lens was designed, there is some residual spherical aberration, which is given by the difference in the two phase functions less an unimportant radially constant factor. The amount of the mode returning into the collimated beam is calculated by finding the overlap of the phase distortion, $\exp[j\Delta\Phi(r)]$, across the beam profile,

$$
\kappa_{\text{lens}} = \frac{2\pi \int_0^{r_{\text{max}}} |E(r)|^2 \exp(j\Delta\Phi) r \, dr}{\left\{ 2\pi \int_0^{r_{\text{max}}} |E(r)|^2 r \, dr \right\}}
$$

The magnitude of this complex coupling factor is squared to allow for the two-pass coupling of the beam into the diffraction-limited mode, as it couples to the focal spot on incidence and to the collimated beam on reflection. In the calculation, the focus displacement inside the disk was treated as the independent variable, and the lens-to-disk separation was adjusted slightly from the paraxial focal condition to minimize the rms phase deviation in the aperture (in a manner similar to using the "circle of least confusion" for aberrated foci). By doing this, a slight amount of defocus partially compensates for the spherical aberration. In Fig. 10 is plotted the two-pass field coupling $|\kappa_{\text{lens}}|^2$ as a function of interior layer offset from the design optimum. Also shown is the residual displacement of the disk to minimize the phase error. The formula above expresses the coupling for any mode shape (e.g., Gaussian). We have used a uniform beam intensity across the lens aperture, which gives a worst-case estimate, because high-angle phase distortion is weighted more heavily. For simple, fixed high numerical aperture lenses, the aberration-induced focal degradation may be the most stringent limit on the available depth of data storage. In more sophisticated systems, a multielement microzoom lens or compensating plate could be used to compensate for this aberration and greatly extend the available depth of storage [22]. In the above example, assuming a usable focal range of 0.2 mm, a layer separation of 20 μm would allow 10 layers with no optics compensation.

Next, we examine two cases of DD systems, the first with 1 mW power (using the same broadband source considered above) and a second with 10 mW power, such as a semiconductor laser. The laser will have much longer coherence length, leading to worse cross-talk problems. For a thermally limited DD receiver using a *pin* photodiode, a detector sensitivity is approximately 10,000 photons/bit. Quantum-limited direct detection can be achieved with low-noise optical amplifiers, but their expense probably precludes their use in the type of systems we envisage,

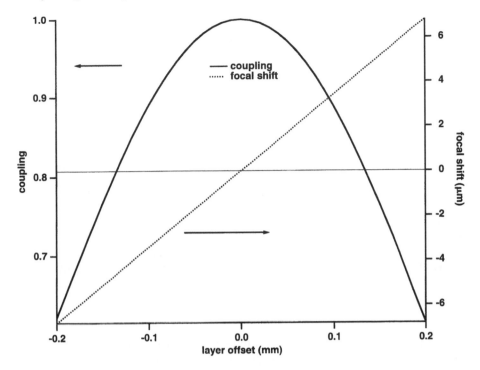

Figure 10 Aberration-induced OCT signal reduction (coupling) and optimized focal shift (right-hand axis) as a function of focal layer offset.

even if low excess noise can be achieved. At the previous bit rate, this sensitivity is equivalent to a minimum detectable power of 1.45×10^{-8} W, which is derated as above to 1.45×10^{-7} W. With the two DD input powers, the minimum Fresnel reflectivities required to achieve the detection limits are 1.45×10^{-4} and 1.45×10^{-5}, respectively. The read-field intensity after going back and forth through N data layers is $(1 - R_{\text{eff}})^{2N}$, which is also required to be greater than 0.9. Note the factor of 2 in the exponent, resulting from intensity, rather than amplitude, attenuation. In the limit of small R, this is equivalent to $NR_{\text{eff}} \leq -0.5 \times \ln(0.9) = 0.053$. Using the smallest values of R from the detection limits (1.45×10^{-4} and 1.45×10^{-5}),
$R_{\text{min,eff}} = 2.85 \times (1.45 \times 10^{-4}, 1.45 \times 10^{-5}) = (4.1 \times 10^{-4}, 4.1 \times 10^{-3})$ respectively, which gives maximum values for N of 1.3×10^2 (1 mW) and 1.3×10^3 (10 mW). These limits on allowable numbers of layers are two and one order(s) of magnitude less than that of the OCT system. All of the previous limit relations are summarized in Table 1.

In general, we note that an OCT system is about 100 times as sensitive as a DD system. In principle, this advantage can be used to achieve ~ 100 times as many layers for the same sensitivity or 100 times the sensitivity for the same number of layers. This sensitivity advantage may also enable the use of lower power sources, particularly in the blue spectral region where only limited power and lifetime have been demonstrated. More important, it is imperative to have low reflectivity per layer to achieve high volume density. Otherwise, the beam quality and point spread

Table 1 System Sensitivity Limits

Parameter	OCT (heterodyne) (incoherent)	Direct detection	
		Incoherent	Coherent
Input power P_{in}	0.5 mW	1 mW	10 mW
Min recd. power,	100 photons/bit	10,000 photons/bit	
P_{min} at 5.7 Mb/s	1.45×10^{-10} W	1.45×10^{-8} W	
Max attenuation,	2.9×10^{-7}	1.45×10^{-5}	1.45×10^{-6}
Min reflectivity:			
P_{min}/P_{in}	2.9×10^{-6}	1.45×10^{-4}	1.45×10^{-5}
(derated): R_{min}			
10% uniformity	$(1 - R_{eff})N \geq 0.9$	$(1 - R_{eff})^{2N} \geq 0.9$	
constraint ($u = 0.9$)			
($R_{eff} \sim 2.85R$)	$NR_{eff} \leq 0.105$	$NR_{eff} \leq 0.053$	
$N_{max} = -\ln u/2.85 R_{min}$	1.3×10^4	1.3×10^2	1.3×10^3

function will degrade from scattering, and interlayer reflective cross-talk will be high. OCT system sensitivity advantages can be used to accommodate these low distortion and cross-talk requirements for low reflectivity interfaces. Finally, as noted above, other practical considerations such as medium thickness and variable aberration at different focal depth may limit the number of layers. Here, too, the OCT method has the advantage of being able to use more closely spaced layers to maximize their number within a fixed depth range in systems where aberration compensation is not used.

14.6 EXPERIMENTAL RESULTS

14.6.1 Experimental Setup

As a first demonstration and verification of OCT and DD readout, we measured small-field images of a standard, single-layer CD-ROM and prototype multilayer disks. A diagram of the experimental apparatus is shown in Fig. 11. The broadband incoherent source is a fiber-coupled superluminescent LED emitting near 830 nm, whose spectrum is shown in Fig. 12a. The spectrum was measured using a commercial optical spectrum analyzer at its maximum resolution, 0.1 nm. Data from several adjacent spectral windows were acquired, stored, and concatenated to provide a large-bandwidth, high resolution spectrum required for accurate Fourier analysis. The coherence function of the source was measured with the apparatus described below by scanning the reference mirror position. The measured LED coherence function is shown in Fig. 12b, with an FWHM scan coherence length of 9.4 μm. There is good agreement between the experimentally measured coherence function and that obtained from the Fourier transform of the measured frequency spectrum. Because the measured scan distance is half the change in reference displacement, the usual coherence length is $2 \times 9.4 \, \mu$m $= 18.8 \, \mu$m. Using the definition of OCT resolution as half the usual coherence length, we see that our measured FWHM scan

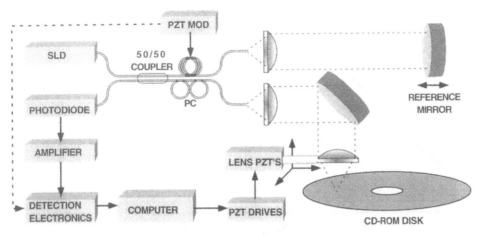

Figure 11 Schematic diagram of version 1 of experimental apparatus for OCT measurements of optical disk, using fiber phase modulation. For direct detection measurements the reference beam is blocked and the signal beam is chopped (intensity modulated). [Adapted from Ref. 11, Fig. 10.]

coherence length is also the OCT resolution. If the spectrum were a pure Gaussian with the same width, the coherence length [from Eq. (42)] would be 24.3 μm. Note that the peak-to-baseline ratio of the correlation function is limited by the broadband spectral shape (particularly its exponential-like tails). This point is discussed in more detail in Ref. 23.

This broadband source is coupled to a single-mode fiber, with a 50/50 fiber coupler serving as the interferometric beamsplitter. In one version of the apparatus, after the splitter the fiber in the reference path is wrapped around a cylindrical piezoelectric (PZ) element that provides phase modulation. The bias to the PZ element is a sawtooth, serrodyne waveform that gives a total linear 2π phase shift per cycle, thereby providing an approximately sinusoidal heterodyne signal at the modulation frequency (except for the brief retrace interval). The reference beam is collimated in free space and retroreflected from a planar reference mirror back into the collimating lens and reference arm fiber. The beam from the signal path fiber is similarly collimated and focused onto the CD-ROM using a standard CD focus objective. The signal is reflected from the CD back into the signal fiber. Spatially recombined signal and reference beams from the fiber coupler exit both ports of the coupler, with one of them leading to a photodiode detector, followed by a transimpendance amplifier. A fiber polarization controller in the signal fiber is used to align the reflected signal and reference polarizations in the detection path to maximize the heterodyne signal. The heterodyne photocurrent signal (at the modulation frequency) is bandpass filtered and detected. The CD objective lens is mounted on an x-y-z translation stage with piezoelectric fine x,y positioners on the attached low-mass lens mount. The z axis (focus) position is controlled by a computer-interfaced stepper motor with 0.1 μm resolution. A two-dimensional image of the CD is created by scanning the lens in a computer-generated rasterlike x,y pattern using the piezoelectric translator while recording the heterodyne signal. A computer data acquisition system is used to control the two-dimensional lens scan and the data A/D conversion, storage, and display. To acquire the DD output, the optical refer-

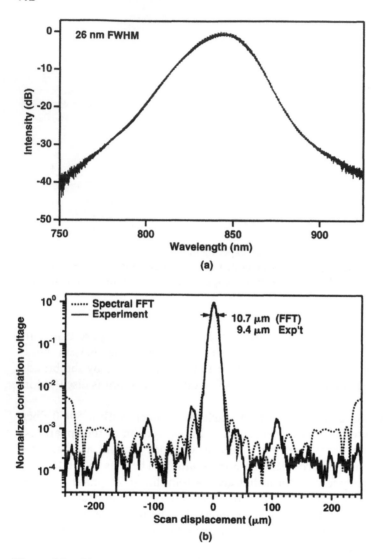

Figure 12 Characteristics of the broadband superluminescent diode used in measurements. (a) The measured optical spectrum. (b) The measured correlation function compared with the Fourier transform of the measured frequency spectrum. [From Ref. 11, Fig. 11.]

ence path is blocked, and the beam in the free-space part of the signal path is detected at base band.

In a second version of the apparatus (shown in Fig. 13), designed to provide a higher modulation frequency and allow faster data acquisition, heterodyne detection was implemented by frequency shifting the reference beam in a fused silica acousto-optic modulator instead of phase-modulating the beam in the optical fiber. The rf drive was at 40 MHz, and double-pass propagation through the modulator imposed an 80 MHz frequency offset on the optical reference. An identical fused silica modulator device (not shown) was placed in the signal path. This device has no rf excitation applied but was used solely to provide dispersion compensation for the

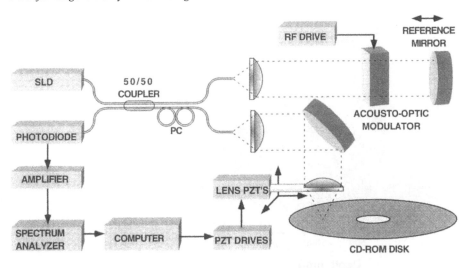

Figure 13 Schematic diagram of version 2 of experimental apparatus for OCT measurements of optical disk, using acousto-optic frequency shifting of reference beam. For direct detection measurements the reference beam is blocked, the signal beam is chopped (intensity modulated), and different detection amplification is used (without the spectrum analyzer).

active modulator so as not to spread the measured coherence function and decrease the depth resolution. The heterodyne signal from the photodiode was fed into an rf spectrum analyzer with sweep frequency fixed at 80 MHz, which provided a baseband signal proportional to the heterodyne rf power from the photodiode.

14.6.2 Multilayer Sandwich

First, to demonstrate the OCT system capability and sensitivity for samples with low interface reflectivity and many layers, we performed a simple multilayer measurement. Using the first apparatus described above, a layered sample was prepared by sandwiching three layers of glycerol between four glass microscope cover slips (nominal 0.009 in. thickness). The Fresnel reflectivity at each glass/glycerol interface is about 0.001. In this instance, a weakly focused beam was used in the sample arm. Figure 14 shows the OCT heterodyne photocurrent signal versus depth and one-dimensional lateral displacement for this multilayer sample, with each peak representing an interface reflection. There is excellent signal-to-noise (greater than 50 dB power) and contrast for the weak reflections. A gray-scale projection of the logarithmic signal is also shown in the lower plane of the figure. As expected, the reflections from the two exterior glass/air interfaces are stronger than those from the interior. Note that this figure shows data on a logarithmic (dB) scale, to emphasize the sensitivity to weak reflections. Later data displays of CD-ROM images will have linear scales.

14.6.3 Conventional CD-ROM

Using the first version of the apparatus, a typical display of the OCT image from a standard single-layer CD-ROM is shown in Fig. 15a, and the DD display of the same region, taken immediately after, is shown in Fig. 15b. The images are shown

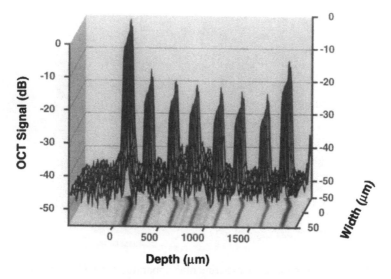

Figure 14 Measured reflectivity profile of a multilayer glass/glycerol structure, scanned in depth and one lateral dimension. The bottom image is a gray-scale projection of the data using the same logarithmic gray scale as the vertical display. [Adapted from Ref. 11, Fig. 13.]

with false-color gray scales ,with signal levels indicated in the corresponding gray-scale bars for each image. To compare the image contrasts more readily, we took the square of the OCT signal before creating its image, as was done mathematically in Eq. (37). The quality of the two images is very similar, as is expected for this relatively simple case of a single data layer. This demonstration [10] was the first to show the feasibility of detecting good CD-ROM signals using either OCT or DD with a low power broadband incoherent source.

14.6.4 Multilayer CD-ROMS

Prototype samples of multilayer CD-ROM media were provided for analysis by the Optical Technology Center of Imation Corporation (formerly part of the 3M Company). These prototypes had conventional CD-ROM exterior dimensions and form. The first two samples had two data layers each, one with 49 μm layer separation (sample 1) and the other with 11 μm separation (sample 2). Recall that the layer separation for a DVD is 30–55 μm. These samples were measured with the rf acousto-optic spectral shift apparatus, enabling image scans to be acquired in 1–2 s (depending on field size and scan resolution). Another experimental feature that was implemented for the multilayer samples was automatic tracking of the reference mirror position with change in stepper motor position of the focusing lens, allowing for the effects on the optical path length of the index of refraction of the disk medium.

Representative gray-scale images for samples 1 and 2 are shown in Figs. 16 and 17, where the OCT images are shown on the left and the DD images are shown on the right. For easy comparison, the gray-scale ranges are autoscaled for each image. To study the amount of cross-talk that might not be visible by eye, we analyzed the OCT images of sample 2, with the smallest layer separation of all the samples. First, two-dimensional autocorrelations of the images from each of the layers were calcu-

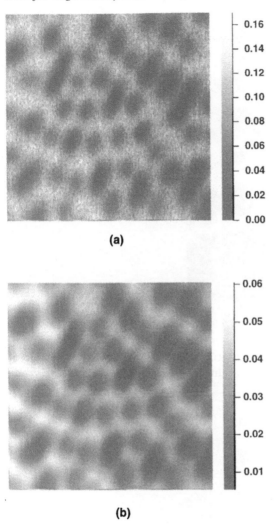

(a)

(b)

Figure 15 Measured images of a single-layer CD-ROM taken using (a) OCT and (b) direct detection. The signal for the OCT image was squared, in accordance with Eq. (34), to provide a direct contrast comparison with image (b). [From Ref. 10, Fig. 4.]

lated, using a Fourier transform method. Then the cross-correlation of these two image signals was performed. All three correlation functions are shown as intensity/gray-scale surfaces in Fig. 18. The autocorrelations each show a strong peak at zero displacement, with lower background coming from the statistical correlation of random data with themselves. Note the periodicity of the background perpendicular to the track direction and low, randomly varying amplitudes along the tracks. The cross-correlation image shows no increased level at the zero-displacement origin, indicating little interference of the signals between the two layers.

A three-layer CD-ROM with layer separations of 20 and 26 μm was measured with the same method as above. The results of the OCT and DD measurements are shown in Fig. 19, where the images are shown in stacked perspective views for a

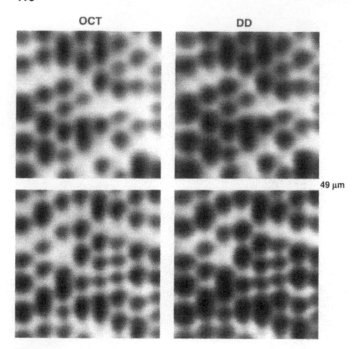

Figure 16 Measured images of a two-layer CD-ROM disk (sample 1) with 49 μm layer separation using OCT (left) and direct detection (right). The images from the two layers are in the upper and lower portions of the figure.

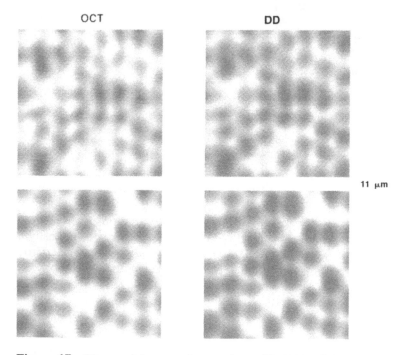

Figure 17 Measured images of a two-layer CD-ROM disk (sample 2) with 11 μm layer separation using OCT (left) and direct detection (right). The images from the two layers are in the upper and lower portions of the figure.

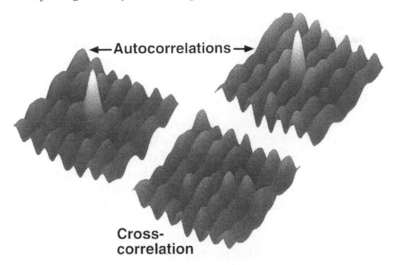

Figure 18 OCT image correlations for data of Fig. 17 (11 μm layer separation). The upper images represent autocorrelation of each layer, and the lower image represents the cross-correlation of the signals from the two layers.

better appreciation of the geometry. As before, the gray scales are determined by the minimum-to-maximum spans of each image.

For all of the multilayer samples, the layer reflectivities were determined by proprietary internal coatings so as to provide large signal levels for the relatively small number of layers. In these instances, the OCT and DD methods provided similar signal quality. We did observe, however, that optimizing the focal conditions with the OCT method was somewhat easier, because the signals in the out-of-focus

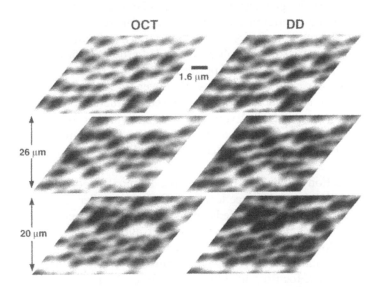

Figure 19 Measured images of a three-layer CD-ROM disk with 26 μm and 20 μm layer separations using OCT (left) and direct detection (right). The gray-scale images from the three layers are stacked vertically above each other.

condition were smaller. Also, the expected quality of the DD signals would degrade more quickly than that of the OCT, as the layer number increases and the data layer reflectivities decrease.

14.7 SUMMARY AND CONCLUSIONS

Optical coherence tomography is a potentially valuable tool for increasing the data storage capacity in optical disks. The high detection sensitivity of OCT permits a low reflectivity at each data interface, which is a prerequisite for extending high transmission of the readout beam to many layers, with minimal beam distortion. This feature combined with the increased depth resolution of OCT should allow optical readout of many closely spaced data layers with technology that is an evolution of today's CD implementations.

Although the discussion here has used disks as an example, it also pertains to other optical media such as tape or cards. Also, the data format can take forms other than the optical phase pit we have discussed. For example, data stored as small regions of material phase change (reflectivity) would be usable as long as transmission through the data layer does not severely distort the beam. Data encoding with more than one bit of information (reflectivity level) per bit region could be accommodated by OCT. Such m-ary storage is another potentially important growth area for optical storage and matches the capabilities of OCT very well. This is because m storage symbols will produce more closely spaced signals than binary levels. The smaller signal separation will therefore be less affected by cross-talk and scattering, which should be reduced in an OCT system.

Even without using the interferometric aspect of OCT, broadband sources with direct detection reduce coherent fluctuations among cross-talk signals from different layers. These fluctuations result from interferometric addition of the fields from nonselected layers, albeit reduced by geometric defocusing. The greater the coherence of the source, the larger the interference effects become. Fluctuations in this cross-talk arise mainly from the random nature of the data patterns affecting reflections. Although these fluctuating parts of the coherently added cross-talk fields can become small, in DD there are always cross-talk power fluctuations from the individual layers. For data-free planar layers, each cross-talk power would be constant, so the cross-talk variation in the low coherence limit is caused by fluctuations from the nonselected data patterns or uncontrolled variation in layer separations on the order of optical wavelengths. Our analysis also showed that reflective interlayer cross-talk is likely to be a more severe problem than beam quality degradation on transmission through many layers.

OCT's range discrimination allows, in principle, the elimination of all the cross-talk power fluctuations. With a coherence length sufficiently smaller than the layer separation, only the field reflected from the layer matching the reference path will be detected. In addition, the heterodyne behavior of OCT allows greater sensitivity, which ultimately can allow more layers with smaller separations.

Ultimately, the maximum number of layers may be limited by system engineering factors. As we have discussed, focusing at different layers in the medium may cause varying focal spot spherical aberration. For large ranges of focal depth, this may be alleviated with dynamic optical compensation, but at the cost of increased system complexity. OCT offers an advantage for this problem, in that it allows a given number of layers to be stored in a smaller thickness. This reduced range of focus may eliminate the need for any spherical aberration compensation. In an OCT system, dynamic tracking of the reference mirror as well as the focal depth will be required, as well as the usual lateral signal tracking. Both reference and focus tracking problems will become more difficult with smaller layer separations. These reduced separations will also impose tighter manufacturing tolerances and possibly require the development of new multilayer disk fabrication procedures for mass production. It may also prove advantageous to incorporate formatting information that identifies each disk layer.

We have presumed the existence of multilayer media and have discussed only the detection aspect of the system. In their simplest form, such disks could be replicated in a process similar to stamping conventional CDs, with sequential layers of alternating materials (having slightly different refractive indices) being deposited and stamped by different master disks.* The use of multilayer optical writing (or erasing) techniques such as those employed in single-layer phase-change or magneto-optical disks presents a much more difficult problem. The need to selectively alter data at a restricted depth in the medium would probably require a highly nonlinear absorption mechanism that will affect the medium only at the writing beam's tightest focus or at the intersection of two different writing beams. Using two writing beams with either short pulse or low coherence could also allow better depth discrimination for the power deposition. For the present, we believe that OCT multilayer disk systems will be best suited to storage applications requiring widely distributed, very large amounts of permanently stored (read-only) data.

We have provided experimental demonstrations of CD-ROM imaging using OCT for one-, two-, and three-layer optical disks. In the course of our investigation, we have also found advantages of broadband incoherent sources for direct detection. Future evaluation of multilayer disks should show the superiority of OCT for read-out of large numbers of densely spaced optical layers.

For this technology to become widely adapted, there are two aspects that must be commercially developed, the media (multilayer CD disks) and the reading instrument (multilayer CD player). Imation Corporation (3M) has fabricated multilayer CD prototypes whose data we have presented, although the disks were not designed or optimized for our technology. With this demonstration of media technology in hand, we see no barriers to fabrication of optimized disks with more layers. The OCT CD player would share most of its technology with existing players, and the addition of the interferometric components and the replacement of the laser by a superluminescent LED ought to be straightforward. Because there are no apparent technological barriers, the main factor in determining implementation will be market forces: Is there a demand for this type of high density CD storage that can justify the further development costs? Some candidate applications may suggest an answer to this: (1) archival storage of imagery (medical, satellite), (2) archival storage of data (e.g., financial records), and (3) mass market entertainment (multiple movies). The advantage of the multilayer technology would be to reduce the number of CDs required and improve the access time over the stored data. Another critical issue is whether a group or consortium of companies could agree on common standards

---

*One concise pictorial description of this process for the two-layer DVD is given in the technical note, "Plain Talk: Dual-Layer Compact Disk," 80-9550-2253-0(85.75)ii, ©3M Company, June 1995.

for multilayer media and players. Such standardization was done in CD and DVD development, and it should be possible in this case once the commitment is made to the OCT data storage technology.

REFERENCES

1. Asthana P, Finkelstein B. Superdense optical storage. IEEE Spectrum 32:25–31, 1995.
2. Lenth B. Optical storage: A growing mass market for lasers. Laser Focus World 30:87–91, 1994.
3. Lubell PD. The gathering storm in high-density compact disks. IEEE Spectrum 32:32–37, 1995.
4. Rubin KA, Rosen HJ, Tang WW, Imaino W, Strand TC. Multilevel volumetric optical storage. SPIE 2338:247–253, 1994.
5. Rosen HJ, Rubin KA, Tang WC, Imaino WI. Multilayer optical recording (MORE). SPIE 2514:14–19, 1995.
6. Immink KAS. Digital versatile disk (DVD). IEE Colloq on New High Capacity Digital Media and Their Applications (Ref. No. 1997/114), IEE, 1997:1/1–6.
7. Wijn JM, Alink RBJM. Digital video disc mastering. SPIE 2931:160–171, 1996.
8. Koop H, Priess K. Mastering and manufacturing of high density optical discs. SPIE 2931:120–124, 1996.
9. Swanson EA, Chinn SR. Apparatus and method for accessing data on multilayered optical media. U.S. Patent 5,784,352 (July 21, 1998).
10. Chinn SR, Swanson EA. Multilayer optical storage by low-coherence reflectometry. Opt Lett 21:899–901, 1996.
11. Chinn SR, Swanson EA. Multi-layer optical readout using direct or interferometric detection and broad-bandwidth light sources. Opt Memory Neural Networks 5:197–218, 1996.
12. Youngquist RC, Carr S, Davies DEN. Optical coherence-domain reflectometry: A new optical evaluation technique. Opt Lett 12:158–160, 1987.
13. Gilgen HH, Novak RP, Salathe RP, Hodel W, Beaud P. Submillimeter optical reflectometry. J Lightwave Technol 7:1225–1233, 1989.
14. Takada K, Himeno A, Yukimatsu K. High sensitivity and submillimeter resolution optical time-domain reflectometry based on low-coherence interference. J Lightwave Technol 10:1998–2005, 1992.
15. Swanson EA, Huang D, Hee MR, Fujimoto JG, Lin CP, Puliafito CA. High-speed optical coherence domain reflectometry. Opt Lett 17:151–153, 1992.
16. Swanson EA, Izatt JA, Hee MR, Huang D, Lin CP, Schuman JS, Puliafito CA, Fujimoto JG. In vivo retinal imaging by optical coherence tomography. Opt Lett 18:1864–1866, 1993.
17. Swanson EA, Chinn SR. Apparatus and methods for reading multilayer storage media using short coherence length sources. U.S. Patent 5,748,598 (May 5, 1998).
18. Lee BS, Strand TC. Profilometry with a coherence scanning microscope. Appl Opt 29:3784–3788, 1990.
19. Milster TD. New way to describe diffraction from optical disks. Appl Opt 37:6878–6883, 1998.
20. Yeh W-H, Li L, Mansuripur M. Vector diffraction and polarization effects in an optical disk system. Appl Opt 37:6983–6988, 1998.
21. Fleck JA, Morris JR, Feit MD. Time-dependent propagation of high energy laser beams through the atmosphere. Appl Phys 10:129–160, 1976.
22. Milster TD, Upton RS, Luo H. Objective lens design for multiple-layer optical data storage. SPIE 3109:142–149, 1997.
23. Chinn SR, Swanson EA. Blindness limitations in optical coherence domain reflectometry. Electron Lett 29:2025–2027, 1993.

15

Applications of Optical Coherence Tomography to the Study of Polymer Matrix Composites

JOY P. DUNKERS

National Institute of Standards and Technology, Gaithersburg, Maryland

15.1 INTRODUCTION

The use of optical coherence tomography (OCT) to study polymer matrix composites (PMCs) is very recent. So recent, in fact, that the full potential and limitations of this technique have yet to be studied completely, because PMCs are a large and varied class of materials. At the onset of this program, OCT was pursued as a technique to nondestructively study PMCs because it offered a combination of spatial resolution and depth of penetration that was not otherwise available. Research efforts have been focused thus far on fiberglass-reinforced composites, although some work has been done on Kevlar.* A comparison of OCT and more traditional nondestructive evaluation (NDE) techniques in the area of PMCs is provided later in this chapter. The discussion will focus on OCT as an NDE tool for microstructural and defect characterization and damage assessment. Because this chapter is a departure from the rest of this book, an introduction to PMCs to provide background and direction is given in the following section.

---

* Identification of a commercial product is made only to facilitate experimental reproducibility to adequately describe experimental procedure. In no case does it imply endorsement by NIST or imply that it is necessarily the best product for the experimental procedure.

15.2 POLYMER MATRIX COMPOSITES

Polymer matrix composites (PMCs) are heterogeneous materials consisting of, in general, a polymer matrix and reinforcing fibers. The fibers provide the load-bearing capability and are generally classified as either inorganic, with glass being the largest category, or organic. Carbon fibers are the most common type of organic reinforcement, but polymeric fibers such as Kevlar are also widely used. Initially, the discussion will be focused on both carbon and glass. Then, the bulk of the discussion will shift to glass reinforcement because OCT cannot image carbon fiber reinforced composites. Since carbon strongly absorbs visible and near-infrared light. The selection of fibers influences the following properties of the PMC: specific gravity, tensile strength and modulus, compressive strength and modulus, fatigue strength, electrical and thermal conductivities, and cost. The reinforcement can exist as short fibers that range from several hundred micrometers long to many millimeters in length or as continuous fibers that are meters long. Continuous fibers can be woven into two- or three-dimensional fabrics, depending on the load-bearing requirements. An example of an application that has load-bearing requirements is the use of glass-reinforced PMC in bridges for decks, reinforcing bars, tendons, cables, beams, columns, and paneling [1]. Figure 1 shows a bridge erected in Scotland with composite cables, towers, and deck [1].

The polymer matrix aids in forming the fibers into a final structure, contributes toughness to the composite by transferring loads between fibers, and protects the fibers from chemical and physical degradation. The choice of matrix material depends upon the desired end-use properties such as adhesion to the fibers, modulus, shrinkage, thermal stability, corrosion resistance, and specific chemical resistance. The matrix for a composite can be thermoplastic or thermoset. A thermoplastic matrix is a fully reacted polymer of several thousand repeat units that can repeatedly be heated and reshaped. In contrast, a thermoset matrix begins as small molecules and reacts during fabrication to form a cross-linked network with virtually infinite molecular mass. This solid is permanent and cannot be reshaped upon heating, but it is more resistant to attack by organic fluid. Composites are usually designed so that fibers carry the loads, leaving the matrix to play a secondary role. The matrix provides resistance to buckling of fibers loaded in compression and transfers load between fibers and around fiber breaks when they are in tension. Even the best designs, however, cannot always avoid loads in directions not dominated by fibers. One example is delamination, where loads perpendicular to the fiber layers cause the layers to separate. For such cases, the properties of the matrix are very important. More basic information about polymer science and technology is available elsewhere [2]. In this chapter, the composites of interest consist of a thermoset matrix and continuous glass fibers.

The fiber/matrix interface region, frequently called the interphase, is also important to composite performance. This region contains interactions, both chemical and physical, between the fibers and the matrix. The quality of the interphase has a substantial effect on the lifetime of the PMC. A good interphase, or interaction, is desired and will efficiently transfer load between fibers and support loads transverse to the fibers. A poor interphase may result in premature failure of the composite. Surface treatment of the fibers promotes adhesion between the fibers and matrix by depositing or generating molecules at the fiber surface [3]. These molecules

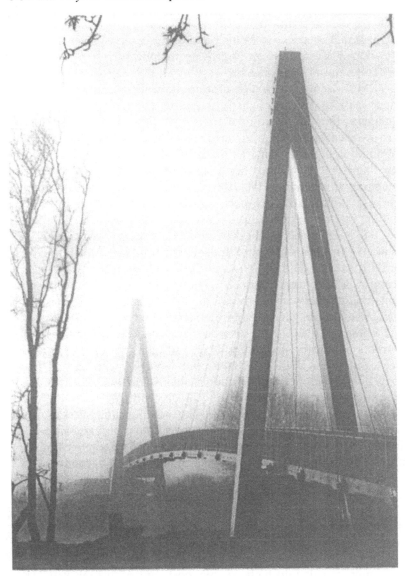

Figure 1 Composite cables, decks, and towers at the Aberfeldy Bridge, Scotland.

wet and may even react with the fiber surface at the same time as they become entangled with or react with the matrix.

There are several reasons why polymer matrix composites are used over more traditional materials such as metal and wood. The biggest advantages are their high strength-to-mass and modulus-to-mass ratios and design flexibility. Other advantages are longer lifetime, mechanical damping, and controllable thermal and electrical conductivity. The biggest disadvantages include the high cost of raw materials and manufacturing, low toughness, environmental degradation, and the lack of standards for testing and long-term performance. Although recycling is an issue in certain applications, the use of recycled PMC as filler in new parts is being implemented [4]. Probably the biggest hurdle that inhibits the breakthrough of composites into high volume, commercial markets is the high cost of the composite which can be brought down by reducing waste through improving manufacturing methods and quality control. OCT can aid in this endeavor.

Traditionally, PMCs were used in high cost applications such as commercial military aircraft and weapons, where weight is of greater concern than cost. Some specific PMC components that have been used are wings, rotors, tails, rudders, fins, and ailerons [5]. In a recent application, a business jet fuselage was built with a carbon fiber honeycomb composite that was made in only two pieces. This PMC fuselage weighs less than 1000 lb and provides more cabin space because of reduced wall thickness compared to aluminum [6]. PMCs are not simply limited to high performance, high cost aircraft and aerospace applications. They have expanded into the transportation, marine, infrastructure, construction, and consumer markets.

For example, the body panels of the Chevrolet Corvette are made of glass-reinforced composites [7]. In 1996, a nylon 6,6 and glass fiber air intake manifold was introduced on the Ford Mustang V8 [8]. Now, all General Motors air intake mani-folds and fuel injector rails are glass-reinforced nylon 6,6. Spoolable composite pipe and tubing products constructed with thermoplastic liners for corrosion resistance and pressure containment are being installed into North Sea oil wells [9]. In addition to motorboats and sailboats, PMCs have also been used in seawalls, pilings, and docks. In the construction industry, decking, roofing, and walkways have been made with PMC. Bridge columns in California have been wrapped with carbon fiber embedded in epoxy to provide additional support against earthquakes [10]. The first composite-reinforced concrete deck on a vehicular bridge was built over Buffalo Creek in McKinleyville, West Virginia [11]. The incorporation of composites in the consumer industry is found mainly in sporting goods and is best known in golf club shafts and fishing rods. Tennis rackets made with carbon fiber composites have the rigidity required to produce a more accurate shot than traditional wood rackets. Stiff composite frames on bicycles prevent twisting on rugged terrain while still affording weight savings, and carbon fiber skis and ski poles are also entering the market [12].

With all of the aforementioned examples of applications of PMCs, why the interest in the nondestructive evaluation of these materials? Although composites have demonstrated superior performance in many applications, their high cost pre-vents them from gaining inroads into high volume, cost-competitive markets. The major obstacle in cutting the cost of PMC lies in increasing the speed of the man-ufacturing process while maintaining or increasing the quality of the resulting com-posite part. This is where NDE plays a role in cutting costs.

The final properties of a composite are highly dependent upon, among other variables, microstructure and defects. Microstructure is defined as any physical characteristic within the PMC that can be identified with some regularity. Defects are physical characteristics that are not planned and prevent the composite from achieving optimal properties. For example, the size and shape of glass tows are considered microstructural characteristics. How the layers of glass orient themselves when the mold is closed is also considered microstructure. Any microscopic or macroscopic void in the reinforcement is considered a defect. Wrinkling of the reinforcement in the final part is considered a defect. Microstructure and defects are highly influenced by the manufacturing or processing of the PMC. For example, in fabrication by resin transfer molding, where the reinforcing fibers are placed in a mold and the matrix resin is then injected, the number, size, and mechanism of voids formed were found to be dependent upon the reinforcement type and injection pressure [13]. The effects of voids on shear, tensile, and flexural strengths have been the subject of much study [14–16]. The final composite properties are heavily, although not solely, dictated by the microstructure and defects. The need for a microstructure and defect characterization tool led to the exploration of OCT of composites.

15.3 NONDESTRUCTIVE EVALUATION OF PMCS

Optical coherence tomography has some advantages and disadvantages over conventional NDE techniques. This discussion of NDE is limited to those techniques that are mainstream or similar to OCT. An analogous optical technique used widely in the biological community is confocal optical microscopy. There is very limited information in the literature about confocal optical microscopy of PMCs [17]. The most likely explanation for this is that the highly scattering nature of composites makes an appreciable depth of field impossible with confocal microscopy. It has already been demonstrated that the resolution, depth of field, and dynamic range of OCT are far superior to those of confocal optical microscopy [18].

Ultrasonic imaging is a good method to compare with OCT because ultrasound is a major NDE technique. Both transducer- and laser-based ultrasonics have been used on composites, although measurements with a transducer are complicated by the requirement of a coupling material between the transducer and composite. The practical resolution of ultrasonics is on the order of hundreds of micrometers with tens of millimeters penetration depth [19,20]. Ultrasound imaging is primarily used to observe defects and works best with planar samples [19]. A major drawback to ultrasonics is that the depth of a feature must be determined by model studies, whereas it is known precisely when OCT is used. Both OCT and ultrasonics suffer from contrast degradation and shadowing through the sample thickness. However, ultrasound can successfully image voids and damage in carbon fiber reinforced composites whereas OCT cannot.

X-ray-based techniques are used extensively to evaluate damage and have been applied less frequently to the examination of voiding and tow placement. Composite damage has been studied with X-ray radiography [21,22]. All X-ray techniques rely on the contrast generated by the differences in the attenuation of the X-ray beam to differentiate heterogeneity from undisturbed material. Unlike ultrasound, this technique is a non-contact one. However, it may be necessary to use a dye tracer to provide contrast between the damage zones and the rest of the composite. Also, superposition of features can confound interpretation with this conventional film radiography. A more recent technique, X-ray computed tomography (CT), relies on the measurement of transmitted radiation from many angles to reconstruct an image of the composite [23]. X-ray CT can be used to detect various heterogeneities such as resin and fiber distribution, anisotropic fiber structure, voiding, and porosity as well as damage events. The X-ray transmission is limited by the density, size, and atomic number of the material and the X-ray source available. Perhaps the biggest drawback is the spatial resolution, which is typically 500 μm. With specialized sources and detectors, the spatial resolution can approach a few tens of micrometers with objects tens of millimeters in maximum dimensions at great cost [23].

Nuclear magnetic resonance (NMR) imaging has been performed on composites with some success [24] but has one major drawback. Imaging of glassy polymers such as epoxy is very difficult because of the very long spin–lattice relaxation time (T_1) that leads to line broadening and a very short spin–spin relaxation time (T_2) that cannot be detected with current electronics. Thus, samples are usually imbibed with a liquid, and it is the relaxations of the liquid that are monitored. The spatial resolution is comparable to that of OCT, reportedly down to $10\,\mu m$ [25]. In addition, carbon fiber composites can be imaged in the majority of cases, except where the plane of the laminate sheets is perpendicular to the radio-frequency (rf) field, because the conductive sheets screen the rf field within the coil [26]. But as with ultrasound, voids and other defects are usually imaged instead of microstructure.

15.4   OCT INSTRUMENTATION

The imaging system used for the experimental work described in this chapter is from the laboratory of Professor James Fujimoto at the Massachusetts Institute of Technology, Cambridge, MA, and is shown schematically in Fig. 2 [27]. A commercial superluminescent light source was used. The source operated at $1.3\,\mu m$ with an output power of up to 15 mW and a spectral bandwidth of 40 nm, corresponding to an axial spatial resolution of $\approx 20\,\mu m$. The laser light was coupled into a single-mode fiber-optic Michelson interferometer and delivered to both the reference mirror and the sample. The reference mirror was mounted on a rotating galvanometer, which was driven with a sawtooth voltage waveform. Transverse scanning was performed using a computer-controlled motorized stage to translate the sample.

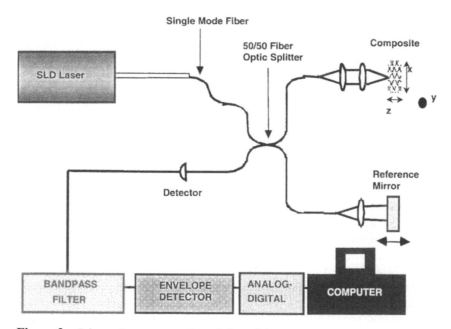

Figure 2   Schematic representation of the solid-state laser and OCT system layout.

The interferometric signal was electronically filtered with a bandpass centered on the fringe or heterodyne frequency. The filtered fringe waveform was then demodulated, digitized, and stored on a computer. The high dynamic range of this system allowed backreflections as low as femtowatts to be detected. Images were displayed by mapping the logarithm of the signal strength to a gray-scale look-up table. The acquisition time for each image was approximate 1 min. The axial (z) measurement range was determined by the distance moved by the reference mirror (4.5 mm) normalized by the refractive index (n) of the sample: 4.5 mm/n. For the epoxy matrix samples discussed here, the refractive index was 1.55. For the vinyl ester matrix sample, the refractive index was 1.55 for the low void sample and 1.46 for the high void sample. The probe beam was focused to a 30 μm diameter spot at a depth of approximately 750–1000 μm below the surface of the sample. For the images presented here, 1.5–2 mm depth can be resolved with good contrast. More recent work indicates that at least 4 mm can be resolved in these samples.

The OCT images were taken for both the epoxy and vinyl ester matrix composites with the fibers oriented perpendicular to the laser as shown in Fig. 3 [28]. For any position along the x axis, reflections that represent heterogeneities are collected as a function of z. The sample is then moved with a motorized stage to image a new x, z slice of the composite, and this process is repeated for various positions along the fiber, or y axis. The transverse resolution along the x axis is estimated to be 40 μm. The transverse resolution is governed by spot size and scan rate: There is an inverse relationship between transverse resolution and sampling depth. The axial resolution along the z axis is 20 μm. The images typically contained 300 × 450 or 350 × 450 pixels. All samples were tilted 4° to avoid collection of the laser reflection from the top surface.

15.5 OCT OF POLYMER MATRIX COMPOSITES

15.5.1 Imaging of Microstructure and Defects

The following discussion focuses on some of the very first results we obtained on PMCs [28]. The composite samples of initial interest for OCT were composed of

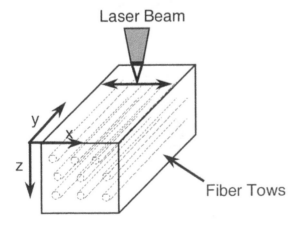

Figure 3 Schematic showing the laser orientation and sampling directions with respect to the composite.

seven layers of a unidirectional E-glass fabric in an epoxy resin. Figure 4 shows an OCT image of the entire cross-section of the composite. The image is 6.0 mm wide (x axis) and 3.7 mm deep (z axis). Each tow is typically 1 mm wide and 550 μm thick. A tow is a bundle of the individual glass filaments. This image is a composite of two images taken from the top and bottom of the sample at the same y position as shown in Fig. 3. The bottom image quality is slightly degraded compared to that of the top image owing to the difference in quality between the top and bottom surfaces. The dark ellipses indicated by an arrow are the polyester threads that are stitched to hold each layer of the fabric together. The light regions outside the tows are identified as resin-rich areas, and the medium gray regions are the fiber tows. The black spots within the fiber tows could be voids from incomplete wetting of the fiber tows and consequent air entrapment. However, care must be taken when interpreting these images for the following reasons.

It is well known that the contrast between features degrades as a function of depth because of the scattering of photons. This contrast degradation is much more pronounced than for biological materials. For this particular figure, because it is a composite of top and bottom images, the noise increases as you move toward the center of the sample thickness. The intensity of the light reaching a particular depth for any position across the sample is affected by how strongly features directly above that position reflect or randomly scatter the light. Although the structure of this sample is somewhat regular, it is difficult to predict its effects on the scattered light. Therefore, for any particular depth within the sample, the intensity of a pixel or group of pixels cannot be assigned to a particular feature upon first inspection. For example, a light area within a tow could result from a resin-rich region, the destructive interference caused by a group of fibers, or shadowing from a strongly reflecting feature from above. In addition to lens and interference effects in the sample, another source of noise arises from the gray vertical lines that project from the black reflection at the air/composite interface. These lines are a result of detector saturation from the signal at that strongly reflecting interface. In fact, the noise from the

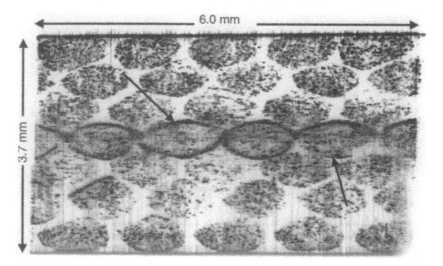

Figure 4 As-collected OCT image of unidirectional E-glass fibers in epoxy resin.

instrumentation is far below the level of noise generated from the sample itself. From the foregoing discussion, it is obvious that the best way to differentiate real features from artifacts is to evaluate a number of slices from a different perspective, perhaps along the xy plane at a particular z position.

The OCT volumetric image of the epoxy/unidirectional E-glass composite has been reconstructed as shown in Fig. 5 so that it can be resliced along any plane of interest for inspection [27]. The image dimensions are 6.00 mm along the x axis, 1.48 mm along the z axis, and 3.85 mm along the y axis. The gray ellipses are the fiber tows, which are approximately 2 mm wide and 750 μm thick and consist of about 2000 glass fibers 10–20 μm in diameter [29]. The long axis of the tows is shown on the xy plane. The polyester stitching that holds a single layer of tows together is indicated by the black arrows. Upon closer inspection, small dark areas are evident inside the fiber tows. These dark areas are high reflectivity regions indicative of individual voids. During the molding process, air can become entrapped as channels in tows if there is insufficient driving pressure, high resin viscosity, or low reinforcement permeability [30]. Also, OCT images provide important information about the permeability of the reinforcement, because the stacking of the layers has a large influence on the infiltration of the resin with the reinforcement, as we will see later. A preform with the tows in a nested configuration has about 50% lower permeability than the same material with the tows in a stacked configuration [31,32].

Figure 6 displays a cross section of the composite along the xy plane at 740 μm from the top that bisects the middle row of tows in Fig. 5 [33]. The dark features of high reflectivity shown by arrows labeled 1 are the polyester threads that hold the layer of tows together. The dark, elongated regions parallel to the y axis are thought to be voids (arrow 2). However, the issue of contrast degradation through the thickness can be assessed with a simple calculation. Power reflectivity for the fiber/resin and resin/void interfaces can be easily calculated: $[(n_1 - n_2)/(n_1 + n_2)]^2$. This equation suggests that the voids will be much more highly backreflecting than the fibers. Therefore, as we lose signal because of scattering attenuation, we should

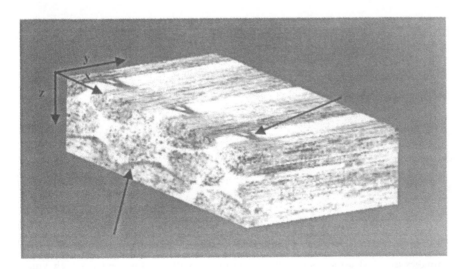

Figure 5   OCT volumetric reconstruction of an epoxy/unidirectional E-glass composite.

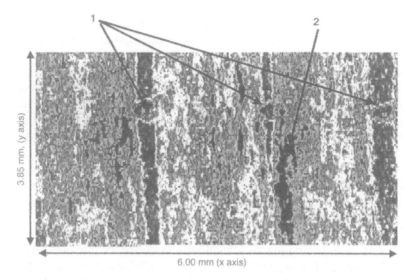

Figure 6 An xy cross section that is 740 μm from the surface. Arrows indicate regions of high reflectivity that correspond to polyester stitching (1) and voids (2).

clearly see the voids much deeper inside the sample than the fibers. There are also geometric effects on the reflectivity that depend on the shape of the reflecting/scattering boundary and can be included in the modeling. Roughly speaking, the back-reflected signal will also be larger if the boundary has less curvature. With known reflectivity and scattering, one could estimate features (i.e., voids) at different positions along the z axis. The correlation between voids and depth of penetration is demonstrated further in the following figures.

Figure 7 contrasts the OCT cross-sectional images of the low (a) and high (b) void content vinyl ester resin and glass samples as discussed in previous work [28].

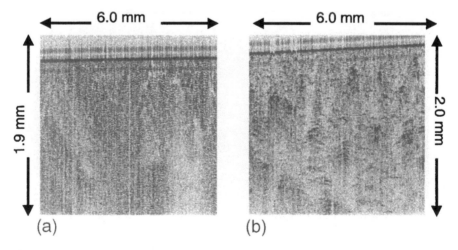

Figure 7 Images of vinyl ester resin/E-glass composites with (a) low and (b) high void content.

These images are uncorrected in the axial direction. In Fig. 7a individual fibers can be discerned near the top of the image. These fibers appear as a speckled pattern. As discussed before, the contrast fades as a function of depth in the images, so fewer of the individual fibers can be discerned. In Fig. 7b, some individual fibers can be identified. More important, there are larger black features that can be correlated with the existence of voids, as shown in the next figure.

Figure 8a is the rescaled Fig. 7b and compares the OCT image of the high void content composite with the corresponding optical micrograph, Fig. 8b. The OCT image was collected at 260 μm in the z direction, whereas the optical micrograph was from a section taken at 270 μm. From multiple optical micrographs, these voids extend from at least 180 to 360 μm, making the comparison valid. The dimensions of Fig. 8a are 5.1 mm wide and 1.9 mm deep, and the dimensions of Fig. 8b are 5.1 mm wide and 1.8 mm deep. The dotted lines show the correspondence of representative voids in the OCT and the optical microscopic images. The voids observed in the micrograph image, Fig. 8b, can be seen in the OCT image, Fig. 8a, but the delineation of the void boundaries are not as pronounced in the latter. The small resin-rich areas in Fig. 8b are not detected in the OCT image.

Figure 9a displays an OCT image of the low void sample, with the corresponding optical micrograph in Fig. 9b. The dimensions of Fig. 9a are 6.0 mm wide and 2.0 mm deep. Although some correspondence can be made at shallow penetration depths, it is difficult to identify the resin-rich areas in Fig. 9a that are so prominent in Fig. 9b. The dimensions of Fig. 9b are 6.2 mm wide and 1.7 mm deep. Figure 9b is

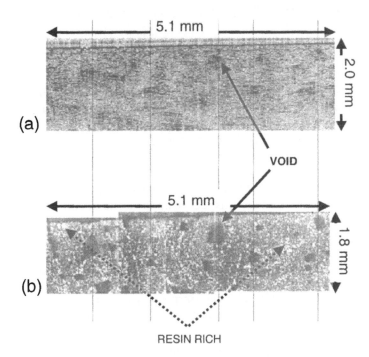

Figure 8 Comparison of (a) OCT image and (b) optical micrograph for high void vinyl ester resin/E-glass sample.

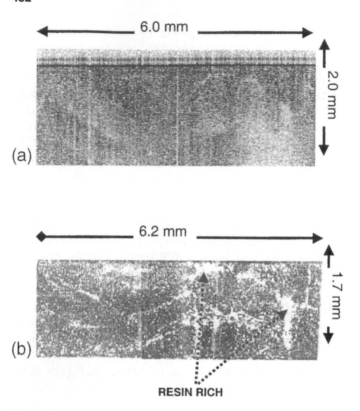

Figure 9 Comparison of (a) OCT image and (b) optical micrograph for high void vinyl ester resin/E-glass sample.

170 μm along the z axis. Multiple OCT images are essentially identical from 180 μm to 2180 μm along the z axis. The OCT image is featureless for two reasons. The first is the previously mentioned attenuation as a function of depth. The second is the fact that small features that do not have large refractive index differences, such as embedded voids, are difficult to detect because boundaries can become blurred in this technique.

Other types of reinforcement were also imaged in previous work [27]. The volumetric reconstruction of the epoxy/0–90° woven composite is shown in Fig. 10. In this image, tows that run along the x axis are positioned above and below tows that are parallel to the y axis. The image dimensions are 6.14 mm along the x axis, 2.13 mm along the z axis, and 4.95 mm along the y axis. Arrow 1 identifies the tows along the x axis that are crossing over the tows along the y axis. Arrow 2 shows the tows along the y axis that are crossing over the tows along the x axis. The layer microstructure has a direct influence on mechanical properties and has been studied elsewhere [34]. Now that we have established that OCT can be used to examine composite microstructure, we present an example of how the microstructure, obtained using OCT, influences real properties.

An important fiber reinforcement property for manufacturing is permeability. Permeability is the factor that controls the rate of fluid flow through the mold during the manufacturing of the PMC. Knowledge of the permeability tensor in liquid

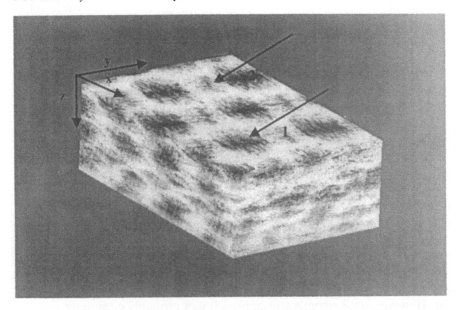

Figure 10 OCT volumetric reconstruction of an epoxy/0–90° woven E-glass composite.

composite molding is important for process optimization. Unfortunately, experimental determination of permeability is difficult and time-consuming [35]. In previous work, binary images were generated from the OCT data and input into a lattice–Boltzmann fluid flow model for permeability prediction [36]. Calculated permeabilities were compared to experimental values for the same fiber volume fraction.

Fluid flow in liquid composite molding (LCM) processes such as resin transfer molding (RTM) is usually modeled using Darcy's law given by

$$v = -\frac{\underline{\underline{K}}}{\mu} \cdot \nabla P \tag{1}$$

where v is the vector of average (superficial) velocity in the medium, P is the pressure, $\underline{\underline{K}}$ is the symmetrical second-order permeability tensor, and μ is the fluid viscosity. Darcy's law is a volume-averaged model in which all the complicated geometry of the fiber preform structure is accounted for through the permeability. Accurate permeability data, therefore, are a critical requirement if a priori modeling efforts based on Darcy's law are to be successfully used in the design and optimization of these processes. Currently, the most reliable and most commonly used technique for obtaining permeability values is experimental measurement in either radial or unidirectional flow configurations [37]. However, experimental characterization is slow, because it involves a large number of carefully controlled experiments over a large range of volume fractions. Another, more serious, limitation is the difficulty conducting experiments on the materials in the deformed states they encounter when placed in LCM tooling, although there have been some recent efforts [38].

In light of these limitations, computational prediction of permeability [32,39–41] offers a potentially accurate and robust alternative to experimental methods. Such calculations consist of imposing a pressure drop across the medium, solving the appropriate transport equations for the detailed flow field, and then back-calculating the permeability by applying Darcy's law. The biggest drawback of this approach has been the inability to determine quickly and accurately the detailed geometry of the fibrous preform materials, which, in addition to many intricate structural features, typically contain statistical variations and defects in their microstructure [42]. Without a precise representation of the media, it is not possible to accurately predict permeability values using computational methods.

There have been two main approaches to the problem of microstructure determination. The first is to perform calculations on small, computationally efficient "unit cell" structures using nominal dimensions that represent the average preform structure. The major problem with this approach is that calculations on the "average" unit cell structure do not, in general, yield an accurate value for the average permeability [42]. A second approach is to determine the microstructure via optical methods (e.g., microscopy) and directly perform the numerical calculation on a discretization of the optical image. This approach has the advantage of exactly representing the media, and, by including large sections of the media in the image, variations and defects in the microstructure are automatically accounted for in the calculation. However, until recently this approach was probably even more tedious to perform than direct experimental measurement of permeability, because the composite specimens typically had to be carefully sectioned, polished, and examined. However, OCT offers a means for rapidly and nondestructively determining the microstructure of fiber-reinforced plastic materials.

15.5.2 Governing Equations

Modeling the flow in fibrous reinforcement is complicated by the existence of an open region outside the tows and micropores created by the individual fibers inside the tows. Following previous studies [32,39–42], the Stokes equation, given by

$$\nabla P = \mu \nabla^2 \boldsymbol{v} \tag{2}$$

is used to model flow in the open regions. The Brinkman equation, given by

$$\nabla \langle P \rangle = \mu \nabla^2 \langle v \rangle - \mu \underline{\underline{K}}^{-1} \cdot \langle \boldsymbol{v} \rangle \tag{3}$$

is used to model flow in the micropores created by the individual fibers inside the tows, where $\underline{\underline{K}}$ is the permeability of the porous tows. In both regions, the continuity equation,

$$\nabla \cdot \boldsymbol{v} = 0 \tag{4}$$

is used to enforce conservation of mass.

15.5.3 Permeability Computation

Permeability for different flow directions was computed by imposing a constant pressure along opposite faces of the lattice in the desired direction and integrating the foregoing system of equations to steady state. Estimates for the intra-tow permeability values were obtained from the formulas given in previous work [32]. The steady-state velocity field at the inlet was integrated over the surface to obtain the flow rate Q, and this was used in the formula

$$K_{\text{eff}} = \frac{\mu Q L}{A \, \Delta P} \tag{5}$$

to obtain the effective permeability, K_{eff}, for the desired direction.

Before permeability could be predicted, the OCT images were converted to binary images in the following manner. An automated image processing program was written using MATLAB 5.1 with the Image Processing Toolbox to convert the raw gray-scale OCT images to binary images of glass fiber and epoxy (Fig. 11). The raw image is first rotated and cropped to eliminate sample tilt and edge effects. An example of this preprocessed image is provided in Fig. 11a, where the darker ellipses correspond to the three cross-sectional layers of fiber tows and the lighter regions are due to the epoxy. The image is then doubled in size by linear interpolation of adjacent pixels to minimize any artificial alteration of the tow size in subsequent image processing. To increase the contrast between the darker tows and the lighter epoxy regions, a variance image is created by replacing the intensity value of a 2×2 cluster of pixels with the standard deviation of that cluster. In the next two steps, spurious light pixels within the tow regions and vertical lines corresponding to detector saturation are eliminated. Using the automated program, the boundaries of the tows are determined and a binary image (Fig. 11b) is formed. Smoothing and filling operations that maintain the area of the tows are being pursued. The resulting binary image is then used as input for the permeability modeling.

The results from the permeability calculation are shown in Table 1. The value for the experimental axial permeability (K) is 5.3×10^{-4} mm^2 and results from one axial flow experiment. The axial K is the K measured along the fiber tows or in the y direction as in Fig. 5. The standard deviation ($\pm$) associated with it is taken from previous work with this reinforcement at higher fiber volume fractions [43]. Image sets for computing K values within this table were processed in two different ways.

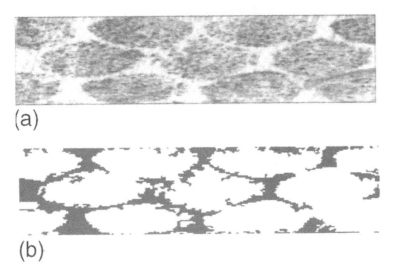

(a)

(b)

Figure 11 (a) Original gray-scale OCT image of the epoxy/unidirectional E-glass composite. (b) Binary OCT image after automated image processing.

Table 1 Values of Experimental and Calculated Permeabilities and Corresponding Brinkman Fraction

Brinkman fraction	Sample name	Type of processing	Image set	Axial $K \times 10^{-4}$ (mm^2)	Transverse $K \times 10^{-4}$ (mm^2)	Anisotropy ratio
0.770	Experimental	—	—	5.3 ± 1.1	—	—
0.767	Data 1	Manual	87–91	4.45	0.882	5.06
0.788 ± 0.021	Data 2	Manual	75–95	3.81	0.992	4.11
0.768 ± 0.021	Data 3	Automated, no smoothing	75–95	2.83	0.654	4.32
0.750 ± 0.027	Data 4	Automated, smoothing	75–95	3.18	0.991	3.21
0.727 ± 0.014	Data 5	Automated, smoothing	4–24	5.09	0.934	5.45
0.795 ± 0.021	Data 6	Manual, roughened	75–95	2.73	0.662	4.12
0.387 ± 0.020	Data 7	Manual, dilated	75–95	2.99	0.767	3.90

For the "manual" method, the tow outlines were drawn by sight and filled in to generate a binary image. Images using the "automated" method were processed as described in the previous paragraph. For Data 2, the axial K of $3.81 \times 10^{-4}\,mm^2$ is considered to be the best possible value because the images are drawn manually. Part of the discrepancy between the experimental value for K and the calculated values may also originate from microscale variations of permeability within the fabric. The 21 images used in these calculations represent a width of only 6.0 mm, a depth of approximately 1.5 mm, and, most important, a length of 1.0 mm. For comparison, the size of the reinforcement used in experimental determination of permeability is 15 cm wide, 1.3 cm deep, and 15 cm long. The effect of microscale variation in the permeability can also be illustrated by comparing K values from Data 1 and Data 2. The K from Data 1 is $4.45 \times 10^{-4}\,mm^2$ and was calculated using five images, whereas the K from Data 2 is $3.81 \times 10^{-4}\,mm^2$ and was calculated using 21 images. Data 5 was calculated on a totally different section of the composite and yields an axial permeability within the experimental error.

For the automatically processed images in Data 3, the axial K of 2.83×10^{-4} mm^2 is much lower than for Data 2. For Table 1, the Brinkman fraction is defined as the area occupied by the tows. The higher the area occupied by the tows (or the higher the Brinkman fraction), the lower the value of K because there is less open space available for fluid flow. If the Brinkman fractions are considered, then the axial K for Data 3 should be higher than for Data 2, because the Brinkman fraction for Data 3 is slightly lower than for Data 2. From these results and from analysis of the fluid velocity data, we conclude that the roughness of the tow boundaries has a large influence on the velocity of the flow because it acts to increase the resistance to flow. This influence propagates to the middle of the channels between the tows, where fluid velocity should be at a maximum.

This conclusion is supported by results from Data 6 compared to those from Data 7. The images from Data 6 are originally from Data 2, the manually processed images. However, a small amount of roughness was introduced in Data 6 while retaining nominally the same Brinkman fraction. For Data 7, the images in Data 2 were dilated to increase the Brinkman fraction, but the roughness was not altered. When the axial K from Data 7 is compared to that from Data 6, the result is initially unexpected. A relative increase of roughly 4% of the Brinkman fraction in Data 7 should lead to a decrease in axial K over that of Data 6, but the result is the opposite. The axial K of Data 7 is higher than that of Data 6. This comparison between the permeabilities from Data 6 and Data 7 means that an increase in roughness will have more of an impact on permeability than a similar increase in Brinkman fraction. These results also highlight the importance of processing the images as close to the actual structure as possible.

15.5.4 Imaging of Damage

Both microstructure and damage in polymer matrix composites are often characterized by using destructive techniques such as microscopy on sectioned samples, which provides detailed information on a small size scale. The capability to measure these features nondestructively, however, is very desirable because that permits monitoring of damage evolution and correlation of the results with microstructural features that can initiate, influence, or even control the damage. It is even more advantageous if these measurements are performed with a single technique because this eliminates the complications involved in combining data from different sources.

Optical coherence tomography has also been used for nondestructive evaluation of damage in composites in previous work [27]. This approach is important in providing an understanding of the initiation of failure because there is little in the literature about the nondestructive evaluation of damage initiation in composites. To illustrate the capability of OCT for imaging damage, an epoxy/unidirectional E-glass composite was subjected to impact damage, and imaging was performed along a surface crack. Figures 12a–16a show the damage along the xy plane through the first layer of composite and are all 5.50 mm wide and 1.98 mm high. Of course, there is always an issue of shadowing of highly reflecting features such as cracks. The resulting shadowing is not a consistent problem and requires further study. Figures 12b–16b are xz images showing the position of the tows designated by the dark-colored crossing thread and are 1.98 mm wide (x axis) and 2.23 mm high (z axis). The arrows on the left of these figures indicate the positions of the image in Figs. 12a–15a with respect to the tow placement.

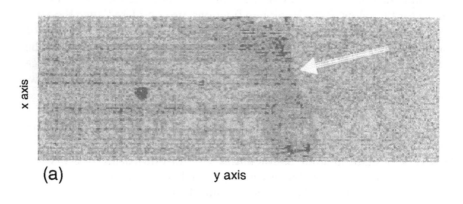

(a)   y axis

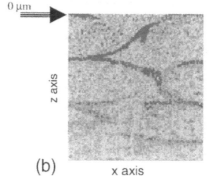

(b)   x axis

Figure 12 OCT images of impact-damaged epoxy/unidirectional E-glass composite (a) 0 μm from surface along the xy plane and (b) along the xz plane, showing placement of tows via polyester stitching.

The damage at the surface of the composite is shown in Fig. 12a by the arrow, which points to the ridge created by the impact. Figure 13a shows a slice of the composite 337 μm below the surface. The black lines are drawn into this and subsequent figures to indicate the path of the tows. Arrows 1 and 2 indicate cracks propagating through the fiber tow. Arrow 3 shows the polyester crossing threads that hold the top layer together. Figure 14a shows images that are 460 μm from the surface. The crack indicated by arrow 1 is beginning to propagate along the tow/resin boundary. It is about 820 μm long and is shown to be approaching the bottom of the tow in Fig. 14b. The crack extends to 1.8 mm long in Fig. 15a and is 550 μm from the surface as shown by arrow 1. The polyester stitching is still evident (arrow 2). Finally, a delamination zone is shown by the white arrow in Fig. 16a at the interface between the bottom of the first tow layer and the resin (Fig. 16b). The delamination is about 1.9 mm wide and 0.5 mm high and is 652 μm from the surface. This crack continues to propagate into the second layer, and a delamination area is found at 1.66 mm as well. Damage in the direction of the tows is consistent with impact damage observed in other composites [44]. Comparison of these results with complementary techniques such as X-ray CT and optical microscopy is the subject of ongoing work.

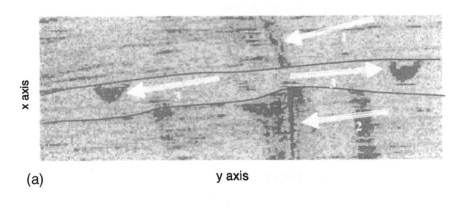

(a)

y axis

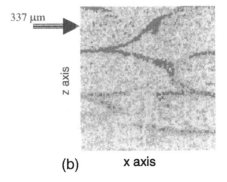

(b)   x axis

Figure 13 OCT images of impact-damaged epoxy/unidirectional E-glass composite (a) 337 μm from the surface along the *xy* plane and (b) along the *xz* plane, showing placement of tows via polyester stitching.

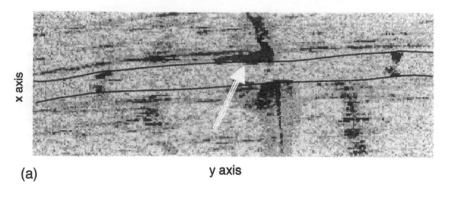

(a)   y axis

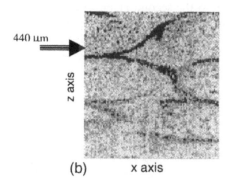

(b)   x axis

Figure 14 OCT images of impact-damaged epoxy/unidirectional E-glass composite (a) 460 μm from the surface along the *xy* plane and (b) along the *xz* plane, showing placement of tows via polyester stitching.

15.6 SUMMARY AND FUTURE DIRECTIONS

This work has demonstrated the potential of OCT as a nondestructive evaluation (NDE) tool for polymer matrix composites. OCT goes beyond typical composite NDE because of its ability to image microstructure in addition to damage and has been shown to yield results in good agreement with those of optical microscopy. For the first time, microstructural information obtained nondestructively was used in the prediction of an important reinforcement property, permeability. A more complex reinforcement was imaged showing the effect of mold compaction on layer placement and orientation, which are also important for permeability considerations. Of equal importance, OCT was used as a rapid nondestructive probe for damage, suggesting the concurrent use of mechanical testing and OCT. OCT provided absolute information on the location and size of the defects with the resolution required to detect damage initiation.

In the immediate future, in-house instrumentation will be used to optimize image collection by varying the confocal parameter, scanning and stage velocity, and bandpass. The potential applications of OCT to the field of PMCs are plentiful. Extending the permeability prediction to OCT images with more complex reinforcement is of great interest. Using OCT coupled with fatigue testing to monitor the

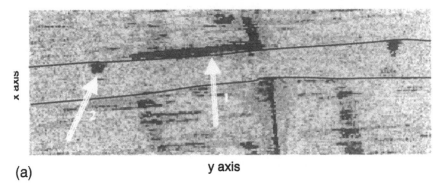

(a)   y axis

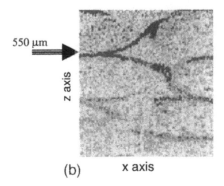

(b)   x axis

Figure 15 OCT images of impact-damaged epoxy/unidirectional E-glass composite (a) 550 μm from the surface along the xy plane and (b) along the xz plane, showing placement of tows via polyester stitching.

initiation and progression of damage is also planned. Imaging of short fiberglass thermoplastic composites is extremely important for determination of fiber orientation distribution, a critical property of this material in a high volume market. However, short fiberglass in thermoplastic composites is nominally 10 μm in diameter and challenges the instrumental resolution. More far-reaching ideas use tunable sources to probe how moisture or other environmental fluids diffuse into the composite. Also, polarized OCT could be used to probe residual stress in composites, which could help in understanding their design and failure.

ACKNOWLEDGMENTS

I am grateful to Professor James Fujimoto for the use of his OCT instrumentation and insightful discussions. A number of members of his laboratory, including Drs. Brett Bouma, Jergen Herrmann and Xingde Li, and Mr. Rohit Prasankumar, kindly shared their time and expertise with us.

    I also thank the people in my group, who contributed so much to the success of my work. I would first like to thank my group leader, Dr. Richard Parnas, for his full support of my work. I am grateful to Dr. Carl Zimba for much of the data collection

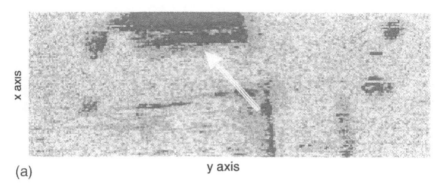

(a)   y axis

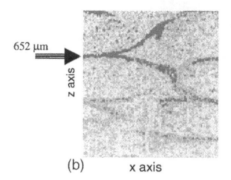

652 μm

(b)   x axis

Figure 16 OCT images of impact-damaged epoxy/unidirectional E-glass composite (a) 652 μm from the surface along the xy plane and (b) along the xz plane, showing placement of tows via polyester stitching.

and for his willingness to mentor me. I also thank many other people who have contributed in their own way—Drs. Frederick Phelan for the modeling, Donald Hunston for his help on the damage aspects of the work, and Richard Peterson for permeability measurements. Special thanks to our technician, Ms. Kathleen Flynn, for doing all of the hard work.

Lastly, I thank Dr. Matt Everett and his group in the Medical Technology Program at Livermore National Laboratory for their continued efforts in helping me build an OCT system.

REFERENCES

1. Bodamer D. Civ Eng 68(1):56, 1998.
2. Billmeyer F Jr. Textbook of Polymer Science. 3rd ed. New York: Wiley, 1984.
3. Plueddemann E. Silane Coupling Agents. 2nd ed. New York: Plenum Press, 1991.
4. Naitove M, Gaspari J. Plastic Technol 43(3):32, 1997.
5. Anonymous. Manuf Eng 12, 1995.
6. Anonymous. Manuf Eng 120(3):48, 1998.
7. Mraz S, Dibble M. Mach Des 65(18):166, 1993.

8. Jost K. Automotive Eng 104:27, 1996.
9. Silverman S. Hart's Petrol Eng Int 71(12):21, 1998.
10. Cercone L, Korff J. Civil Eng 67(7):60, 1997.
11. Thippeswamy H, Franco J, GangaRao H. Concrete Int: Des Construct 20(6):47, 1998.
12. Larson M. Quality 37(9):30, 1998.
13. Patel N, Lee J. Polym Compos 16(5):386, 1995.
14. Patel N, Rohatgi V, Lee J. Proc 49th Annu SPI Compos Inst Conf, Session 10-D, 1994.
15. Patel N, Rohatgi V, Lee J. Polym Compos 14:161, 1993.
16. Ghlorse S. SAMPE Quart 24:54, 1993.
17. Thomason J, Knoester A. J Mater Sci Lett 9:258, 1990.
18. Izatt J, Hee M, Owen G, Swanson E, Fujimoto J. Opt Lett 19(8):590, 1994.
19. Wooh S, Daniel I. Mater Eval 52(10):1199, 1994.
20. Dewhurst RJ, He R, Shan Q. Defect visualization in carbon fiber composite using laser ultrasound. Mater Eval 51(8):935–940, 1993.
21. Highsmith A, Keshav S. J Compos Tech Res 19(1):10, 1997.
22. Kortschot M, Zhang C. Compos Sci Tech 53(2):175, 1995.
23. Bossi R, Georgeson G. Mater Eval 53(10):1198, 1995.
24. Hoh, K-P, Ishida H, Koenig J. Polym Compos 11(3):192, 1990.
25. Blumich B. Adv Mater 3(5):237, 1991.
26. Jezzard P, Wiggins C, Carpenter T, Hall L, Barnes J, Jackson P, Clayden N. J Mater Sci 27(23):6365, 1992.
27. Dunkers J, Zimba C, Flynn K, Hunston D, Prasankumar R, Li X, Fujimoto J. Proc SPIE Int Symp on Nondestructive Evaluation Techniques for Aging Infrastructure and Manufacturing, 1999: Volume 3585, page 208.
28. Dunkers JP, Parnas RS, Zimba CG, Peterson RS, Flynn KM, Fujimoto JG, Bouma BE. Composites A 30(2):139, 1999.
29. Ranganathan S, Wise G, Phelan F Jr, Parnas R, Advani S. Advanced Composites X: Proc 10th Annu ASM/ESD Adv Compos Conf and Exposition (ACCE94), ASM Int 1994: 309.
30. Lundström TS. Thesis, Luleå Univ Technology, Luleå, Sweden, 1996.
31. Phelan FR, Leung Y, Parnas RS. J Thermoplast Compos Mater 7:208, 1994.
32. Ranganathan S, Wise G, Phelan F Jr, Parnas R, Advani S. Advanced Composites X: Proc 10th Annu ASM/ESD Adv Compos Confer and Exposition (ACCE94), ASM Int 1994:309.
33. Dunkers J, Zimba C, Hunston D. Flynn K, Parnas R, Fujimoto J, Herrmann J. Proc ASC 13th Tech Conf Compos Mat 1998:1626.
34. Bradley DJ, Adams DO, Gascoigne HE. J Reinf Plast Compos 17(11):989, 1998.
35. Parnas RS. Preform permeability. In: TK Kruckenberg, ed. RTM for Aerospace Applications. London: Chapman & Hall, 1999, Chap. 8.
36. Dunkers J, Phelan F, Zimba C, Flynn K, Peterson R, Prasankumar R, Fujimoto J. Proc 57th Annu ANTEC Conf, May 2–6, 1999, New York.
37. Parnas R, Salem A. Polym Compos 14(5):383, 1993.
38. Friedman H, Johnson R, Miller B, Salem D, Parnas R. Polym Compos 18(5):663, 1997.
39. Phelan F Jr, Wise G. Composites 27A(1):25, 1996.
40. Spaid M, Phelan F Jr. Phys Fluids 9(9):2468, 1997.
41. Spaid M, Phelan F Jr. Composites 29A:749, 1998.
42. Ranganathan S, Easterling R, Advani S, Phelan F Jr. Polym Polym Compos 6(2):63, 1998.
43. Parnas R, Flynn K, Dal-Favero M. Polym Compos 18(5):623, 1997.
44. Blodget ED, Miller JG, Freeman SM. In: DO Thompson, SE Chimenti, eds. Review of Progress in Quantitative Nondestructive Evaluation. New York: Plenum, 1986:1227.

16

Relationship Between Tissue Microscopic Structure and Scattering Properties: Implications for OCT Imaging

REBEKAH DREZEK, ANDRÉS F. ZULUAGA, and REBECCA RICHARDS-KORTUM

The University of Texas at Austin, Austin, Texas

16.1 INTRODUCTION

Optical coherence tomography (OCT) provides a sensitive tool to measure spatially resolved backscattering events in highly turbid media. OCT images provide detailed views of tissue structure with near-microscopic resolution. To use these images to identify the presence of pathophysiology and diagnose the presence of disease, it is necessary to more fully understand the relationship between the microscopic structure of tissue and its scattering properties. In this chapter we review several theoretical descriptions of light propagation in tissue, beginning at the macroscopic level and progressing to the microscopic level.

Computational approaches based on numerical solution of Maxwell's equations can provide considerable insight into the connection between the microscopic structure of tissue and the resulting optical properties. This insight can be used to understand important features in OCT images of turbid tissues. Simple contrast agents can perturb the scattering properties of tissues and may play an important role in improving the ability to recognize disease in OCT images.

16.2 MODELS OF LIGHT PROPAGATION: MACROSCOPIC APPROACHES

Neglecting polarization, interference, and diffraction, the propagation of light through tissue can be modeled as neutral particle transport. At the macroscopic level, tissue can be characterized by three spatially varying, wavelength-dependent parameters [1]: the absorption coefficient (μ_a), the scattering coefficient (μ_s), and the scattering phase function [$p(\mathbf{s}, \mathbf{s}')$]. $\mu_a \Delta s$ denotes the probability of photon absorption for a Δs pathlength, $\mu_s \Delta s$ denotes the probability of photon elastic scattering for a Δs pathlength, and the phase function is the probability density function that describes the likelihood of scattering from direction $\mathbf{s}$ to direction $\mathbf{s}'$ per unit solid angle. In a multiple scattering medium, photon particle transport can be described by the time-dependent Boltzmann equation [2],

$$\frac{1}{c}\frac{\partial L(\mathbf{r}, \hat{s})}{\partial t} + \hat{s} \cdot \nabla L(\mathbf{r}, \hat{s}) + [\mu_a(\mathbf{r}) + \mu_s(\mathbf{r})]L(\mathbf{r}, \hat{s}) = \int_{4\pi} d\Omega' \mu_s(\mathbf{r})p(\hat{s}, \hat{s}')L(\mathbf{r}, \hat{s}')$$

$$+ S(\mathbf{r}, \hat{s})$$

$$(1)$$

Here $L(\mathbf{r}, \hat{s})$ represents the local angular photon flux at position $\mathbf{r}$ at time t in unit direction $\hat{s}$, $S(\mathbf{r}, \hat{s})$ represents the source of photons generated at $\mathbf{r}$ and t in direction $\hat{s}$ and $d\Omega'$ is an element of solid angle. This equation can be solved, subject to appropriate boundary conditions [2]; its solution can be used to estimate homogeneous tissue scattering and absorption properties from measurements of steady-state tissue reflectance and transmission [3].

The angular flux, $L(\mathbf{r}, \hat{s})$, can be expanded as a sum of Legendre polynomials, and when scattering dominates absorption all but the first two terms in the expansion can be dropped. In this case, the transport equation reduces to the optical diffusion equation for the angle-independent photon flux, $\Phi(\mathbf{r})$ [4].

$$\frac{1}{c}\frac{\partial \Phi(\mathbf{r})}{\partial t} - D\nabla^2\Phi(\mathbf{r}) + \mu_a\Phi(\mathbf{r}) = S(\mathbf{r})$$

$$(2)$$

Here, D is the optical diffusion coefficient, $D = [3(\mu_a + (1-g)\mu_s)]^{-1} \cdot g$ is the anisotropy parameter, defined as

$$g = \int_{4\pi} p(\hat{s}, \hat{s}')(\hat{s} \cdot \hat{s}') \, d\Omega'$$

and represents the average cosine of the scattering angle. Closed-form analytical solutions can be obtained for the diffusion approximation to the radiative transport equation in both one and three dimensions for cases with a high degree of symmetry [2,4]. Alternatively, they can be solved numerically.

Another approach is to use Monte Carlo methods to simulate the random walk of photons within an absorbing and scattering tissue [5]. This approach offers a flexible, rigorous approach to describe photon transport in tissue according to the rules of radiative transport [6]. Monte Carlo based approaches are particularly useful for describing the propagation of light in heterogeneous tissues and close to boundaries. Welch and colleagues described a Monte Carlo technique to permit optical modeling that takes into account knowledge of complex three-dimensional anatomical structures such as small blood vessels [7]. Monte Carlo methods are used to describe the propagation of photons through a tissue where the optical properties, stored in a material grid array, can vary arbitrarily in three dimensions [7].

Monte Carlo techniques have also been used to simulate the signal collected in OCT [8–10]. Pan et al. [8] described a Monte Carlo simulation of pathlength-resolved reflectance from multilayer tissues. This model assumed that all waveforms collected by the detector with a pathlength difference ΔL less than the source coherence length will produce interference. Using this model, they predict that OCT signals are most sensitive to changes in index of refraction and least sensitive to changes in absorption coefficient over the range of optical properties found in tissue [8]. A similar approach was presented by Ducros [11]. Milner and colleagues extended this concept for OCT and optical Doppler tomography (ODT) [9,10]. Three-dimensional Monte Carlo models of accumulated photon pathlength were combined with a geometrical optics model of the probe geometry with low coherence interferometric detection [9]. They found that at depths of less than three mean free paths in highly scattering media, backscatter position of photons corresponded well with the focus position of the probe, but at greater depths localization of backscattering was lost due to detection of stray photons [9].

A drawback of Monte Carlo models is the computational time required to process the large number of photons required to yield good statistics. Several analytical models have been proposed to predict OCT signals in turbid media. The first analytical models [12–14] assumed that only light that has undergone a single backscattering event in the sample arm generates a heterodyne signal. However, light in the sample arm can be attenuated by scattering out of the detector collection path or by absorption events in the sample. The tissue optical properties incorporated in this model are the depth-dependent sample reflectivity, which is a function of the radar backscattering cross section of the scatterers in the sample volume (μ_b), and the extinction coefficient (μ_{ext}), which is related to the single-particle scattering cross section, the particle density, and the absorption coefficient. This model was shown experimentally to be accurate only at very small probing depths; beyond this, multiple scattering effects have an observable effect on the measured OCT signal [15,16].

Multiple scattering events detected in OCT are mostly *forward*-scattering events, which significantly degrade the signal due to beam spread and loss of spatial coherence. To incorporate these effects, the extended Huygens–Fresnel formulation of Yura [17] was adapted to OCT by Knuttel et al. [18] and then extended by Schmitt and Knuttel [17]. In this representation, loss of spatial coherence due to turbidity is characterized by the mutual coherence function (MCF) of the probing beam. The MCF is the cross-correlation of two optical, electric field vectors separated by a certain distance on a plane perpendicular to wave propagation. The lateral coherence length (ρ_0) is the characteristic separation at which the MCF falls to $1/e$ of its maximum value. Under certain conditions [19] the lateral coherence length can be expressed as

$$\rho_0 = \sqrt{\frac{3}{\mu_s z}\left(\frac{2}{k\theta_{rms}}\right)} \tag{3}$$

where $\mu_s z$ characterizes the loss of coherence as the wave moves deeper into the medium, $k = 2\pi/\lambda$ is the optical frequency, and θ_{rms} is the mean scattering angle of the scatterers in the tissue. All of these parameters depend on the scattering properties of the sample; these can be approximated using Mie theory if it is assumed that scattering is produced by a combination of individual spherical particles with a fractal size distribution as described in Ref. 20. With these assumptions, this model gives a reasonable approximation of the maximum tissue depth that can be probed with OCT.

In summary, analytical and computational models both indicate that OCT measurements are extremely sensitive to small changes in refractive index; a Δn as small as 0.01 can produce a significant interference modulation [8]. In most models of tissue optics, the index of refraction has been assumed to be homogeneous and nearly that of water and tissue scattering is characterized by a single scattering coefficient and anisotropy. However, the signal measured in OCT images (backscattering) is produced by local heterogeneities in refractive index. In order to understanding the microscopic and biological basis of OCT signals, tissue cannot be modeled as a homogeneous medium characterized simply by a scattering coefficient but must be considered an optically heterogeneous composite of microstructural segments with different refractive indices [8].

16.3 MODELS OF LIGHT PROPAGATION: MICROSCOPIC APPROACHES

16.3.1 Background

To facilitate interpretation of data obtained using OCT or other scattering-based optical diagnostic techniques, mathematical models of light transport that account for refractive index fluctuations on a microscopic scale are needed. The initial step in developing such a model is to examine the interaction of light with a single cell, by considering the electromagnetic interaction of light with an arbitrarily heterogeneous biological cell. This approach allows investigation of how factors such as nuclear size and structure, organelle content, medium surrounding the cell, and incident light wavelength affect how light scatters from a cell.

Due to the size of scatterers in cells relative to the wavelengths used in optical imaging, electromagnetic methods are required to describe scattering. Mie theory has been used extensively to approximate scattering but generally requires modeling a cell as a homogeneous sphere. Schmitt and Kumar [21] presented a useful expansion of this idea by applying Mie theory to a volume of spheres with various sizes distributions. In addition, anomalous diffraction approximations [22], multiple solutions [23], and T-matrix computations [24] have been proposed and implemented. Each of these techniques offers significant advantages over conventional Mie theory; however, all require limiting geometrical and refractive index assumptions.

A more flexible approach is provided by a three-dimensional finite-difference time-domain (FDTD) model of cellular scattering [25]. Although computationally intensive, this model allows the computation of scattering patterns from inhomogeneous cells of arbitrary shape. The aim of the work described in this chapter is to develop an increased understanding of how light interacts with tissue on a cellular level using the FDTD model to predict cellular scattering patterns.

16.3.2 Origins of Cellular Scattering

Because scattering arises from mismatches in refractive index, when considering a cell from the perspective of how it will interact with light, the cell is viewed more appropriately as a continuum of refractive index fluctuations than as a single object containing a number of discrete particles. The magnitude and spatial extent of the index of refraction fluctuations arise from the physical composition and size of the components that make up the cell. Organelles and subcomponents of organelles having indices different from those of their surroundings are expected to be the primary sources of cellular scattering. The cell itself may be a significant source of small-angle scatter in applications such as flow cytometry in which cells are measured individually; however, for in vivo scattering-based diagnostics, the cell as an entity is not as important, because cells will be surrounded by other cells or tissue structures of similar index.

Certain organelles in cells are important potential sources of scattering. The nucleus is significant because it is often the largest organelle in the cell, and in diagnostic applications its size increases relative to the rest of the cell throughout neoplastic progression. Other potential scatterers include organelles whose size relative to the wavelength of light suggest that they may be important backscatterers. These include mitochondria (0.5–$1.5\,\mu$m), lysosomes ($0.5\,\mu$m), and peroxisomes ($0.5\,\mu$m). Mitochondria may be particularly influential in those cells that contain significant mitochondrial volume fractions because of the unique folded membrane structure of mitochondria. For instance, Chance and coworkers [26] found that mitochondria contribute 73% of the scattering from hepatocytes. Additionally, melanin, traditionally thought of as an absorber, must be considered an important scatterer owing to its size and high refractive index. Finally, structures consisting of membrane layers such as the endoplasmic reticulum or Golgi apparatus may prove significant because they will contain index fluctuations of high frequency and amplitude. Although the work presented here primarily concerns cells, to understand scattering from tissue, fibrous components such as collagen and elastin must be considered in addition to cellular matter. The relative importance of fibrous and cellular components depends upon tissue type.

16.3.3 Methods

Yee's Method

Yee's method [27] can be used to solve Maxwell's curl equations using the finite-difference time-domain (FDTD) technique. The algorithm takes Maxwell's curl equations and discretizes them in time and space, yielding six coupled finite-difference equations. The six electric and magnetic field components ($E_x, E_y, E_z, H_x, H_y, H_z$) are spatially and temporally offset on a three-dimensional grid. The grid spacing must be less than $\lambda/10$ to yield accurate results. Except when otherwise noted, a $\lambda/20$ grid was used for the simulations presented here. As the six finite-difference equations are stepped in time, the electric and magnetic fields are updated for each grid point. To simulate propagation in an unbounded medium, boundary conditions must be applied to the tangential electric field components along the edges of the computational boundary at each time step. The Liao boundary condition [28] is used. The incident wave is a sinusoidal plane wave source.

The FDTD method computes the fields in a region around the cell that lies in the near field, which is then transformed to the far field. Parameters such as anisotropy and scattering cross section can be computed from the scattering pattern. The details of the FDTD model used in this work and the relevant calculations can be found in Ref. 25.

Simulation Parameters

The cell is constructed by assigning a permittivity value to each cell component. If desired, a range of permittivity values may be assigned to one component if that component, for example, the nucleus, is inhomogeneous. For a purely real refractive index, the dielectric constant is simply the square of the refractive index.

To accurately determine scattering patterns, it is necessary to model the cells in as physically realistic a manner as possible. Information about the size, quantity, and dielectric structure of cellular organelles was obtained from the literature and by examining phase contrast images and electron micrographs of cells and organelles of interest. Refractive index is a function of the concentration of macromolecules in a particular organelle. However, an organelle's composition can vary significantly among different types of cells. For instance, it has been reported that the refractive index of the nucleus is higher than that of the cytoplasm in Chinese hamster ovary cells [29] and breast epithelial cells [30], whereas the cytoplasm was found to have a higher index than the nucleoid in *E. coli* [31]. Thus, accurate modeling of dielectric structure requires specific knowledge of organelle composition for the cell type of interest. Because this information is not readily available, refractive index values from the literature were assembled as a starting point for the simulations. The nucleus was always modeled with some inhomogeneities in refractive index. The distribution of index variations employed in the simulations was based on Fourier analysis of 100× phase contrast images of normal and cancerous human breast epithelial cells. The general ranges of refractive index values used in the FDTD simulations are shown in Table 1 [29,32–34].

16.3.4 Results

Verification

The simulation program was verified by computing the scattering patterns of homogeneous spheres ranging in diameter from 5 to 10 μm and comparing the results to Mie theory. For small spheres, the two curves agree closely for all angles at horizontal and vertical polarizations For larger spheres, the FDTD pattern agrees very well for most angles but is somewhat greater than the Mie pattern for angles higher than 160°. The artificial increase is due to imperfect boundary conditions, resulting in artificial reflections at the edges of the computational domain. The scattering pattern of a 5 μm sphere is shown in Fig. 1. The anisotropy parameter g and scattering cross section differ from theoretical values by less than 0.2% despite the artificial reflections.

Model output is presented in several ways: (1) scattering patterns, which illustrate the scattered intensity as a function of angle; (2) normalized scattering patterns, where the scattered power is normalized to the value at 0°; and (3) scattering phase functions, $P(\theta)$, which present the scattered power versus angle, where the area under the curve has been normalized to 1. In the scattering pattern, it is visually easier to

Table 1 Index of Refraction Values Obtained from the Literature

Organelle	Refractive index	Reference
Extracellular fluid	1.35–1.36	32
Cytoplasm	1.36–1.375	29
Nucleus	1.38–1.41	29
Mitochondria/organelles	1.38–1.41	33
Melanin	1.6–1.7	34

assess the relative magnitude of scattered power at particular angles when comparing results from multiple simulations. However, when comparing FDTD data to Mie theory or Henyey–Greenstein phase functions, data must first be normalized to an area of 1.

Influence of the Nucleus

It is important to understand the effect of nuclear morphology on scattering properties, because nuclear morphology is dramatically altered in cancerous cells. In general, cancerous cells have an increased nuclear-to-cytoplasmic ratio [35]. Additionally, because cancerous cells divide more rapidly than normal cells and often have extra chromosomes, the protein concentration of the nucleus may be higher, altering the nuclear refractive index. Also, there are changes in nuclear shape and texture as cells become cancerous [35].

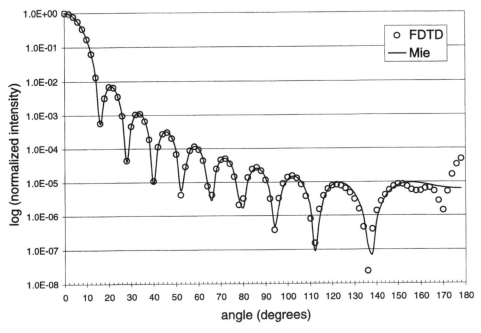

Figure 1 Validation of FDTD code. Comparison of FDTD results to Mie theory predictions for a 5 μm sphere ($m = 1.04$; $\lambda = 900$ nm).

The FDTD model was used to study the relationship between the physical structure of the nucleus and its scattering properties, examining, separately, the effects of nuclear size and nuclear refractive index on scattering pattern. Unless otherwise specified, all simulations presented here involved a 15 μm diameter spherical cell containing cytoplasm, a nucleus, and organelles of multiple sizes and shapes. The wavelength of light was 900 nm. To isolate changes due to the nucleus, the volume fraction of other organelles was kept low (0.02%) and a small mismatch between cytoplasm and extracellular fluid ($m = 1.014$) was employed. Note that m is defined to be a relative index of refraction (in this case, between cyto-

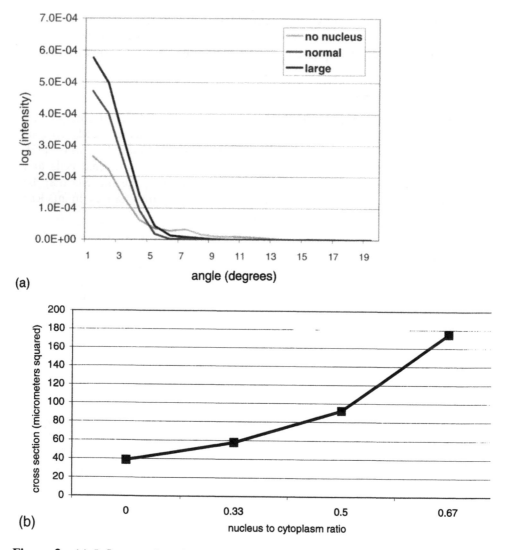

(a)

(b)

Figure 2 (a) Influence of nuclear structure on scattering pattern. Small-angle scatter is shown on a linear scale. There were no visible differences in scattering patterns at angles over 20°. (b) Influence of nuclear-to-cytoplasmic ratio on scattering cross section. (c) Influence of relative nucleus/cytoplasm refractive index on scattering cross section.

plasm and extracellular fluid), and n is defined to be an absolute index of refraction. Nuclear index variations were uniformly distributed between $\Delta n = \pm 0.03$ about the mean nuclear index, $n = 1.39$, at spatial frequencies ranging from 2 to $20\,\mu m^{-1}$.

Scattering patterns were calculated for cells with nuclei with diameters of 0, 5, 7.5, and $10\,\mu m$. Increases in nuclear size create noticeable changes in the scattering pattern at small angles. Figure 2a shows the small-angle scattering patterns of a 15 μm cell with no nucleus, a small (normal) nucleus ($5\,\mu m$ diameter), and a large nucleus ($10\,\mu m$ diameter). The most noticeable changes in scattering were at low angles. The higher angle (over $20°$) scattering of cells containing nuclei of various sizes is highly dependent on factors such as incident wavelength and refractive index structure of the nuclei. For instance, when cells are modeled with homogeneous nuclei, large-angle scattering is not significantly altered as nuclear size is increased [36]. However, when the nucleus is modeled as a heterogeneous structure, large-angle scattering increases with increasing nuclear size [36].

The scattering cross section significantly increases as the nuclear-to-cytoplasm (N/C) ratio increases (Fig. 2b). The N/C ratio is defined as the diameter of the nucleus divided by the diameter of the cytoplasm. Scattering cross section also increases as the relative nuclear/cytoplasm refractive index is increased (Fig. 2c). For nuclear sizes and index of refraction values within the ranges expected for biological cells, there appears to be a linear relationship between relative nuclear/cytoplasmic refractive index and scattering cross section; the relationship between N/C ratio and scattering cross section is of higher order.

Influence of Organelles

To investigate the effect of small cytoplasmic organelles, three simulations were conducted. For each of the three cases, a $15\,\mu m$ spherical cell with a $5\,\mu m$ nucleus (mean $m = 1.02$; spatial fluctuations of 2–$20\,\mu m^{-1}$) was created. In addition to the nucleus, the first cell contained an 8.5% volume fraction (v.f.) of melanin ($n = 1.65$;

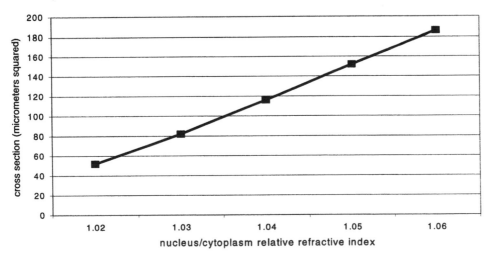

(c)

Figure 2 *(continued)*

1 μm sphere). Melanin was modeled with and without absorption. There was little difference in results when absorption was incorporated as an imaginary component of the refractive index. Despite its high absorption coefficient, melanin causes little attenuation within a cell because pathlengths are very small. To compare the effects of melanin to an organelle of lower refractive index, a second cell was modeled containing an 8.5% volume fraction of organelles similar in size, shape, and refractive index to mitochondria (ellipsoids $\sim 0.5\,\mu$m $\times$ 0.5 μm $\times$ 1.5 μm; $n = 1.41$). A third cell (amelanotic) was constructed similarly to the second cell but contained only a 3% organelle volume fraction. The scattering patterns from these simulations are shown in Fig. 3.

Figure 3 demonstrates that internal structure can have a strong influence on scattering pattern, particularly for angles over 40°. In the cells containing melanin and mitochondria, the total volumes of organelles in the cell are identical. The difference in the two curves is due to the higher index of melanin relative to mitochondria. The melanin results in a scattering pattern that covers a smaller magnitude range than the other two curves. The magnitude range of a scattering pattern is defined as the scattering pattern's maximum intensity value divided by the minimum intensity value (I_{max}/I_{min}). Scattering cross section was also larger for a cell containing melanin rather than lower index organelles. Scattering cross sections of cells containing melanin and mitochondria (8.5% v.f.) and the amelanotic cell (3% v.f.) were 861, 729, and 639 μm^2, respectively. In general, increasing organelle volume

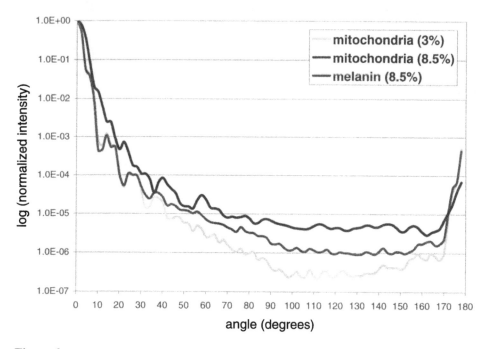

Figure 3 Influence of internal structure on scattering pattern. Three simulations are shown: a cell containing organelles of refractive index and size consistent with melanin (8.5% volume fraction), a cell containing organelles with index and size of mitochondria (8.5% volume fraction), and an amelanotic cell containing organelles with index and size of mitochondria but smaller volume fraction (3%).

fraction increases scattering cross section and makes the scattering pattern more isotropic.

Influence of Morphology

The FDTD model was used to investigate the influence of morphology on scattering patterns. For example, does it matter whether a cell is constructed by placing a certain number of organelles of specific size and refractive index at explicit locations rather than randomly generating a dielectric structure, using a range of refractive indices and a chosen frequency of index fluctuations? To examine the difference between these two cases, the scattering pattern of a cell generated with specific morphology was compared to the scattering pattern of a cell constructed using random refractive index assignments. To generate the cell without morphological structure, all grid points within the sphere were assigned refractive index values, based on the desired frequency of spatial fluctuations in refractive index (2–20 μm^{-1}) and a chosen range of refractive index values uniformly distributed about a mean index ($n = 1.40 \pm 0.05$). The cell with known morphology is similar to the melanotic cell described in the previous section. Results are shown in Fig. 4. The overall shape and range of the scattering pattern are similar for a cell with random dielectric structure and a cell with specific morphology.

Figure 5 demonstrates the effect of changing the frequency of spatial variations while keeping the mean refractive index value constant for a cell with randomly generated dielectric structure. The normalized scattering patterns for two cells are plotted. Both cells have a mean index of $n = 1.4$, with uniform distributed variations between $n = 1.35$ and $n = 1.45$. In one cell, the spatial frequency of the index variations ranges from 5 to 20 μm^{-1}; in the other cell, the spatial frequency of the varia-

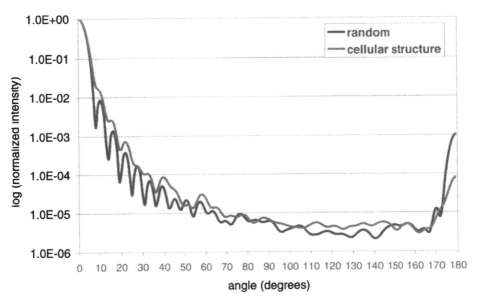

Figure 4 Comparison of scattering pattern from cell with specified internal structure (cytoplasm, nucleus, and organelles) to that of a cell with randomly assigned dielectric structure. Mean indices of both cells are identical, $n = 1.4$.

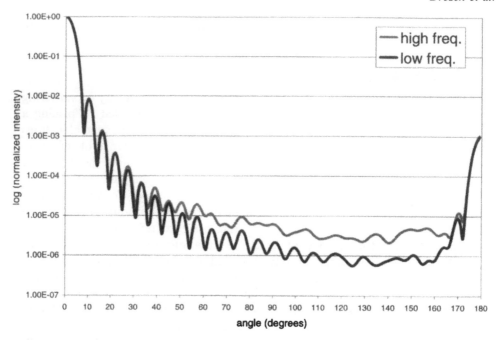

Figure 5 Scattering pattern of two cells with randomly assigned dielectric structure. The spatial frequency of index fluctuations is higher in the top curve (labeled high freq.) than in the lower curve (labeled low freq.). Mean refractive index is the same for both cells.

tions ranges from 2 to $10\,\mu m^{-1}$. The curves demonstrate that as the frequency of refractive index fluctuations is increased, the scattering intensity becomes higher at large angles.

Influence of Extracellular Medium

Typically, in published simulations of cell scattering or goniometric measurements, the cell is surrounded by a low index medium such as extracellular fluid ($n = 1.35$), blood ($n = 1.345$), growth medium ($n = 1.34$), or phosphate-buffered saline ($n = 1.33$) [24,29,30,37]. However, in tissue, cells are likely surrounded by other cells or tissue structures of higher index of refraction. When an object is bordered by other objects of similar index rather than a medium of significantly lower index, scattering will be reduced due to index matching. To demonstrate this concept, we repeated an experiment first performed by Barer and Joseph in the 1950s [38]. Figure 6a shows two images of cuvettes filled with equal concentrations of breast cancer cells ($10^6\,mL^{-1}$). In the cuvette on the left, the cells are immersed in saline solution ($n = 1.33$). Because of scattering from the cells, it is not possible to read the text behind the cuvette. In the cuvette on the right, the cells are immersed in an albumin solution ($n = 1.37$). Scattering is reduced, and the text is readable.

The FDTD model predicts the index-matching effect. Figure 6b shows the scattering pattern of an ovarian cancer cell immersed in solutions of different indices of refraction: $n = 1.35$ and $n = 1.37$. When the index of the medium surrounding the cytoplasm is increased to more closely match that of the cytoplasm ($n = 1.37$), scattering at the smallest angles is reduced by almost an order of magnitude relative

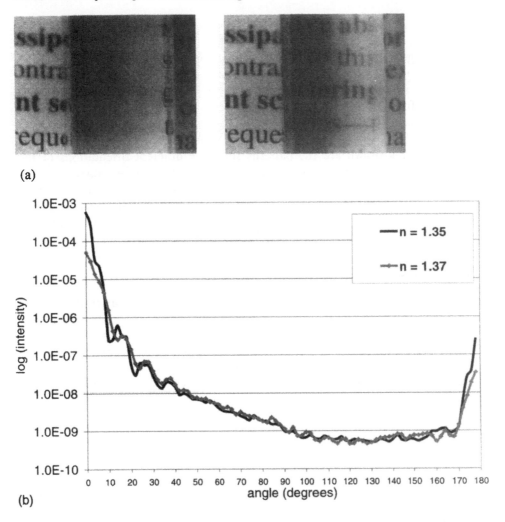

(a)

(b)

Figure 6 (a) As a visible demonstration of the reduction in scattering achievable by immersing cells in a solution of like index, two cuvettes are shown with equal concentrations of cells. In the cuvette on the left, cells are immersed in saline ($n = 1.33$); in the cuvette on the right, cells are immersed in a higher index albumin solution ($n = 1.38$). Index matching reduces the scattering, and the text behind the cuvette is readable. (b) Influence of external medium on scattering pattern. The scattering patterns of the same cell immersed in media of varying index ($n = 1.35$, $n = 1.37$) are compared.

to the $n = 1.35$ case. Scattering cross section is reduced from $729\,\mu m^2$ to $192\,\mu m^2$ simply by decreasing the index mismatch by $\Delta n = 0.02$.

Scattering from a Collagen Fiber

To investigate the scattering pattern of collagen, a collagen fiber was modeled using a cylindrical geometry ($3\,\mu m$ diameter, $20\,\mu m$ length). The collagen fiber was composed of a number of fibrils oriented along the long axis of the cylinder. The diameter of the fibrils ranged from 60 to 240 nm. The fibrils contained cross-striations approximately every 60 nm along the length. These cross-striations were implemented through refractive index fluctuations. The refractive index of collagen has been measured to be between $n = 1.46$ and $n = 1.55$ [39]. The high end of this range was measured using dried collagen and is not realistic for in vivo tissues. The simulation reported here used a mean value for collagen of $n = 1.46$ ($\Delta n = \pm 0.04$. The extra-cellular matrix surrounding collagen can vary from watery to a gel-like consistency, altering its refractive index. For this experiment, the index of refraction of the extracellular matrix was set at $n = 1.36$.

The calculated scattering pattern of a collagen fiber is shown in Fig. 7. The scattering patterns shown are the patterns for three different orientations of the collagen fiber with respect to an incoming plane wave in the $+z$ direction. The collagen fiber was placed along the x axis, the y axis, and the z axis for the three trials. As is the case for cells, the scattering pattern is highly peaked in the forward direction. The number of orders of magnitude covered by the scattering partern (I_{max}/I_{min}) is lower for collagen than for a cell by one to two orders of magnitude.

Wavelength Dependence of Scattering Pattern

To investigate the wavelength dependence of cellular scattering, scattering from the same cell was simulated for wavelengths of 514 mm, 780 nm, and $2\,\mu$m. The results are shown in Fig. 8. As evidenced by Fig. 8, changes in wavelength, even in the visible portion of the spectrum, produce significant changes in the scattering. As the wavelength increases with respect to the size of the scatterers, the number of peaks in the curves decreases. This can be qualitatively predicted from a decrease in the average Mie size parameter.

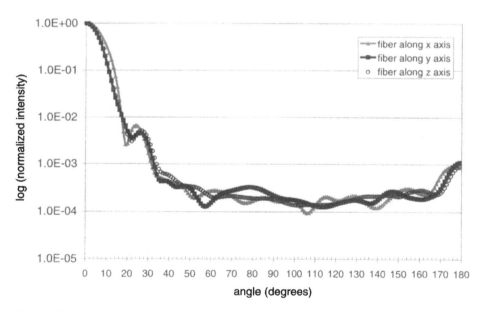

Figure 7   Scattering pattern of a collagen fiber. Curves shown are for three orientations of the collagen fiber with respect to an incoming plane wave along the $+z$ axis. The collagen fiber was oriented along the x axis, y axis, and z axis, respectively.

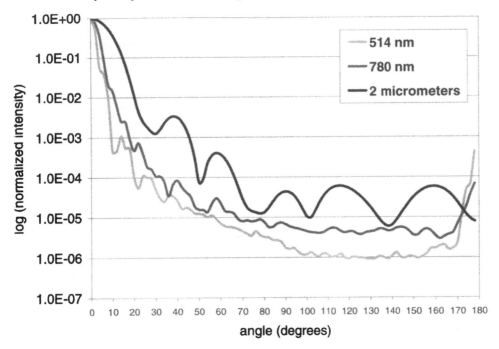

Figure 8 Wavelength dependence of scattering pattern. The normalized scattering pattern of one cell is shown for three wavelengths (514 nm, 780 nm, 2 μm).

The FDTD model was also used to investigate the wavelength dependence of scattering cross section. Recently, Perelman et al. [40] presented a technique for extracting nuclear size distributions from measurements of tissue backscattering. A fundamental assumption of the technique is that the optical scattering cross section, $\sigma_s(\lambda, l)$, of the nucleus of a cell can be predicted using the van de Hulst (anomalous diffraction) approximation [41],

$$\sigma_s(\lambda, l) = \frac{1}{2}\pi l^2 \left[1 - \frac{\sin(2\delta/\lambda)}{\delta/\lambda} + \left(\frac{\sin(\delta/\lambda)}{\delta/\lambda}\right)^2 \right] \tag{4}$$

where $\delta = \pi n_c l(m-1)$, n_c being the refractive index of cytoplasm, m is the refractive index of the nucleus relative to that of cytoplasm, and l the diameter of the nucleus. The van de Hulst approximation assumes that the nucleus of a cell can be modeled as a homogeneous sphere.

Finite-difference time-domain predictions for optical scattering cross section for inhomogeneous nuclei were compared to results obtained using the van de Hulst approximation for wavelengths between 500 and 900 nm. The van de Hulst approximation was computed for 5 μm diameter nucleus, $m = 1.04$, surrounded by cytoplasm, $n_c = 1.36$. Two sets of FDTD computations were considered. First, the nucleus was modeled as a 5 μm sphere, $m = 1.04$, surrounded by cytoplasm, $n_c = 1.36$. This produces the same results that would be predicted by Mie theory. The comparison of FDTD homogeneous sphere results to results from the van de Hulst approximation (Fig. 9) demonstrate that the van de Hulst

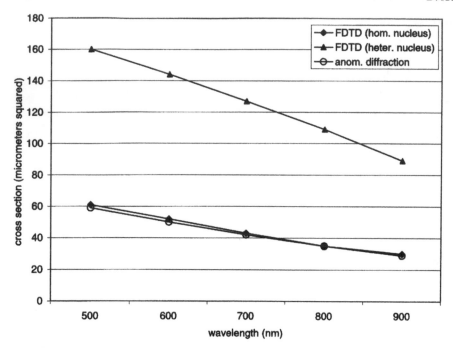

Figure 9 Scattering cross section versus wavelength for nucleus surrounded by cytoplasm. Three cases are shown. First, the van de Hulst approximation (anomalous diffraction approximation) is used to calculate scattering for a $5\,\mu$m nucleus ($m = 1.04$; $n_{\text{cytoplasm}} = 1.36$). Second, the FDTD model is used to calculate scattering for a homogeneous $5\,\mu$m nucleus ($m = 1.04$; $n_{\text{cytoplasm}} = 1.36$). Third, the FDTD model is used to calculate scattering for a heterogeneous $5\,\mu$m nucleus, with mean relative refractive index identical to the homogeneous case and spatial fluctuations ranging from 2 to 30, μm^{-1}.

approximation is valid in this wavelength and particle diameter region. For the second set of FDTD simulations, the nucleus was modeled as an inhomogeneous sphere surrounded by cytoplasm, with nuclear index uniformly distributed between $m = 1.01$ and $m = 1.07$ (mean $m = 1.04$). The frequency of spatial variations ranged from 2 to 30 μm^{-1}. A 33 nm grid spacing was used for all wavelengths so that the same spatial frequency fluctuations could be simulated for all cases. As shown in Fig. 9, FDTD results for an inhomogeneous cell predict a cross section versus wavelength trend similar to that predicted by the van de Hulst approximations. However, the cross section values predicted for an inhomogeneous nucleus are a factor of 2–3 higher.

16.3.5 Discussion

An obvious question about a model as computationally intensive as the FDTD method is whether such an approach is really necessary. Are simple analytical descriptions of phase function such as those provided through Mie theory or Henyey–Greenstein approximations sufficient? It is our belief that simple analytical descriptions of cellular scattering are adequate for only some purposes. For instance, if a Monte Carlo model is used to calculate total tissue reflectance or transmittance, approximations such as Henyey–Greenstein or Mie theory are likely to produce acceptable results. However, if the same Monte Carlo model is used to simulate a typical endoscopic situation, in which the light delivery and collection fibers are very near to each other, the choice of phase function will significantly affect the number of photons collected. The influence of phase function on light transport for small source–detector separations was demonstrated previously by Mourant et al. [42]. The results of their simulations demonstrate the necessity of choosing a phase function that accurately reflects the probability of large-angle scatter when small source–detector separations are used. Accurate information about large-angle scattering is particularly critical in understanding the subcellular sources of OCT signals because most of the photons collected have been scattered through large angles.

We believe that a more flexible and more realistic approach such as that provided by the FDTD solution is the only way to estimate the accuracy of current Mie theory and Henyey–Greenstein approximations. In addition, we believe that there is valuable information about the interaction of light with a single cell that can be obtained from our more complicated approach. For instance, we find that the overall shape of the nucleus influences small-angle scattering whereas the effects of small intracellular organelles, or high frequency index of refraction fluctuations, are more evident at larger angles. We believe that understanding these types of trends not only develops fundamental knowledge of the interaction of light with a single cell but also serves a practical purpose in facilitating the design of more effective optical diagnostic systems, by allowing prediction of changes in scattering as a function of cell morphology.

Currently, limitations in the knowledge of cellular composition and dielectric structure make it difficult to construct a specific type of cell, simulate it, and conclude that the obtained scattering pattern is exactly what would be obtained through experimental measurements of the scattering from that kind of cell. However, the simulations presented in this chapter clearly establish that scattering patterns change significantly depending on the cell's internal structure, the surrounding environment, and the wavelength of the illuminating light. Thus, the use of one phase function such as the Henyey–Greenstein phase function or a Mie theory approximation to represent a "typical" cell is probably unrealistic. Henyey–Greenstein phase functions have been shown to poorly describe large-angle scattering. This was documented by Mourant et al. [37] and is further supported by the experimental measurements presented in this work. Mie theory approximations are severely limited because they do not account for internal structures, which are expected to be the primary source of cellular scattering in in vivo measurements.

The FDTD simulations document the influence of organelle volume fraction and refractive index on cellular scattering. Both volume fraction and refractive index of cell components will be highly variable in biological cells and will depend upon cell type. Although it is possible to qualitatively predict trends in phase function or scattering cross section as refractive index and volume fraction are varied, the FDTD method provides more quantitative information. The simulations suggest that it is possible to consider that increasing the size and spatial variations of the nucleus is analogous to changing organelle volume fraction. The similarity of cells simulated with specific morphology to those with randomly generated dielectric structure suggest that it is the overall frequency and magnitude of index of refraction fluctuations, rather than a particular spatial arrangement of cell components, that has the more crucial effect on a cell's scattering pattern. The effect of high frequency fluctuations, which can be viewed as small scatterers, is particularly apparent at large angles. In a cell, high frequency fluctuations in refractive index might created by components such as microtubules, membranes, chromatin, or other organelle constituents.

In summary, although computationally intensive, the FDTD method places no limitations on the geometry or index structure of the objects under question. The model can be used to study the effect of changes of wavelength and of cellular biochemical and morphological structure. The data obtained from the model can be used to obtain phase functions, scattering cross section, and anisotropy. As the data demonstrate, relatively small changes in internal structure, external medium, and wavelength can impact both phase function and scattering cross section. These changes in phase function and scattering cross section significantly influence the appearance of OCT images.

16.4 THE INFLUENCE OF TISSUE MICROSTRUCTURE ON OCT IMAGES

We now consider how changes in tissue microstructure affect OCT images. Most sources used in OCT have coherence lengths that limit the depth resolution to tens of micrometers. Even using high-powered, ultrafast laser sources of the shortest coherence length, the obtainable resolution is on the order of a few micrometers. With these specifications it is difficult to directly image even the largest organelle in a single (human) cell, the nucleus, which ranges between 5 and 15 μm. However, the effects of subresolution particles have been experimentally observed in OCT images, in ways that are consistent with the predictions of the FDTD model presented in Section 16.3 [43 45].

Sergeev and colleagues [43] studied the effect of melanin on light scattering in tissue and the effect it had on OCT images. The FDTD model predicts increased scattering for a cell with melanin at all angles with respect to an amelanotic cell. This increase is most significant at large angles, where predicted scattering is increased by three to four orders of magnitude. The effect of this change in the scattering properties on OCT images was studied by imaging a pigmented nevus [43]. Although individual cells cannot be resolved in the OCT images obtained, they showed that by properly segmenting the image the regions of cells with melanin could be isolated. The isolated regions corresponded to areas of increased brightness in the OCT image.

The effects of increased nuclear size in epithelial cells are also evident in measured OCT images. The groups of Feldchtein [44] and Pitris [45] have shown images of cervical epithelium as it transitions from a normal region to a cancerous region. Figure 10 (see color plate) shows an image taken from Ref. 44 that illustrates this transition. At the left of the image, a layered structure is observed. The top layer, corresponding to the epithelium, shows characteristic relatively low backscatter with respect to the second connective tissue layer. To the right of the image, an invasive cancer of the uterine cervix is observed. Not only is the layered structure lost, but the backscatter of the epithelium is seen to increase with respect to the normal epithelium. This observation is consistent with the increased scattering cross section from cells with higher nuclear-to-cytoplasmic ratios.

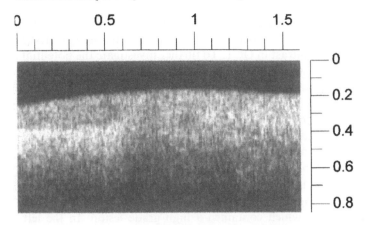

Figure 10 Optical coherence tomographic image of the transition from normal epithelium (left) to pathological epithelium (right). (See color plate.) (Adapted from Ref. 44.)

16.5 METHODS TO ENHANCE INTRINSIC CONTRAST

Scattering properties may be modulated in an attempt to enhance optical differentiation between normal and diseased tissue. In this section we consider one particularly promising approach to induce changes in scattering properties: the application of acetic acid as an optical contrast agent. Acetic acid is already in routine clinical use as a contrast agent during colposcopic examination to identify atypical areas of the cervix that require biopsy. Addition of 1–6% acetic acid causes acetowhitening of many cervical epithelial abnormalities including cervical intraepithelial neoplasia, adenocarcinoma, invasive squamous cell carcinoma, and inflammation [46]. Numerous studies have documented the use of acetic acid to improve the detection of dysplastic regions of the cervix [47,48].

Although acetic acid can augment detection of cervical dysplasia missed by Papanicolau screening [49], the mechanism through which acetic acid produces selective tissue whitening has never been fully elucidated. It has been suggested that acetic acid causes cross-linking of proteins, preventing light from passing through the epithelium. Because light does not penetrate to the underlying vessels, the epithelium appears white rather than pink. The effect is more pronounced in abnormal regions because these regions have a higher nuclear density and consequently a higher concentration of protein [46]. We hypothesize that some of the same mechanisms that cause the visual whitening effect of acetic acid may also help improve contrast in optical imaging techniques based on single backscattering such as OCT and reflected light confocal microscopy.

Smithpeter et al. [50] reported that acetic acid increases nuclear contrast in reflected light confocal images of human breast epithelial cells. Based on phase contrast microscopic experiments, we demonstrated that acetic acid induces spatial fluctuations in the nuclear refractive index. We hypothesized that these fluctuations increased backscattering from the nuclear region, resulting in clearer delineation of nuclear structure when cells were viewed using a reflected light confocal imaging system. Because both confocal microscopy and OCT rely on fluctuations of refractive index to generate image contrast, the confocal imaging results are relevant to

OCT imaging techniques as well. Because confocal methods provide subcellular resolution, confocal images can provide useful insight into the microscopic tissue structures responsible for image contrast in OCT. To further investigate the potential of acetic acid as a contrast agent, we imaged normal and dysplastic cervical biopsies before and after acetic acid application.

The confocal imaging system ($\lambda = 808$ nm) used to obtain the images presented in this section provides high contrast reflected light images of unstained biological samples at near video rate. Details of the instrumentation have been previously described [50]. The confocal system was used to obtain images of a colposcopically normal and a colposcopically abnormal biopsy from the same patient before and after addition of acetic acid. Results are shown in Fig. 11. The top row shows images of the colposcopically normal biopsy, and the bottom row contains images of the colposcopically abnormal biopsy, which contained a high grade lesion. In the left panel, the pre-acetic acid images of the abnormal biopsy show the cell outlines and

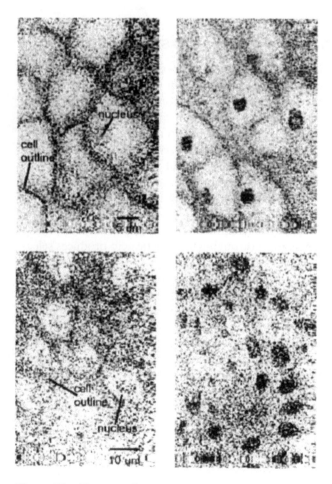

Figure 11 Top row: Images of normal cervical biopsy before (left) and after (right) application of 6% acetic acid. Bottom row: Images of colposcopically abnormal cervical biopsy before (left) and after (right) addition of 6% acetic acid. Illumination wavelength was 808 nm.

an occasional nucleus. The pre-acetic acid images of the abnormal biopsy show increased reflectivity of both the cell membranes and the nuclei. In addition, the cells are more crowded and irregularly spaced. Post-acetic acid images show increased signal from the nuclei in both the normal and abnormal biopsies. After confocal imaging, transverse frozen sections were cut and stained with hemotoxylin and eosin and were sent to an experienced pathologist for histological examination. Pathological diagnosis confirmed clinical expressions at the time of colposcopy.

The results show that after the addition of acetic acid, images of tissue can be obtained that illustrate characteristic differences between normal and neoplastic tissue. Without the application of acetic acid, it is difficult to distinguish the nucleus from the cytoplasm of a cell because of low contrast. This suggests that to develop diagnostic applications of confocal microscopy, enhanced visualization of the nucleus may be required to facilitate the identification of morphological changes indicative of dysplasia such as increased nuclear size and irregular shape. We have achieved similar results using acetic acid on multiple cell lines and tissue types in both in vitro and in vivo situations, so we suspect that acetic acid will be useful for improving nuclear contrast in a variety of organ sites.

Further work is needed to elucidate the underlying physical mechanisms responsible for the changes caused by acetic acid. Goniometric measurements have indicated increased scattering from cells after the addition of acetic acid [51]. Measurements of scattering cross section of cells before and after exposure to acetic acid also offer further evidence of enhanced scattering [36]. In addition, finite-difference time-domain simulations of light scattering from inhomogeneous cells indicate increased scattering when cells are modeled with alterations in nuclear refractive index structure, based on phase contrast microscope images of cells before and after the addition of acetic acid [30]. Despite all of the evidence suggestive of heightened scattering due to acetic acid, the particular biochemical and morphological alterations caused by acetic acid that are responsible for the increase in scattering are not known.

Although further work is necessary to elucidate the precise mechanisms responsible for acetowhitening, it is evident that contrast agents such as acetic acid may offer a simple, inexpensive means to enhance the diagnostic utility of scattering-based imaging modalities. The encouraging preliminary results achieved using acetic acid to enhance contrast in confocal reflected light images suggest that acetic acid might be a valuable contrast agent for OCT as well.

Because the resolution of an OCT system is typically 10–20 μm, whereas the resolution of a confocal microscope is closer to 1–2 μm, the expected effect of acetic acid on an OCT image would be an apparent enhancement in brightness of those regions where scattering from nuclei had increased. It is important to recognize that changes in scattering, such as those induced by acetic acid, occur on a microscopic spatial scale well below the resolution of OCT imaging systems. However, these changes still impact OCT images.

It is possible to observe the enhanced backscattering induced by the addition of acetic acid in OCT images. Figures 12 and 13 (see color plates) show the effect of the exposure of normal buccal mucosa in vivo to 6% acetic acid for 3 min. Figure 12 shows the measurement site before the application of acetic acid, and Fig. 13 shows the same site after treatment with acetic acid. The figures were acquired with a fiber-optic probe–based system detailed in Ref. 52. For these measurements the system

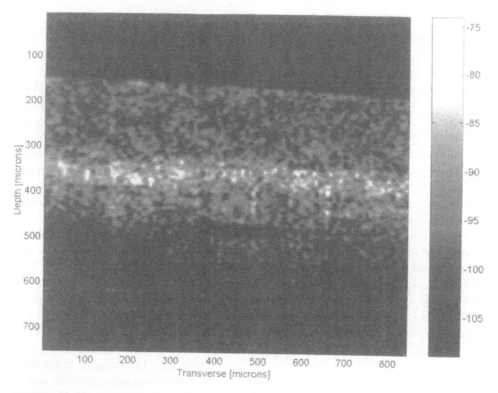

Figure 12 In vivo OCT image of normal buccal mucosa. The intensity scale is in decibels of sample reflectivity. The figure shows a layered structure corresponding to the epithelium and connective tissue layers. (See color plate.)

had a shot noise limited sensitivity of −102 dB, with a measured axial resolution of 24 μm. The dimensions of the images are 750 μm (depth) by 840 μm (transverse). The intensity scale is in decibels of sample reflectivity. Figure 12 illustrates the typical layered structure of the buccal mucosa. The top layer corresponds to the epithelium, which is weakly scattering. It has a uniform depth of about 150 μm. Immediately below the epithelium there is a thin layer of dense connective tissue. This layer measures about 75 μm and is observed as a bright band across the width of the image. Underneath the dense connective tissue lies a layer of softer connective tissue. This layer is less scattering in the image. Blood vessels, an example of which 500 μm deep and 400–500 μm across is shown in Fig. 12, are often observed in the soft connective tissue layer. The depth of this layer exceeds the total imaging depth of the system. Figure 13 shows the same site as Fig. 12 after the application of 6% acetic acid for a period of 3 min. Note that the intensity scales in both figures are the same. Increased backscatter is observed from the epithelial layer, making it difficult to discern from the underlying connective tissue. A faint demarcation is observed at a depth of 300 μm. This increased scattering is consistent with the simulations and measurements mentioned above. Increased scattering from the epithelial layer significantly reduces the maximum imaging depth. Figure 13 shows that OCT imaging is sensitive to changes induced by exogenous agents, even when these changes are of a scale smaller than the resolution of the technique.

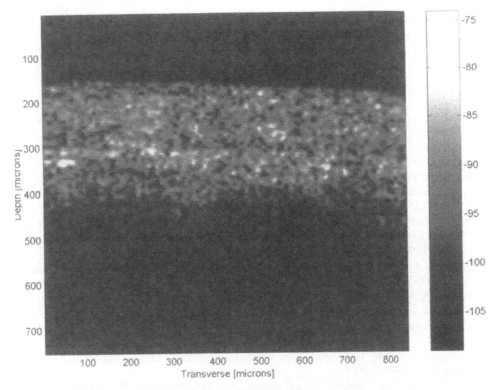

Figure 13 In vivo OCT image of normal buccal mucosa (same site as Fig. 12) after exposure to 6% acetic acid for 3 min. The epithelium shows enhanced scattering, consistent with FDTD modeling, goniometric measurements, and confocal imaging. (See color plate.)

16.6 SUMMARY

Although it is clear that the large-scale, bulk optical parameters of a medium are important in the acquisition of OCT images, subresolution fluctuations of these parameters also affect the images significantly. Finite-difference time-domain modeling of the scattering characteristics of different tissues and tissue components provides a powerful tool with which to investigate their effect on OCT images. It also is an effective tool to investigate the changes in scattering induced by exogenous agents. The spatial resolution afforded by the technique has the added benefit of allowing the modeling of structures that closely resemble the morphological changes that occur throughout disease progression. FDTD modeling of these changes provides a bridge between subresolution morphological changes and the scattering properties of cells and tissue. The information gained from simulations of changes in tissue microstructure can then be applied to predict changes in the signal detected in OCT.

ACKNOWLEDGMENTS

The authors gratefully acknowledge financial support from NSF (BES-9872829). In addition, the contributions of Tom Collier, Benoit de Pradier, Peggy Shen, Anais

Malpica, and Michele Follen in collecting and analyzing the confocal microscopy images are gratefully acknowledged.

REFERENCES

1. Welch A, van Gemert M. Overview of optical and thermal laser-tissue interaction and nomenclature. In: A Welch, M van Gemert, eds. Optical-Thermal Response of Laser-Irradiated Tissue. New York: Plenum Press, 1995.
2. Ishimaru A. Wave Propagation and Scattering in Random Media, Vol 1. San Diego, CA: Academic Press, 1978:572.
3. Prahl S, Jacques S, Welch A. A Monte Carlo model of light propagation in tissue. SPIE 5:102–111, 1989.
4. Star W. Diffusion theory of light transport. In: A. Welch, M van Gemert, eds. Optical-Thermal Response of Laser-Irradiated Tissue. New York: Plenum Press, 1995.
5. Jacques S, Wang L. Monte Carlo modeling of light transport in tissue. In: A Welch, M Gemert, eds. Optical-Thermal Response of Laser-Irradiated Tissue. New York: Plenum Press, 1995:1–5.
6. Jacques S, Wang L, Hielscher A. Time resolved photon propagation in tissue. In: A Welch, M van Gemert, eds. Optical-Thermal Response of Laser-Irradiated Tissue. New York: Plenum Press, 1995.
7. Pfefer TJ, et al. A three dimensional modula adaptable grid numerical model for light propagation during laser irradiation of skin tissue. IEEE J Selected Topics Quant Electron 2:934–942, 1996.
8. Pan Y, et al. Low-coherence optical tomography in turbid issue: Theoretical analysis. Appl Opt 34:6564–6574, 1995.
9. Smithies DJ, et al. Signal attenuation and localization in optical coherence tomography studied by Monte Carlo simulation. Phys Med Biol 43:3025–3044, 1998.
10. Lindmo T, Chen Z, Nelson J, Milner T. Accuracy and noise in ODT studied by Monte Carlo simulation. Phys Med Biol 43:3045–3064, 1998.
11. Ducros MG. Design and construction of an optical coherence microscope prototype, PhD. Thesis, Department of Electrical and Computer Engineering, The University of Texas at Austin, Austin, TX, 1996, p. 84.
12. Schmitt JM, et al. Optical characterization of dense tissues using low-coherence interferometry. Proc Soc Photo-Opt Instrum Eng 1889:197, 1993.
13. Schmitt JM, et al. Optical-coherence tomography of a dense tissue: Statistics of attenuation and backscattering. Phys Med Biol 39(10):1705–1720, 1994.
14. Schmitt JM, Knuttel A, Bonner RF. Measurement of optical properties of biological tissues by low-coherence reflectometry. Appl Opt 32:6032–6042, 1993.
15. Yadlowsky MJ, Schmitt JM, Bonner RF. Multiple scattering in optical coherence microscopy. Appl Opt 34(25):5699–5707, 1995.
16. Pan Y, Birngruber R, Engelhardt R. Optical coherence-gated imaging in biological tissues. Proc SPIE Int Soc Opt Eng 2678:165–171, 1996.
17. Schmitt JM, Knuttel A. Model of optical coherence tomography of heterogeneous tissue. J Opt Soc Am A. Opt Image Sci 14(6):1231–1242, 1997.
18. Knuttel A, Schork R, Bocker D. Analytical modeling of spatial resolution curves in turbid media acquired with optical coherence tomography (OCT). In: Three-Dimensional Microscopy: Image Acquisition and Processing III. Bellingham, WA: (C. Cogswell, G. Kino, and T. Wilson, eds.) Proc. SPIE 2655, p. 258–270 (1996).
19. Lutomirski RF. Atmospheric degradation of electrooptic system performance. Appl Opt 17:3915–3921, 1978.

20. Schmitt J, Kumar G. Turbulent nature of refractive index variations in biological tissue. Opt Lett 21:1310–1312, 1996.
21. Schmitt JM, Kumar G. Optical scattering properties of soft tissue: A discrete particle model. Appl Opt 37(13):2788–2797, 1998.
22. Streekstra GJ, Hoekstra AG, Nijhof EJ, Heethaar RM. Light scattering by red blood cells in ektacytometry: Fraunhofer versus anomalous diffraction. Appl Opt 32:2266–2272, 1993.
23. Videen G, Ngo D. Light scattering multipole solution for a cell. J Biomed Opt 3:212–220, 1998.
24. Nillson A, Alsholm A, Karllson A, Andersson-Engels S. T-matrix computations of light scattering by red blood cells. Appl Opt 3:2735–2748, 1998.
25. Dunn A, Richards-Kortum R. Three-dimensional computational of light scattering from cells. IEEE J Spec Topics Quant Electron 1997:1997.
26. Beauvoit B, Kitai T, Chance B. Time-resolved spectroscopy of mitochondria, cells, and rat tissue under normal and pathological conditions. In Photon Transport in Highly Scattering Tissue (S. Aurillier, B. Chance, G. Mueller, A. Priezzhev, and V. Tuchin, eds.) Proc. SPIE 2326, 127–136. 1995.
27. Yee K. Numerical solutions of initial boundary value problems involving Maxwell's equations in isotropic media. IEEE Trans Antennas Propagation AP-14:302–307, 1966.
28. Liao Z, Wong B, Yang B, Yuan Y. A transmitting boundary for transient wave analysis. Sci Sin Ser A 27:1063–1076, 1984.
29. Brunsting A. Differential light scattering from spherical mammalian cells. Biophysic J 14:439–453, 1974.
30. Drezek R. Finite difference time domain simulations and goniometric measurements of light scattering from cells. PhD Thesis, Electrical and Computer Engineering. Austin, TX: University of Texas at Austin, 1998.
31. Valkenburg J, Woldringh C. Phase separation between nucleoid and cytoplasm in E. coli as defined by immersive refractometry. J Bacteriol 160:1151–1157, 1984.
32. Maier J, Walker S, Fantini S, Franceschini, Gratton E. Possible correlation between blood glucose concentration and the reduced scattering coefficient of tissues in the near infrared. Opt Lett 19:2062–2064, 1994.
33. Liu H, Beauvoit B, Kimura M, Chance B. Dependence of tissue optical properties on solute-induced changes in refractive index and osmolarity. J Biomed Opt 1:200–211, 1996.
34. Vitkin I, Woolsey J, Wilson B, Anderson R. Optical and thermal characterization of natural (Sepia oficinalis) melanin. Photochem Photobiol 59:455–462, 1994.
35. Boone C, Kelloff G, Steele H. The natural history of intraepithelial neoplasia: Relevance to the search for intermediate endpoint biomarkers. Cell Biochem 16G:23–26, 1992.
36. Dunn A. Light scattering properties of cells. PhD Thesis, Electrical and Computer Engineering. Austin, TX: University of Texas at Austin, 1997.
37. Mourant J, Freyer J, Hielscher A, Eick A, Shen D, Johnson T. Mechanisms of light scattering from biological cells relevant to noninvasive optical tissue diagnostics. Appl Opt 37:3586–3593, 1998.
38. Barer R, Joseph S. Refractometry of living cells. Quart J Microsc Sci 95:399–423, 1954.
39. Yarker Y, Aspden R, Hukins D. Birefringence of articular cartilage and the distribution of collagen fibril orientations. Connect Tissue Res 11:207–213, 1983.
40. Perelman L, Backman V, Wallace M, Zonios G, Manoharan R, Nustrat A, Shields S, Seiler M, Lima C, Hamano T, Itzkan I, Van Dam J, Crawford J, Feld M. Observation of periodic fine structure in reflectance from biological tissue: A new technique for measuring nuclear size distribution. Phys Rev Lett 80:627–630, 1998.
41. van de Hulst HV. Light Scattering by Small Particles. New York: Dover, 1981.

42. Mourant J, Boyer J, Hielscher A, Bigio I. Influence of the scattering phase function on light transport measurements in turbid media performed with small source-detector separations. Opt Lett 21:546–548, 1996.
43. Sergeev A, et al. Melanin effect on light scattering in tissues: From electrodynamics of living cell to OCT imaging. In: Coherence Domain Optical Methods in Biomedical Science and Clinical Applications. V. Tuchin, H. Podbielska, and B. Ovyrn, eds. Proc. SPIE 2981, 58–63 (1997).
44. Feldchtein FI, et al. Endoscopic applications of optical coherence tomography. Opt Express 3(6):257–270, 1998.
45. Pitris C. et al. High resolution imaging of gynecologic neoplasms using optical coherence tomography. Obstet Gynecol 93(1):135–139, 1999.
46. Anderson M, Jordon J, Morse A, Sharp F. A Text and Atlas of Integrated Colposcopy. St. Louis: Mosby, 1993.
47. Ottaviano M, La Torre P. Examination of the cervix with the naked eye using the acetic acid test. Am J Obstet Gynecol 143:139–142, 1987.
48. Van Le L, Broekhuizen F, Janzer-Steele R, Behar M, Samter T. Acetic acid visualization of the cervix to detect cervical dysplasia. Obstet Gynecol 81:293–295, 1993.
49. Fiscor G, Fuller S, Jeromin J, Beyer D, Janca F. Enhancing cervical cancer detection using nucleic acid hybridization and acetic acid tests. Nurse Practitioner 15:26–30, 1990.
50. Smithpeter C, Dunn A, Drezek R, Collier T, Richards-Kortum R. Near real time confocal microscopy of in situ amelanotic cells. Sources of signal, contrast agents, and limits of contrast. J Biomed Opt 3:429–436, 1998.
51. Drezek R, Dunn A, Richards-Kortum R. Light scattering from cells: FDTD simulations and goniometric measurements. Appl Opt 38:3651–3661, 1999.
52. Zuluaga AF. Development of a cervical probe for optical coherence imaging in-vivo. PhD. Thesis, Dept Electrical and Computer Engineering. Austin, TX: Univ Texas at Austin, 1998:49.

17

Optical Coherence Tomography in the Diagnosis and Management of Posterior Segment Disorders

MARK J. RIVELLESE

Tufts University School of Medicine, Boston, Massachusetts

CARMEN A. PULIAFITO

University of Miami School of Medicine, Miami, Florida

17.1 INTRODUCTION

The use of optical coherence tomography (OCT) to diagnose posterior segment disorders is the most mature clinical application of OCT. Approximately 120 OCT machines are in use in the United States. At our institution thousands of patients have been imaged, and OCT has improved our ability to accurately diagnose and document pathological conditions of the posterior segment. OCT has contributed to a better understanding of the pathogenesis of macular holes and vitreomacular traction and has provided a quantitative method of accurately detecting changes in retinal thickness due to diabetes, epiretinal membrane, and cystoid macular edema.

The anatomy of the eye is well suited for transpupillary examination of the posterior segment using OCT. OCT has proven to be useful in the evaluation and management of a variety of disorders of the posterior segment. The application of OCT to these disorders will be discussed.

The OCT images presented in this chapter were generated with a prototype OCT imager with the following specifications: center wavelength 800 nm; FWHM spectral bandwidth 30 nm; FWHM axial resolution 10 μm; FWHM lateral resolution 40 μm; reference arm scanning mechanism, galvanometric scanning; frame rate 0.5 Hz; axial scan rate 50 Hz; axial scan length 3 mm; sample arm probe type, slitlamp biomicroscope.

17.2 OPTICAL COHERENCE TOMOGRAPHY OF THE NORMAL POSTERIOR SEGMENT

One of the most attractive features of optical coherence tomography is the relative ease and rapidity with which the scans are performed and interpreted. The recognition of pathology on OCT images requires familiarity with the OCT representation of the normal posterior segment. Figure 1a (see color plate) is an OCT image of a normal retina through the optic nerve and fovea. The posterior boundary of the neurosensory retina is well delineated by a highly reflective red layer corresponding to the retinal pigment epithelium and the choriocapillaris. The outer segments of the photoreceptors are represented by a dark layer of minimal reflectivity just anterior to the highly reflective band of the RPE and choriocapillaris. The inner margin of the retina, the nerve fiber layer, is represented by a red band due to bright backscatter that is easily seen in contrast to the nonreflective vitreous. Intervening structures between the highly reflective red bands of the RPE and nerve fiber layer are represented as alternating layers of moderate and low reflectivity. This is due to the stratified structure of the retina with moderate backscatter from the fibrous inner and outer plexiform layers that are oriented perpendicular to the incident beam [1,2]. The nuclear layers have cell bodies that are oriented parallel to the incident beam and therefore have minimal backscatter and are represented by dark bands [1,2]. The retinal blood vessels are identified by their shadowing of deeper structures.

Longitudinal surveillance of patients with macular disease is accomplished by obtaining six radial scans centered at the fovea [3]. Retinal thickness is then computed for 600 macular locations and displayed as a false color topographic map (Fig. 1b). Retinal thickness is also reported as a numerical average in nine regions. Evaluation of the entire macular region is possible using the retinal thickness map. Tomograms of the optic nerve are obtained by scanning the nerve head around two radii of curvature (2.25 and 3.37 mm). The nerve fiber layer is then plotted schematically (Fig. 1c). The nerve fiber layer is thickest in the superior and inferior quadrants. Normal nerve fiber layer thickness is a mean of 148.6 μm superiorly, 143.5 μm inferiorly, 66.9 μm temporally, and 117.2 μm nasally [4].

17.3 MACULAR DISEASE

Optical coherence tomography (OCT) has become a valuable tool for a number of macular diseases, particularly those involving the vitreoretinal interface. OCT has led us to a better understanding of the anatomical relationships and pathogenesis of macular holes and epiretinal membranes and has also proven useful in the management of patients with age-related macular degeneration. The high resolution imaging of OCT also allows accurate longitudinal monitoring of patients with diabetic macular edema and central serous chorioretinopathy.

17.3.1 Macular Holes

Traditionally, the diagnosis and staging of macular holes have been accomplished by using contact lens slitlamp biomicroscopy. There are a number of lesions such as partial thickness or lamellar holes, pseudoholes, and macular cysts that may be difficult to distinguish from full thickness macular holes. OCT facilitates the identification of macular holes and aids in the staging according to the Gass classification

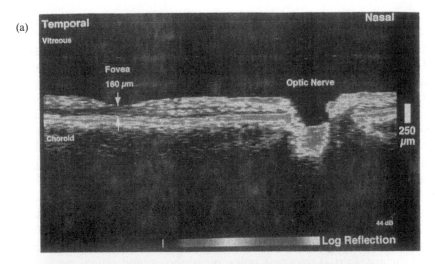

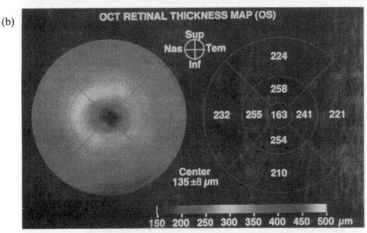

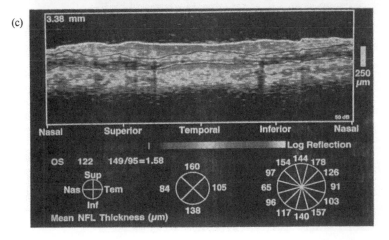

Figure 1 (a) Cross-sectional OCT image through the optic nerve and fovea of a normal subject. (b) Retinal thickness map of a normal macula. The numerical values are represented in micrometers and represent the average value of six radial scans centered at the fovea. (c) Tomogram of the optic nerve head with nerve fiber layer thickness represented in false color and numerically. (See color plate.)

of idiopathic macular holes: stage I, foveal detachment; Stage II, small full thickness hole; Stage III, fully developed, full thickness hole; and stage IV, fully developed hole with posterior vitreous detachment [5].

On OCT, a stage I macular hole appears as a decreased foveal depression with an abnormal, minimally reflective space beneath the neurosensory retina in the fovea (Fig. 2a) (see color plate). The foveolar detachment is consistent with Gass' stage I hole. Vitreous fibrils may be demonstrated inserting obliquely onto the fovea. An OCT image of a stage II hole demonstrates a flask-shaped full thickness defect (Fig. 2b). The retinal defect in stage II holes is small, and eccentric stage II holes may have a flap of retina attached to their surface. Stage III holes demonstrate a larger full thickness defect without a retinal flap (Fig. 2c). OCT images of stage IV macular holes demonstrates a full thickness defect with complete separation of the vitreous (Fig. 2d). This is in contrast to stages I–III, where the vitreous is usually seen inserting onto the retinal surface. Partial thickness holes, pseudoholes, and retinal cysts are readily distinguished from macular holes by using OCT. All of these disorders lack the full thickness defect and fluid cuff with its classic flask-shaped appearance.

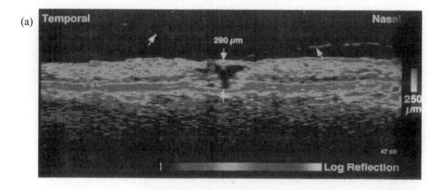

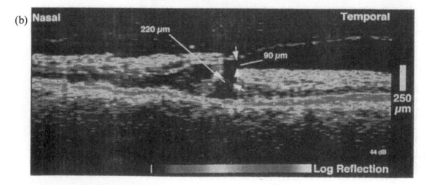

Figure 2 (a) OCT image of a stage I macular hole with loss of the foveal depression but no full thickness defect. (b) OCT image of a stage II macular hole showing a small full thickness macular hole with an eccentric flap of retinal tissue. (c) OCT image of a stage III macular hole with a larger full thickness flask-shaped retinal defect. (d) OCT image of stage IV macular hole with posterior vitreous detachment. (See color plate.)

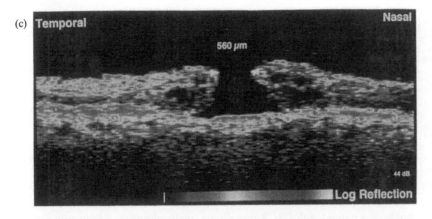

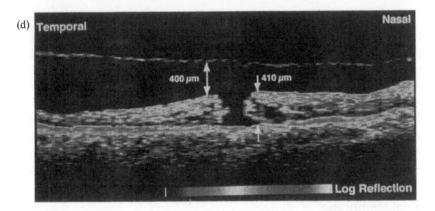

Figure 2 (*continued*)

Optical coherence tomography is also valuable for the longitudinal documentation of the progression of macular holes and can aid in the timing of surgical intervention. Approximately 50% of stage I macular holes will spontaneously improve, whereas the majority of stage II holes will progress to stage III [6]. This progression or resolution is easily demonstrated on OCT images. Additionally, patients with an idiopathic macular hole in one eye may be at increased risk for developing a macular hole in the fellow eye, and OCT may be used to evaluate the vitreoretinal interface and identify impending macular holes in fellow eyes [7].

17.3.2 Central Serous Chorioretinopathy

Central serous chorioretinopathy (CSCR) is a common retinal disorder characterized by idiopathic detachments of the neurosensory retina in the macular region [8]. OCT has proven useful for multiple purposes in CSCR. Small or shallow neurosensory detachments may be difficult to see clinically. Because of micrometer-scale resolution, OCT is capable of detecting neurosensory detachments that are difficult to detect by slitlamp biomicroscopy (Fig. 3) (see color plate). The contrast in optical

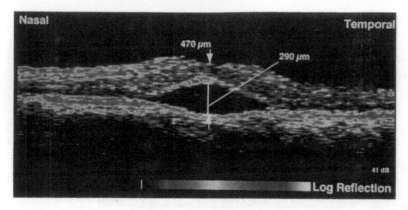

Figure 3 OCT image of a patient with CSCR revealing a small collection of fluid seen as an optically empty area beneath the highly reflective red RPE band. (See color plate.)

reflectivity between the nonreflective serous fluid and the more highly reflective posterior boundary of the neurosensory retina allows detection of small amounts of subneurosensory fluid. OCT is also capable of imaging the same retinal area over time, making it a noninvasive method of monitoring the clinical course of patients longitudinally [9]. A frequent problem arises when CSCR is present in older patients or patients with drusen or pigmentary changes in the macula. OCT images may document the absence of subretinal neovascular complexes or detect abnormalities in the choriocapillaris and RPE and aid in distinguishing between subretinal neo-vascularization and CSCR.

17.3.3 Epiretinal Membrane

Epiretinal membrane is a preretinal proliferation of fibrocellular material that may occur in healthy eyes or eyes with a pathological condition such as inflammation or retinal breaks [10]. OCT is well suited for imaging epiretinal membranes regardless of their etiology and has been used to characterize epiretinal membranes secondary to trauma, inflammatory disease, proliferative disease, intraocular surgery, and idiopathic causes [11]. The appearance of epiretinal membranes on OCT images is variable, depending on how tightly adherent the membrane is to the retinal surface. Membranes that are tightly adherent to the retinal surface may appear as a contrast in reflectivity between the membrane and the surface of the retina. Some adherent membranes may show only a deepening of the foveal pit or the formation of a pseudohole (Fig. 4a) (see color plate). A tuft or edge of membrane may be seen in some cases. Occasionally, epiretinal membranes are clearly visible on OCT as reflective tissue anterior to the retinal surface (Fig. 4b). Membranes of this type are distinguished from the posterior hyaloid by the difference in thickness of the anterior reflective band, with epiretinal membranes having a thickener reflective band.

Measurements of retinal thickness related to epiretinal membranes have shown correlation with visual acuity [11]. Furthermore, OCT images may be useful in predicting membranes that may be difficult to treat surgically and therefore aid in the timing of surgical intervention.

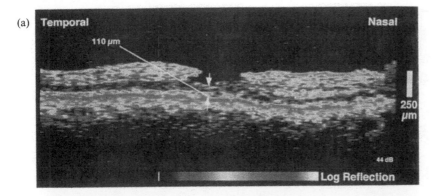

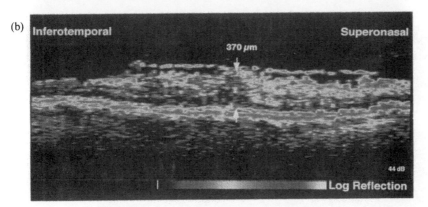

Figure 4 (a) OCT image of a pseudomacular hole with deepening of the foveal pit. Note that retinal tissue at the trough of the pseudohole. (b) OCT image of an epiretinal membrane showing skip areas of retinal adherence. (See color plate.)

17.3.4 Age-Related Macular Degeneration

Optical coherence tomographic images are useful in several aspects of age-related macular degeneration (ARMD). OCT has been used in nonexudative ARMD to characterize soft drusen and retinal pigment epithelial atrophy [12]. OCT has also been used to image detachments of the retinal pigment epithelium, detachments of the neurosensory retina, and subretinal neovascularization [12,13]. Soft drusen appear as focal elevations of the retinal pigment epithelial layer (Fig. 5a) (see color plate). Retinal pigment epithelial atrophy appears as enhanced backscatter from the choroid (Fig. 5b). In exudative ARMD, common pathologies such as serous pigment epithelial detachment (PED), hemorrhagic PED, fibrovascular PED, and neurosensory detachment have characteristic appearances. Serous PED presents as a focal elevation of the reflective RPE band over an optically empty clear space (Fig. 6a) (see color plate). The angle of elevation of the detachment is typically acute, possibly secondary to the tight adherence of the RPE cells to Bruch's membrane at the edge of the detachment. Hemorrhagic PED can be distinguished by the presence of a reflective band beneath the RPE reflective layer corresponding to the sub-RPE blood (Fig. 6b). OCT images of fibrovascular PED show a moderately reflective layer throughout the sub-RPE space beneath the detachment (Fig. 6c).

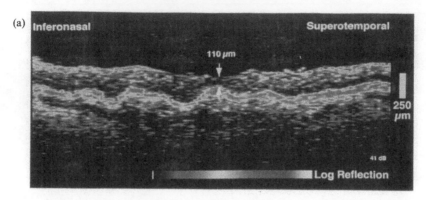

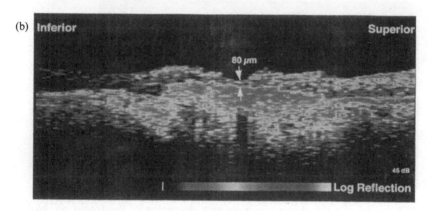

Figure 5 (a) Optical coherence tomographic image of soft drusen showing focal elevations of the RPE layer. (b) OCT image of RPE atrophy beneath the fovea. Note the increased reflectivity of the choroidal band in bright red. (See color plate.)

Optical coherence tomography may also be useful in identifying subretinal neo-vascular complexes. For this purpose, OCT is used in conjunction with fluorescein and indocyanine green angiography. Subretinal neovascularization may be represented as a fibrovascular pigment epithelial detachment or as a well-defined or poorly defined membrane. Membranes that are well defined on fluorescein angiography typically appear as fusiform or discoid thickening of the reflective band of the RPE/chorioca-pillaris that extends anteriorly, elevating the RPE (Fig. 7) (see color plate). Membranes that are poorly defined on fluorescein appear as diffuse areas of reflectivity beneath the RPE without discernible borders. A potential use for OCT is to localize choroidal neovascular membranes to either the sub-RPE space or the subretinal space. In such cases, OCT may be useful in identifying appropriate surgical candidates.

17.3.5 Macular Edema

Macular edema is a common complication of a number of retinal disorders such as diabetic retinopathy and retinal vascular disease as well as uveitis and intraocular surgery. Fluorescein angiography is the current gold standard for qualitative detection of leakage from retinal vessels. It does have several limitations: It is minimally

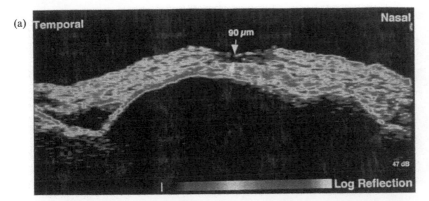

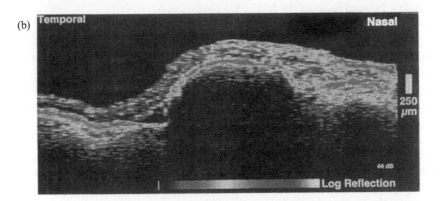

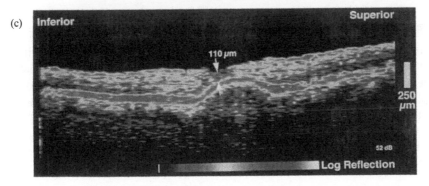

Figure 6 (a) Optical coherence tomographic image of a serous pigment epithelium detachment (PED) showing the optically empty space beneath the RPE band. (b) OCT image of a hemorrhagic PED showing a reflective band beneath the retinal pigment epithelium. (c) OCT image of a fibrous PED showing moderate backscatter beneath the RPE, which is elevated. (See color plate.)

invasive with known morbidity, results are difficult to reproduce, quantitative comparison between subsequent angiograms is difficult, and the extent of leakage does not correlate with visual function [14]. OCT has the advantage of being a noninvasive, objective, reproducible, and quantitative method of measuring retinal thickness [15]. Furthermore, retinal thickness measurements through the central fovea have

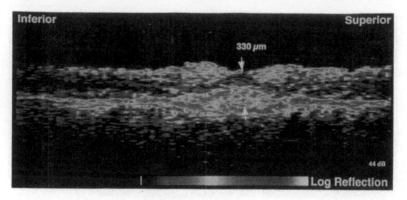

Figure 7 Optical coherence tomographic image of a well-defined subretinal neovascular membrane protruding forward beneath the RPE. (See color plate.)

been shown to correlate with visual acuity [15]. This is clinically useful for a number of reasons. First, OCT images can display early retinal thickening before it is clinically evident to the average observer. Second, OCT images can be used to direct laser treatment of intraretinal thickening. Finally, OCT can be used to follow patients longitudinally either for worsening of edema or resolution of thickening after laser treatment.

Macular edema is characterized on OCT by retinal thickening. Intraretinal areas of decreased reflectivity secondary to fluid accumulation may be present (Fig. 8a) (see color plate). Cystoid macular edema is classified by round, optically clear regions within the neurosensory retina (Fig. 8b).

17.3.6 Vitreomacular Traction

Vitreomacular traction is characterized by persistent vitreous attachment in the center of the macular causing traction on the retina. This may cause a cystoid configuration and result in decreased vision. OCT images of vitreomacular traction show incomplete detachment of the vitreous with persistent attachment to the inner retina in the macula (Fig. 9) (see color plate). Varying degrees of retinal involvement can be present, ranging from loss of the normal foveal pit to intraretinal thickening with a cystoid appearance. Longitudinal examinations may provide information as to the appropriate timing of surgical intervention.

17.4 PERIPHERAL RETINAL DISORDERS

The main clinical utility of optical coherence tomography in peripheral retinal disorders is the differentiation between retinal detachment and retinoschisis. These two entities may appear similar clinically. Optical coherence tomography is an objective and reproducible test capable of differentiating between these two disorders.

Retinoschisis is a splitting of the layers of the retina in the outer plexiform layer that has an appearance similar to retinal detachment. In most cases, these two entities are distinguishable clinically. In cases where the diagnosis is not clear on the basis of clinical appearance, ancillary tests such as perimetry, laser photocoagulation, or B-scan ultrasound may be helpful. OCT is a reliable and objective method of distinguish-

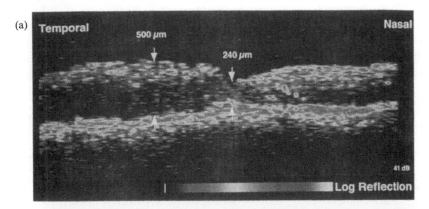

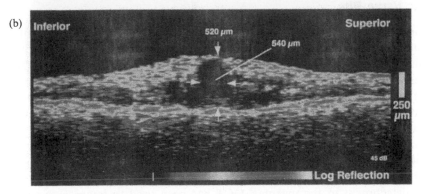

Figure 8 (a) Optical coherence tomographic image through the fovea of a patient with diabetic macular edema. There is distortion of the retinal contour and retinal thickening. (b) OCT image of a patient with cystoid macular edema. Note the intraretinal cysts represented by optically empty areas within the retina. (See color plate.)

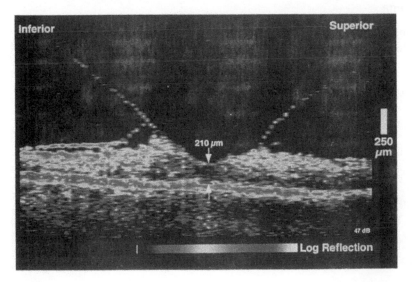

Figure 9 Optical coherence tomographic image of a patient with severe vitreomacular traction and intraretinal edema. The vitreous is displayed attached to the macula. (See color plate.)

ing schisis from retinal detachment, although lesions anterior to the equator cannot be imaged unless there is a posterior component [16]. The appearance of retinoschisis is consistent with the known histopathology. The images display splitting of the neurosensory retina at the outer plexiform layer (Fig. 10) (see color plate). Retinal detachment appears as a detachment of the entire neurosensory retina from the RPE.

17.5   OPTIC NERVE DISEASE

Optical coherence tomography has provided a better understanding of optic nerve disorders, particularly optic nerve pits. Additionally, OCT may yet prove useful for the early diagnosis and monitoring of patients with glaucoma.

17.5.1   Optic Nerve Pits

Congenital pits of the optic nerve head occur in approximately one in 11,000 patients [17]. They consist of round or oval depressions in the optic disc, usually temporally. Serous macular retinal detachment complicates 25–75% of optic disc pits [18]. OCT images of eyes with optic nerve pits and serous macular retinal detachments show a retinoschisis type of cavity that appears to communicate with the optic pit (Fig. 11) (see color plate). OCT images of eyes with resolved serous detachments show deep excavations corresponding to the optic pit and frequently display cystoid and schisis types of retinal changes. Lincoff and coworkers [19] suggested that fluid emanated from the optic disc through a communication with the subarachnoid space, causing the formation of a retinoschisis-like cavity and the secondary development of a serous retinal detachment in the macular. OCT has been used to image eyes with optic nerve pits with and without serous macular detachments [20,21]. The images obtained suggest the development of cystoid- and schisis-like changes preceding serous macular detachment.

17.5.2   Glaucoma

The early diagnosis and early detection of glaucomatous progression are challenges that the ophthalmologist must face. Significant axon loss may precede the develop-

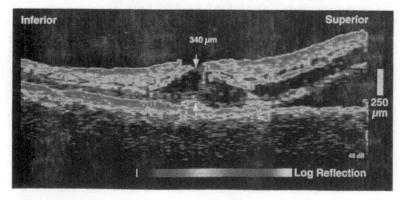

Figure 10   Optical coherence tomographic image of a patient with retinoschisis. Splitting of the retina as the outer plexiform layer is evident. (See color plate.)

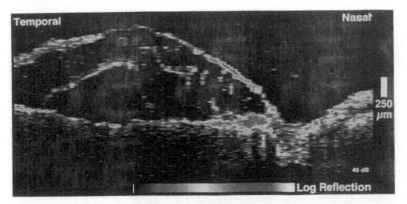

Figure 11 Optical coherence tomographic image of a patient with an optic nerve pit with a retinoschisis-like cavity within the retina. The schisis cavity communicates with the optic nerve pit. (See color plate.)

ment of visual field defects and identifiable cupping [21]. Optical coherence tomography is a noninvasive modality that is capable of obtaining high resolution cross-sectional images of the optic nerve head (Fig. 12) (see color plate). Because of its high resolution, OCT is capable of detecting nerve fiber layer thinning before the onset of visual changes [4]. Reproducibility results for nerve fiber layer measurements are good, with a standard deviation of 10–20 μm [23]. Nerve fiber layer thickness measurements have been shown to have good correlation to histology and also to correspond to visual function [4]. Longitudinal use of nerve fiber layer measurements is an objective method of detecting early nerve fiber layer changes before they are evident by examination or visual field study.

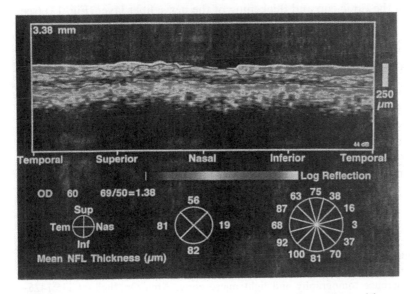

Figure 12 Optical coherence tomographic image of a patient with severe glaucoma and thinning of the nerve fiber layer. Compare the numerical values to those of Fig. 1c. (See color plate.)

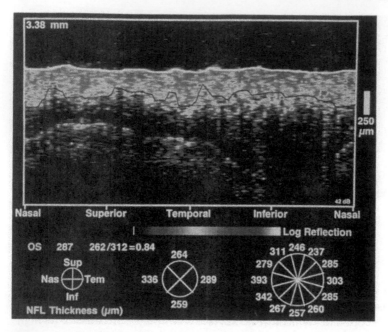

Figure 13   Optical coherence tomographic image of a patient with papilledema. Note the increase in nerve fiber layer thickness. (See color plate.)

17.5.3 Papilledema

Optical coherence tomography has utility both in the evaluation of papilledema and in monitoring patients with papilledema for improvement. OCT images of papilledema show loss of the optic cup and thickening of the nerve fiber layer (Fig. 13) (see color plate).

17.6 SUMMARY

The use of optical coherence tomography in the posterior segment has contributed to our understanding of the pathology of a number of disorders, particularly macular holes, vitreomacular traction, and optic nerve pits. OCT has found use in the evaluation of patients with ARMD, CSCR, epiretinal membranes, macular edema, retinoschisis, and glaucoma. Furthermore, OCT is helpful in the longitudinal management of patients with many disorders of the posterior segment.

REFERENCES

1. Puliafito CA, Hee MR, Schuman JS, et al. Optical coherence Tomography of Ocular Diseases. Thorofare, NJ: Slack, 1996.
2. Toth CA, Narayan DG, Bappart SA, et al. A comparison of retinal morphology viewed by optical coherence tomography and light microscopy. Arch Ophthalmol 115:1425–2428, 1997.
3. Hee MR, Puliafito CA, Duker JS, et al. Topography of diabetic macular edema with optical coherence tomography. Ophthalmology 105:360–370, 1998.

4. Schuman JS, Hee MR, Puliafito CA, et al. Quantification of nerve fiber layer thickness in normal and glaucomatous eyes using optical coherence tomography. Arch Ophthalmol 113:586–596, 1995.

5. Gass JDM. Idiopathic senile macular hole: Its early stages and pathogenesis. Arch Ophthalmol 106:629–639, 1988.

6. Gass JDB, Jooneph BC. Observations concerning patients with suspected impending macular holes. Am J Ophthalmol 109:638–646, 1990.

7. Hee MR, Puliafito CA, Wong C, et al. Optical coherence tomography of macular holes. Ophthalmology 102:748–756, 1995.

8. Gass JDM. Pathogenesis of disciform detachment of the neuroepithelium, II: idiopathic central serous choroidopathy. Am J Ophthalmol 63:587–615, 1967.

9. Hee MR, Puliafito CA, Wong C, et al. Optical coherence tomography of central serous chorioretinopathy. Am J Ophthalmol 120:65–74, 1995.

10. Johnson MW. Epiretinal membrane. In: M. Yanoff, JS Duker, eds. Ophthalmology. London: Mosby, 1999: 8.32.1

11. Wilkins JR, Puliafito CA, Hee MR, et al. Characterization of epiretinal membranes using optical coherence tomography. Ophthalmology 103:2142–2151, 1995.

12. Hee MR. Baumal C, Puliafito CA, et al. Optical coherence tomography of age-related macular degeneration and choroidal neovascularization. Ophthalmology 103:1260–1270, 1996.

13. Puliafito CA, Hee MR, Lin CP, et al. Imaging of macular diseases with optical coherence tomography. Ophthalmology 102:217–229, 1995.

14. Nussenblatt R, Kaufman S, Palestine A, et al. Macular thickening and visual acuity. Ophthalmology 94:1134–1139, 1987.

15. Hee MR, Puliafito CA, Wong C, et al. Quantitative assessment of macular edema with optical coherence tomography. Arch Ophthalmol 113:1019–2029, 1995.

16. Ip M, Garza-Karren C, Duker JS, et al. Differentiation of retinoschisis from retinal detachment using optical coherence tomography. Ophthalmology 105:600–605, 1999.

17. Kranenburg EQ. Craterlike holes in the optic disc and central serous retinopathy. Arch Ophthalmol 64:912–924, 1960.

18. Brown GC, Shields JA, Goldberg RE. Congenital pits of the optic nerve head, II: Clinical studies in humans. Ophthalmology 87:51–65, 1980.

19. Lincoff H, Lopez, Kreissig I, et al. Retinoschisis associated with optic nerve pits. Arch Ophthalmol 109:61–67, 1988.

20. Krivoy D, Gentile R, Liebmann M, et al. Imaging congenital optic disc pits and associated maculopathy using optical coherence tomography. Arch Ophthalmol 114:165–170, 1996.

21. Rutlege BK, Puliafito CA, Duker JS, et al. Optical coherence tomography of the macular lesions associated with optic nerve head pits. Ophthalmology 103:1047–1053, 1996.

22. Quigley HA, Addicks EM, Green WR. Optic nerve damage in human glaucoma, III: Quantitative correlation of nerve fiber loss and visual field defect in glaucoma, ischemic neuropathy, papilledema, and toxic neuropathy. Arch Ophthalmol 100:135–146, 1982.

23. Schuman JS, Pedut-Kloizman T, Hertzmark E, et al. Reproducibility of nerve fiber layer thickness measurements using optical coherence tomography. Ophthalmology 103:1889–1898, 1996.

18

Optical Coherence Tomography in the Anterior Segment of the Eye

HANS HOERAUF

Medical University of Lübeck, Lübeck, Germany

REGINALD BIRNGRUBER

Medical Laser Center Lübeck, Lübeck, Germany

18.1 INTRODUCTION

Since optical coherence tomography (OCT) was introduced as a new imaging method in ophthalmology [1], many studies have been published on OCT investigations of the posterior segment of the eye [2–7]. However, OCT can also be a useful tool in examining the anterior segment of the eye at microscopic resolution. It can be helpful to image and measure complex details of corneal pathologies and structural changes of the chamber angle and the iris. The ability to define the relationship of angle structures in cross section allows a new morphometric gonioscopy and imaging of these structures at high resolution, which may be potentially helpful in glaucoma research and treatment. Corneal thickness measurements by OCT can provide therapeutic control in refractive laser surgery. Because the commercially available OCT system is based on the fundus camera, it does not allow routine examinations of the anterior segment. Therefore only a few experimental studies of OCT measurements of the anterior segment have been published [8–10]. In these studies high two-dimensional resolution and excellent sensitivity have been demonstrated. To use examination techniques familiar to ophthalmologists, OCT was adapted to a slitlamp, which allows comfortable and rapid measurements in routine clinical use of the anterior segment [11] and with a handheld 78 dpt lens of the posterior segment as well.

18.2 METHODS

The images presented in this chapter were generated by a newly developed slitlamp-adapted OCT system. They demonstrate the potential and limitations of this technique as a diagnostic and biometric tool for measurements of the anterior segment in healthy subjects and in patients with pathological changes. The slitlamp-adapted OCT system used a scanning module with a lateral scan range of 7 mm, attached to a normal slitlamp (see Figs. 1 and 2). The source was a superluminescent diode with a power of 1 mW and a center wavelength of 830 nm. The axial resolution achieved with this source was 13.5 μm. Images were acquired using 100–400 A-scans with an axial scan frequency of 100 Hz. The total axial depth in the OCT images was 1.5 mm.

18.2.1 Cornea

The slitlamp-adapted OCT system is capable of differentiating three corneal layers. The highest reflectivity is found at the epithelial-Bowman layer and at the Descemet-endothelial layer, whereas lower reflectivity is observed in the corneal stroma. An OCT image of a section of normal human cornea is shown in Fig. 3. It cannot be further differentiated between the epithelial layer and the Bowman's membrane or between the Descemet's membrane and the endothelial layer. In the corneoscleral junction the different arrangements of the collagen fibers in the cornea and sclera are responsible for the different optical properties in the two adjacent tissues, leading to a dramatic change in reflectivity. Conjunctiva, tenon, and sclera appear as only one highly reflective complex due to the highly scattering sclera, which limits OCT imaging of deeper structures.

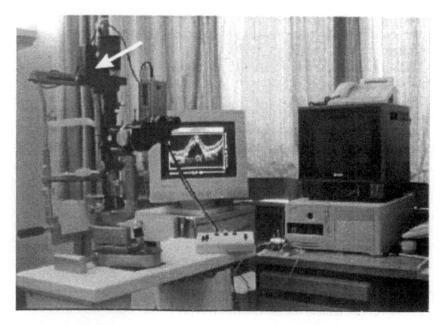

Figure 1   Photograph of a prototype of the slitlamp-adapted OCT system. The scanning module is integrated in a Haag-Streit (BQ 900) slitlamp (arrow).

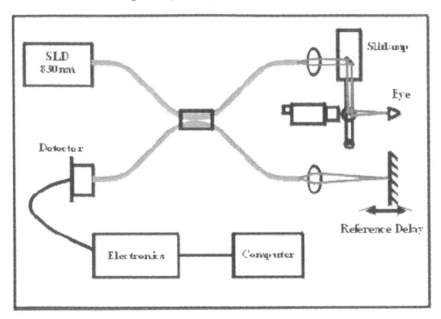

Figure 2   Schematic diagram of the slitlamp-adapted OCT. The sample arm of the inter-ferometer is coupled into the slitlamp illumination.

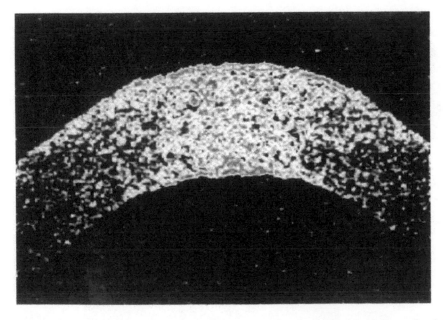

Figure 3   OCT image of a healthy human cornea in vivo with higher reflectivity of the epithelium and endothelium and lower reflectivity in the corneal stroma. The higher signal in the central area is caused by the perpendicular angle of the OCT beam to the arrangement of the collagen fibers in the cornea (100 Hz scanning rate, 200 axial scans, 5.5 mm × 2 mm).

18.2.2 Pachymetric Analysis and Photorefractive Laser Surgery

Photorefractive laser surgery has proven successful correcting myopia, hyperopia, and astigmatism in recent years. An exact corneal thickness measurement prior to refractive ablation is essential to avoid over- or undercorrection; the corneal thickness measurement is called pachymetric analysis. OCT offers the possibility to perform two-dimensional morphometric measurements of the cornea. An example is given in Fig. 4. Scanning the incident beam perpendicular to the surface of the cornea results in a central specular reflection in the OCT image. On the other hand, off-axis reflectivity drops rapidly. To measure the corneal thickness precisely, the OCT beam was directed perpendicularly to the corneal surface. Calibration was performed with a glass plate of defined thickness (148 μm). The achievable precision of central pachymetry is less than 3 μm.

The optical path through the cornea is defined as the distance between the endothelial and epithelial maxima of the axial profile. The geometric thickness of the cornea equals the optical pathlengths divided by the group refractive index of the cornea, which was assumed to be 1.376 [12]. Measurements were performed in the center of the cornea, and the diameter of the scanning beam waist was 20 μm. The center of the pupil was taken as reference. Preliminary results of corneal thickness OCT measurements showed good agreement with ultrasonic pachymetry. The median central corneal thickness measured by OCT and by ultrasonic pachymetry was 540 μm and 546 μm, respectively. The median difference was only 6 μm, which corresponds to a systematic underestimation with the corneal OCT of 1.2%. The double standard deviation of corneal thickness was 22 μm, which resulted in an error ($2\,\mathrm{SD}/x_{\mathrm{mean}}$) of 4.1%.

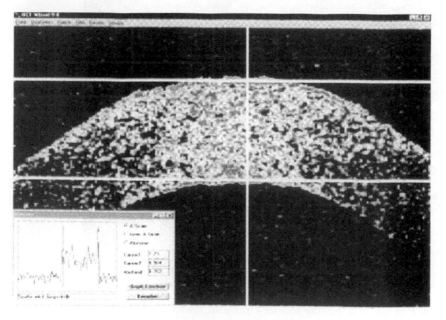

Figure 4 Pachymetric measurement of a healthy human cornea in vivo showed an optical path of 776 μm, which results in a corneal thickness of 562 μm considering a refractive index of 1.38 (100 Hz, 200 scans, 5.5 mm $\times$ 2 mm).

Pachymetric analysis during photorefractive laser therapy by OCT may improve the results of the therapy. OCT measurements demonstrated thinning of the cornea after removal of the epithelium and photorefractive excimer laser keratectomy (PRK) in myopic patients (Fig. 5). The amount of the ablation thickness could be quantified reproducibly by calculating the difference of pre- and postoperative measurements. In myopic patients a flattening of the corneal profile could be observed after PRK. By spherical fitting of the surface profile measured by OCT before and after PRK the change in corneal refraction (ÆD) can be calculated using the formula $\text{ÆD/dpt} = 337.5 \, (\text{mm}/R_0 - \text{mm}/R_1)$ with R_0 and R_1 being the radius of curvature before and after PRK, respectively (Fig. 6). A limiting factor for the accuracy of corneal thickness measurements by OCT is the assumption of a constant refractive index of the human cornea before and after treatment. Interestingly, the contrast between corneal epithelium and stroma improves after PRK because of the slight haze, which means an increased opacity of the corneal stroma due to the wound healing process. Strong haze formation can be responsible for limited results in photorefractive laser treatment causing glare, particularly at night. It can occur centrally, sectorally, or arcuately, and the risk of haze increases with the thickness of cornea ablated. OCT may improve the investigation and quantitation of haze and haze formation. Future studies by OCT should analyze the posterior corneal surface as well, to improve the diagnosis of corneal changes such as keratectasies induced by PRK.

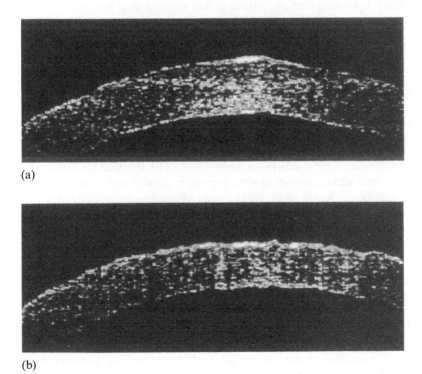

(a)

(b)

Figure 5 Corneal OCT before and after PRK in a myopic patient (-5.5 diopters) showing corneal thinning and flattening after treatment.

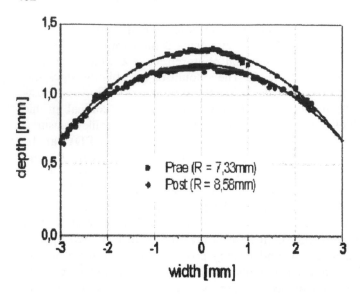

Figure 6 Mathematical analysis of the surface profile shown in Fig. 3. Spherical fitting results in a flattening of the radius of curvature of 1.0 mm.

Another alternative approach in photorefractive laser treatment is laser in situ keratomileusis (LASIK). During this procedure a thin corneal flap is created by a microkeratome, and the corneal stroma is treated by an excimer laser. OCT could allow non-contact in vivo control of the thickness of these corneal flaps during LASIK.

A third refractive laser treatment is laser thermokeratoplasty (LTK), which was performed earlier by pulsed holmium-YAG lasers and replaced later by a cw infrared diode laser. In this treatment precise coagulation of the peripheral corneal stroma leads to a refractive correction. OCT was able to determine the location and the exact extent of lesions as shown in an image of a patient after treatment by LTK for hyperopia (Fig.7). A precise biometric evaluation and documentation of the lesions and their dimensions were made possible by OCT. The thermal LTK effects were highly reflective, extending through almost the entire cornea and nearly reaching the endothelial cell layer. Koop et al. [10] compared morphological changes of the cornea measured by OCT with histological sections in enucleated porcine eyes after laser thermokeratoplasty and showed that OCT is able to deliver additional information without artificial changes caused by histological preparation. They concluded that OCT may be able to provide online control of the LTK parameters to improve the postoperative results and to avoid under- or overcorrection.

In summary, our first results indicate that the slitlamp-adapted OCT system could become an important tool to improve and control photorefractive laser treatment and may offer the possibility to give new information about corneal wound healing after these procedures. OCT may also be able to deliver more information about wound healing processes in the cornea after phototherapeutic keratectomy (PTK), which is performed in patients with recurrent epithelial defects or pterygium, which resembles fibrovascular tissue arising from the conjunctiva extending onto the cornea.

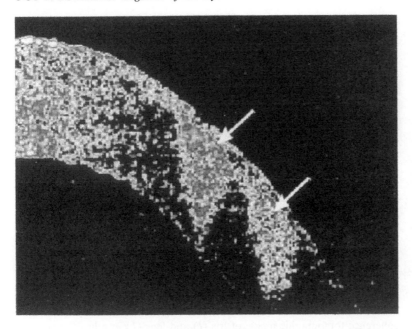

Figure 7 Slitlamp-adapted OCT allowed visualization of laser effects in the cornea in a patient one week after holmium laser thermokeratoplasty. The laser effects (arrows) are hyperreflective and extend through almost the whole of the corneal thickness, nearly reaching the endothelium (100 Hz, 200 scans, 5.5 mm × 2 mm).

With the existing OCT system it would also be possible to perform topographical measurements of the cornea, analyze corneal curvature, and calculate corneal refraction. Limiting factors for corneal topography at the moment are the relatively long acquisition time for multiple images with resulting motion artifacts, often caused by patients' poor compliance, oculomotor dysfunctions, or reduced fixation. Further technical developments should aim to overcome these problems.

18.2.3 Iris

Optical coherence tomography could resolve the iris into three different layers—a highly reflective thick superficial layer, a lower reflective stroma, and a thin highly reflective posterior layer of iris pigment epithelium (Fig. 8). Changes in the superficial layers and in the configuration of the iris could be evaluated precisely as demonstrated in a patient with an anterior synechia, which is an incarceration of the iris in the cornea (Fig. 9). In this case OCT could deliver additional information by visualizing the separation of the iris layers, which could not be identified by the slitlamp examination alone. Another example is the channel of a Nd:YAG laser iridotomy, which could be clearly identified as open by OCT in a markedly higher resolution than by slitlamp microscopy (Fig. 10). Iridotomies are usually performed in glaucoma patients with acute angle closure or a narrow chamber angle to guarantee better circulation of aqueous from its production site, the ciliary body epithelium, to the site of outflow, which is the trabecular meshwork and Schlemm's canal located in the anterior chamber angle.

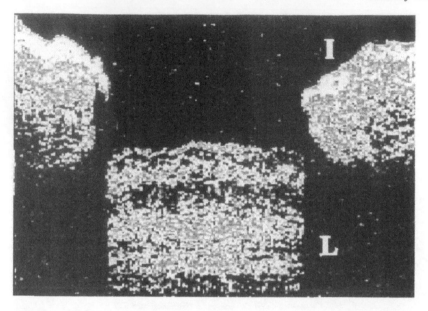

Figure 8 Optical coherence tomographic image of iris (*I*) and lens (*L*) in a healthy young patient in miosis. The highly reflective iris is shadowing structures located posterior to it. The lens capsule and nuclear region shows a higher reflectivity, whereas the cortex is hyporeflective (100 Hz, 200 scans, 5.5 mm × 2 mm).

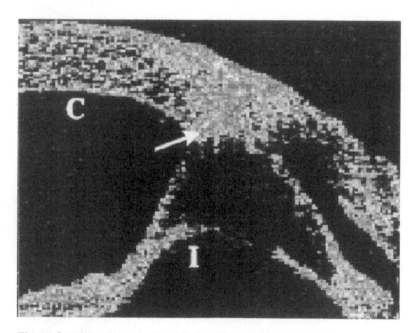

Figure 9 Patient after perforating eye injury with an anterior synechia (arrow) and separation of the iris layers (*C* = cornea, *I* = iris). This is one of the first images and was performed at 54 Hz, with 100 lateral scans resulting in reduced resolution (5.5 mm × 2 mm).

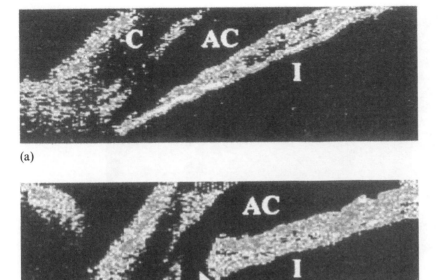

(a)

(b)

Figure 10 Optical coherence tomographic image (100 Hz, 200 scans, 5.5 mm × 2 mm) of an acute angle glaucoma (I = iris, C = cornea, AC = anterior chamber). (a) Pretreatment with a narrow chamber angle, (b) after YAG iridotomy with demonstration of the opening in the iris (arrow) and deepening of the anterior chamber.

Other interesting ocular structures, which are clinically scarcely observable or not observable at all, such as the ciliary body, the zonular fibers located at the equator of the lens, the pars plicata, and the pars plana, were shadowed in OCT by the highly reflecting iris pigment epithelium, attenuating the incident light of an 830 nm light source (Fig. 8). However, changes within the iris such as iris cysts and iris tumors can be visualized, monitored, and documented objectively to measure their size and control their possible growth.

18.2.4 Anterior Chamber Angle

As mentioned before, the anterior chamber angle is a very important structure in the eye. A narrow angle increases the risk of acute angle glaucoma. Also, structural changes in this area, such as fibrotic scar formation or new vessel growth, can cause a rise in intraocular pressure and may be detected earlier by OCT. Clinical examination and classification of the chamber angle is routinely performed by direct visualization using a gonioscopic lens. The classification according to Shaffer or Becker [14] is widely used but depends on the experience and subjective estimation of the individual examiner. Therefore, it is often difficult, if not impossible, to quantitatively compare follow-up examinations in glaucoma patients. Hence, there is a need for an objective method to measure and document the chamber angle pre- and post-treatment as seen in a patient after Nd:YAG laser iridotomy with post-operative deepening of the anterior chamber (Fig. 10).

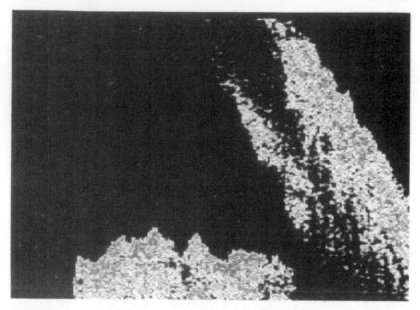

Figure 11   Optical coherence tomographic image (100 Hz, 200 scans, 5.5 mm × 2 mm) of an open chamber angle and corneoscleral region. Shadowing of the most peripheral part of the angle and iris by the highly backscattering anterior part of the sclera.

With the slitlamp-adapted OCT, the chamber angle could be visualized without using a gonioscopic lens and was demonstrated in high resolution cross-sectional images. This OCT system is an ideal device for the morphometry of the chamber angle in vivo, similar to histological sections but without artificial changes. OCT images can be taken in each position, and it seems reasonable to measure the angle at the 3, 6, 9, and 12 o'clock positions. An OCT image of an open angle is shown in Fig. 11. The ability of OCT to show the angle region in cross section allows quantitative measurements (Fig. 12). However, due to the curvature of the cornea it is not possible to get a perpendicular incident light beam over the whole scanning range. The OCT beam is refracted by the air/cornea interface if the incident angle of the beam is not perpendicular. To correct this refraction, the knowledge of the refractive index, the corneal curvature, and the distance from the cornea to the iris is needed. In the OCT system discussed here it was difficult to acquire this information because of the limited axial image depth of 2 mm.

One more general limitation of this method so far is that the peripheral part of the iris and the anterior chamber angle region, essential for classification of the chamber angle, are shadowed by the anteriorly located highly backscattering part of the sclera (Fig. 11). To overcome this problem, measurements were performed at oblique incident angles. When the incident OCT beam was directed more obliquely, the chamber angle could be visualized completely, but the resulting distortion of the OCT images made it more difficult to quantify the chamber angle (Fig. 13). Another drawback is that structures like the trabecular meshwork and Schlemm's canal could not be identified because of shadowing properties of the anterior sclera.

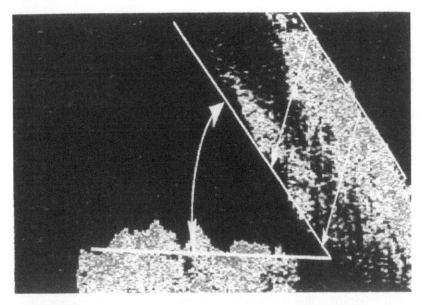

Figure 12 OCT measurement of an open chamber angle (100 Hz, 200 scans, 5.5 mm × 2 mm). Limitations are the missing reference point due to shadowing of the peripheral iris and the uneven iris configuration. The refraction causes distortion of the OCT image, thus, quantitative measurements require mathematical correction (I = iris, C = cornea).

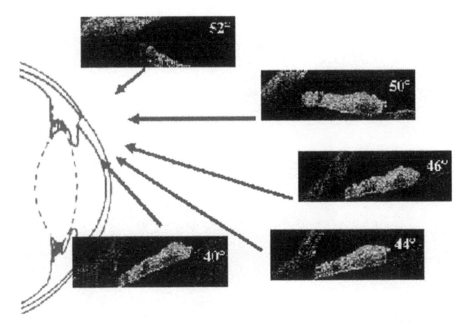

Figure 13 Optical coherence tomographic image of an open chamber angle from oblique incident angles. The values shown in the figure were measured directly from the scaled OCT images. Mathematical correction of the distortion was performed for each image, and the resulting value for each measurement was approximately 38°.

18.2.5 Transscleral OCT

To penetrate highly reflective tissues like the sclera, the scleral spur, the iris pigment epithelium, or other hazy media such as corneal opacification, light sources with a wavelength longer than 830 nm could be useful. OCT images generated by an experimental prototype using a handheld applicator for dermatological examinations and a superluminiscent diode emitting at a wavelength of 1310 nm were promising. The number of lateral scans was varied between 100 and 400. In enucleated pig and human eyes the chamber angle could be fully visualized without shadowing by the anterior part of the sclera (Fig. 14) and were compared to histological sections. Furthermore, the ciliary body could be identified (Fig. 15). By the use of a 1310 nm light source the scleral-choroidal-retinal complex could be demonstrated and penetrated, enabling visualization of the vitreous (Fig. 16). With this experimental setup in vivo measurements of the complete anterior chamber angle in healthy volunteers could also be performed successfully (Fig. 17).

18.2.6 Normal Lens and Cataract

Optical coherence tomographic imaging of the lens, capsular bag and anterior vitreous was possible within the pupillary opening. OCT measurements of the human lens in a young healthy adult revealed a slightly increased reflectivity in the nuclear region and the lens capsule (Fig. 8). In patients with a nuclear cataract, the lens nucleus revealed markedly higher reflectivity than the cortex (Fig. 18). Because of the limited lateral depth of 2 mm, the entire thickness of the lens could not be visualized

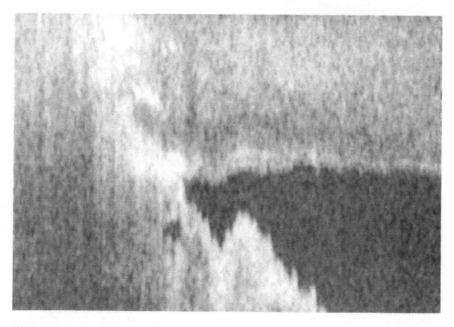

Figure 14 Optical coherence tomographic image of the chamber angle of an enucleated porcine eye using a light source of 1310 nm wavelength. Complete visualization without shadowing is possible.

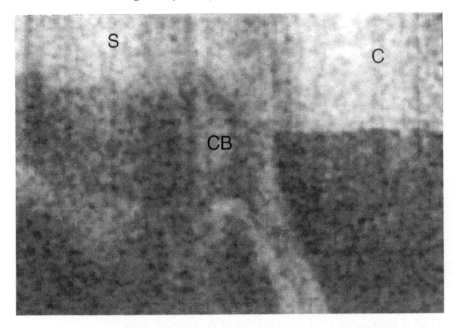

Figure 15 Transscleral OCT image of an enucleated phtitic human eye showing an atrophic ciliary body (CB). The high reflective sclera can be penetrated by 1310 nm OCT. (Cornea = C, sclera = S).

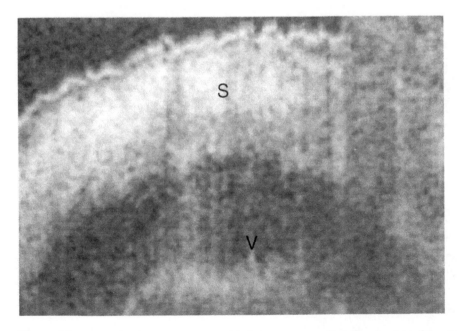

Figure 16 Optical coherence tomographic image measured on the equator of an enucleated porcine eye (1310 nm) showing hyporeflective zones that correspond to vitreous vacuoles in histological sections. (V = vitreous, S = sclera).

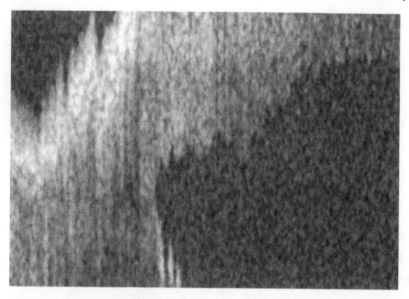

Figure 17 In vivo transscleral OCT measurement in a healthy human eye with a prototype of a 1310 nm OCT allowing complete visualization of the chamber angle.

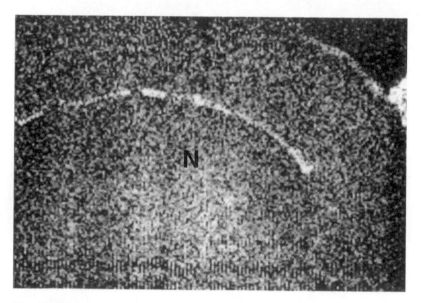

Figure 18 Optical coherence tomographic image of a senile nuclear cataract. The lens nucleus (*N*) corresponded to a higher reflectivity and appeared well demarcated in the OCT, whereas the lens cortex is hyporeflective (100 Hz, 200 scans, 5.5 mm × 2 mm).

in one OCT image. Combining several OCT images, however, measurement of the lens thickness was possible.

The slitlamp-adapted OCT can serve as an important diagnostic tool by densitometric analyses of the human lens, correlating the reflectivity of lens opacities to morphological changes. This may offer an objective classification and a new grading system for cataract development which is otherwise possible only with the Scheimpflug camera system [15] or with a subjective method, the LOCS III test [16]. The latter test is a classification system based on a set of standard color photographic transparencies of cataract that can be used as references to classify lens opacities at the slitlamp. In a cataract model OCT was able to detect induced nuclear cataracts in enucleated calf eyes [8]. Experimental in vivo measurements in monkeys were performed by DiCarlo et al. [9], who converted the reflectivity to a qualitative grading system and correlated the results with the LOCS III test.

18.2.7 Intraocular Lenses and Secondary Cataract

The capsular bag, particularly if secondary cataract formation was present, could be visualized in vivo by OCT as a well-defined slightly hyperreflective bandlike structure (Fig. 19). Reflectivity of the bag increased with the thickness of secondary cataract formation and could be quantified by OCT. Also, the anterior vitreous could be examined by the slitlamp-adapted OCT system.

Optical coherence tomographic measurements of lens, secondary cataract, and anterior vitreous are possible only within the pupillary opening and are very limited in eyes with small pupils. We examined patients with intraocular lenses of

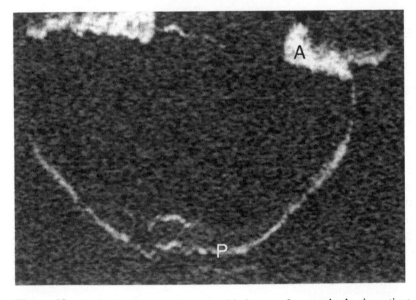

Figure 19 Optical coherence tomographic image of a pseudophacic patient with secondary cataract formation (100 Hz, 200 scans, 5.5 mm × 2 mm). Capsular bag showed hyperreflectivity of the anterior (*A*) and posterior (*P*) capsular opacification in the OCT. The intraocular lens could not be visualized.

the three different materials, PMMA, acrylic, and silicone, which are the most common materials in use today in cataract surgery. The capsular bag could be identified but in no case could the intraocular lens itself be visualized by the OCT. The reason for this phenomenon is probably the homogeneous and extremely translucent material of the lenses and their smooth surface. Therefore only a punctate specular reflection could be detected, and no structure could be visualized within the OCT image.

18.2.8 Potential and Limitations of OCT in the Anterior Segment

Imaging in ophthalmology has considerably improved over recent years, but only selected techniques allow high resolution imaging of the anterior segment [15,17]. The first clinical experiences with the slitlamp-adapted OCT system, which was developed for routine clinical examinations of the anterior and posterior segments, are promising. OCT measurements performed with this system deliver high resolution cross-sectional images of intraocular structures using the familiar slitlamp examination technique, thus extending the use of OCT to the anterior globe. It allows a quick change between anterior and posterior segment examinations and provides exact and rapid biometric analyses of structures and dimensions in the anterior globe without direct contact or immersion techniques. Important clinical measurements include corneal thickness, corneal surface profile, corneal refraction, iris thickness, anterior chamber angle, lens thickness, and thickness of secondary cataract formation. A drawback is that direct morphometric analysis is possible only for axial measurements. Off-axis measurements need further correction. For this correction, knowledge of the profile of the ocular structures anteriorly to the structure of interest is required.

18.3 PERSPECTIVES

Our preliminary results suggest a wide range of potential clinical and scientific applications for the slitlamp-adapted OCT system presented here for examination of the anterior segment of the eye. Further technical improvements will shorten the acquisition time and reduce motion artifacts. Optimization of the coherence signal demodulation and image processing can improve the sensitivity and contrast of the OCT images. Increasing the length of the lateral scans will provide a better analysis of the complete anterior segment. Simultaneous documentation of the scanned area in related color photographs will further improve the reproducibility of measurements and orientation within the images.

Further studies will have to investigate the infrared OCT technique, which has the potential to replace ultrasound biomicroscopy. Current technical refinements and the slitlamp adaptation of OCT will improve imaging quality for the examination of the anterior segment of the eye.

REFERENCES

1. Fujimoto JG, Brezinski ME, Tearney GJ, Boppart SA, Bouma B, Hee MR, Southern JF, Swanson EA. Optical biopsy and imaging using optical coherence tomography. Nature Med 1:970–972, 1995.

2. Hee MR, Puliafito CA, Duker JS, Reichel E, Coker JG, Wilkins JR, Schuman JS, Swanson EA, Fujimoto JG. Topography of diabetic macular edema with optical coherence tomography. Ophthalmology 105:360–370, 1998.

3. Puliafito CA, Hee MR, Schuman JS, Fujimoto JG. Optical Coherence Tomography of Ocular Diseases. Thorofare, NJ: Slack Inc, 1996.

4. Rutledge BK, Puliafito CA, Duker JS, Hee MR, Cox MS. Optical coherence tomography of macular lesions associated with optic nerve head pits. Ophthalmology 103:104–105, 1996.

5. Schuman JS, Hee MR, Puliafito CA, Wong C, Pedut-Kloizman T, Lin CP, Hertzmark E, Izatt JA, Swanson EA, Fujimoto JG. Quantification of nerve fiber layer thickness in normal and glaucomatous eyes using optical coherence tomography. Arch Ophthalmol 113:586–596, 1995.

6. Toth CA, Birngruber R, Boppart SA, Hee MR, Fujimoto JG, DiCarlo CD, Swanson EA, Cain CP, Narayan DG, Noojin GD, Roach WP. Argon laser retinal lesions evaluated in vivo by optical coherence tomography. Am J Ophthalmol 123:188–198, 1997.

7. Wilkins JR, Puliafito CA, Hee MR, Duker JS, Reichel E, Coker JG, Schuman JS, Swanson EA, Fujimoto JG. Characterization of epiretinal membranes using optical coherence tomography. Ophthalmology 103:2142–2151, 1996.

8. Izatt JA, Hee MR, Swanson EA, Lin CP, Huang D, Schuman JS, Puliafito CA, Fujimoto JG. Micrometer-scale resolution imaging of the anterior eye in vivo with optical coherence tomography. Arch Ophthalmol 112:1584–1589, 1994.

9. DiCarlo CD, Boppart S, Gagliano DA, Amnotte R, Smith AB, Hammer DX, Cox AB, Hee MR, Fujimoto J, Swanson E, Roach WP. A new noninvasive imaging technique for cataract evaluation in the rheus monkey. In: Proceedings of Lasers in Surgery: Advanced Characterization, Therapeutics, and Systems V, 1995. SPIE 2395: 636–643.

10. Koop N, Brinkman R, Lankenau E, Flache S, Engelhardt R, Birngruber R. Optische Kohärenztomographie der Kornea and des vorderen Augenabschnitts. Ophthalmologe 94:481–486, 1997.

11. Hoerauf H, Wirbelauer C, Scholz C, Engelhardt R, Koch P, Laqua H, Birngruber R. Slitlamp-adapted optical coherence tomography (OCT) of the anterior segment. Graefe's Arch Clin Exp Ophthalmol 1999.

12. Snell RS, Lemp MA. Clinical Anatomy of the eye. Oxford, UK: Blackwell Scientific, 1989:119–194.

13. Huebscher HJ, Genth U, Seiler T. Determination of excimer laser ablation rate of the human cornea using in vivo Scheimpflug videography. Invest Ophthalmol Vis Sci 1996:37–42.

14. Becker SC. Gonioscopic grading of the angle. In: Becker SC, ed. Clinical Gonioscopy. A Test and Stereoscopic Atlas. St. Louis: Mosby, 1972:73–80.

15. Hockwin O, Wergekin E, Laser H, Dragonmirescu V. Scheimpflug photography. Ophthalmic Res 15:102–108, 1983.

16. Chylack LT, Wolfe JK, Singer DM, Leske C, Bullimore MA, Bailey IL, Friend J, McCarthy D, Suh-Yuh W. The lens opacities classification system III. Arch Ophthalmol 111:831–836, 1993.

17. Pavlin CJ, Harasiewicz K, Sherar MD, Foster FS. Clinical use of ultrasound biomicroscopy. Ophthalmology 98:287–295, 1991.

19

Optical Coherence Tomography and Developmental Biology

STEPHEN A. BOPPART and JAMES G. FUJIMOTO

Massachusetts Institute of Technology, Cambridge, Massachusetts

MARK E. BREZINSKI

Harvard Medical School, Massachusetts General Hospital, Boston, Massachusetts

19.1 INTRODUCTION

Developmental biology is a research field that has exploded within recent years due to advances in molecular biological techniques. The field seeks to answer fundamental questions of how a single fertilized egg can develop into a multicellular complex organism. Developmental processes are directed via the expression of genes within the animal genome. If the expression of the genetic program is understood, then researchers can determine when and why failure occurs and how failure can be avoided. Aside from the inherent quest for this scientific knowledge, the research has long-ranging clinical applications to humans such as gene therapy, cloning research, and the treatment of genetic diseases.

Optical coherence tomography (OCT) can produce high resolution cross-sectional images of biological issues in vivo and in real time [1–4]. OCT has been demonstrated for high resolution in vivo imaging of developmental processes, including morphological abnormalities and functional parameters [5–8]. With the advent of molecular biology and genetic techniques that can site-specifically modify the genome of animal models, OCT has been shown to be a useful tool for imaging and tracing the morphological and functional expression of the genetic code. OCT fills a niche between confocal microscopy and imaging modalities such at magnetic resonance imaging (MRI) and ultrasound. High image resolutions (2–10 μm) with 2–3 mm imaging penetration depths in scattering tissue permit the microscopic visualization of dynamic changes that occur during all stages of embryonic development. High speed OCT imaging enables functional assessment of developmental changes such as those within the cardiovascular system. By imaging developing specimens in vivo at near-histological resolutions, fewer animals will have to be killed at single time points for longitudinal studies. OCT permits the longitudinal tracking of morphological and functional development in single specimens. Thus, OCT promises to become a powerful and unique investigative tool for developmental biology.

19.2 DEVELOPMENTAL BIOLOGY ANIMAL MODELS

The field of developmental biology uses several common animal models ranging from prokaryotic bacteria and eukaryotic yeast to increasingly more advanced nematodes (worm, *Caenorhabditis elegans*), fish (zebra fish, *Brachydanio rerio*), insects (fruit fly, *Drosophila melanogaster*), amphibians (African frog, *Xenopus laevis*), birds (chicken, *Gallus domesticus*), and small mammals (mouse, *Mus musculus*; rat, *Rattus norvegicus*). The lower species on the evolutionary tree are preferred for their ease of care and handling and their rapid reproductive cycles. Mice and rats are preferred for their close homology to humans, although even the single-cell yeast has a significant degree of homology. The advancements in molecular biological techniques have permitted researchers to site-specifically modify the genomes of these animal models. By modifying the genome and observing how mutations are expressed within the developing organism, locations and functions of specific genes can be determined. OCT can be applied to developmental biology to observe the expression of genes in vivo.

The high resolution and high speed imaging capabilities of OCT make it well suited for imaging the small animal models used in developmental biology. These animal models are also interesting for demonstrating OCT because of their small size, ease of care and handling, variations in optical transparency, intact in vivo functioning organ systems, and high cellular mitotic rates. Common developmental animal models, namely amphibians and fish, are used in a series of experiments that not only demonstrate the capabilities of OCT as an imaging modality for biological microscopy and developmental biology but also demonstrate the principles of high resolution OCT imaging.

19.3 IDENTIFICATION OF TISSUE MORPHOLOGY

Improved imaging of morphological changes has the potential for offering new insight into the complex process of embryonic development. Imaging embryonic morphology that results from cellular differentiation is important for the understanding of genetic expression, regulation and control. Several well-recognized imaging technologies are currently used to provide structural information about microscopic specimens. These include magnetic resonance imaging, computer tomography, ultrasound, and confocal microscopy. High resolution magnetic resonance imaging has been used to image the mouse embryonic cardiovascular system [9] as well as to produce in vivo cross-sectional images of early *Xenopus laevis* development [10,11] with resolutions of 12 μm. Because the static and gradient magnetic fields required to obtain these resolutions are orders of magnitude greater than those found in most clinical systems, this modality represents a technically challenging option that requires considerable skill from its operator in order to achieve high resolution images. High resolution computed tomographic imaging of fixed insect specimens revealed internal microstructure with 8–12 μm resolution yet required an elaborate microfocusing instrument and image reconstruction algorithms [12]. Ultrasound backscatter microscopy using high frequencies (40–100 MHz) is capable of 50 μm resolutions to depths of 4–5 mm and has been applied to the analysis of early embryonic development in the mouse [13]. To effectively image with ultrasound, probes require contact with the tissue.

The invention of the confocal microscope [14] and laser-scanning confocal microscopy has advanced the understanding of biological systems and their development largely due to the ability to selectively visualize biological specimens, cells, and subcellular constituents [15]. Transverse resolutions of 0.5 μm with 1 μm optical sections are possible [16]. Although confocal microscopy is superb for optically sectioning a specimen, imaging depths are limited to less than 500 μm in nontransparent tissue [17]. Recent advances in confocal microscopy have successfully shown that in vivo confocal imaging is possible. Examples include the imaging of calcium dynamics in sea urchin eggs [18] as well as *Xenopus* oocytes [19] during fertilization. Obtaining in vivo images is difficult, however, primarily due to the toxicity of the products that are released when the fluorophores are excited by the incident laser radiation. This limitation, as well as limited imaging penetration, prevents biologists from imaging structures over time, at later developmental stages, and in highly scattering, optically opaque specimens. Currently, internal morphological changes occurring in later stages can be studied only with histological preparations at discrete time points.

An in vivo means of imaging morphology is frequently needed to help identify the expressions of genes. Furthermore, observing and tracking morphological changes throughout development is useful for characterizing all aspects of genetic expression. OCT can perform high resolution, non-contact, cross-sectional tomographic imaging in vivo with the potential to analyze the morphological changes in both semitransparent and highly scattering specimens during normal and abnormal development. Optical coherence tomographic imaging was performed on several of the commonly used animal models in order to establish baselines and demonstrate the domains of application for this technology [5–8]. To verify image representation of morphology, OCT images were correlated with standard histological observations of the specimen, the current gold standard for identifying morphological features during development.

Optical coherence tomography has the ability to image specimens that are opaque to visible light because it uses wavelengths of light in the near-infrared region. Although most tissues appear opaque under visible light, they are relatively nonabsorbing in the near-infrared. Imaging depth using near-infrared light is limited by attenuation from optical scattering rather than absorption. All of the OCT imaging described in this chapter employed low coherence light sources with center wavelengths around 1300 nm. In general, a superluminescent diode was used for imaging stationary tissue structures. However, to achieve a sufficient signal-to-noise ratio (SNR), acquisition times were slow, ranging from 10 to 30 s depending on the image size. Because the SNR is proportional to the incident optical power, faster

OCT image acquisition requires higher optical powers. A solid-state Kerr lens mode-locked Cr^{4+}:forsterite laser was used for high speed OCT imaging [20]. For both of these low coherence light sources, OCT imaging depths up to 3 mm were possible. Although this imaging depth is not as great as that of ultrasound, it is sufficient for imaging many anatomical features of interest in most developing embryos. Throughout this chapter, OCT imaging parameters specific to each study will be described.

The first investigation of OCT in developmental biology examined the morphology of developing tadpoles [5]. For these studies, a superluminescent diode was used with a free-space longitudinal spatial resolution of 16 μm (as determined by the 50 nm optical bandwidth of the low coherence light source). The transverse resolution was set to be 30 μm (as determined by the spot size of the light beam). Within the specimen, a longitudinal resolution of $\sim$ 12 μm was determined by dividing the free-space resolution by the measured average index of refraction of the specimen [21], $n = 1.35$.

The transverse resolution for the following OCT images was 30 μm with a corresponding confocal parameter of 1.1 mm. The SNR was 109 dB. The fact that OCT uses low coherence light and detects light at selected echo time delays greatly discriminates against the detection of light that is multiply scattered. Whereas confocal microscopy discriminates against unwanted light by using spatial filtering, photons can be multiply scattered into the spatial mode that is detected and degrade image quality [22].

Imaging studies were performed on several standard biological animal models commonly employed in developmental biology investigations. The animals used in these research studies were cared for and maintained under the established and approved protocols of the Committee on Animal Care, Massachusetts Institute of Technology, Cambridge, MA. OCT imaging was performed in *Rana pipiens* tadpoles (in vitro), *Brachydanio rerio* embryos and eggs (in vivo), and *Xenopus laevis* tadpoles (in vivo). Tadpoles were anesthetized by immersion in 0.5% Tricaine until they no longer responded to touch. Specimens were oriented for imaging with the optical beam incident from either the dorsal or ventral sides. After imaging, specimens for histology were euthanized in 0.05% Benzocaine for 30 min until no cardiac activity was observed. Specimens were fixed in 10% buffered formalin for 24 h, embedded in paraffin, sectioned, and stained with hematoxylin and eosin.

To facilitate the registration between OCT images and corresponding histology, numerous OCT images were first acquired as desired anatomical locations at 25–50 μm intervals. Serial sectioning at 20 μm intervals was performed during histological processing. Following light microscopic observations of the histology, OCT images from the same transverse plane in the specimen were selected in correspondence with the histological sections.

To illustrate the ability of OCT to image developing internal morphology in optically opaque specimens, a series of cross-sectional images were acquired in vitro from the dorsal and ventral sides of a stage 49 (12 day) [23] *Rana pipiens* tadpole. The plane of the OCT image was perpendicular to the anteroposterior axis. Figure 1 shows representative OCT images displayed in gray scale. The gray scale indicates the logarithm of the intensity of optical backscattering and spans a range of approximately -60 dB to -110 dB of the incident optical intensity. These images were 7 mm $\times$ 3 mm, corresponding to 500 $\times$ 250 pixels with 12-bit resolution.

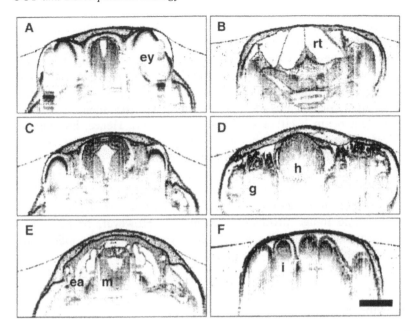

Figure 1 *Rana pipiens* tadpole. Images in left and right columns acquired from the dorsal and ventral sides, respectively. ea, ear; ey, eye; g, gills; h, heart; i, intestinal tract; m, medulla; rt, respiratory tract. Bar represents 1 mm. (From Ref. 5.)

Features of internal architectural morphology can be clearly identified in the images. Identifiable structures in Fig. 1e include the midbrain, fourth ventricle of the brain, and medulla as well as the ear vesicle. The horizontal semicircular canal and developing labyrinths are observed. Internal morphology not accessible in one orientation due to the specimen size or shadowing effects was imaged by reorienting the specimen and scanning in the same cross-sectional image plane. The images in Figs 1b, 1d, and 1f were acquired with the OCT beam incident from the ventral side to image the ventricle of the heart, internal gills, and gastrointestinal tract. The image of the eye (Fig. 1a) differentiates structures corresponding to the cornea, lens, and iris. The corneal thickness, measured to be on the order of $10\,\mu m$, was resolved due to the differences in index of refraction between the water and the cornea. By imaging through the transparent lens, the incident OCT beam imaged several of the posterior ocular layers, including the ganglion cell layer, retinal neuroblasts, and choroid. The thickness of these layers were measured from the corresponding histology by using a microscope with a calibrated reticule. The thicknesses of the ganglion cell, retinal neuroblast, and choroid layers were $10\,\mu m$, $80\,\mu m$, and $26\,\mu m$, respectively, and demonstrate the high imaging resolution of the OCT system.

Retinal layers were not imaged throughout the entire globe because of shadowing effects from the highly backscattering iris and sclera, which attenuate the transmission of light to deeper structures directly below. A sharp vertical boundary demarcated the regions where light was transmitted through the lens and where light was shadowed. Variation of the specimen orientation will vary the shadow orientation and permit the imaging of different internal structures.

Optical coherence tomographic image contrast results from the different optical backscattering properties between different structures. Tissue structures are differentiated according to their varying degrees of optical backscattering, whereas the fluid-filled cavities within the specimen have low backscattering. The cartilaginous skeletal system of the tadpole appears highly scattering and is clearly identified in Fig. 1a. As light propagates deeper through the specimen, a larger percentage of the incident beam is either scattered or absorbed. Hence, less signal is available from deeper structures and the shades of gray become lighter as the signal-to-noise ratio is reduced. Morphology located directly below a highly backscattering structure can be shadowed from the structure above. These effects are analogous to the attenuation and shadowing observed in ultrasound. If the biological specimen is relatively homogeneous, the signal attenuation with depth can be compensated for by simple image processing techniques. However, because the morphology of the specimens used in this study is highly complex, the application of these techniques is problematic.

19.3.1 Neural Morphology

The study of neural development is important because even slight aberrations, particularly during early stages, can be lethal to the organism. OCT is well suited for imaging the complex processes that occur during neural development because micrometer-scale morphological changes in semitransparent and opaque specimens must be visualized in vivo. Because OCT can detect subtle changes in the optical properties of tissue, developing neural morphology can be clearly identified in specimens that appear relatively homogeneous under light microscopy. The dynamic organization of the nervous system is complex. OCT may be uniquely suitable for imaging longitudinally over relatively long periods of time in order to capture these organizational events. OCT was used to image developing neural morphology in *Xenopus laevis* (African clawed frog) specimens [6]. A sagittal section through a *Xenopus* brain is shown in Fig. 2. This image was of a 2 mm × 6 mm field with 250 × 500 pixels and represents a 30 μm thick (spot size) optical slice of the specimen. This image shows high resolution detail of internal brain morphology. Structures corresponding to the cerebellum, choroid plexus, and medulla oblongata are identified as well as a longitudinal section of the nasal tube and olfactory nerve as it enters the nasal placode. The white internal regions correspond to the low-backscattering cerebral spinal fluid within the lateral, third, and fourth ventricles. Posteriorly, a longitudinal section of the spinal cord is observed.

The vertical labeled lines in Fig. 2 correspond to planes where cross-sectional OCT images were acquired from this same specimen. These images, shown in Fig. 3, are each 1.5 mm × 1.5 mm with 200 × 200 pixels and were acquired perpendicular to the anteroposterior axis of the specimen. These represent a normal developing *Xenopus* nervous system. In each image, distinct regions of the brain can be identified. Figure 3a shows the paired cerebral hemispheres of the telencephalon and the two lateral ventricles. Figure 3D illustrates the narrowing of the aqueduct of Sylvius connecting the diocoel with the rhombocoel. The posterior choroid plexus, which is on the order of 50–100 μm, is clearly resolved in the fourth ventricle in Fig. 3g.

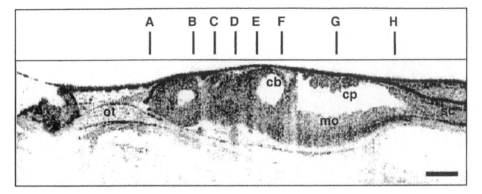

Figure 2 Sagittal section of *Xenopus laevis* neural tube. Labeled lines correspond to cross-sectional images in Fig. 3. cb, cerebellum; cp, choroid plexus; mo, medulla oblongata; ot, olfactory tract; sc, spinal cord. Bar represents 500 μm. (From Ref. 6.)

19.3.2 Cardiovascular Morphology

The developing cardiovascular system presents a technical challenge because of the inherent dynamic motion. A comparison was first made between in vitro acquired OCT images and the corresponding histology (stained with hematoxylin and eosin) from a stage 47 (7-day) specimen. In Fig. 4, representative data from three different cross-sectional planes are shown from the same specimen that illustrate the strong correlation throughout various regions of the developing cardiovascular system. The OCT image in Fig. 4a (histology, Fig. 4b) is a cross-sectional image of the two major branches of the ventral aorta anterior to the bifurcation. The muscular walls, as thin as three or four cell layers, are clearly distinguished from the larger lumens and

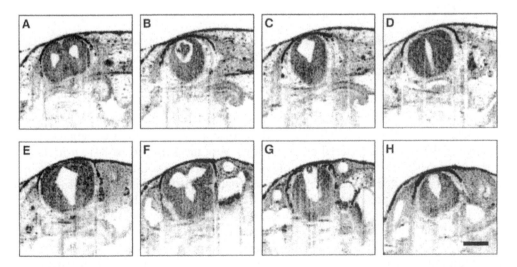

Figure 3 *Xenopus* neural tube cross sections. Images correspond to labeled lines in Fig. 2. Bar represents 500 μm. (From Ref. 6.)

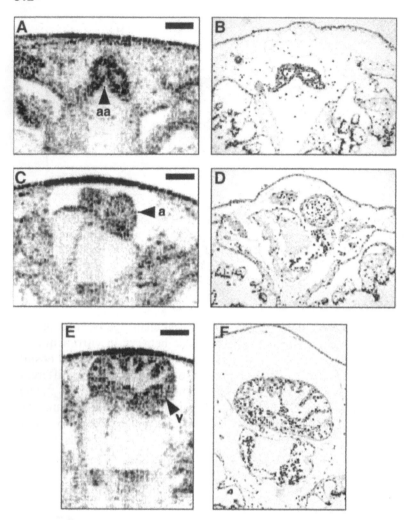

Figure 4 *Xenopus* cardiovascular histology. Excellent correspondence exists between the OCT images in the left column and the histology in the right column. a, atrium; aa, arteries; v, ventricle. Bar represents 250 μm. (From Ref. 7.)

surrounding tissue. However, in Fig. 4a, the smaller arterial lumens were not clearly identified on the OCT image. Using a light microscope with a calibrated reticule, the lumens of these smaller arterial cross sections were measured to be 8–15 μm. This diameter is below the 16 μm resolution of the superluminescent diode-based OCT system. In Fig. 4e, the internal trabeculae carneae network and papillary muscles of the ventricular wall are easily identified in the OCT image and histology.

Figure 5 is a selection from 22 cross-sectional images that were acquired from a stage 47 (7-day) *Xenopus* tadpole. This sequence demonstrates the ability of OCT imaging to delineate fine cardiovascular microstructure along the axis of the embryo and maintain registration between images for three-dimensional reconstruction. These OCT scans were acquired at planes perpendicular to the anteroposterior axis of the embryo. The image most anterior to the heart (Fig. 5a) includes two

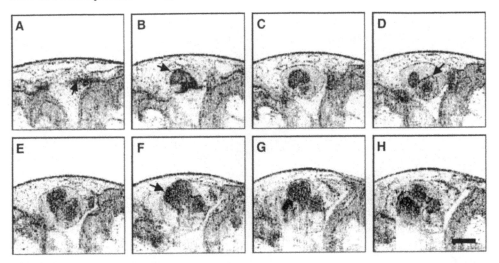

Figure 5 OCT cross sections of in vitro *Xenopus* heart. Arrows indicate (A) branch of ventral aorta, (B) pericardial sac, (D) atrium, (F) ventricle. Bar represents 500 μm. (From Ref. 7.)

branches of the ventral aorta leaving the heart, one of which is noted by the arrow. Figure 5b was acquired 200 μm posterior and coplanar to Fig. 5a. This image shows the bifurcation of the ventral aorta as it exits the truncus arteriosus. Other cardiac structures noted in the three-chamber amphibian heart include an atrium, shown in Fig. 5d, and the ventricle indicated in Fig. 5f. Both atria and the ventricle can be identified in many of the images in this sequence. The pericardial sac is also readily apparent in Figs. 5b–5h.

Spatially acquired OCT images can be used to assemble three-dimensional data sets of developing specimens that can then be displayed as either 3-D projections or surface renderings. Examples of 3-D OCT projections on a developing *Xenopus* heart are shown in Fig. 6. Data were processed on a Macintosh 9500/200 using Image 1.60 (National Institutes of Health). Computer-controlled stages with micrometer step size were used to position the specimen under the imaging beam. A series of 45 images were acquired every 25 μm from a stage 49 (12-day) tadpole and used to produce the 3-D projections. Four projections of this 3-D data set illustrate the 3-D morphological arrangement of developing cardiac structure, which is often difficult to envision from a series of 2-D images. Two major branches of the ventral aorta, one atrium, and the ventricle are distinguishable. The second atrium is difficult to visualize near the ventricle. A cutaway section of the ventricle allows the internal trabeculae carneae network and papillary muscles to be visualized.

The ability of OCT to assess cardiovascular anatomy and function in three dimensions could also represent a powerful tool for the developmental and molecular biologist. Morphological abnormalities may not clearly be identified or appreciated in two dimensions, particularly those involving misorientation of cardiovascular structures. Three-dimensional reconstruction may extend the sensitivity of analysis. As shown in Fig. 6, an advantage of reconstruction is that rotation of the volume around any axis is possible, preventing the limitations associated with interpretation based on a single viewing plane.

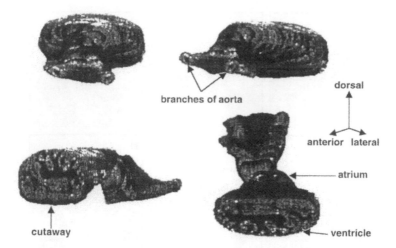

Figure 6 Three-dimensional projections of a *Xenopus* heart. Four projections are shown to illustrate the 3-D spatial orientation of an atrium, the ventricle, and the branches of the aorta. A cutaway of the ventricle reveals the internal trabeculae carneae network. Bar represents 500 μm. (From Ref. 7.)

19.3.3 Histological Correlations

Strong correlations exist between the tissue architectural morphology observed with histology and the features found in OCT images. However, it is important to note that OCT images tissue properties in a completely different manner than histology. Histology relies on the differences in the transmission of light through stained tissue sections, whereas OCT relies on differences in optical backscattering.

The presence of histological processing artifacts is common. High quality histology, especially serial sectioning, is often difficult, time-consuming, and costly. It is especially difficult to histologically prepare the large numbers of specimens typically needed for genetic and developmental studies. OCT technology offers a promising alternative for rapidly assessing changes in architectural morphology. Because the position of the OCT optical beam on the specimen is precisely controlled by micrometer stepping motor stages and galvanometric scanners, the registration of the OCT images with respect to the specimen is precisely established. Repeated serial OCT sectional images can easily be acquired to construct a three-dimensional representation of specimen morphology in analogy with MRI. In contrast, alignment of sectioned planes in histology is often difficult and not repeatable. The major discrepancy in registration between OCT images and histology occurs as the result of small discrepancies in the tilt angle of the angle planes rather than axial (anterior–posterior) registration.

A number of comparisons and contrasts can be drawn between the OCT images and histological preparations. Histology with light and electron microscopy offers unprecedented resolution on the cellular and subcellular levels. OCT does not have comparable resolution but has the ability to rapidly and repeatedly perform imaging in vivo. Histological images have artifacts due to tissue dehydration, shrinkage, and stretching during processing. OCT images have artifacts that arise from optical attenuation with depth, shadowing, and refractive index effects. The axial distances measured in OCT images represent the echo time delay of light, and thus in order to convert this information into physical dimensions it is necessary to know the index of refraction of the tissue. The index of most tissues varies between 1.35 and 1.45; thus, possible errors in longitudinal range can be on the order of only 5–10% if the index is unknown.

In addition to axial scale changes, the index of refraction also produces refraction of light rays when they traverse boundaries with different indices. This effect is most significant at the proximal boundary of the specimen where the OCT beam is incident on the specimen from air. This refraction effect can cause internal features to appear as if they were angularly displaced. Refraction depends on the mismatch of the index across a boundary. It is negligible if the light enters the tissue perpendicular to the boundary and becomes larger when the light ray is more oblique. These errors can be minimized by either partially or fully submerging the specimens in liquid that produces refractive index matching. It is important to note that these same scale uncertainties and refractive effects are also present in ultrasound imaging. However, if measurements are performed in a consistent manner, these effects are considered part of the baseline. The diagnostic power of the imaging technique is not compromised because it relies on detecting deviations from the baseline.

Image scale and distortion effects are also present in both ultrasound and MRI images although they arise from slightly different physical principles. Histology suffers to some extent from similar problems in obtaining measurements from preparations due to tissue preservation, dehydration, and sectioning. Tissue configuration following preparation may not always reflect the in vivo orientation, making quantification difficult. Despite the artifacts in these techniques, these artifacts are reproducible and can be treated as the baseline. The differences in calibrating histopathology against real tissue dimensions usually does no compromise diagnostic utility.

19.4 MORPHOLOGICAL ABNORMALITIES

The application of OCT in developmental biology, and biomedical imaging in general, is advantageous if the technique is sensitive enough to detect subtle changes in tissue microstructure compared to a normal baseline. This is demonstrated using developmental biology animal models by distinguishing internal structural abnormalities from normal morphology [12]. Figures 7a–7f compare and contrast in vivo morphology between normal and abnormal *Xenopus* with OCT images (3 mm × 3 mm, 300 × 300 pixels) and corresponding histology. These developmental abnormalities are believed to be spontaneous and not the result of mutagenic agents. The normal *Xenopus* OCT image (Fig. 7a) correlates well with histology (Fig. 7d). The neural tube shows normal formation as well as symmetrically placed and correctly oriented eyes. Internal gills are observed in both OCT and histology. Shadowing of the clay-lined dish is evident below the highly scattering ocular structure. In striking contrast, the abnormal specimen (Figs. 7b and 7e), at the same stage, has an irregularly shaped neural tube and abnormally large orbits that contain small, poorly formed optic cups. The optic cups are oriented asymmetrically. In this image plane, a longitudinal section of the left optic nerve and ocular muscles are noted by the arrow in Fig. 7b. An OCT image acquired more posterior in the abnormal specimen reveals the continuation of the poorly formed neural tube with morpho-

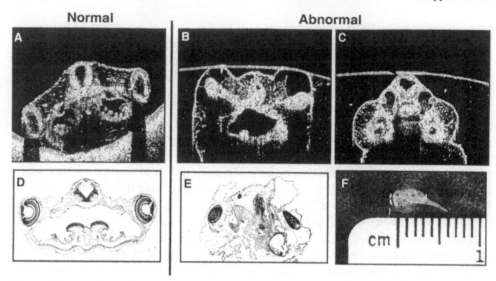

Figure 7 Identification of abnormal *Xenopus* development. Normal specimen in A with corresponding histology in D can be compared to an abnormal specimen in B and E. Arrow in B indicates longitudinal section of left optic nerve and ocular muscles. Subtle neural tube abnormality is shown in C. Bar represents 500 μm. (From Ref. 5.)

logical variations occurring on the scale of 50 μm (Fig. 7c). These images show that both gross and microscopic structural differences are clearly identifiable.

The molecular pathways involved in heart development are complex, requiring the interaction of multiple genes at precise time points during development [24]. Because of this, cardiovascular malformations are common. Abnormal developing cardiovascular structures were imaged in in vitro *Xenopus* specimens. The images in Fig. 8 illustrate abnormal vasculature (arrows in Figs. 8a and 8b) and poorly formed cardiac chambers (arrows in Figs. 8c and 8d). Prior to OCT imaging, the stage 43 (3-day) specimen was active, but future development is likely to be retarded due to the

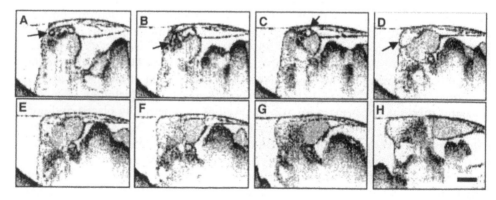

Figure 8 Abnormal cardiovascular development. Arrows in A and B indicate abnormal vasculature; arrows in C and D indicate poorly formed cardiac chambers. Bar represents 500 μm. (From Ref. 36.)

poorly functioning circulatory system. Because the cardiovascular system is inherently dynamic, a later section will describe in detail the application of OCT to imaging and measuring functional heart parameters from the developing cardiovascular system.

19.5 TRACKING DEVELOPMENT

The non-contact nature of OCT and the use of low-power near-infrared radiation for imaging causes few harmful effects on living cells. However, the higher power focused beams of 800 nm light from lasers used in optical tweezers, optical traps, and two-photon microscopes have been shown to induce irreversible damage within the cellular DNA [25,26]. This is highly significant if such techniques are to be used to assist in vitro fertilization procedures in humans. OCT imaging does not require the addition of fluorophores, dyes, or stains to improve contrast in images. OCT relies on the inherent optical contrast generated from variations in optical scattering and index of refraction. All of these advantages contribute to the use of OCT for extended imaging of development over the course of hours, days, or weeks.

Figure 9 demonstrates the application of OCT for sequential imaging of development in vivo. Images (3 mm × 3 mm, 300 × 300 pixels) of a developing zebrafish embryo within its egg were acquired every 15 min beginning at 1 h post-fertilization and continuing for 24 h. Images were acquired from the same cross-sectional plane within the specimen. The egg was suspended in low temperature gelling agar to

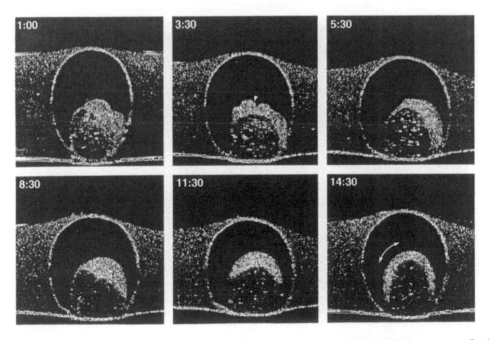

Figure 9 Early embryonic zebrafish development. Times are indicated in hours post-fertilization. At 3:30 h, cells have migrated to the dorsal pole (arrow). At 14:30 h, the anteroposterior axis has been established (arrow). Bar represents 500 μm. (From Ref. 5.)

prevent egg movement and to maintain a uniform state of hydration. Developmental changes illustrate early cleavage beginning at the eight-cell stage, 1 h post-fertilization. Because of the high mitotic rate of the embryo, results of cellular division and migration were observed as well as the establishment of the anteroposterior axis. In this example, the zebrafish egg and embryo were semitransparent and the use of OCT significantly complemented observations made using light microscopy. By imaging subtle differences in backscattering intensity, interfacial structural layers millimeters deep within specimens can be clearly delineated. In Figs. 10a and 10b, images of a second zebrafish embryo are shown at the two- and four-cell stage, must minutes after fertilization. Images of a zebrafish embryo prior and immediately after hatching are shown in Figs. 10c and 10d.

A fundamental question in developmental biology is the establishment of patterns within the developing embryo and the interaction of genes that control this process. The *hox* gene is a member of the homeobox domain, which governs anteropostero segmentation and limb development [27]. The development of *Xenopus* limb buds was followed with OCT. In Fig. 11, early images reveal a small limb bud that extends and develops into individual digits. A larger developing hindlimb, shown in Fig. 12, reveals internal vascular and skeletal development. A cross section of the lower leg reveals the internal formation of the tibia and fibula. Genes responsible for limb development are a common site for genetic manipulation. OCT can be used to track the morphological expression of these genes without sacrificing the specimens for histological processing.

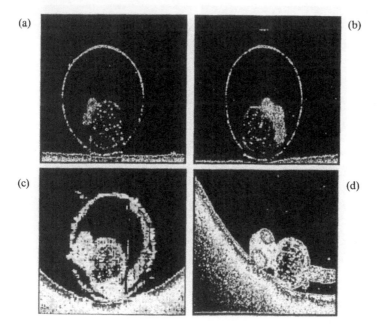

Figure 10 Early and late zebrafish development. (a,b) Two- and four-cell stages 1 and 1.75 h after fertilization, respectively. (c,d) Embryo before (24 h) and after (48 h) hatching. Bar represents 500 μm. (From Ref. 36.)

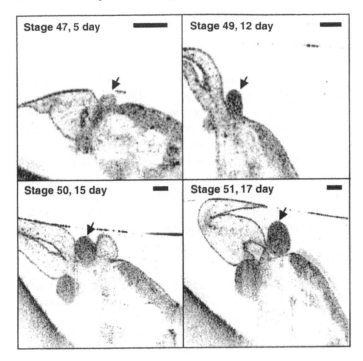

Figure 11 Early *Xenopus* hindlimb bud development. Arrow in each image indicates right hindlimb bud. Bar represents 500 μm. (From Ref. 36.)

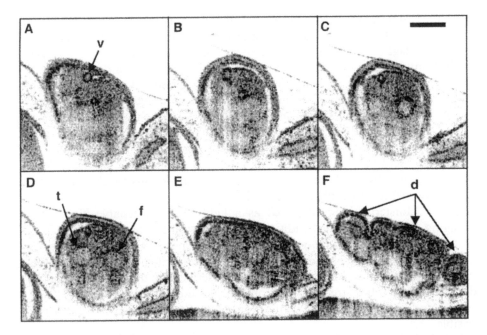

Figure 12 Cross sections of internal hindlimb structures. Images were acquired proximal-to-distal along the length of one hindlimb. d, digits; f, fibula; t, tibia; v, vasculature. Bar represents 500 μm. (From Ref. 36.)

19.6 FUNCTIONAL IMAGING

Previous OCT images characterized morphological features within biological specimens. These structures are static even though they may have been acquired from in vivo specimens. In vivo imaging in living specimens, particularly in larger organisms and humans, must incorporate fast acquisition techniques to eliminate motion artifacts within the images. In vivo imaging is necessary but not sufficient to perform functional imaging. Functional imaging is the quantification of in vivo images that yield information characterizing the functional properties of the organ system or organism. Prime examples include the use of functional MRI (fMRI) to characterize brain activity during various states of consciousness, thought, or motor control, and determining cardiac performance using ultrasound, computed tomography, or MRI. Developmental biology animal models represent a nearly ideal functioning system to demonstrate both high speed and functional OCT imaging.

19.6.1 Cardiovascular System

Abnormal cardiac function remains a leading cause of morbidity and mortality worldwide. Developmental animals models have been used to assess molecular and physiological mechanisms of not only congenital cardiac abnormalities but also the genetic predisposition to acquired abnormalities. However, although imaging technologies exist that allow the progression of human adult cardiac function to be followed with time, comparable imaging does not exist for following cardiac function in the developing animal embryo. Video light microscopy has been used to acquire real-time images of the developing beating heart. However, it is limited to *en face*, views, and only surface morphology is visible. Therefore, investigators are either confined to using embryos that are transparent during early stages of development, exposing the heart via surgical intervention, or killing the animal at a predetermined stage.

Studies investigating normal and abnormal cardiac development are frequently limited by an inability to access cardiovascular function within the intact organism. OCT has been used for the high resolution assessment of structure and function in the developing *Xenopus laevis* cardiovascular system [7]. Unlike technologies such as computed tomography and magnetic resonance imaging that require gated-image acquisition, OCT provides real-time, high speed in vivo imaging. This allows quantitative dynamic activity, such as ventricular ejection fraction, to be assessed. Axial OCT scanning and 2-D OCT imaging techniques are analogous to ultrasound M-mode and 2-D echocardiography, respectively.

The Cr^{4+}:forsterite laser was used as a light source to enable high speed OCT imaging. The laser provided additional optical power incident on the specimen to maintain a high signal-to-noise ratio during high speed imaging. Other modifications to the OCT system include the incorporation of a fast axial scanning mechanism. Fast axial scanning mechanisms, described in detail in Chapter 5, include piezoelectric fiber stretchers and optical phase control delay lines [28–32]. With these modifications, real-time acquisition rates of 4–8 frames per second (fps) are possible.

Though the relatively slow data acquisition rate of a superluminescent diode–based system is adequate for in vitro imaging of microstructure, two-dimensional in vivo imaging of the rapidly beating heart requires considerably faster imaging

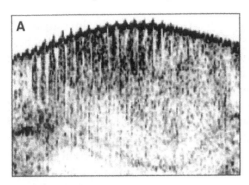
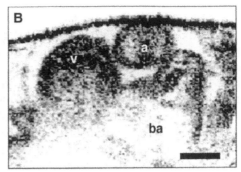

Figure 13 Comparison of slow and fast OCT imaging. Images of beating *Xenopus* heart were acquired in (A) 30 s and (B) 250 ms. a, atrium; ba, bulbous arteriosis; v, ventricle. Bar represents 500 μm. (From Ref. 7.)

speeds. To illustrate the presence of motion artifacts, an in vivo image of a beating heart acquired with the diode-based system is shown in Fig. 13a. The periodic bands within the image correspond to the movement of the cardiac chamber walls during the cardiac cycle. In contrast, in Fig. 13b, an image of the same heart was generated at 4 fps. The morphology of the in vivo cardiac chambers is clearly delineated at this faster imaging speed. Image acquisition was fast enough to capture the cardiac chambers in midcycle. With this capability, in vivo images 2.5 mm × 2.0 mm and 300 × 300 pixels were acquired in 250 ms from multiple beats and at various times during the cardiac cycle. A sequence of six frames is shown in Fig. 14 that represent a complete beat. These frames were assembled to produce a movie illustrating the dynamic, functional behavior of the developing heart.

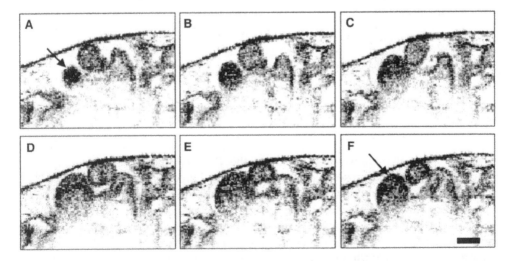

Figure 14 Single *Xenopus* heartbeat sequence. Each image was acquired in vivo in 250 ms but from different cycles. Sequence from (A) beginning of diastole with emptied ventricle (arrow) to (F) beginning of systole with filled ventricle (arrow). Bar represents 500 μm. (From Ref. 7.)

Although high speed OCT imaging is possible, this study investigated whether any dynamic information, other than two-dimensional imaging, can be obtained with the slower diode light source based OCT system. In particular, because a single axial scan can be acquired in approximately 100 ms with the diode-based system, an OCT optical cardiogram, analogous to an M-mode echocardiogram, can be obtained with this slower system. Characteristic oscillations corresponding to movement of the embryonic cardiovascular structure were observed. Both the ventral and dorsal walls of the ventricle, in addition to the ventricular lumen, were identified as well as the oscillatory nature inherent during the cardiac cycle. To capture OCT optical cardiograms, the beam was positioned in one location over the ventricle (which corresponded to the center of the OCT image) and held stationary as data from this single location were acquired over time. In Fig. 15a, the OCT beam was positioned over the ventricle at the site corresponding to the center of the image (arrow). Axial (depth) scans from this location were acquired over time. Figure 15c is an OCT optical cardiogram of a normal functioning anesthetized heart.

Optical coherence tomography optical cardiograms permitted quantitative measurements of chamber function and allowed assessment of changes over time. Measurements were recorded from optical cardiograms as illustrated in Fig. 15c. For each beat within these cardiograms, four points were recorded by a blinded observer (using IP Lab 3.0, Spectrum Analytics) that corresponded to the locations of the dorsal and ventral ventricular walls. The end of systole was defined as the maximum ventricular dimension, and the end of diastole was defined as the minimum ventricular dimension. No micropipet electrode was used to obtain an electrocardiogram from the specimens, because this would have interfered with cardiac performance and optical imaging. Measurements were obtained for the heart rate (HR), end diastolic and systolic dimensions (EDD, ESD), and ejection and fill times (ET, FT). The ventral wall velocity (VWV) was calculated as

$$VWW = \frac{EDD - ESD}{2ET}$$

and the fractional shortening (FS) was calculated as

$$FS = \frac{EDD - ESD}{EDD} \times 100$$

Although many algorithms exist, such as the Pappus rule, summated ellipsoid method, and biplane Simpson's rule for modeling human ventricle volumes [33–35], few studies have modeled the developing amphibian heart. On the basis of OCT image data of these embryonic hearts, the ellipsoid model most accurately represented the in vivo ventricle. Therefore, to determine the volume, an ellipsoid model was used, assuming that the two minor axes (a) were equal and the major axis was twice the length of a minor axis ($2a$) [33]. Hence, the volume of the ventricle is

$$Volume = \frac{8}{3}\pi a^3$$

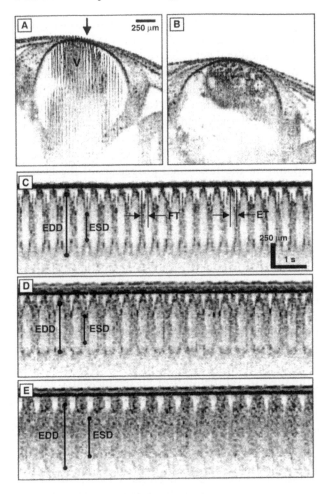

Figure 15 Optical coherence tomography optical cardiogram variations following verapamil dose. (A) OCT image of beating *Xenopus* heart. Arrow indicates ventricle (v) site of optical cardiogram acquisition. (C, D, E) Optical cardiograms acquired at 0, 1, and 4 min, respectively, following verapamil dose. Lines indicate measurements of end-diastolic (EDD), end-systolic dimension (ESD), fill time (FT), and ejection time (ET) used to evaluate functional parameters. Image in (B) was acquired 10 min after dose when heart had stopped. (From Ref. 7.)

The ejection fraction (EF) can then be determined as

$$EF = \frac{V_D - V_S}{V_D} \times 1000$$

where V_D is the diastolic volume and V_S is the systolic volume.

19.6.2 Response to Pharmacological Agents

High speed OCT imaging and OCT optical cardiograms are useful for determining the pharmacological response to drugs. In addition, these imaging techniques may have application in toxicological studies for determining dose–response curves. To demonstrate this concept, verapamil, an inotropic drug, was administered to vary the functional behavior of the embryonic heart as well as to determine the sensitivity of OCT optical cardiograms for assessing functional changes. A 25 ng dose was administered to a specimen by placing drops on the ventral side of the tadpole as the specimen rested in the optical imaging setup. This permitted data acquisition prior to and immediately following administration and the observation of the transient effects of the drug as it diffused from the external membrane to the heart.

An image of the beating heart prior to the verapamil dose is shown in Fig. 15a, with a normal optical cardiogram in Fig. 15c. In Figs. 15d and 15e, optical cardiograms illustrate the effects of verapamil on the functional properties of the heart. These optical cardiograms were acquired at 1 and 4 min, respectively, following administration of verapamil. Figure 15b is an image of the ventricle 10 min following the verapamil dose. Here, cardiac motion is minimal and dilation of the ventricular chamber is evident.

Cardiac measurements and heart parameters were obtained as described for the initial optical cardiograms. From each OCT optical cardiogram, dynamic indices (heart rate, end diastolic and systolic dimensions, ejection and filling times) were measured. Measurement averages and standard deviations were obtained from 16 beats present in each optical cardiogram. Paired t-tests were performed on all the measured data (heart rate, end diastolic and systolic dimensions, ejection and filling times) to determine if there were statistically significant changes between successive recording times. The results of these statistics are listed in Tables 1 and 2, which compare the responses following the dose of verapamil. For all the measured parameters, only 3 out of 20 paired t-tests failed to have a p-value below 0.05. In addition, 13 out of 20 had p-values less than 0.005. No significant change in heart rate occurred after 2 min, and no significant change in filling time was noted between the initial measurement and 1 min after the verapamil dose. All other changes were statistically significant ($p < 0.05$).

As shown in Tables 1 and 2, OCT demonstrated a decrease in heart rate after verapamil administration in addition to reductions in fractional shortening and ejection fraction. The EF reached a minimum of $56 \pm 8\%$ at 2 min before beginning to recover. The administration of an inotropic drug via diffusion from the external ventral membrane to the heart was chosen to minimize side effects that would result from micropipet injections. Although diffusion does not result in a bolus of drug

Table 1 Measured Parameters of Verapamil Effects[a]

Time	HR (bpm)	EDD (μm)	ESD (μm)	ET (ms)	FT (ms)
Initial	128 ± 4	666 ± 18	398 ± 35	217 ± 22	251 ± 27
1 min	124 ± 5^{b}	616 ± 13^{c}	371 ± 27^{c}	236 ± 20^{b}	251 ± 20
2 min	119 ± 4^{b}	537 ± 13^{c}	413 ± 30^{c}	268 ± 11^{c}	236 ± 19^{d}
3 min	117 ± 5	710 ± 19^{c}	507 ± 22^{c}	223 ± 41^{c}	288 ± 34^{c}
4 min	115 ± 7	741 ± 17^{c}	478 ± 20^{c}	279 ± 31^{c}	240 ± 17^{c}

[a] HR, heart rate; EDD, end diastolic dimension; ESD, end systolic dimension; ET, ejection time; FT, filling time. Significant differences: [b] $p < 0.05$; [c] $p < 0.01$; [d] $p < 0.005$.
Source: Ref. 7.

Table 2 Calculated Parameters of Verapamil Effects[a]

Time	VWV (μm/s)	FS (%)	EF (%)
Initial	630 ± 86	40 ± 6	77 ± 6
1 min	572 ± 109	40 ± 5	77 ± 6
2 min	366 ± 69	23 ± 5	56 ± 8
3 min	504 ± 104	29 ± 4	63 ± 7
4 min	585 ± 66	35 ± 3	73 ± 4

[a] VWV, ventral wall velocity; FS, fractional shortening; EF, ejection fraction
Source: Ref. 7.

delivery, the emphasis of this research was to demonstrate the use of the OCT technology for noninvasively assessing changes in cardiac function, not to determine the specific effects of precise doses on the amphibian heart.

Incorporating high speed OCT to assess the functional behavioral response to pharmacological drugs provided rapid feedback on the organism's state of health. The high speed image sequence of the beating *Xenopus* heart shown in Fig. 14 was assembled from several beats. Although each 300×300 pixel image was acquired in 250 ms (four frames per second), the images were not sequential in time. This was a limitation of the data acquisition system and computer memory used at that time. The development of rapid optical delay line scanning and direct data storage on Super-VHS video tape enabled the acquisition of sequential 256×256 pixel images at 8 fps [32,36]. A stereomicroscope outfitted with orthogonal OCT beam scanning galvanometers was used for high speed transverse scanning. The Cr^{4+}:forsterite laser was used to provide high incident optical power. The high speed acquisition enabled immediate feedback of scan location within the tadpole. Transverse, oblique, and sagittal orientations of the in vivo cardiovascular system were explored. Heart valves and multiple arterial branches were identified and observed in real time.

The administration of verapamil produced dramatic changes in the functional performance of the heart. Changes in heart rhythm from a 1 : 1 atrial-to-ventricle conduction to a 2 : 1 heart block were observed. A toxic dose of verapamil converted a normal ventricular rhythm heart into ventricular fibrillation. A series of this conversion is shown in Fig. 16. The initial image shows the ventricle and atrium. Over time, the ventricle dilates and begins fibrillating.

Optical measurements with OCT can be applied to the assessment of other variables such as cardiac output and flow velocity. To achieve this, OCT can be configured to measure the velocity of moving tissue and flowing blood using laser Doppler velocimetry [37–41]. Rather than having a fixed specimen in the sample arm and a moving reference arm mirror, the reference arm mirror may remain fixed and the moving sample produces Doppler-shifted backscatter. Other variations involving a moving reference arm mirror are also possible. The frequency of this Doppler-shifted light can be used to calculate the velocity of the moving tissue or blood. This is analogous to Doppler ultrasonography.

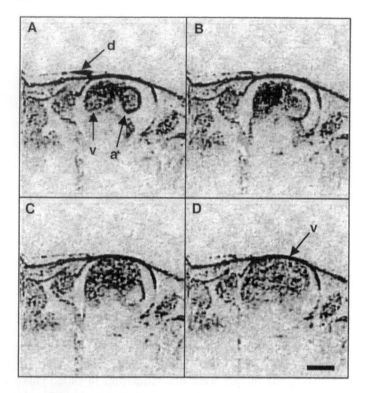

Figure 16 Verapamil-induced ventricular fibrillation. Drug (d) was applied on outer membrane. Atrium (a) was displaced from imaging plane by dilating ventricle (v). Bar represents 500 μm. (From Ref. 36.)

The investigation of cardiovascular development in animal models, using the powerful technologies of molecular and cellular biology, has been aggressively pursued to understand the mechanisms underlying cardiac dysfunction. However, severe limitations exist with current methods for assessing cardiac structure and dynamics in these animal models, frequently forcing investigators to analyze phenotypes with postmortem histopathology. The disadvantages of this approach include an inability to assess dynamic information and the sacrificing of mutants that typically are in limited supply. These research results have demonstrated the feasibility of OCT for overcoming the limitations associated with both histopathology and current methods of imaging through its assessment of structural and dynamic information at micrometer scale resolutions.

Though organisms were anesthetized prior to imaging, higher acquisition speeds and image stabilization algorithms may offer the potential for images to be obtained without the need to anesthetize specimens. Improved acquisition rates will also enable 3-D images to be rapidly acquired and processed, permitting the four-dimensional (x, y, z, time) analysis of the dynamic functioning of the heart as well as morphological changes that occur during development. The high resolution, high speed imaging provided by OCT should represent a powerful tool for assessing and understanding the molecular basis of abnormal cardiovascular development.

19.7 CELLULAR AND SUBCELLULAR IMAGING

Optical coherence tomography is capable of cellular resolution imaging that may ultimately have a role in the early diagnosis of human malignancies. Neoplasias are most responsive to medical intervention at early stages, prior to undergoing metastasis. When these disorders arise from known premalignant states, and if a detection method exists, high risk populations can be screened to reduce patient mortality. Organs where these premalignant conditions occur at relatively high frequency include the esophagus, uterus, bladder, colon, and stomach. The ability to image these organs in real time at cellular and subcellular resolutions could be a powerful tool for the early identification of neoplasms.

19.7.1 Technical Considerations

Imaging at cellular and subcellular resolutions with OCT is a major technical challenge. This is particularly difficult for human cells, which vary in size from 5 to 20 μm. For example, the stratified squamous epithelium of the cervix has 10–20 μm diameter cells with 5–15 μm diameter nuclei. Larger cells include megakaryocytes at 30 μm and tumor giant cells as large as 100 μm. There are significant structural changes in tissue that begin immediately after the tissue is separated from its in vivo blood supply. Cells rapidly lose the oxygen and nutrients necessary to maintain ionic gradients, and cell death begins within minutes to hours. The hydrated state of in vivo tissue improves OCT image contrast, enabling smaller microstructure to be resolved.

Optical contrast can arise from changes in absorption, fluorescence, refraction, reflection, phase shifts, scattering, and polarization changes. One study found that for confocal reflectance imaging, changes in index of refraction contributed most to image contrast, followed by absorption then scattering [42]. Assessment of indices of refraction for cellular components can be used to determine which structures are likely to provide contrast in OCT images [43]. High contrast should particularly be present with melanin granules, mitochondria, and structural fibers because of their relatively high indices of refraction.

The *Xenopus* developmental animal model was selected because it is relatively easy to care for and handle. This model also provides a variety of cell types with high mitotic indices. The Cr^{4+}:forsterite laser was used for imaging with axial and transverse resolutions of 5 and 9 μm, respectively. Many of the cells observed were as large as 100 μm in diameter, but cells ranged in size down to dimensions below the resolution of current OCT systems. Images of mesenchymal cells of various sizes are shown in Fig. 17. These images provide an evaluation of cell size limits for future human investigations. Cells as small as 15 μm in diameter could be imaged with this OCT system [8]. The size of most malignant cells in humans varies dramatically, showing an approximate correlation with the degree of differentiation As a general rule, cell dimensions found in human neoplasias are typically in the range of 10–40 μm and therefore similar to those of the cells images in this animal model. With low grade dysplasias, cell size tends to be smaller and will be more difficult to resolve with OCT at 5 μm resolution.

The use of broader bandwidth laser sources at other wavelengths in the near-IR can be used to increase image resolution. Shorter coherence length laser sources have been used to achieve higher axial resolutions [44,45], on the order of 2–4 μm.

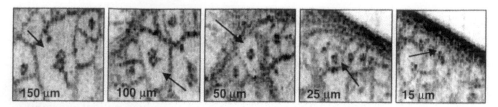

Figure 17   In vivo cell sizes imaged with OCT. Dimensions refer to diameter of cell indicated by the arrow. (From Ref. 36.)

OCT can be performed using a high numerical aperture lens to achieve high transverse resolutions, as in confocal microscopy, at the expense of reducing the depth of field [22]. With these higher resolutions, in vivo imaging of individual human cells may be possible.

Cellular imaging in in vivo human tissue, however, may not be absolutely necessary to extract useful information regarding the state of differentiation of the cells within the tissue. The nuclear-to-cytoplasmic (N/C) ratio of a cell is a histopathological indicator of the state of differentiation. Cells with high N/C ratios are less differentiated, often indicating a high degree of cellular division or rapid tumor growth. In addition, the degree of pleomorphism, the variation of differentiated and undifferentiated cells within a tissue, can indicate possible early neoplastic changes. Examples of these two types of cells are shown in Fig. 18. The images shown were acquired from regions that, at this developmental stage, were considered differentiated and undifferentiated [23]. However, no molecular techniques were performed to validate the precise state of cell differentiation. Area measurements of the nucleus and cytoplasm were taken from each image using Image 1.60 (NIH). The comparison is shown in Table 3. The left-hand image in Fig. 18 was acquired from a more differentiated region of the *Xenopus* ventral membrane. The N/C ratio and the degree of pleomorphism are low compared to those of the undifferentiated image on the right, which was acquired from a rapidly developing region near the dorsal neural tube. In human cells, the N/C rate approaches 1 : 1 for undifferentiated cells. The larger N/C ratio subsequently implies less cytoplasm, which results in higher scattering coefficients. Studies have shown that a 100 nm decrease in the radius of a

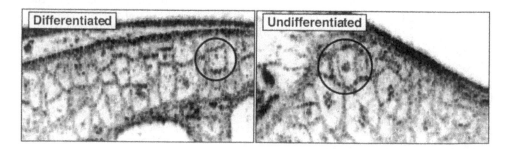

Figure 18   Differentiated and undifferentiated cells. Encircled cells represent two states of cellular differentiation. Differentiated cells (left) have small nuclear-to-cytoplasmic (N/C) ratios, whereas undifferentiated cells (right) have larger N/C ratios. (From Ref. 36.)

Table 3 Comparison of Cell Area Measurements Obtained from Images in Fig. 18

	Differentiated cells	Undifferentiated cells
Nuclear area	$216 \, \mu m^2$	$832 \, \mu m^2$
Cytoplasmic area	$7488 \, \mu m^2$	$12012 \, \mu m^2$
Nuclear cytoplasm ratio	Low, $1:35$	High, $1:14$
Pleomorphism	Low	High

Source: Ref. 36.

cell will affect the reduced scattering coefficients by as much as 37% [46]. This suggests that changes in cell size or N/C ratios may be detectable with OCT.

19.7.2 In Vivo Subcellular Imaging

Although previous studies have demonstrated in vivo OCT imaging of tissue morphology, most have imaged tissue at ~ 10–$15 \, \mu m$ resolutions, which does not allow differentiation of cellular structure. The *Xenopus laevis* (African frog) tadpole has been used to demonstrate the feasibility of OCT for in vivo cellular and subcellular imaging [8]. In this study, the ability of OCT to identify the mitotic activity, the nuclear-to-cytoplasmic ratio, and the migration of cells were evaluated. OCT images were compared to corresponding histology to verify identified structures. These results have implications for OCT imaging of in vivo cellular morphology, which, on extension to humans, could represent a powerful tool for the early evaluation of neoplastic changes.

Xenopus laevis specimens used to demonstrate in vivo subcellular imaging ranged in age from 14 to 28 days (stages 25–30). Drops of housing-tank medium were placed over the specimen at 5 min intervals to prevent dehydration during imaging. Multiple two-dimensional crossections ($900 \, \mu m \times 600 \, \mu m$, 300×300 pixels) were acquired perpendicular to the anteroposterior axis. Fifteen two-dimensional sections acquired at $5 \, \mu m$ intervals were assembled to produce a 3-D data set. Three-dimensional volumes were acquired every 10 min from the region posterior to the eyes and lateral to the neural tube of the specimen.

Immediately following image acquisition, the locations of the image planes were marked with India ink for registration between OCT images and histology. Specimens were euthanized by immersion in 0.05% Benzocaine for 1 h and then placed in a 10% buffered solution of formaldehyde for standard histological preparation. Histological sections, $5 \, \mu m$ thick, were sectioned and stained with hematoxylin and eosin for comparison with acquired OCT images. Correspondence was determined by matching the acquired OCT images with light microscopic observations of the histology. Images were processed using IP Lab 3.0 (Signal Analytics) on a Power Macintosh 9500/200. The 3-D volumes were analyzed to identify individual cells and track these cells within the acquired volumes over time. Cell position was determined by measuring distances from two internal reference points—the neural tube and the outer membrane.

A comparison between OCT images and corresponding histology is shown in Fig. 19. The comparison between Figs. 19a and 19b confirms the presence of multiple nuclei and cell membranes. The seemingly wide cell membranes in the OCT images are actually composed of membranes and extracellular matrix. The variation in correspondence between the OCT image and histology in Figs. 19a and 19b is likely due to small angular deviations in the histological sectioning plane or cell movement prior to fixation. The OCT image in Fig. 19a illustrates cells with varying size and nuclear-to-cytoplasmic ratios. Based on image measurements, cells as small as 15 μm in diameter can be imaged. An OCT image of a dividing cell was enlarged and is shown in Fig. 19c with the corresponding histology in Fig. 19d. Two distinct nuclei are clearly observed. To the right of the nuclei, the membrane had begun to pinch in. The OCT image in Fig. 19e demonstrates the high backscatter from melanin contained within neural crest melanocytes and tissue structures. Two melanocytes, indicated by black arrows, were located within the superficial membrane along with a melanin layer (white arrow) from the pigmentation pattern. The corresponding histology in Fig. 19f verified these observations.

Precise image registration with histology can be more problematic at the cellular level. The cellular level correlation of *Xenopus* cardiac structures in Fig. 4 and

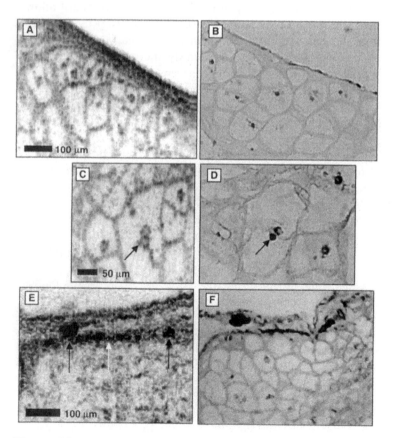

Figure 19 Cellular histological correlation. (A–D) *Xenopus* mesenchymal cells; (E,F) *Xenopus* melanocytes (black arrows) and pigmentation pattern (white arrow). (From Ref. 8.)

mesenchymal cells in Fig. 19 represent successful examples. These correlations with histology are strong, despite the likelihood that the cells divided, enlarged, and migrated between the time the cells were imaged and the time the specimen was euthanized and fixed for processing.

19.7.3 Cell Mitosis

Mitosis is the process by which a parent cell replicates DNA and physically divides into two daughter cells [47]. This process contributes to the growth of an organism and the differentiation of progenitor cells into specific tissue types. Abnormal mitotic activity can result in unregulated growth, poor differentiation, and the growth of neoplasms. The ability to assess the mitotic stage of cells in vivo and to determine their state of differentiation will provide a key diagnostic for the early detection of neoplasms in humans.

To confirm the ability of OCT to identify cell division, a sequence of OCT images following the mitotic activity of a single cell was acquired; these images are shown in Fig. 20. A number of mesenchymal cells are observed within each image. These undifferentiated cells range in size from $100 \mu m$ down to sizes below the current resolution of OCT. Cell nuclei and cell membranes are readily apparent as regions of high backscatter compared with the low backscattering cytoplasm. A number of cells in Fig. 20a show subnuclear morphology, such as the regions of

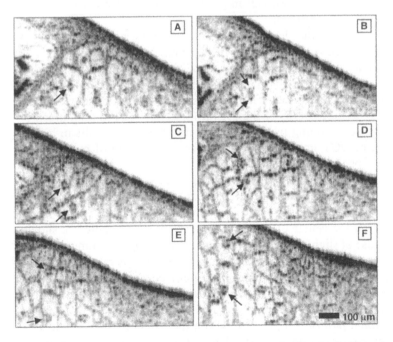

Figure 20 OCT imaging of *Xenopus* mesenchymal cell mitosis. Parent cell indicated by the arrow in (A) undergoes mitosis and divides into two daughter cells indicated by the two arrows in (B–F). Following cell division, daughter cells migrate apart and increase in size, preparing for subsequent cell division. Images were from 3-D data sets acquired at 10 min intervals. (From Ref. 8.)

increased optical backscatter within the nucleus. One possibility is that these are regions of varying chromatin concentration, indicative of high mitotic activity.

Within each image, cells are found in various stages of mitosis and exhibit a high degree of pleomorphism. Mitotic activity of one parent mesenchymal cell and the migration of the two daughter cells are shown in the sequence in Fig. 20. The parent cell (arrow) in Fig. 20a is in telophase as the chromosomes appear to have reached the mitotic poles. The membrane in the upper left of this cell has begun to pinch in. Fig. 20b, acquired 10 min later, more distinct separation has occurred and two adjacent nuclei are observed. After an additional 10 min, the two daughter cells in Fig. 20c have a distinct membrane separating them. The remaining figures (d–f) show the increasing separation of the nuclei and the growth in cell size.

19.7.4 Cell Migration

Cell migration, like mitosis, has a positive role in development as well as a negative role in the spread of neoplasms. The capability of monitoring cell migration through an organism would be a powerful tool in a variety of developmental and molecular models and may have clinical applications in oncology. In developing embryos, neural crest cells originate from the newly formed neural tube and migrate to differentiate into cardiovascular and epidermal tissue. In neoplasms, tumor cells will migrate through tissue, contributing to the growth and spread of the tumor. When a tumor metastasizes, tumor cells typically spread over great distances, usually through the circulatory system. Tumor cell migration occurs before the cell enters and after the cell exits the bloodstream.

The neural crest cells of the developing embryo migrate along two distinct pathways [47]. Progenitor cells that migrate to the dermal layers follow a superficial pathway, whereas cardiac progenitor cells follow a path more internal to the embryo. The neural crest cells migrating to the dermal layers are also called melanocytes because of their high concentration of melanin. These cells are also responsible for establishing the pigmentation patterns of the organism. Melanin has a high index of refraction compared to surrounding tissue structures and therefore results in higher optical backscattering in OCT images. This facilitates the tracking of melanocytes deep within scattering specimens.

The ability of OCT to track individual cell movement is illustrated in Fig. 21. A neural crest melanocyte in Fig. 21a was imaged at 10 min intervals by acquiring three-dimensional volumes containing the cell. From each volume, the 2-D cross section acquired through the center of the cell was identified, and these are shown in Figs. 21a–21f. Because of slight changes in specimen movement over time, internal morphological features and markers within the images were used as reference points. The arrow at the top right in Fig. 21a indicates the outer membrane of the specimen, and the arrow at the left edge of the figure indicates a melanin layer covering the dorsal neural tube. Each was used as an internal reference point.

A three-dimensional plot of cell position within the specimen is shown in Fig. 22. The X and Y Cartesian coordinates were determined from the image measurements obtained in Figs. 21a–21f. The Z coordinate was determined from the cell movement between planes of the three-dimensional volume. The points labeled $A–F$ correspond to the images shown in Fig. 21. The cell migration between labeled points corresponds to 10 min intervals. This plot indicates that the cell migrated along a

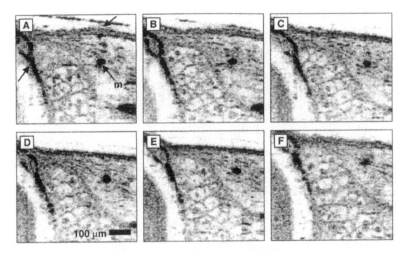

Figure 21 OCT tracking of neural crest cell (melanocyte) migration. A single migrating melanocyte (m) was tracked by acquiring 3-D data sets at 10 min intervals. (A) Unlabeled arrows indicate internal points from which migration measurements were referenced. (From Ref. 8.)

curved path, progressing first dorsolaterally and then dorsomedially. Projections of the migration in the transverse, coronal, and sagittal planes of the tadpole are also shown in Fig. 22. Although the specimen was repeatedly hydrated during imaging, drying and motion artifacts may be present in these data. Measured cell migrations of 20–60 μm were not significantly larger than the resolutions of the system. The movement in Fig. 22 from point D to point E is large and inconsistent compared to the movements during other intervals, suggesting a possible artifact. However, these results demonstrate a general protocol for tracking cell migration. More precise results will be possible with higher image resolutions and longer tracking times.

19.8 SIGNIFICANCE FOR DEVELOPMENTAL BIOLOGY

The studies described here demonstrate the fundamental principles of applying optical coherence tomography in developmental biology and microscopy. The results are significant because they demonstrate the feasibility of using OCT as a research microscopy technique to enable the in vivo, real-time, repeated imaging of developing morphology and functional behavior. In situations where it can be applied, OCT imaging could result in a significant reduction in the time, complexity, and cost over conventional histology for imaging developing morphology. For these reasons, developmental biology promises to become one of the major application areas for optical coherence tomography.

The cross-sectional imaging in nontransparent embryos at near-histological resolutions enables repeatable in vivo imaging without having to kill the specimen. This is particularly useful with established mutant specimens, which are often difficult to produce and are limited in number. The non-contact, noninvasive imaging of OCT can be used to track the development of single specimens over time. The use of high speed OCT imaging of cardiac structures enabled functional imaging to be

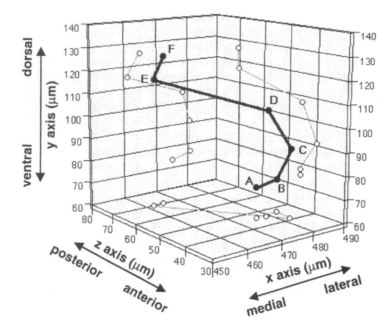

Figure 22 Three-dimensional plot of neural crest cell (melanocyte) migration. Labeled data points refer to images in Fig. 21 from which *X*, *Y* measurements were obtained. *Z* measurements were obtained from position of OCT image plane within 3-D data set. (From Ref. 8.)

performed in these specimens where previously this had been unattainable. OCT imaging will enable developmental research on genes that are expressed functionally as well as morphologically.

The dynamic nature of living cells may require a means of tracking cells in tissue. For these experiments, three-dimensional OCT imaging was performed over time to enable subtle cell movements to be recorded within the acquired volume. A series of 2-D OCT cross-sectional images were acquired at intervals that ensured oversampling in the third dimension. Hence, the nuclei of the cells were imaged in at least one of the 2-D images contained within the 3-D volume. Such 3-D imaging may be necessary in humans. However, high speed imaging at cellular resolutions may permit real-time tracking of a cell by positioning the OCT imaging plane at arbitrary angles. The ability to position the OCT imaging plane at arbitrary angles will be advantageous when cell divisions are observed, because the division of a parent cell into two daughter cells may not always occur in the same OCT imaging plane. The subcellular OCT imaging techniques demonstrated using *Xenopus* mesenchymal cells have helped to establish the necessary protocols for future in vivo cellular imaging in humans.

19.9 CLINICAL APPLICATIONS

Subcellular imaging was demonstrated in a living, nontransparent, organism with OCT. This suggests the feasibility of its use for assessing neoplastic changes in humans. Of greatest clinical relevance, with these OCT images it was possible to identify active cell division and assess nuclear-to-cytoplasmic ratios, two important markers of malignant transformation. In addition, to further confirm the ability to identify cell division, a single cell was followed through a single division cycle and changes in morphology were noted. A change in the backscattering intensity from nuclei was also noted as a function of time. This is postulated to represent a change in the concentration or packing of chromatin, which may be of diagnostic relevance.

The ability to track single cells as they migrate through tissue has future clinical relevance. Following malignant cells in vivo in animal models may help researchers understand the mechanisms of cancer. In many cases, the resection of tumors and tumor cells must be complete, because even single cells may continue to divide, resulting in recurrence of the tumor. OCT imaging at the cellular level may have the potential to identify tumor cells that have migrated away from the central tumor. The first stage of tumor metastasis is the penetration of tumor cells through the basement membrane of epithelial tissue. This process may be monitored in vivo to further understand mechanisms and characterize treatment effectiveness.

The investigation of development biology animal models using OCT serves as a clear demonstration that OCT is valuable for imaging tissue microstructure. Imaging at high cellular resolutions in these models identifies the future challenges for imaging at the cellular level in human tissue. With this fundamental information, OCT images can be characterized and OCT imaging techniques can be applied to clinical applications.

19.10 CONCLUSIONS

The ability of OCT to image tissue microstructure has been demonstrated using developmental biology animal models. These frog and fish embryos provide an excellent in vivo model because of the variety of organ systems, morphological variations, and cellular structures that develop over time. Morphological abnormalities during development can be identified and compared with histology. The non-contact, noninvasive nature of OCT permits repeatable imaging over extended periods of time at resolutions that approach the level of histology. Unlike laser-scanning confocal microscopy, no contrast agents that would limit the viability of cells are necessary. OCT can be used to track the morphological and functional expression of genes without having to sacrifice specimens for histological observations. The first demonstration of functional OCT imaging was performed in the developing *Xenopus* cardiovascular system. Optical cardiograms and high speed OCT imaging were used to assess functional parameters of the normal heart and one affected by an inotropic agent. The Cr^{4+}:forsterite laser was used as a high resolution source ($\approx 5\,\mu$m axial resolution) to image cell nuclei and membranes. Cell mitosis and migration were tracked in these animal models. Cellular imaging studies in these animal models provide insight into the relevant issues for cellular imaging in humans.

The future potential of OCT in developmental biology is extremely promising. Visualizing and studying many developmental processes, those known as well as those yet undiscovered, may be possible only with the unique imaging capabilities of this technology. Ultimately, OCT can contribute to the scientific understanding of how a single fertilized egg can develop into a complex, multisystem organism. Beyond this scientific investigation, OCT can contribute to the understanding of developmental processes that have the long-term potential to improve clinical therapies and patient care.

ACKNOWLEDGMENTS

The material in this chapter is excerpted in apart from the doctoral dissertation of Stephen A. Boppart, entitled "Surgical Diagnostics, Guidance, and Intervention Using Optical Coherence Tomography," which was submitted to the Harvard-MIT Division of Health Sciences and Technology and the Massachusetts Institute of Technology in May 1998. These studies were performed in the Department of Electrical Engineering and Computer Science and the Research Laboratory of Electronics at the Massachusetts Institute of Technology. We are grateful to Dr. Hazel Sive and her associates at MIT for advice and support as well to Dr. James Southern for his contributions. We also thank Drs. Gary Tearney and Brett Bouma for their invaluable scientific contributions. This research is sponsored in part by the National Institutes of Health Contracts NIH-9-RO1-EY11289-12 (JGF), NIH-1-RO1-CA75289-02 (JGF and MEB), NIH-1-R29-HL55686-01A1 (MEB), NIH-1-RO1-AR44812-01 (MEB); the Medical Free electron Laser Program, Office of Naval Research Contract N00014-94-1-0717 (JGF); the Air Force Office of Scientific Research Contract F4920-98-1-0139 (JGF); and the Whitaker Foundation Contract 96-0205 (MEB). Dr. Stephen Boppart gratefully acknowledges the support of the Air Force Palace Knight Program.

REFERENCES

1. Huang D, Swanson EA, Lin CP, Schuman JS, Stinson WG, Chang W, Hee MR, Flotte T, Gregory K, Puliafito CA, Fujimoto JG. Optical coherence tomography. Science 254:1178–1181, 1991.
2. Schmitt JM, Yadlowsky MJ, Bonner RF. Subsurface imaging of living skin with optical coherence microscopy. Dermatology 191:93–98, 1995.
3. Brezinski ME, Tearney GJ, Bouma BE, Izatt JA, Hee MR, Swanson EA, Southern JF, Fujimoto JG. Optical coherence tomography for optical biopsy: Properties and demonstration of vascular pathology. Circulation 93:1206–1213, 1996.
4. Fujimoto JG, Brezinski ME, Tearney GJ, Boppart SA, Bouma BE, Hee MR, Southern JF, Swanson EA. Biomedical imaging and optical biopsy using optical coherence tomography. Nature Med 1:970–972, 1995.
5. Boppart SA, Brezinski ME, Bouma BE, Tearney GJ, Fujimoto JG. Investigation of developing embryonic morphology using optical coherence tomography. Dev Biol 177:54–63, 1996.
6. Boppart SA, Brezinski ME, Tearney GJ, Bouma BE, Fujimoto JG. Imaging developing neural morphology using optical coherence tomography. J Neurosci Meth 70:65–72, 1996.
7. Boppart SA, Tearney GJ, Bouma BE, Southern JF, Brezinski ME, Fujimoto JG. Noninvasive assessment of the developing *Xenopus* cardiovascular system using optical coherence tomography. Proc Natl Acad Sci USA 94:4256–4261, 1997.
8. Boppart SA, Bouma Be, Pitris C, Southern JF, Brezinski ME, Fujimoto JG. In vivo cellular optical coherence tomography imaging. Nature Med 4:861–864, 1998.
9. Smith BR, Johnson GA, Groman EV, Linney E. Magnetic resonance microscopy of mouse embryos. Proc Natl Acad Sci USA 91:3530–3533, 1994.

10. Jacobs RE, Fraser SE. Magnetic resonance microscopy of embryonic cell lineages and movements. Science 263:691–684, 1994.
11. Jacobs RE, Fraser SE. Imaging neuronal development with magnetic resonance imaging (MRI) microscopy. J Neurosci Methods 54:189–196, 1994.
12. Morton EJ, Webb S, Bateman JE, Clarke LJ, Shelton CG. Three-dimensional x-ray microtomography for medical and biological applications. Phys Med Biol 35:805–820, 1990.
13. Turnbull DH, Bloomfield TS, Baldwin HS, Foster FS, Joyner AL. Ultrasound backscatter microscopy analysis of early mouse embryonic brain development. Proc Natl Acad Sci USA 92:2239–2243, 1995.
14. Minsky M. Memoir on inventing the confocal scanning microscope. Scanning 10:128–138, 1988.
15. White JG, Amos WB, Fordham M. An evaluation of confocal versus conventional imaging of biological structures by fluorescence light microscopy. J Cell Biol 105:41–48, 1987.
16. Webb WW, Wells KS, Sandison DR, Strickler J. Criteria for quantitative dynamical confocal fluorescence imaging. In: B Herman, K Jacobson, eds. Optical Microscopy for Biology. New York: Wiley-Liss, 1990:73–108.
17. Jester JV, Andrews PM, Petroll WM, Lemp MA, Cavanagh HD. In vivo, real-time confocal imaging. J. Electron Microsc Technol 18:50–60, 1991.
18. Stricker SA, Centonze VE, Paddock SW, Schatten G. Confocal microscopy of fertilisation-induced calcium dynamics in sea urchin eggs. Dev Biol 149:370–380, 1992.
19. Girard S, Clapham D. Acceleration of intracellular calcium waves in *Xenopus* oocytes by calcium influx. Science 260:229–232, 1993.
20. Bouma BE, Tearney GJ, Bilinsky IP, Golubovic B, Fujimoto JG. A self-phase-modulated Kerr-lens-modelocked Cr:forsterite laser source for optical coherence tomography. Opt Lett 21:1839–1841, 1996.
21. Tearney GJ, Brezinsky ME, Southern JF, Bouma BE, Hee MR, Fujimoto JG. Determination of the refractive index of highly scattering human tissue by optical coherence tomography. Opt Lett 20:2258–2260, 1995.
22. Izatt JA, Hee MR, Owen GM, Swanson EA, Fujimoto JG. Optical coherence microscopy in scattering media. Opt Lett 19:590–592, 1993.
23. Nieuwkoop PD, Faber J. Normal Table of *Xenopus laevis*. New York: Garland, 1994.
24. Olson EN, Strivastava D. Molecular pathways controlling heart development. Science 272:671–676, 1996.
25. Konig K, So PTC, Mantulin WW, Gratton E. Cellular response to near-infrared femtosecond laser pulses in two-photon microscopes. Opt Lett 22:135–137, 1997.
26. Konig K, Liang H, Berns MW, Tromberg BJ. Cell damage in near-infrared multimode optical traps as a result of multiphoton absorption. Opt Lett 21:1090–1092, 1996.
27. Burke AC, Nelson CE, Morgan BA, Tabin C. *Hox* genes and the evolution of vertebrate axial morphology. Development 121:333–346, 1995.
28. Sergeev A, Gelikonov V, Gelikonov A. High-spatial-resolutuion optical-coherence tomography of human skin and mucous membranes. Conference on Lasers and Electro-Optics, Anaheim, CA, May 21–26, 1995.
29. Tearney GJ, Bouma BE, Bopparts SA, Golubovic B, Swanson EA, Fujimoto JG. Rapid acquisition of in vivo biological images by use of optical coherence tomography. Opt Lett 21:1408–1410, 1996.
30. Ballif J, Gianotti R, Chavanne P, Walti R, Salathe RP. Rapid and scalable scans at 21 m/s in optical low-coherence reflectometry. Opt Lett 22:757–759, 1997.
31. Su CB. Achieving variation of the optical path length by a few millimeters at millisecond rates for imaging of turbid media and optical interferometry: A new technique. Opt Lett 22:665–667, 1997.

32. Tearney GJ, Bouma BE, Fujimoto JG. High-speed phase- and group-delay scanning with a grating-based phase control delay. Opt Lett 22:1811–1813, 1997.
33. American Society of Echocardiography Committee on Standards. Recommendations of quantitation of the left ventricle by two-dimensional echocardiography. J Am Soc Echocardiogr 2:358–367, 1989.
34. Schmidt KG, Silverman NH, Van Hare GF, Hawkins JA, Cloez J-L, Rudolph AM. Two-dimensional echocardiographic determination of ventricular volumes in the fetal heart. Circulation 81:325–333, 1990.
35. Stewart WJ, Rodkey SM, Gunawardena S, White RD, Luvisi B, Klein AL, Salcedo E. Left ventricular volume calculation with integrated backscatter from echocardiography. J Am Soc Echocardiogr 6:553–563, 1993.
36. Boppart SA. Surgical diagnostics, guidance, and intervention using optical coherence tomography. PhD Dissertation, Harvard-MIT Division of Health Sciences and Technology, Massachusetts Institute of Technology, May 1998.
37. Wang XJ, Milner TE, Nelson JS. Characterization of fluid flow velocity by optical Doppler tomography. Opt Lett 20:1337–1339, 1995.
38. Chen Z, Milner TE, Dave D, Nelson JS. Optical Doppler tomographic imaging of fluid flow velocity in highly scattering media. Opt Lett 22:64–66, 1997.
39. Chen Z, Milner TE, Srinivas S, Wang X. Noninvasive imaging of in vivo blood flow velocity using optical Doppler tomography. Opt Lett 22:1119–1121, 1997.
40. Wang X-J, Milner TE, Chen Z, Nelson JS. Measurement of fluid-flow-velocity profile in turbid media by the use of optical Doppler tomography. Appl Opt 36:144–149, 1997.
41. Yazdanfar S, Kulkarni MD, Izatt JA. High resolution imaging of in vivo cardiac dynamics using color Doppler optical coherence tomography. Opt Express 1:424–431, 1997.
42. Dunn AK, Smithpeter C, Welch AJ, Richards-Kortum R. Sources of contrast in confocal reflectance imaging Appl Opt 35:3441–3446, 1996.
43. Beuthan J, Minet O, Helfmann J, Herrig M, Muller G. The spatial variation of the refractive index in biological cells. Phys Med Biol 41:369–382, 1996.
44. Clivaz X, Marquis-Weible F, Salathe RP. Optical low coherence reflectometry with 1.9 μm spatial resolution. Electron Lett 28:1553–1555, 1992.
45. Bouma BE, Tearney GJ, Boppart SA, Hee MR, Brezinski ME, Fujimoto JG. High resolution optical coherence tomographic imaging using a modelocked Ti:Al$_2$O$_3$ laser. Opt Lett 20:1486–1488, 1995.
46. Liu H, Beauvoit B,Kimura M, Chance B. Dependence of tissue optical properties on solute-induced changes in refractive index and osmolarity. J. Biomed Opt 1:200–211, 1996.
47. Gilbert SF. Developmental Biology. 4th ed. Sunderland, MA: Sinauer Assoc, 1994.

20

Optical Coherence Tomography in Dermatology

JULIA WELZEL

Medical University of Lübeck, Lübeck, Germany

JOACHIM NOACK, EVA LANKENAU, and RALF ENGELHARDT

Medical Laser Center Lübeck, Lübeck, Germany

20.1 INTRODUCTION

Today three major diagnostic methods prevail in dermatology: visual inspection, high frequency ultrasound (> 15 MHz), and histology. Visual inspection allows investigation of only the uppermost layers of the human skin, but it is an inexpensive, noninvasive, and fast diagnostic method. Ultrasound, in contrast, enables the clinician to perform noninvasive depth-resolved imaging with a resolution of about 100 μm up to depth of 6 mm, but requires an ultrasonic transducer to be placed in contact with the skin. Finally, there is the gold standard, histology, which in conjunction with light microscopy allows depth-resolved imaging with a resolution on the order of 1 μm but relies on the excision of the area of interest and is time-consuming and expensive. Furthermore, histology is unsuitable for follow-up studies due to its invasive nature.

Obviously it would be advantageous to have a diagnostic method that is noninvasive but yields information with a resolution similar to that of histology, i.e., if it were possible to perform noninvasive biopsies. Even if this method did not reach microscopic resolution, it would be helpful for assessment of the architecture of a lesion or for quantification and monitoring of superficial skin changes. A method that allows such noninvasive biopsies is optical coherence tomography, a technique that analyzes light scattered from the different layers of the skin.

539

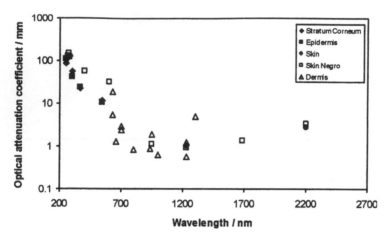

Figure 1 Wavelength dependence of scattering and absorption coefficients of skin and available light sources. (From Refs. 2, 4, and 7.)

20.2 OCT SYSTEM FOR DERMATOLOGY

20.2.1 Light Sources

A good light source for OCT in dermatology should have a short coherence length to achieve high depth resolution. Additionally it should have a wavelength that penetrates deep into the skin to have a large imaging depth, and it should provide sufficient output power to obtain detectable backscattered signals.

Figure 1 shows an overview of the wavelength dependence of the total attenuation coefficiency for different dermatological tissue types compiles form the literature [3,5,11]. Even though the reported values at comparable wavelengths vary considerably due to different tissue origin, tissue preparation, and measurement technique, a clear trend is observable: High attenuation total coefficients prevail in the ultraviolet (UV) due to the high absorption of tissue proteins and water in this wavelength region. The total attenuation decreases rapidly from around $100 \, \text{mm}^{-1}$ in the UV to around $10 \, \text{mm}^{-1}$ for visible wavelengths because both scattering and water absorption decrease with increasing wavelength. A minimum of the total attenuation coefficient is observed for wavelengths between 700 and 1000 nm. Even though the scattering coefficient of tissue decreases even further for even longer wavelengths [10], the total attenuation coefficient starts to increase again, due to the strong absorption of water molecules in the infrared.

Because the penetration depth is inversely proportional to the total attenuation coefficient, any wavelength between 700 and 1000 nm appears to be a good choice for OCT in dermatology. We have used fiber-coupled light sources with wavelengths of 830 nm (superluminescence diode, 1.5 mW, Superlum) and 1300 nm (fiber-optic light source, 10 mW, AFC Technologies) and Ti : sapphire laser tunable between 750 and 850 nm (up to 100 mW). All those light sources had a coherence length of 15–20 μm.

Typical OCT images obtained at two different body locations with four different wavelengths are shown in Fig. 2. At both locations, the images obtained with a wavelength between 750 and 850 nm differ only slightly, which is to be expected

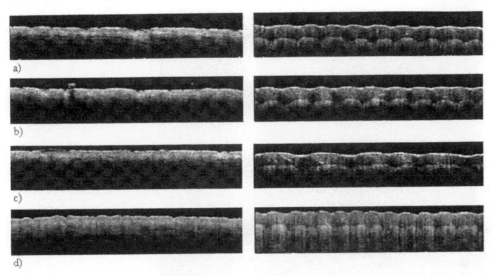

Figure 2 OCT images of the inner side of the forearm (left) and the thumb (right) at wavelengths of (a) 750, (b) 800, (c) 850, and (d) 1300 nm.

because the wavelength dependence of the scattering and the absorption coefficient over this 100 nm range is small (Fig. 1).

Figure 3a gives an impression of the size of the whole OCT system. The box below the computer monitor contains all the electronics, the fiber-optic interferometer, and the reference scanner. The light source is the box at the right, and the computer is below. All components have a modular design to facilitate upgrading and modifications of the system.

20.2.2 Applicator

The first OCT images of human skin were generated with laboratory setups on optical tables. This limited the body locations where OCT measurements were possible to relatively few locations, mostly on the extremities. For widespread clinical use, however, lightweight, compact handpieces of the size of ultrasonic transducers are required that can easily be connected to the interferometer by a fiber-optic cable.

The handpiece must contain imaging optics that emit light directly from the single-mode optical fiber onto the skin and collect the reflected light. Because the light passes through each optical element on its way to the sample as well as on its way back, only high quality lenses should be used. Otherwise, spatial aberrations will cause a disturbance of the beam, which results in a drastic decrease in detected backscattered signal because only a small fraction of the backscattered light can be coupled back into the single-mode fiber.

In our optimized handheld applicator, light emitted form a single-mode optical fiber with a numerical aperture of 0.11 is collimated using a 20 mm achromat and focused by a 40 mm triplet onto the surface of the skin.

To obtain images rather than just individual depth scans, the applicator also contains a galvanometric scanner with its axis of rotation placed in the focus of the triplet. That is, the scanning is performed telecentrically, which implies that all depth

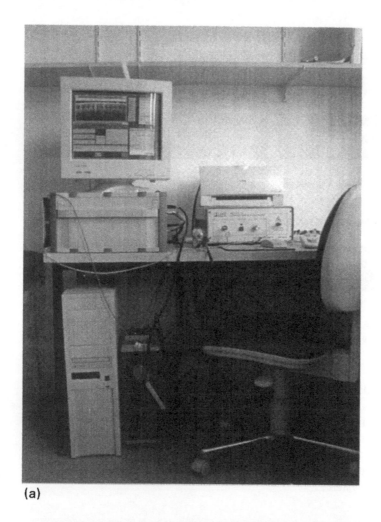

(a)

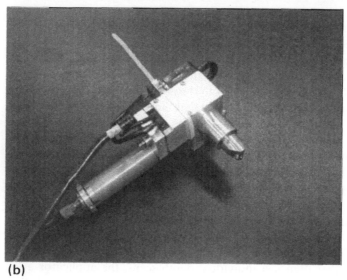

(b)

Figure 3 Image of (a) the OCT system and (b) the OCT handpiece.

scans are parallel to the optical axis. The lateral scanning rage is limited to approximately 7 mm by the aperture.

20.3 IMAGE ANALYSIS

20.3.1 Thickness Measurements

Even though currently most OCT images in dermatology are used to get a qualitative impression of a lesion, OCT can also be used to gain quantitative data about a pathology. The most obvious measurements are thickness measurements of the upper skin layers in vivo. This might be useful additional information to judge the healing of wounds or the effect of cosmetics as outlined in Section 20.4.4.

There is, however, a certain pitfall in those thickness measurements: Depth information in OCT images is usually plotted as optical pathlength. To obtain physical distances that can be compared to other thickness measurements by histology, for example, optical pathlength has to be divided by the refractive index of the tissue. Considering the large concentration of water in living tissue, it is reasonable to approximate the refractive index of the tissue by the refractive index of water, which is 1.33 in the 700–1400 nm wavelength range [6,9].

20.3.2 Digital Image Processing

At the moment there is no established image processing technique that can remove or suppress the speckle noise without compromising lateral resolution. We have therefore experimented with a different approach: The OCT signal measured from a certain depth is a coherent superposition of the scattered waves from all particles that are illuminated by the probe beam and that are located within one coherence length of the sampled depth. The signal amplitude depends on the phase distribution of the individual scattered waves and is assumed to be random. Thus, the speckle can be interpreted as a random noise that modulates the "true" signal. To get an estimate of the underlying image, a weighted average of the signal from all points within one coherence length was calculated, i.e., the image was convolved with the two-dimensional point spread function. Because we use a focused geometry, this point spread function $\mathrm{psf}_{\bar{z}}(z, r)$ is depth-dependent:

$$\mathrm{psf}_{\bar{z}}(z, r) = \exp\left[-\left(\frac{r}{w(z)}\right)^2\right] \times \mathrm{Corr}(z - \bar{z})$$

where

$$w(z) = w_0\left[1 + \left(\frac{\lambda(z - z_0)}{\pi w_0^2}\right)^2\right]^{1/2}$$

denotes the depth around which the point spread function is to be calculated, z_0 is the depth location of the focus (usually the surface), and r is the lateral distance from the optical axis. Deviations from Gaussian beam propagation caused by scattering were neglected.

The convolution with the point spread function does introduce some blurring, but it is kept at a minimum, because the point spread function dimensions are small

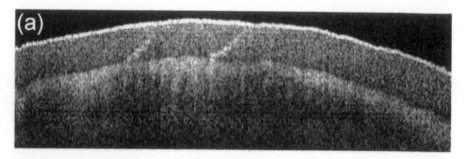

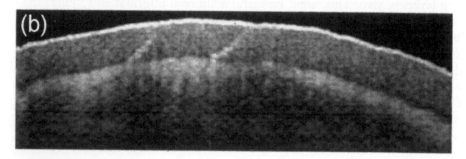

Figure 4 OCT image (a) before and (b) after convolution with the point spread function.

relative to the architectural features of interest. Figure 4 shows an example of an OCT image before and after processing with the point spread function. Processing clearly reduces the coherent speckle at the expense of some lateral and axial resolution. Note that the sweat gland and layers are much better defined in the processed image—a feature that will become particularly important if segmentation techniques are to be applied for cutaway views of 3D OCT images in the future. For the other OCT images demonstrated in this chapter no processing was performed.

20.4 APPLICATIONS IN DERMATOLOGY

20.4.1 OCT Imaging of Healthy Skin In Vivo

Normal Anatomy of Human Skin

Human skin is composed of different layers. The superficial layer is the stratified epidermis, consisting of keratinocytes. In the basal cell layer, some melanocytes are distributed among these cells, producing melanin pigment, which causes the visible color of the skin. In higher layers the keratinocytes undergo a differentiation, resulting in the horny layer, the so-called stratum corneum, as the uppermost layer, consisting of dead corneocytes.

The dermis is composed mainly of dense collagen bundles with a few fibroblasts among them. Additionally, blood vessels, nerves, hair follicles, and sebaceous and sweat glands are found in the dermis.

The thickness of these structures varies depending on the anatomic location. The epidermis on the extremities, the face, and the trunk is about 100 μm thick, whereas on the palms and soles the thickness can reach more than 500 μm, mainly due to the very thick and dense stratum corneum at these locations. The thickness of the dermis varies from about 1 mm on the flexural sides of the arms to about 5 mm on the back.

Location-Dependent Differences

Optical coherence tomographic images of healthy skin show differences depending on the anatomic location. The skin of the inner forearm has a thin stratum corneum of about 10 μm that cannot be distinguished in OCT. The first layer is the epidermis. The lower stratum spinosum and the stratum basale are signal-poor. The border to the dermis is characterized by a second intensity peak in the averaged A-scans (Fig. 5). The dermis is signal-intense with several less intense structures corresponding to blood vessels. If the dermis is thinner than about 1 mm, the border to the subcutaneous fat is detectable in the lower part of the OCT image. The subcutis is signal-poor.

The skin of the cheek has many hair follicles, which are seen in the OCT image. The hair is signal intense. The epidermis shows a retraction in the infundibulum region. Deeper parts of the hair bulb appear as dark areas. The sebaceous glands are round signal-poor structures located in the middle of the dermis next to the hair bulb. The center of the glands is more signal-intense than the margin (Fig. 6).

On the external surface of the lip the epidermis is relatively thick. The border to the dermis is poorly demarcated from the epidermis. The second intensity peak in the averaged A-scans is much lower than the peak of the skin surface. Numerous dilated blood vessels are seen in the upper dermis (Fig. 7).

On palmoplantar skin, the surface is wavy because of the ridge pattern of the dermatoglyphics. The thick stratum corneum of about 450 μm is the first signal-poor layer. Sweat gland ducts are seen as spiral structures in the horny layer. The epidermis is more signal-intense. The border to the dermis is poorly demarcated because epidermis and dermis are more toothed in the palmoplantar region. The dermis is less signal-intense than that of the forearm skin (Fig. 8).

Influence of Skin Treatment

Treatment of the skin surface with ointments leads to an immediate reduction of the light attenuation coefficient and therefore to an increase in the detection depth of the signal. This effect is due to a reduction of the light reflection from the skin surface. Hydrating agents like glycerol show this effect too (Fig. 9). In this case, it may be caused by an increase in the water content of the stratum corneum [11].

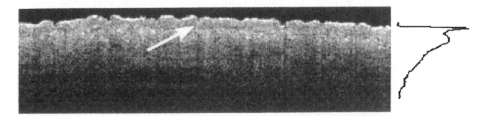

Figure 5 OCT image of healthy forearm skin. The superficial layer is the epidermis. The border to the dermis (arrow) is represented by a second intensity peak in the average A-scan on the right. The averaged A-scan is calculated over the whole scan length. 830 nm OCT; 4 mm × 1.3 mm.

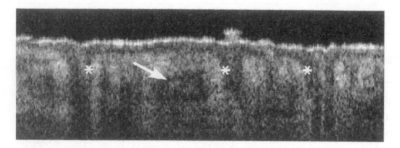

Figure 6 Healthy skin of the cheek. Hair follicles (stars) and sebaceous glands (arrow) are visible. 1300 nm OCT; 4 mm × 1.4 mm.

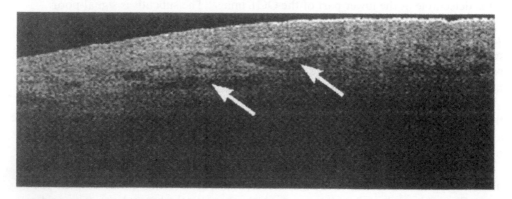

Figure 7 Optical coherence tomography of the lip demonstrates many blood vessels (arrows). 830 nm OCT; 4 mm × 1.8 mm.

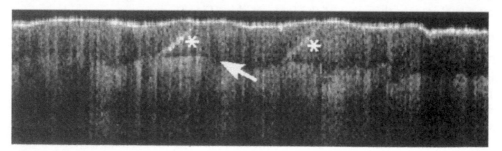

Figure 8 Healthy skin of the finger tip shows a thick stratum corneum with spiral sweat gland ducts (stars). The border to the living epidermis is marked by an arrow. 1300 nm OCT; 4 mm × 1.1 mm.

Tape stripping removes layers of the stratum corneum. The actual thickness of the horny layer can be visualized and quantified by OCT (Fig. 10).

To investigate the influence of blood circulation on OCT images, an erythema was induced by topical application of nicotinic acid. This treatment leads to dilation of vessels. These vessels are visualized in OCT as signal-free cavities in the dermis (Fig. 11). The light attenuation coefficient is decreased due to the higher water content of the dermis. Experimentally induced edema, caused by intradermal injection of histamine, also leads to a decrease of light attenuation.

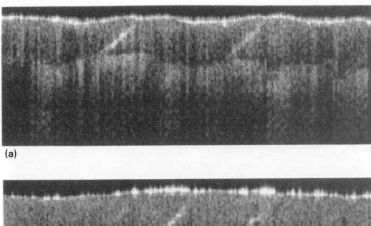

(a)

(b)

Figure 9 Healthy skin of the finger tip (a) before and (b) after the application of glycerole onto the skin surface. The treatment leads to a decrease of the reflectivity of the surface and to an increase of the penetration depth of the signal. 1300 nm OCT; 4 mm × 1.1 mm.

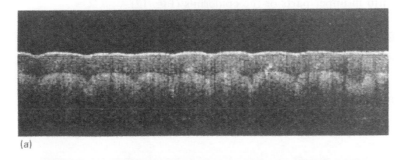

(a)

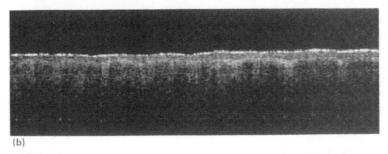

(b)

Figure 10 Fingertip skin (a) before and (b) after repeated tape stripping. The treatment leads to a thinning of the stratum corneum from an average of 666 μm to 235 μm. 830 nm OCT; 4 mm × 1.1 mm.

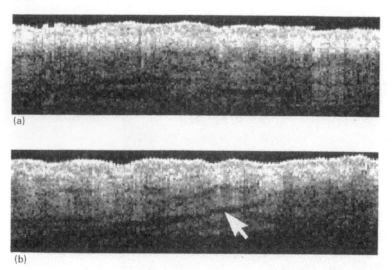

Figure 11 OCT image of the forearm skin (a) before and (b) 20 minutes after application of an ointment stimulating the blood circulation (nicotinate). The treatment leads to a dilation of the dermal blood vessels (arrow) and to a slight increase in the penetration depth of the signal. 1300 nm OCT; 4 mm × 1.1 mm.

In black skin, the melanin content in the epidermis is higher. In OCT images of black skin, the second intensity peak corresponding to the border between epidermis and dermis is replaced by a plateau of the signal due to the more homogeneous distribution of melanin in upper parts of the epidermis (Fig. 12).

20.4.2 OCT Imaging of Skin Tumors In Vivo

Melanocytic Tumors

A malignant melanoma is a malignant tumor of the melanocytes developing at first in the epidermis and then infiltrating the dermis. Most such tumors show a high degree of pigmentation. The tumor cell aggregates lead to destruction of the normal architecture of the basal epidermis.

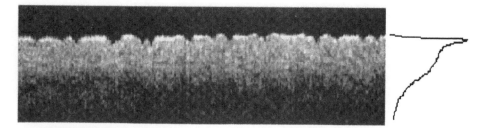

Figure 12 OCT image of black forearm skin. The epidermis is not as well demarcated from the dermis as in non-black skin. In the average A-scan (right), the second intensity peak corresponding to the basal membrane zone is replaced by a plateau. 1300 nm OCT; 4 mm × 1.1 mm.

In OCT images of malignant melanoma, the light scattering is more intense and more homogeneous than in healthy skin. The second peak, which represents an intact basal epidermis, is not found in the tumor region (Fig. 13). In thin tumors the limiting to the depth is detectable in some cases. For thickness measurement of melanomas thicker than 1 mm the detection depth of OCT is not high enough. The architecture of the whole lesion and larger cell aggregates in the epidermis is visible in OCT.

In some benign melanocytic nevi, especially in dermal nevi, a second peak appears in the average A-scan as in healthy skin (Fig. 14). However, due to the inability of OCT to resolve cellular features, reliable differentiation between melanomas and benign nevi is not currently possible with our system.

Epithelial Tumors

Basal cell carcinomas are superficial skin tumors consisting of keratinocytes and surrounded by a fibrous stroma. The tumor aggregates derive from the epidermis and infiltrate the dermis. Basal cell carcinomas are represented in OCT as homogeneous regions in the upper dermis. In most cases, the light scattering in the tumor is higher than in healthy skin. In some cases, the tumor cell aggregates can be distinguished from the stroma (Fig. 15).

Squamous cell carcinomas also derive from the epidermis but develop a higher degree of differentiation into keratinization. Therefore, the tumors have scales and keratosis on the surface. In OCT, squamous cell carcinomas show a multilayered surface reflectivity due to the hyperkeratosis with a high light scattering (Fig. 16).

Other Tumors

A hemangioma is a very common benign tumor of the blood vessels located in the dermis. OCT of a hemangioma shows signal-poor cavities in the upper dermis that correspond to the dilated capillaries (Fig. 17). A hypertrophic scar is caused by a trauma if the repair of the collagen defect does not lead to a network-like arrangement of collagen as in healthy dermis but to dense parallel bundles. In OCT, a scar exhibits parallel signal-poor and signal-rich layers in the dermis, representing the stratified sclerotic collagen bundles (Fig. 18). A seborrheic keratosis is a common benign tumor of the epidermis consisting of a thickened epithelium with some cysts of horn. In the OCT image, the tumor shows irregular structures corresponding to these cysts and is sharply demarcated from the dermis (Fig. 19).

20.4.3   OCT Imaging of Inflammatory Skin Diseases In Vivo

Eczema

Skin irritation, e.g., after treatment with sodium lauryl sulfate, leads to parakeratosis, acanthosis of the epidermis, and inflammatory infiltrates around the blood vessels. In OCT images of irritant contact dermatitis, the surface reflectivity is stronger due to the parakeratosis. The light scattering in the upper dermis is lower because of the higher water content caused by the edema (Fig. 20). The changes can be monitored over time. The degree of acanthosis can be quantified by measurement of the epidermal thickness in the averaged A-scan.

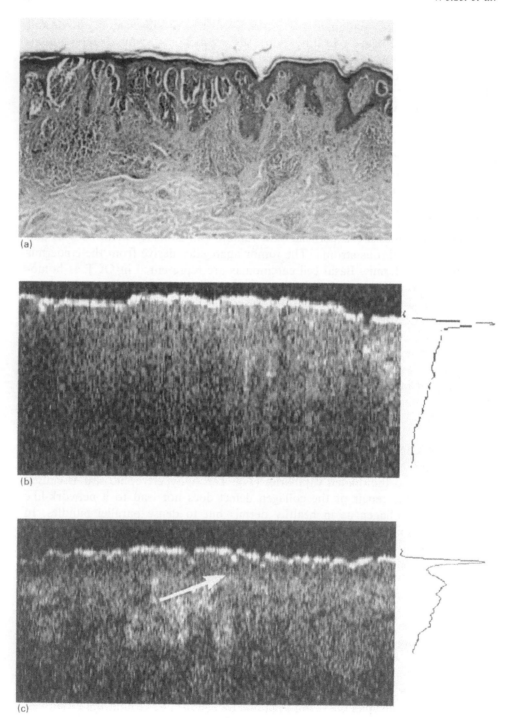

Figure 13 (a) Histology and (b) OCT image of a malignant melanoma on the shoulder. In contrast to the healthy adjacent skin (c), where the border between epidermis and dermis is well demarcated (arrow), the second peak is not detectable in the averaged A-scan. The light scattering is increased. 1300 nm OCT; 4 mm × 1.8 mm.

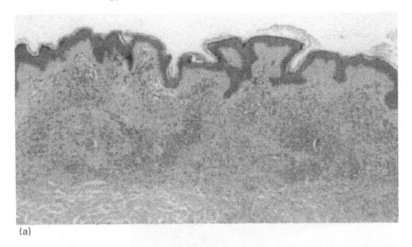

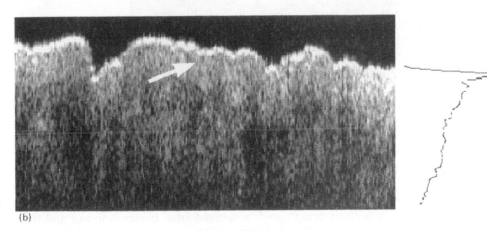

Figure 14   (a) Histology and (b) OCT image of a congenital dermal nevus on the forearm. The averaged A-scan shows a second peak corresponding to the border between epidermis and dermis (arrow). 1300 nm OCT; 4 mm × 1.8 mm.

Psoriasis

Psoriasis is a chronic inflammatory skin disease characterized by massive scaling, a thickening of the epidermis, and inflammatory infiltrates around the dilated blood vessels in the upper dermis. In OCT of psoriasis, the entrance peak is higher and broader than in healthy skin. This can be explained by the severe parakeratosis in psoriatic plaques (Fig. 21). The epidermis is thickened. The blood vessels in the upper dermis are dilated. The light scattering in the upper dermis is lower than in the healthy adjacent skin (Fig. 22). In pustular psoriasis, intraepidermal cavities are seen filled with inhomogeneous material corresponding to the pustules (Fig. 23).

Bullous Diseases

Bullae are represented in OCT as signal-free cavities. The cleft can be located in the OCT images. Thus, a differential diagnosis between autoimmune bullous diseases

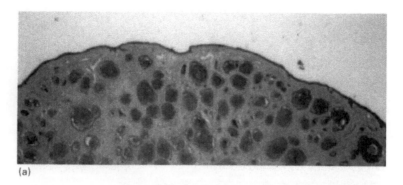

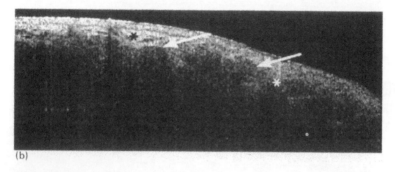

Figure 15 (a) Histology and (b) OCT image of a basal cell carcinoma on the nose. The globular tumor cell aggregates (arrows) can be distinguished from the stroma (stars). 830 nm OCT; 4 mm × 1.5 mm.

can be done by using OCT. In pemphigus vulgaris, the cleft is located within the epidermis, whereas in bullous pemphigoid, a subepidermal blister is found and the whole epidermis is elevated (Fig. 24). In blisters of herpes, aggregations of acantholytic cells in the edges of the intraepidermal blister are seen (Fig. 25).

Other Inflammatory Skin Diseases

Porokeratosis is a disorder of keratinization leading to a small, chimney-like hyperkeratosis on the skin surface, the so-called cornoid lamellae. In lesions of porokeratosis, the cornoid lamellae are characteristic in the OCT image (Fig. 26).

20.4.4 Application in Pharmacology and Cosmetology

Influence of Moisturizers

The best location for investigating the effect of topical treatment using OCT is palmoplantar skin because of the thick stratum corneum. Directly after application of an ointment, a signal-rich layer on the surface is visible representing the amount of cream applied. This highly scattering layer leads to light attenuation in the stratum corneum. After some minutes, the ointment penetrates into the horny layer. This can be observed with OCT. The sharp border between the ointment and the surface becomes less demarcated. Application of moisturizing agents such as urea leads to a swelling of the stratum corneum due to hydration. This can be quantified using

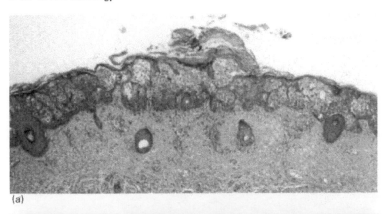

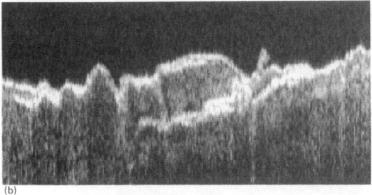

Figure 16 (a) Histology and (b) OCT image of a superficial squamous cell carcinoma (Bowen's disease) on the cheek. The layers of hyper- and parakeratosis are represented as multiple signal strong lines. 1300 nm OCT; 4 mm × 1.8 mm.

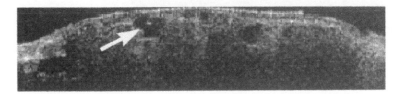

Figure 17 OCT image of a hemangioma on the trunk. The blood vessels are visible as signal-poor cavities in the upper dermis (arrow). 1300 nm OCT; 4 mm × 1.1 mm.

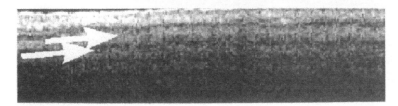

Figure 18 A hypertrophic scar shows parallel layers in the dermis corresponding to enlarged collagen bundles (arrows). 1300 nm OCT; 4 mm × 1.1 mm.

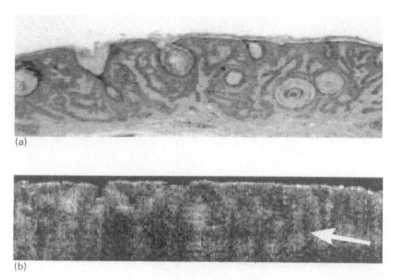

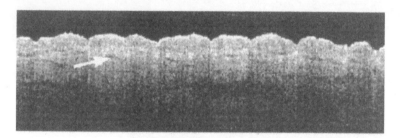

Figure 19 (a) Histology and (b) OCT image of a seborrheic keratosis on the trunk. The tumor shows irregular signal-rich and signal-poor areas corresponding to the horn cysts and is sharply demarcated from the dermis (arrow). 1300 nm OCT; 4 mm × 1.1 mm.

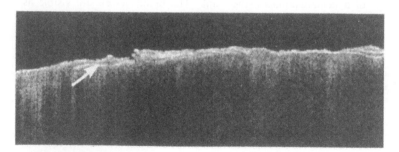

Figure 20 Experimentally induced irritant contact dermatitis on the forearm 4 days after irritation. Compared to the healthy skin of the same subject (Fig. 5), a thickening of the epidermis and a dilation of blood vessels (arrow) is observed. 830 nm OCT; 4 mm × 1.8 mm.

Figure 21 Parakeratosis in psoriatic plaques is represented by a thick, multilayered surface reflectivity (arrow). 1300 nm OCT; 4 mm × 1.8 mm.

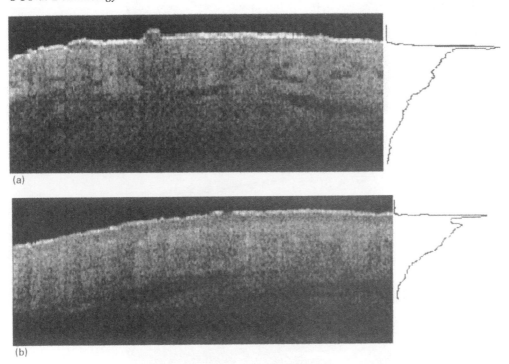

Figure 22   (a) Psoriasis and (b) adjacent healthy skin on the forearm. In the averaged A-scan, a thickened epidermis (407 μm versus 177 μm in healthy skin), a lower second peak, and a lower light scattering ($\mu = 2.3\,\mathrm{mm}^{-1}$ versus $\mu = 4.4\,\mathrm{mm}^{-1}$ in healthy skin) in the dermis is observed in psoriasis. 1300 nm OCT; 4 mm × 1.8 mm.

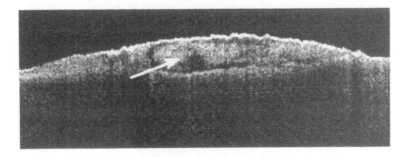

Figure 23   Intraepidermal pustule (arrow) in psoriasis pustulosa.

OCT by measuring the thickness of the horny layer. A 10% urea preparation induces a swelling of about 15% (Fig. 27).

Influence of Soaps and Synthetic Detergents

Prolonged contact with water results in an immediate swelling effect, followed by dehydration. These effects are more pronounced when soap or synthetic detergent solutions are applied. After a 15 min bath in such a solution, the stratum corneum is severely thickened. The light scattering in the upper stratum corneum is increased

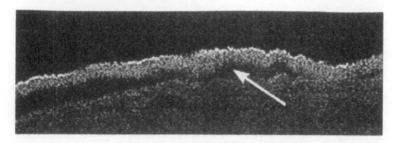

Figure 24 OCT image of a bullous pemphigoid shows a subepidermal blister. The cleft is marked by an arrow. The whole epidermis is elevated. 1300 nm OCT; 4 mm × 1.8 mm.

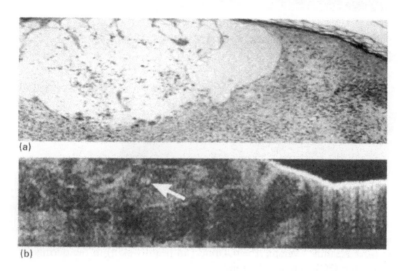

Figure 25 (a) Histology and (b) OCT image of an intraepidermal blister in herpes zoster on the trunk. The blister with acantholytic cells (arrow) is on the left side of the image. 1300 nm OCT; 4 mm × 1.1 mm.

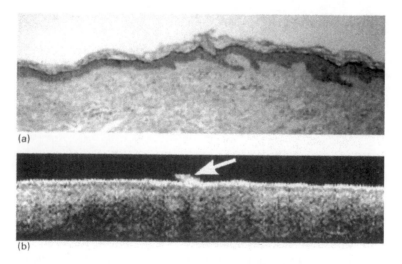

Figure 26 (a) Histology and (b) OCT image of porokeratosis on the lower leg with a chimney-like parakeratotic column in the center of the image. 1300 nm OCT; 4 mm × 1.1 mm.

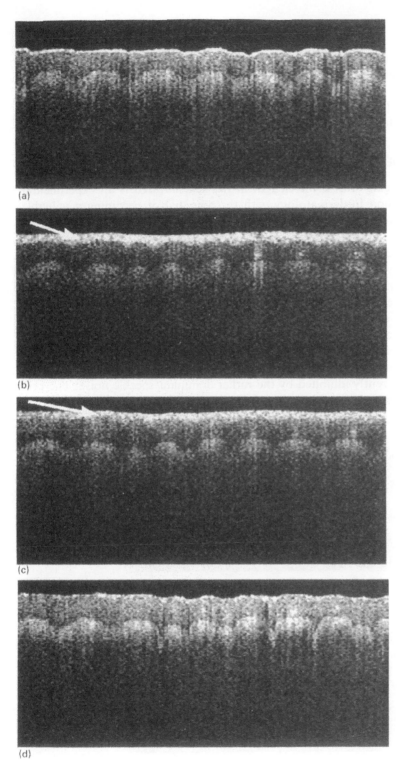

Figure 27 Healthy skin on the fingertip (a) before treatment, (b) directly after application of an ointment containing 10% urea, (c) after 35 min, and, (d) after 45 min after wiping off the ointment. Compared to (a), the stratum corneum is thickened in (d) due to the increase of water content. 830 nm OCT; 4 mm × 1.8 mm.

which might be caused by the swelling of the corneocytes (Fig. 28). After some minutes, the stratum corneum thickness decreases again. Compared to this soap effect, the changes after treatment with synthetic detergents are less pronounced. This might be due to the lower pH value of the products. The OCT allows quantification and comparison of treatment effects.

20.5 FUTURE DEVELOPMENTS

To date, OCT imaging with a wavelength in the near-infrared is an experimental morphological method in dermatology with the potential of becoming a valuable diagnostic tool. Interpretation of the images produced, however, requires a great deal of experience. As the systems start to approach TV imaging rates [10], it becomes possible to examine the structure of a lesion in real time. Thus, adjacent sections can be viewed on larger structures such as vessels, or hair follicles can be traced over adjacent sections. This leads quite naturally to the concept of 3-D OCT, where many adjacent OCT images spaced a few micrometers apart are used to reconstruct tissue volumes rather than tissue sections. This is a challenge not only for the scanning speed but also for data processing and display. The large amounts of data associated with three-dimensional imaging require dedicated image processing and display routines. Segmentation in different features required for useful image display is currently inhibited by the rather dominant speckle noise. The first 3-D OCT results were obtained in an animal model [1]. Figure 29 is an in vivo 3-D

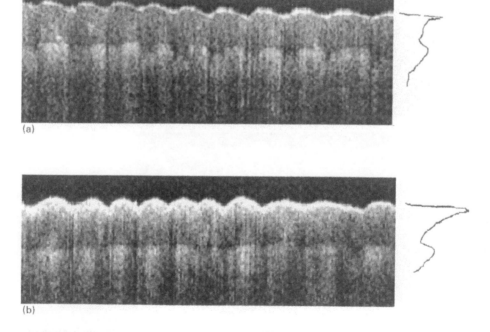

(a)

(b)

Figure 28   Healthy skin of the fingertip (a) before and (b) 15 min directly after a bath in a solution of a synthetic detergent. After treatment, the stratum corneum is thickened and the scattering in upper layers is higher. 1300 nm OCT; 4 mm × 1.1 mm.

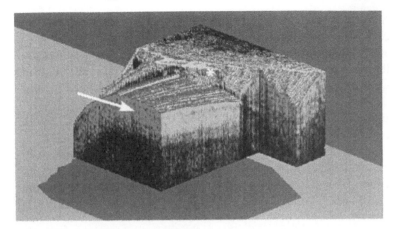

Figure 29 In vivo 3-D OCT image of the nail region of the little finger. In the front, the dome-shaped nail plate is visible (arrow; the proximal nail fold with the small cuticle is in the background (star). A section is taken out of the image to allow a view into deeper regions of the nail plate and matrix region. 1300 nm OCT; 4.2 mm × 4 mm × 1.4 mm.

OCT image of human skin that demonstrates the nail plate and nail fold region of the little finger.

Another potentially useful extension to OCT in dermatology could be the use of polarized light, where not only the amplitude but also the direction of polarization of the backscattered light is detected. This is potentially useful because tissues containing collagen are birefringent. Tissue coagulation causes changes in the birefringence that could be detected by polarized OCT. Even though this technique has been demonstrated [8], its clinical usefulness remains to be seen.

The simultaneous acquisition of OCT images using different wavelengths [3] could provide additional imaging contrast. It may be possible to trace specific substances as they penetrate into the skin by the use of differential imaging at two wavelengths if the absorption bands of the marker substance are sufficiently wide ($\sim$ 30 nm). An OCT system operating of 1.3 μm and 1.55 μm, for example, might be suitable for the measurement of the water content of the skin. This might be particularly interesting for pharmaceutical and cosmetic applications.

20.6 SUMMARY

Optical coherence tomography is an interesting new method for noninvasive investigation of the skin. Compared to other noninvasive morphological methods such as high frequency ultrasound, OCT offers a higher resolution and therefore the possibility of visualization of changes within the stratum corneum, the epidermis, or the upper dermis [5,12–14].

Location-dependent differences are found especially in palmoplantar skin with a thick stratum corneum and in regions with many hair follicles that are detectable in the OCT images. OCT images of skin tumors correspond well to histological sections and exhibit marked changes from the adjacent healthy skin. The light scattering in the tumor region is higher and often more homogeneous than in unaffected skin. For differential diagnosis between different tumors, the resolution of OCT is currently not high enough. The architecture of a lesion and cell aggregates are visible, but the detection of single cells is not possible.

Optical coherence tomography is a suitable method for monitoring inflammatory diseases. The degree of parakeratosis, acanthosis of the epidermis, and dilation of blood vessels as well as treatment effects can be monitored and quantified in vivo over time.

Skin surface treatment influences the OCT image. After application of oil, the detection depth of the light signal is increased due to reduction of scattering from the surface. Hydrating or dehydrating effects of topically applied substances can be quantified. Therefore, OCT is a completion of bioengineering methods for studies on the effectiveness and tolerance of topical treatments and cosmetics.

REFERENCES

1. Barton JK, Izatt JA, Kulkarni MD. Welch AJ. Three-dimensional reconstruction of a rat dermal blood vessel in vivo. Proc SPIE 2970:266–275, 197.
2. Duck FA. Physical Properties of Tissue. London: Academic Press, 1990: 47–51.
3. Gelnikonov G, Gelikonov V, Feldchtein F, Stepanov J, Sergeev A, Antoniou I, Ionnovich J, Reitze D, Dawson W (1997). Two-color-in-one-interferometer OCT system for bioimaging. In: Summaries of papers presented at the conference on lasers and electro-optics, 17:211, 1997.
4. Graaff R, Dassel AMC, Koelink MH, de Mul FFM, Aarnoudse JG, Zijlstra WG. Optical properties of human dermis in vitro and in vivo. Appl Opt 32:437–447, 1993.
5. Hoffmann K, Happe M, Fricke B, Knüttel A, Böcker D, Stücker M, Altmeyer P, von Düring M. Optical coherence tomography (OCT) in der Dermatologie. In: C Garbe, G Rassner, eds. Dermatologie—Leitlinien und Qualitätssicherung für Diagnostik und herapie. Berlin: Springer, 1998: 3–8.
6. Roggan A, Dörschel K, Minet O, Wolff D, Müller D. The optical properties of biological tissue in the near infrared wavelength range—Review and measurements. In: G. Mueller, A Roggan eds. Laser-Induced Interstitial Thermotherapy. Bellingham, WA: SPIE Opt Eng Press, 1995:11–43,
7. Schmitt JM, Liang Z. Deconvolution and enhancement of optical coherence tomograms. Proc SPIE 2981:46–57, 197.
8. Schmitt JM, Xiang SH. Cross-polarized backscatter in optical coherence tomography of biological tissue. Opt Lett 23:1060–1062, 1998.
9. Tearney GJ, Brezinski ME, Southern JF, Bouma BE, Hee MR, Fujimoto JG. Determination of the refractive index of highly scattering human tissue by optical coherence tomography. Opt Lett 20:2258–2261, 1995.
10. Tearney GJ, Boppart SA, Bouma BE, Pitris C, Brezinski ME, Southern JF, Swanson EA, Fujimoto JG. High speed catheter/endoscope optical coherence tomography for the optical biopsies of in vivo tissues. In: Summaries of papers presented at the conference on lasers and electro-optics 17:211, 1997.
11. Vargas G, Chan EK, Barton JK, Rylander HG, Welch AJ. Use of an agent to reduce scattering in skin. Lasers Surg Med 24:133–141, 1999.
12. Welzel J, Lankenau E, Birngruber R, Engelhardt R. Optical coherence tomography of the human skin. J Am Acad Dermatol 37:958–963, 1997.

13. Welzel J, Lankenau E, Pan Y, Birngruber R, Engelhardt R. Optical coherence tomography of the skin. In: P Elsner, AO Barel, E Beradesca, B Gabard, S. Serup, eds. Skin Bioengineering. Techniques and Applications in Dermatology and Cosmetology. Curr Probl Dermatol Vol. 26. Basel: Karger, 1998:27–37.
14. Welzel J, Lankenau E, Engelhardt R. Optische Kohärenztomographie als ein neues Verfhren zur nicht-invasiven Diagnostik oberflächennaher Strukturen der Haut. In: Garbe C, Rassner G, eds. Dermatologie—Leitlinien und Qualitätssicherung für Diagnostik und Therapie.

21

Imaging Neoplasia

CONSTANTINOS PITRIS and JAMES G. FUJIMOTO

Massachusetts Institute of Technology, Cambridge, Massachusetts

MARK E. BREZINSKI

Harvard Medical School, Massachusetts General Hospital, Boston, Massachusetts

21.1 INTRODUCTION

Every year 1.2 million new cases of cancer are detected in the United States alone, resulting in 560,000 deaths, with lung, prostate, breast, and colon cancer leading in mortality [1]. These numbers are double those of 30 years ago and are surpassed only by the number of deaths due to cardiovascular disease [2]. These alarming statistics have prompted much research effort in the diagnosis and treatment of cancer, with a clear understanding that early diagnosis is paramount to increasing the survival chances of the patient. A number of imaging techniques have been employed in the fight against cancer to better understand the disease process, features, and consequences and to more effectively guide diagnosis and treatment. Optical coherence tomography (OCT), which can image tissue microstructure in vivo and in situ, could be a powerful addition to the armamentarium of diagnostic tools for early detection of cancer [3,4].

21.1.1 Biology and Management of Cancer

The current understanding is that cancer begins at the level of individual cells and is a multistep process leading to abnormal, incomplete, and uncontrolled proliferation and differentiation. Genetic factors, chemical carcinogens, radiation, and viruses have all been implicated in the development of cancer [5]. Colonies of mutated, ever-growing, abnormal cells expand first around capillaries. Neovascularization, the proliferation of a new vascular supply initiated and promoted by growth factors secreted by the neoplastic cells, subsequently allows the tumor to grow in size to more than 2 mm [6]. Detachment of tumor cells leads to invasion of adjacent blood and lymph vessels and metastasis to distant organs [7]. Survival rates significantly decrease once metastasis has occurred. Although heredity does play a role in the development of cancer (accounting for about 5% of all cancer cases), a large fraction of malignancies are actually due to avoidable factors [8].

Cancer management involves more than treatment. Rather it refers to a spectrum of care that includes prevention, screening, detection, diagnosis, counseling, psychosocial support, specific therapeutic interventions, rehabilitation, and terminal care. Cancer prevention is by far the easiest and most effective way to fight cancer. Diet and smoking habits and hormone control and/or replacement have all been implicated in enhancing the carcinogenic process and can all be modified to minimize the risk of disease. Where prevention fails, screening can be employed to detect cancer at an early and treatable if not curable stage [9]. However, for a screening test to be successful it must detect cancer earlier and there must be evidence that earlier diagnosis will result in an improved outcome [7]. Unfortunately, to this date, only cancers of the breast, cervix, skin, colon-rectum, prostate, and testes have widely accepted screening interventions, and there is still controversy over some aspects of each [10].

In cancer diagnosis, signs, symptoms, cytological and imaging tests have all been employed, but the medical community still feels that the diagnosis of cancer can be confirmed only by histological investigation of a representative sample of the lesion [11]. To that end, a variety of biopsy techniques have been developed to confirm the diagnosis of malignancy. The choice of technique depends on the amount of tissue required by the pathologist and the location of the tumor. Once a histological cross section is available, an attempt is made to grade the lesion and classify the cellular proliferation as benign or malignant. The histopathological grade is a measure of the degree to which the tumor resembles normal tissue of its type, referred to as "differentiation," as well as the number of mitoses, which presumably correlates with the tumor's aggressiveness. One of the signs of abnormal differentiation is pleomorphism (i.e., variation in cell size and shape) characterized by cells ranging from giant cells to small, primitive-looking cells with disproportionally large nuclei and nuclear-to-cytoplasmic ratios (NCRs) approaching $1:1$ instead of the normal $1:4$ to $1:6$. A large degree of cell division and proliferation is also a sign of abnormal differentiation. Metastases, tumor implants discontinuous with the primary tumor, unequivocally mark a tumor as malignant, because benign neoplasms do not metastasize [12]. For malignant tumors, one of the more pivotal determinants of behavior is the tumor cell lineage identified from morphological criteria and lately immunohistochemistry. A significant proportion of tumors defy classification and are relegated to the "undifferentiated" category [11].

Histopathological grading may be the gold standard of cancer diagnosis, but it suffers from certain limitations. The success of the diagnosis depends on adequately sampling the tissue under investigation and providing a representative sample to the pathologist. If the number of biopsies is inadequate or if they are poorly located, the result will be a false negative reading, with the ramifications that follow a missed diagnosis [13,14]. Research has been motivated by the need to improve the performance of biopsy-based diagnosis, including studying the optimal number of biopsies required to maximize the likelihood of correct diagnosis of certain malignancies, the amount of tissue material required, and the effect of proper personnel training [15,16]. Some imaging modalities are also employed to more effectively guide biopsies to suspect areas, if such areas have been identified. Endoscopy, ultrasound, computed tomography (CT) and magnetic resonance imaging (MRI) are now routinely used to direct the harvest of tissue from neoplastic areas [17]. Another area that imaging is influencing is the effort to minimize the number of biopsies taken from each site. This effort is driven by financial and resource constraints but also by the need to minimize the damage to the normal tissue, especially when sampling cardiovascular or neural organs [18,19].

Once a tumor is detected and graded, there is an attempt to determine the stage of the disease. The objective of staging cancer is to provide a basis for planning appropriate therapy, estimating prognosis, evaluating the results of therapy, and determining the biological behavior of tumors and also to provide a common framework for comparing patient populations and outcomes between different centers [11]. The tumor's anticipated behavior, histological type, and grade and the patient's overall medical condition are also documented and are taken into consideration in determining the patient's life expectancy and deciding on the most suitable treatment [11,20]. Most therapies, however, have been empirical, and we are just now discovering the biological basis of their action.

21.1.2 Imaging Techniques in Cancer Management

Several imaging modalities have become mainstays in cancer diagnosis and management. Unfortunately, the only technology that has been proven effective enough for screening and that is now widely accepted as such is plain film radiography of the female breast (mammography). Other modalities are, however, routinely used for staging cancer in affected individuals. Most are used for detecting or delineating the disease locus and have developed to the point where they have a significant impact on patient management. The diagnostic accuracy of each technique varies depending on the type of neoplasia being imaged and also on expertise and equipment. Surveillance imaging studies are also becoming more common in an attempt to monitor tumor response to treatment, guard against relapse, and detect the presence of residual disease. A common problem that plagues all the currently available imaging systems is their inability to detect the tissue origin and grade the lesion, mass, cyst, or other architectural anomaly that they have detected. Some imaging modalities have, however, emerged as powerful diagnostic tools and are briefly described below, indicating the limitations of each that a high resolution imaging technique such as OCT may address.

Endoscopy

Endoscopy, the direct imaging of the surface of luminal structures, is an expanding field that has revolutionized the diagnostic ability of clinicians to identify and treat more effectively respiratory and gastrointestinal malignancy. The utilization of state-of-the-art video and fiber-optic technology allows detailed survey of luminal surfaces and, in association with biopsies, can lead to diagnostic accuracy of 95% in the case of some gastrointestinal cancers [21]. However, the effectiveness of endoscopy depends on the number of biopsies taken, which sometimes has to be quite high, and on other factors such as personnel training and expertise [22,23]. Endoscopy also fails to detect the subsurface margins of tumors, rendering a complete evaluation of the degree of infiltration of the disease in real time impossible [24]. The effectiveness of endoscopy also relies on the superficial features of the lesion, resulting in high yields for raised lesions but poor performance for other types [25,26]. The size of the endoscope is also prohibitive when it comes to the investigation of small lumens such as the finer branches of the bronchial tree [27]. Laparoscopy is the minimally invasive use of an endoscope, usually solid, to probe into internal body cavities via small incisions on the surface. It is used extensively in surgical interventions, but diagnostic laparoscopy is indicated in only a small number of cases, which include suspected liver tumors and metastases, palpable abdominal masses, staging of tumors, and ascites of unknown origin [28].

Endoscopic Ultrasonography

The development of miniature ultrasound transducers in the late 1980s led to the introduction of endoscopic ultrasonography (EUS). Ultrasound probes with diameters less than 3 mm are introduced through the accessory port of an endoscope, and cross-sectional images of the tissue layer structure are obtained. The source of contrast, as in regular ultrasound, is the density of the layer. EUS was applied extensively in the gastrointestinal tract with an accuracy of preoperative tumor depth of invasion staging in the rage of 80–90%, which even surpassed that of CT [29]. The recent introduction of high frequency (20 MHz) ultrasound transducers with improved resolution could further improve the diagnostic utility of EUS [30]. Unfortunately, EUS relies on the presence of a transducing medium, and the presence of air renders the technique totally ineffective. This limitation is particularly restrictive in the pulmonary tract, where the introduction of a transducing medium may be detrimental to an already compromised patient and limits the application of EUS to the imaging of lung tissue from the mediastinal site [31]. Inflammation and scarring make the interpretation of the EUS images more difficult and make the use of EUS as a tool to monitor tumor response to therapy problematic [32]. EUS is also unable to differentiate between mucosal and submucosal tumors because of its inadequate resolution [33]. EUS is also very user-dependent, although recent advances in technology and the introduction of more complete databases of abnormal findings have made the interpretation of the images less difficult [34].

Imaging Techniques with Whole Body Penetration

The advent of imaging apparatus that can penetrate through several layers of tissue and image the entire human body has revolutionized cancer management and diagnosis. Plain radiography and X-ray computed tomography (CT) are the imaging modalities of choice when it comes to cancer diagnosis [35]. Plain radiography is very effective in certain cases and is also very cost-effective and widely available. CT combines the benefits of radiographs with higher resolution, lower radiation doses, and three-dimensional spatial information. Unfortunately, those systems are still quite expensive and are not available at small, rural hospitals. The place of magnetic resonance imaging (MRI) remains to be clearly defined. At present, it is probably the imaging modality of choice for the central nervous system and for staging some musculoskeletal tumors [36]. Ultrasonography (US) is a target-oriented imaging technique that is very effective for detecting biliary or renal obstruction, abdominal masses, and ascites. It is also efficient in guiding percutaneous biopsy and drainage. This modality is very safe but very operator-dependent and cannot be used whenever there is gas, bone, or previous surgical scarring present or where the probe cannot come into contact with the tissue [11]. Lack of organ-specific contrast agents further limits US applications. Nucleotide imaging, like PET, has found only limited application in bone and thyroid tumor visualization.

All the above techniques offer a unique advantage in their ability to aid staging and investigate and determine nodal involvement. Although OCT has shallow imaging depths and will not image the deep tissues that these modalities can image, OCT has significantly higher resolution and provides a powerful adjunct modality [37].

21.2 OCT IMAGE PROPERTIES AND EARLY NEOPLASTIC CHANGES

Several features of optical coherence tomography suggest that it will be a powerful imaging technology for the diagnosis of a wide range of pathologies [38–40].

1. OCT can image with axial resolutions of $2-10\,\mu m$, one to two orders of magnitude higher than conventional ultrasound. This resolution approaches that of histopathology, allowing architectural morphology as well as cellular features to be resolved. Unlike ultrasound, imaging can be performed directly through air without requiring direct contact with the tissue or a transducing medium.
2. Imaging can be performed in situ, without the need to excise a specimen. This enable imaging of structures in which biopsy would be hazardous or impossible. It also allows better coverage, reducing the sampling errors associated with excisional biopsy.
3. Imaging can be performed in real time, without the need to process a specimen as in conventional biopsy and histopathology. This allows pathology to be monitored on screen and stored on high resolution video tape. Real-time imaging can enable real-time diagnosis, and coupling this information with surgery can enable surgical guidance.
4. Optical coherence tomography is fiber-optically based and can be interfaced to a wide range of instruments, including catheters, endoscopes, laparoscopes, and surgical probes. This enables imaging of organ systems inside the body.
5. Finally, optical coherence tomography is compact and portable, an important consideration for a clinically viable device.

There are three general application scenarios that are envisioned for OCT in neoplastic diagnosis. First, it can be useful for guiding standard excisional biopsy to reduce sampling errors and false negative results. This can improve the accuracy of biopsy and reduce the number of biopsies that are taken, resulting in a cost savings. Second, after more extensive clinical studies have been performed, it may be possible to use OCT to directly diagnose or grade early neoplastic changes. This application will be more challenging, because it implies making a diagnosis on the basis of OCT rather than conventional pathology. Other applications include situations where OCT might be used to grade early neoplastic changes or determine the depth of neoplastic invasion. Third, we hope to find scenarios where diagnosis can be made by OCT alone, enabling diagnosis and surgical guidance to be performed in real time. This would enable OCT diagnostic information to be immediately coupled to treatment decisions. The integration of diagnosis and treatment could reduce the number of patient visits, yielding a significant reduction in health care cost and improving patient compliance.

Each of these application scenarios requires a different level of OCT performance, not only to image tissue pathology, but also to achieve the required level of sensitivity and specificity in clinical trials for a given clinical situation. Generally speaking, OCT can be used to resolve morphological features on several dimensional scales ranging from architectural morphology or glandular organization (10–20 μm) to the cellular level (2–10 μm). Because cancer is a highly heterogeneous disease characterized by a spectrum of morphological changes, etiologies, etc., we expect the viability of OCT to be highly dependent upon the details of the specific clinical application. In the following sections we consider some examples of neoplasias in various tissues and organ systems where we believe OCT promises to have a clinical impact.

21.2.1 Imaging Epithelial Surfaces and Mucosal Layers

Cells in tissue form organized structures that serve various functional purposes. Some cells specialize in forming epithelial layers. These are arranged on luminal sides of organs and play a role in the maintenance and equilibrium of the external milicu, serving as a barrier between the environment and the body. Epithelial surfaces are usually squamous, columnar, or cuboidal. Squamous epithelium is characterized by flattened, plate-like cells and can be multilayered (stratified) and sometimes keratinized. Columnar epithelium is composed of tall cells and can be stratified or pseudostratified (i.e., nuclei are at different levels and cells are variable in shape, giving the appearance of stratified epithelium). Epithelial structures of columnar origin exhibit another degree of variability between tissues. They may form crypts or villi that increase the surface area of the organ or form glands with secretory properties. These glands sometimes become occluded, and when filled with fluids they form cysts. Cuboidal epithelium, as the name implies, is made up of cells that have a cubic shape. These are cases, some physiological and some malignant, when epithelium changes from squamous to columnar, a stage described as transitional epithelium. This process is referred to as metaplasia. Most epithelial structures sit on a collagenous layer called the basal membrane. Cell proliferation and differentiation usually start at the basal membrane, and as cells mature they migrate toward the luminal surface. Below the epithelium usually lies a loose connective tissue layer, the lamina proporia, followed by layers of muscle and connective tissue that vary from organ to organ. Within those layers run vessels and nerves, and different types of lymphoid or inflammatory cells may also reside there. Necrotic tissue and scar formation are usually present in areas of injury. The high mitotic activity close to the basal layer and exposure to the environment make epithelia a prime location for the development of cancer.

A very common histological type of carcinoma is what is referred to as adenocarcinoma. Adenocarcinoma is derived from glandular or other tissue in which tumor cells form recognizable glandular structures. Adenocarcinomas may be classified according to the predominant pattern of cell arrangement, as papillary, alveolar, etc., or according to a particular product of the cells, e.g., as mucinous adenocarcinomas. Squamous carcinoma develops from squamous epithelia, has cuboid cells, and is characterized by keratinization and often by preservation of intercellular bridges but lacks glandular or cystic features.

The ability of OCT to accurately delineate and perhaps grade cancers will be partly based on its ability to detect the structural changes associated with neoplasia. The thickness of squamous epithelium can vary from organ to organ, but it is not unusual to see epithelial layers of up to 0.5 mm thick. Those structures are within the imaging capabilities of OCT, and their thickness, as it relates to abnormal proliferation and differentiation, should be readily assessed (Fig. 1). Even more important is the evaluation of the basal membrane. Its integrity is often used as the defining feature of in situ versus invasive carcinoma, and the distinction between the two types changes both the management of the disease and the prognosis of the patient. Although that membrane is less than a few micrometers thick, it may be possible to evaluate the interface between the epithelium and the underlying lamina propria and deduce the membrane integrity. Several investigators have successfully explored OCT imaging of squamous epithelia in tissues such as skin and the gastrointestinal and female reproductive tracts [41–43]. Columnar epithelium is very difficult to evaluate because it is usually only one cell layer thick. (See discussion below on cellular imaging.) However, it is possible to image and evaluate the microstructure, the glands and crypts, which are usually associated with columnar epithelium (Fig. 2). These structures can have dimensions up to a few millimeters, so changes in tissue

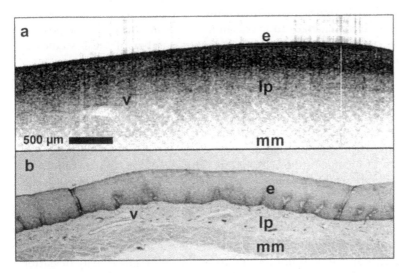

Figure 1 Examples of OCT images of a tissue with a squamous epithelial layer. Normal esophagus imaged in vitro (a) with associated histology (b). The epithelium (e), lamina propria (lp), and muscularis mucosae layers (mm) are visible. Vessels (v) are also present. Resolution: 15 μm axial × 30 μm transverse.

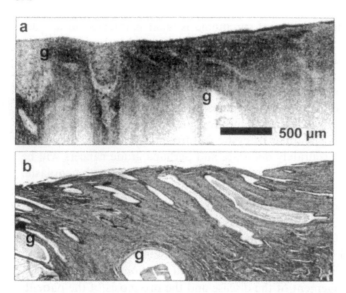

Figure 2 Examples of OCT images of a tissue with a columnar epithelial layer. The image depicts the microstructure of the endocervix imaged in vitro, which is characterized by deep endocervical glands (g), some of which have developed into fluid-filled cysts. The associated histology is also presented. Resolution: $6\,\mu m$ axial $\times$ $15\,\mu m$ transverse.

architecture are well within the resolution limits of OCT systems. There have already been a large number of studies investigating microstructural changes in tissues encompassing the respiratory, gastrointestinal, urinary, and reproductive tracts [44–46]. An epithelial variation that may actually prove more challenging, but that is very important to identify when establishing the diagnostic capabilities of OCT, is metaplasia. The epithelial changes associated with metaplasia have to be differentiated from early neoplastic changes to avoid an increased number of false positive diagnoses. To date, there have not been an adequate number of OCT studies to evaluate such situations.

21.2.2 Imaging Cellular Features

Although there is great variability in cell and nuclear sizes and shapes among different tissue types, each tissue is usually characterized by a unique cell population with defined morphological characteristics. These attributes may be common to all cells in a population or change as the cells mature. However, size, shape, and orientation are conserved and exhibit common variational patterns between similar cells. The nuclear microstructure, such as degree of granularity or presence of nucleoli, should also be similar. The rate of differentiation and proliferation of cells in certain tissues is also well defined. The number of mitoses (the presence of condensed DNA chromatin and the division of the nuclei and cells) is characteristic of the proliferative activity of the cells and should not deviate from the tissue norm. Any deviation in these morphological characteristics coupled with mitotic failure, i.e., incomplete or abnormal cell division, is usually an indicator of uncontrolled proliferation and differentiation and abnormal transcriptional activity. These features are indicative of either the presence of neoplasia or a response to injury. Although changes in architectural morphology and other larger scale features are often used as a first-order diagnostic criterion for cancer, cellular and subcellular features are used to confirm the diagnosis. It is therefore important for OCT to prove its capability to image cellular and subcellular changes to increase its potential as a diagnostic tool and better aid the grading of malignancies.

Studies have been performed in an animal model (*Xenopus laevis*) that demonstrate the capability of OCT to perform cellular level imaging in cells with an average size of 50 μm using an 800 nm, high resolution system based on a mode-locked Ti:Al$_2$O$_3$ laser, imaging at $\sim 1 \mu$m resolution in tissue [47,48]. The observations of greatest clinical relevance were the ability to identify active cell division and assess nuclear-to-cytoplasmic ratios, two important markers of malignant transformation. Figure 3 confirms the presence of multiple nuclei and cell membranes. Cell nuclei and

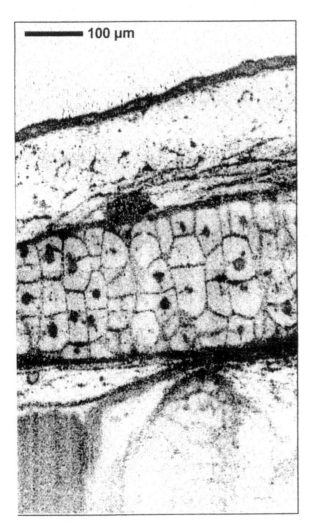

Figure 3 In vivo OCT images of an African frog (*Xenopus laevis*) tadpole. Mesenchymal cells actively dividing are present in both figures. Subcellular microstructures is also appreciable. OT, olfactory tube; M, melanin. Resolution: 1 μm axial $\times$ 3 μm transverse.

cell membranes are readily apparent as regions of high backscatter compared with the low-backscattering cytoplasm. A number of cells show subnuclear morphology such as regions of increased optical backscatter within both the nucleus and the cytoplasm. One possibility is that these are regions of varying chromatin concentration, indicative of high mitotic activity, or cellular organelles. Within each image, cells can be found in various stages of mitosis. Using OCT, the mitotic activity of one parent mesenchymal cell and the migration of the two daughter cells can be followed over time [47]. The OCT image in Fig. 3 also demonstrates the high backscattering observed from neural crest melanocytes and tissue structures. Future studies and improved resolution are necessary to further clarify these observations.

21.2.3 Limitations of OCT

A very important shortcoming of OCT is its limited penetration depth. Attenuation and multiple scattering will probably limit the penetration to only a few millimeters for most scattering tissues, imposing an important constraint on OCT applications for the assessment of cancer. Superficial imaging will probably be adequate for the evaluation of most epithelial cancers, because early neoplastic changes begin in the superficial layers. The evaluation of deep invasion, though, may prove more challenging. The determination of invasion, especially beyond the submucosa/muscularis interface, changes both the patient prognosis and the aggressiveness of management considerably. It is very important for any diagnostic utility, including OCT, to be able to make that distinction. The limited penetration depth of OCT implies that its application will be limited to a specific class of diagnostic scenarios.

The current limits of resolution of most OCT systems are adequate for the evaluation of tissue microstructure but do not allow evaluation of subcellular features. Because these features are of paramount importance for the identification and correct classification of cancer, the resolution of OCT has to be improved. Recent technological advances in laser technology have allowed resolution on the order of $\sim 1\,\mu$m and may prove adequate for high resolution imaging of neoplasias. However, implementing even smaller resolution becomes exceedingly difficult and the technological requirements exceedingly more severe. New, novel techniques must be developed to allow better visualization of cellular characteristics.

The current OCT systems are also limited in speed of acquisition and delivery devices. Because these are related to instrumentation and are not fundamental limitations of the technique, we are hopeful that these problems will be overcome in the near future. The details regarding these aspects of OCT are beyond the scope of this chapter since they have already been discussed in previous chapters.

21.3 APPLICATIONS OF OCT

Optical coherence tomography was first applied in ophthalmology to image retinal morphology at high resolution [49]. Extensive clinical studies have been performed on thousands of patients to examine a wide range of ophthalmic diseases, including glaucoma, diabetic retinopathy, and age-related macular degeneration [50,51]. OCT promises to become a powerful diagnostic tool for a wide range of retinal diseases. More recently, OCT imaging was extended to tissues that are nontransparent, including neoplastic pathologies [52–54]. The data reviewed in this chapter represent some of the first applications of OCT imaging to nonophthalmic tissues. Most of these initial imaging studies focused on in vitro imaging of excised specimens in an effort to assess the performance of OCT imaging as well as to correlate OCT images with histology, the gold standard. Recent OCT imaging studies in animal and human subjects suggest that even better image contrast and differentiation of tissue morphology can be obtained in vivo. The application of OCT for neoplastic imaging is still at an early stage, and extensive studies remain to be done. Nevertheless, the unique features and performance of this new imaging modality suggest that it could have widespread application.

21.3.1 Imaging of the Gastrointestinal Tract

The tissue structure of most of the gastrointestinal tract is quite similar and follows the same histological paradigm. It consists of a *mucosa* with an epithelial layer, lamina propria, and muscularis mucosae; a *submucosa* with loose connective tissue, blood vessels, lymphatics, and glands; a *muscularis propria* with inner circular and outer longitudinal smooth muscle; and an *adventitia*. There are differences, however, in some organs. For example, the esophageal and ductal lumens are covered with a layer of squamous epithelium; most other structures in the gastrointestinal tract are covered with columnar epithelium. The morphology of the epithelium also varies, especially in the stomach and small and large intestine, where the function of those organs necessitates and depends on the presence of villi, crypts, and/or pits. The great variability of gastrointestinal tissue, its continuous exposure to the external environment and rough enzymatic activity, and the cyclical and rapid cell proliferation and epithelial turnover result in an increased number and variety of malignancies.

Most esophageal cancers fall within two histological types, squamous carcinomas and adenocarcinomas, with some occurrences of other rare cancers and metastases. The initial diagnosis is usually based on the findings of chest X-rays (CXR) and/or a barium swallow study, but endoscopy and biopsy are always used to confirm the findings. A group at high risk for esophageal cancer are patients with Barrett's esophagus, a form of esophageal metaplasia, who have at least a 30-fold greater chance of developing adenocarcinoma of the esophagus than the general population [55]. These patients are advised to seek regular endoscopic evaluations to monitor for the development of dysplasia and to ensure that they receive treatment at the earliest stage of the disease if needed.

Approximately 95% of all malignant gastric neoplasms are adenocarcinomas, with some other rare tumors comprising the remaining 5% [56]. In Asian and South American countries the incidence of gastric cancer is very high, reaching epidemic proportions in Japan (100 : 100,000) [57]. The evaluation of gastric cancer can be performed with a barium study or flexible upper endoscopy. EUS has been studied extensively for the evaluation of depth of penetration and was proven more effective than CT in identifying primary tumors but not in establishing nodal involvement [29]. Mass screening programs have been successful in Japan, but gastric cancer remains the number one cause of death [58].

The high proliferation rate and the environment of the intestines make them prime locations for the development of cancer. Colon cancers can be classified according to gross appearance or on a histological basis [59]. Grading of colon cancer is based on histological type, overall cell differentiation, nuclear polarity, tubule configuration, pattern of growth, lymphocytic infiltration, and amount of fibrosis [60]. Endoscopy with biopsies is commonly applied to evaluate colon cancer. If there is occlusion or edema, which block access to the cancer, a barium enema X-ray evaluation can be performed. Endoscopic screening for colon cancer is recommended for high risk populations, such as patients suffering from ulcerative colitis, and for asymptomatic individuals over the age of 50 [61,62]. Although there are more than 35 histological variants of small bowel neoplasms, small intestinal malignancies are rare considering the size and surface area of the small intestine [63]. The evaluation of patients presenting with these malignancies consists of upper GI series and CT.

Cancers may also arise in other organs of the gastrointestinal tract. The normal pancreatic architecture, for example, is markedly altered in carcinoma, which is difficult to diagnose and very aggressive. The evaluation of the disease depends mainly on CT. Unfortunately, there are no good therapies, and sometimes the treatment is worse than the disease and offers little benefit [64]. Cancer can also appear along the biliary tree in the forms of carcinoma of the gallbladder and cholangiocarcinoma, i.e., carcinoma of the bile duct, manifested mainly as adenocarcinoma [65]. The incidence of gallbladder cancer is very high in some Latin American countries and Japan. American Indians, and Israelis have a five- to sevenfold greater incidence of cholangiocarcinomas than the general world population. Evaluation of biliary tree carcinomas is based on ultrasonography, CT, MRI, cholangiography, and angiography, but there is no good screening technique. Prognosis for gallbladder carcinoma is poor because most patients have unresectable tumors at presentation.

Optical coherence tomographic imaging of the esophagus is being investigated actively by several groups, and the initial results appear to be very promising [66,67]. The stratified squamous epithelium of the normal esophagus is clearly visible in OCT images (Fig. 4a). It presents as a uniform, highly backscattering layer, as would be expected for that epithelial structure. The submucosa appears loose and less optically backscattering. Blood vessels in the submucosa are also identified. In the case of esophageal metaplasia (Barrett's esophagus), the uniformly layered structure is destroyed and is replaced by columnar epithelium (Fig. 4b). OCT images of Barrett's esophagus clearly demonstrate the disorganized and nonuniform nature of the mucosal layers. Squamous cell carcinoma of the esophagus can also be visualized using OCT (Fig. 4c). The tumors appear as abnormal growths that interrupt the normal structure of the esophageal layers. The formation of malignant cell nodules is evident. These images were acquired in vitro with a 1300 nm system, based on an amplified semiconductor source, imaging at $\sim 15\,\mu$m resolution in air.

Imaging of the small intestine and the colon is another area of OCT that has attracted a lot of interest [44,67]. The data acquired in vitro and in vivo clearly delineate the layers characteristic of intestinal microstructure. The mucosa of the normal colon is clearly visible, although its columnar epithelium cannot be resolved with the current OCT systems (Fig. 5a). Ordered, narrow crypts, glands, and villi are present as expected and confirmed by histological cross-sectioning. The submucosa appears as a loose, less backscattering layer. Imaging of the colon also demonstrates the capability of OCT to delineate pathological microstructure.

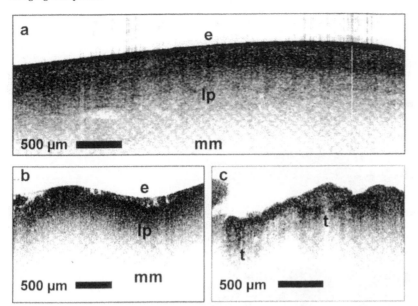

Figure 4 In vitro OCT images of (a) normal esophagus, (b) Barrett's esophagus, and (c) esophageal cancer. The epithelium (e), lamina proporia (lp) and muscularis mucosae layers (mm) are visible. Tumor nodules (t) are also present. Resolution: $15\,\mu$m axial $\times$ $30\,\mu$m transverse.

Destruction of the normal mucosal layers and ulcerative lesions were identified in cases of ulcerative colitis, a condition that can increase a patient's risk of developing colon cancer (Fig. 5b). In the case of adenocarcinoma of the colon and ampullary carcinoma of the duodenum, OCT was able to detect changes in the mucosal/submucosal microstructure (Figs. 5c and 5d). There was a marked proliferation of the glandular structure, and the crypts appeared dilated and/or disorganized in sharp contrast to the normal appearance of those tissues. The images described above were collected in vitro with a system similar to the one described earlier, with the exception that a superluminescent diode source ($500\,\mu$W output power) was used for the samples shown in Figs. 5a and 5d instead of the amplified semiconductor source.

It is improbable that an imaging technology such as optical coherence tomography would be cost-effective for screening the general patient population for early neoplasias. However, future applications of OCT could be identified in screening high risk populations. One such target population could be patients who have been diagnosed with esophageal metaplasia (Barrett's esophagus). By using OCT to guide conventional biopsy, sampling errors can be reduced and higher sensitivity may be achieved using fewer biopsies, thus increasing the diagnostic yield of endoscopy and histology [22]. OCT could also play a role in the screening of asymptomatic individuals over the age of 50 and patients with chronic ulcerative colitis for colon cancer according to current recommendations. Furthermore, OCT could perhaps aid in identifying invading tumors and in monitoring tumor response to therapy, functions not possible with endoscopic ultrasonography (EUS), the clinical imaging modality with the highest resolution at the present time [68].

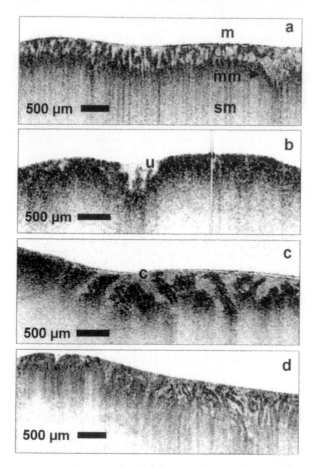

Figure 5 In vitro OCT images of (a) normal colon, (b) ulcerative colitis, (c) adenocarcinoma of the colon, and (d) ampullary carcinoma of the duodenum. The mucosal (m), muscularis mucosal (mm), and submucosal layers of the normal colon are identifiable in the OCT images. Ulcerative lesions (u) were identified in cases of ulcerative colitis. Dilated and disorganized crypts (c) are present in the case of colon carcinoma. Resolution: $15\,\mu m$ axial $\times\ 30\,\mu m$ transverse. [(a,d) From Ref. 44.]

21.3.2 Imaging of the Reproductive Tract

Most cancers of the cervix are squamous cell carcinomas(80–90%) and adenocarcinomas (10–16%) [69]. The current understanding is that the malignancy starts from the squamocolumnar junction and is preceded by cervical dysplasia and carcinoma in situ [70]. Cervical cancer precursors can be divided into mild, moderate, and severe dysplasias or, using an alternative scheme, into intraepithelial neoplasias ranging from CIN I, with minimal morphological changes, to CIN III, where the entire epithelium from the basal membrane to the surface is composed of malignant cells. Invasion is defined as the spread of malignant cells below the basal membrane. Screening for cervical cancer is performed by periodic cytology, the Papanicolaou smear, and annual gynecological examinations [71,72]. Once atypical cells are seen in the cytological smear the cervix is further evaluated with colposcopy and biopsies and also with CT scans if macroinvasion is suspected. It is interesting to note that all deaths due to cervical cancer are preventable but screening is less frequent in under-served groups, resulting in a higher percentage of fatalities from the disease in that population.

Cancer of the uterus, the most common manifestation of which is adenocarci-noma, is the most common female genital cancer, with a peak incidence between 55 and 60 years of age. It has been shown that it is closely associated with and preceded by hyperplasia of the endometrium [73]. The diagnosis of endometrial cancer is based on dilatation and curettage, with chest X-ray, CT, and cystoscopy recom-mended for staging and discovering distant metastases. The 5-year survival rate for uterine cancer is high, in the range of 80–95%, mainly due to early diagnosis of the abnormal bleeding associated with 70–75% of all cases, which is easily iden-tifiable, especially if the patient is postmenopausal [74].

Fallopian tube cancer is very rare, comprising only 0.5–1.1% of gynecological malignancies [75]. Most cancers fall in the pathological category of adenocarcinomas and present as dilated tubes with papillary and solid tumor. Degeneration with hemorrhage and necrosis may also be present [75]. The cancer is evaluated and treated following the same guidelines that apply to ovarian cancer.

Ovarian carcinoma can be epithelial carcinoma (80–90%) or germ or stromal cell carcinomas (10–20%). Of all ovarian cancers 60% are adenocarcinomas, 17% are undifferentiated, 15% are endometrioid carcinoma, and 6% are clear cell carci-noma [76]. Extraovarian spread by transperitoneal insemination is common. Once ovarian cancer is suspected, X-rays, ultrasound, or transvaginal ultrasound may be employed for the evaluation of the pelvic area [77]. Despite the relatively low inci-dence of ovarian cancer, more women die from this cancer than from cervical and endometrial cancers combined. In 1998, more than 50% of the deaths from cancers of the female reproductive system were due to ovarian cancer [1]. The high mortality rate is largely due to poor techniques for early detection. The 5-year survival rate drops from 74–98% for benign to 91–93% for borderline malignant to a dramatic 29–34% for malignant, making the need for early diagnosis all the more obvious [78].

Reproductive structures can be access by using either a colposcope or a hys-teroscope from a vaginal approach or by using a laparoscope during a minimally invasive laparoscopic procedure. Each technique offers access to different sides of the reproductive tract, allowing the investigation of various pathologies that may localize to different areas. Structures that would be visible in a vaginal approach scheme include the ectocervix, endocervix, uterine mucosa, and fallopian tubes. Approaching the reproductive tract transabdominally allows access to the pelvical side of the reproductive organs, including the ovaries, the myometrium, and the serosal layer of the fallopian tubes.

Vaginal Approach

Imaging of the human cervix in vitro has demonstrated the possibility of OCT colposcope-based evaluation [79,80]. The microstructure associated with both the ectocervix and the endocervix was clearly demonstrated. The epithelial layer of the ectocervix and the basal membrane were identified. Deep endocervical glands, some of which developed into fluid-filled cysts, a finding common in postmenopausal women, were also visible (Fig. 2). Carcinoma in situ and poorly differentiated carcinoma of the cervix were also examined and compared with the normal findings. Carcinoma in situ was characterized by a thick, irregular epithelial layer in addition to what appeared to be increased backscattering from the cells of the basal layers (Fig. 6a). In cases of invasive carcinoma, the tissue was more heterogeneous, and the basement membrane was no longer defined (Fig. 6b). Areas of necrotic tissue were identified in more advanced cases (Fig. 6c). These images were taken in vitro using a 1300 nm, high resolution system based on a mode-locked Cr : forsterite laser imaging at ~ 6 μm resolution in air. In vivo imaging of the human cervix resulted in images confirming the conclusions drawn from the in vitro experiments Fig. 7. The in vivo images were acquired with an 800 nm system equipped with a forward-imaging OCT endoscope.

In vitro experiments to examine the possibility of hysteroscopically based OCT examination of uterine tissue also concluded with positive results [79,80]. OCT images of postmenopausal endometrium demonstrated sparse uterine glands and larger fluid-filled cysts, consistent with postmenopausal uterine atrophy (Fig. 8a). Images of neoplastic changes in uterine endometrial adenocarcinoma are demonstrated in Fig. 8b. Defined epithelial layers and glands were no longer present. The interlacing of cellular and noncellular tissues resulted in a layered appearance, with the presence of rare hyperplastic glands.

By integrating optical coherence tomography with small imaging endoscopes, the uterine surface could be scanned and the pathology imaged in situ at high resolution and in real time. This suggests the potential for future applications in screening patients for endometrial carcinoma. Endometrial cancer is one of the most common neoplasms of women in many industrialized societies. The majority of

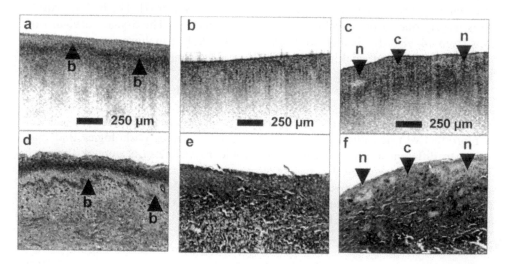

Figure 6   Cervical disease imaged in vitro (a,d) Carcinoma in situ (OCT image and associated histology) characterized by a thick, irregular epithelial layer in addition thickening of the basement layer (b). (b,e; c,f) Invasive carcinoma (OCT image and associated histology). the tissue surface is now heterogeneous, and the basement membrane is no longer defined. Distinct backscattering patterns can be noted in cellular (c) and noncellular (n) regions. Resolution: 6 μm axial × 10 μm transverse. (From Ref. 79.)

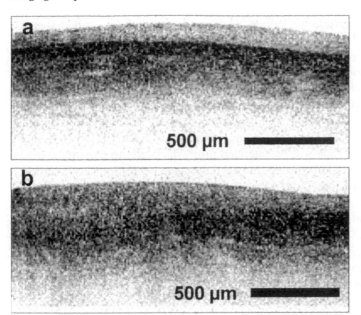

Figure 7 (a) Normal cervix and (b) cervical carcinoma imaged in vivo. Cervical epithelium appears as a layer of low backscattering tissue with a sharp border separating it from the deeper layers. The uniformity and clear demarcation between layers are lost in the presence of cervical cancer. Resolution: $10\,\mu m$ axial $\times\ 20\,\mu m$ transverse. (Courtesy of A. Sergeev and F. I. Feldchtein, Russian Academy of Science, Institute of Applied Physics Nonlinear Dynamics and Optics, Nizhny Novgorod.)

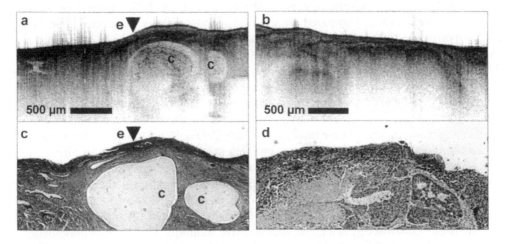

Figure 8 (a,b) Normal postmenopausal endometrium and (c,d) endometrial adenocarcinoma imaged in vitro, with associated histology. Sparse uterine glands, consistent with postmenopausal uterine atrophy, the epithelial layer (e), and larger fluid-filled cysts (c) can be identified in the image of normal endometrium. Defined epithelial layers and glands are no longer present in neoplastic tissue. The interlacing of cellular and noncellular tissue results in a layered appearance. Resolution: $6\,\mu m$ axial $\times\ 10\,\mu m$ transverse. (From Ref. 79.)

patients have postmenopausal bleeding and are identified at early stages. Unfortunately, 90% of dilatation and curettage procedures performed for postmenopausal bleedings show no abnormality. A minimally invasive technique with a high sensitivity but low false positive rate would be a powerful modality in selecting patients who would benefit from invasive investigation. This is particularly relevant to patients on tamoxifen, who demonstrate an increase incidence of endometrial abnormalities, 6.3 per 1000 women at 5 years, a factor of 2–3 increase over the general population [81]. Therefore a screening approach is needed for this patient population, especially if therapy will be extended prophylactically to patients at high risk for breast cancer. It should be noted that current recommendations leave screening to the discretion of the individual gynecologist [82].

It is improbable that an imaging technology such as optical coherence tomography would be cost-effective for screening the general patient population for early cervical neoplasias. The development of the Papanicolaou smear has reduced the number of cases of cervical cancers per year in the United States to 12,000 and the number of deaths to approximately 3000. The Papanicolaou smear has also significantly reduced the cost of screening by making such a test available to a broad range within the general public. However, a role for optical coherence tomography is envisioned in scenarios such as the follow-up management of cervical intraepithelial neoplasia (CIN) I lesions in addition to its potential for the reduction of cone biopsies in patients with CIN II, CIN III, and microinvasive lesions.

Laparoscopic Approach

The peritoneal surface of the ovaries and uterus can also exhibit abnormal tissue morphology. High resolution OCT imaging from the external surface of the ovary can identify atypical morphology as is shown in Fig. 9a [83]. Normal ovary is relatively homogeneous compared to the cystic and papillary structures observed in the ovarian serous papillary cystadenocarcinoma. The OCT image in Fig. 9b is that of an ovarian adenoma that had spread to the peritoneal surface of the uterus. This likely resulted from contact between the two organs or intra-abdominal spread. The normal uterus is relatively homogeneous with serosal tissue adjacent to the uterus myometrium. The ovarian adenoma showed characteristic glandular morphology. A subserosal leiomyoma was also observed adjacent to the glandular morphology of the adenoma. These images were collected with a 1300 nm system, based on an amplified semiconductor source, imaging at $\sim 15\,\mu$m resolution in air.

The use of OCT to identify subtle morphological changes such as those seen here, can become a powerful diagnostic application. In addition, the use of OCT laparoscopy can guide the surgical ablation of suspect tissue sites or the placement of biopsy forceps when tissue specimens are physically respected for histopathological examination. Laparoscopy is a minimally invasive technique that enables diagnostics and surgery to be performed with decreased morbidity. Although laparoscopy offers exceptional visualization of remote, internal tissue, imaging is limited to surface features. OCT enables cross-sectional, subsurface imaging of biological structure. The combination of these two techniques has the potential for significantly improving the ability to nonexcisionally sample suspect gynecological tissue at high resolutions.

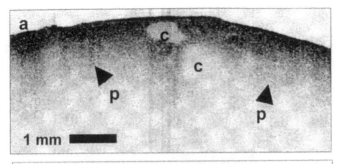

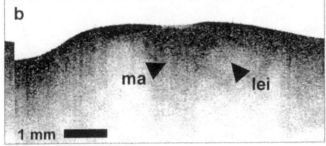

Figure 9 Optical coherence tomographic images of (a) ovarian serous papillary cystadeno-carcinoma and (b) ovarian adenoma spread to the uterus, with associated histology, c, cystic cavities; p, papillary structures; lei, subserosal leiomyoma; ma, metastatic adenoma. Resolution: 15 μm axial × 30 μm transverse.

21.3.3 Imaging of the Urinary Tract

Bladder cancers usually fall into the pathological categories of transitional cell carcinomas (95%), squamous cell carcinomas (3%) and adenocarcinomas (2%) and can be multifocal or superficial [84]. The depth of penetration is very important in staging, because it directly correlates with metastatic potential [85]. There were 54,400 new cases and 12,500 deaths per year in the United States, with a peak incidence in the seventh decade of life and a male/female ratio of 3 : 1, although the disparity is not as great in populations where smoking is equally prevalent in men and women. Evaluation consists of X-ray or CT imaging and cystoscopy. Therapy is usually transurethral resection (TUR) or partial or total cystectomy with radiation and chemotherapy depending on the degree of invasion [86]. Despite high recurrence, early bladder cancer is completely treatable. Unfortunately, the 5-year survival rate of muscle invasive cancer is only 20–50% [86].

The bladder has also been an area of investigation using OCT [87]. Images of bladder in vitro appear to contain structural information that could be diagnostic of significance. The mucosa/submucosal interface as well as the submucosa/muscularis interface were differentiated in OCT images of normal bladder obtained from postsurgical resection (Fig. 10a). High muscle bundles (m) and vessels (v), such as capillaries within the submucosa, were also noted. In OCT images of invasive transitional cell carcinoma, the mucosa/submucosal and submucosal/muscularis boundaries were no longer observed (Fig. 10b). In addition, there were no capillaries, which were present in all normal images. The distorted sections of muscle bundles and area of fat

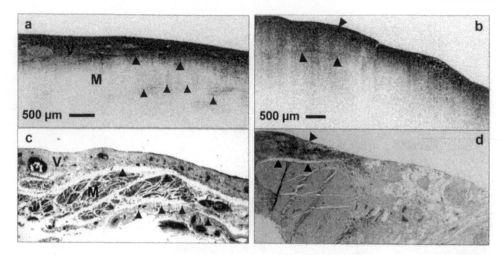

Figure 10 (a,c) Optical coherence tomographic images of normal bladder and corresponding histology. The top row of arrows identifies the mucosa/submucosal interface, and the lower row identifies the submucosa/muscularis interface. High muscle bundles (m) and vessels (v) are also noted. (b,d) OCT images of invasive transitional cell carcinoma (top arrow) and corresponding histology reveal that the mucosa/submucosal and submucosal muscularis boundaries are no longer observed. In addition, there are no capillaries noted, which were presented in all normal images. There are also distorted sections of muscle bundles (arrows) and an area of fat (arrow) from the outer edge of the sample. Resolution: 15 μm axial × 30 μm transverse.

from the outer edge of the sample completed a set of indications usually associated with cancer of the bladder. These images were collected with a 1300 nm system similar to the one described in the previous section.

21.3.4 Metastases and Staging

Although the limited penetration of OCT precludes its use for large-area, whole-body surveying for cancer staging and metastases, a role can be foreseen for OCT in the identification and evaluation of individual metastases and lymph nodes. OCT could assess, in a minimally invasive fashion, nodules that were initially identified by CT or X-rays. This could help both to reduce the number of biopsies necessary for the complete staging of cancer and to guide, in real time, the surgical resection nor chemoradiative destruction of the neoplastic tissue. Tumor metastases have already been under investigation by some groups.

One possible application of OCT could be to aid the complete and precise resection of cancerous tissue in organs such as the central nervous system, where precise intraoperative identification of the tumor margin is vital both for the complete resection of the neoplasm and the prevention of iatrogenic injury. Various imaging modalities, including ultrasound, CT, and MRI, have already been used in an attempt to improve patient morbidity [88]. Unfortunately, the resolutions of such modalities are often hundreds of micrometers, thereby poorly resolving small tumors and reducing the sharp definition of the tumor margin. Furthermore, the registration of images with tissue at the submillimeter level is problematic, and extensive research and development have explored means of stereotactically aligning the two [89]. Optical techniques including fluorescence and Raman spectroscopy have enabled quantitative identification of brain tumor cells and tumor margins based on detected spectra [90,91]. Image representation of tumors based on these techniques is limited to surface features without cross-sectional imaging or optical ranging into the tissue. High resolution video imaging for discrimination of brain tissues has been effective but requires the administration of topical or systemic fluorescent dyes [91].

In order to evaluate OCT for the detection of brain tumors and their interfaces with normal brain parenchyma, metastatic melanoma with multiple small ($< 500\,\mu$m) metastases surrounding a larger lesion was imaged. More information as well as the resulting images from that study are included in Chapter 23.

21.4 CONCLUSION

Optical coherence tomography can function as a type of optical biopsy to yield image information with resolutions approaching that of conventional histopathology. It can also perform micrometer-scale, real-time imaging of tissue pathology in situ, without the need for excision and processing. OCT can be integrated to a wide range of clinical instruments, including endoscopes, catheters, laparascopes, and surgical probes The ability of OCT to image epithelial and other architectural morphology and the possibility of cellular level imaging can be used to identify and grade many types of early neoplastic changes. The features and performance of OCT imaging technology suggest that it will become a powerful modality for the diagnosis and management of cancer.

In summary, we believe that there are three general application scenarios that are envisioned for OCT in neoplastic diagnosis.

1. Guiding standard excisional biopsy. Because excisional biopsy is a sampling procedure, there are many cases where it suffers from sampling errors and yields false negative results. We believe that the initial applications of OCT will focus on guiding conventional excisional biopsy. Its use can improve the accuracy of the procedures and also reduce the number of biopsies that are taken, resulting in cost savings. In addition, diagnosis and decisions about treatment are still made on the basis of the gold standard, biopsy and pathology.

2. Screening or direct diagnosis. After more extensive clinical studies have been performed and more data are available, it may be possible to use OCT to directly diagnose or grade early neoplastic changes. This application will be possible only for certain types of neoplasias where OCT would demonstrate sufficient sensitivity and specificity. It will also be more challenging because it implies making a diagnosis on the basis of OCT rather than conventional pathology. Perhaps the most intriguing application of OCT in this scenario is screening. In screening, the initial OCT finding can be followed up and confirmed by using standard excisional biopsy and pathology, thus avoiding the demanding requirement that the diagnosis be made on the basis of OCT imaging alone. Other applications include situations where OCT might be used to grade early

neoplastic changes or determine the depth of neoplastic invasion. In these cases, treatment decisions would be made on the basis of OCT information, placing stringent requirements on its sensitivity and specificity.

3. Real-time diagnosis and surgical intervention and guidance. After more extensive clinical studies, we hope to find scenarios where diagnosis can be made by OCT alone, enabling the diagnosis to be performed in real time. This would provide the means for OCT diagnostic information to be immediately coupled to patient management decisions. The immediate availability of this information could reduce the number of patient visits, yielding a significant reduction in health care costs and improving patient compliance. Finally, the highest level of OCT application would be for real-time guidance of surgical or other intervention. In this case OCT imaging information could be coupled directly with interventional procedures to show the extent of neoplastic or dysplastic tissue that should be surgically resectioned or otherwise removed.

As with any other diagnostic tool, technique, or method, the ultimate proof of effectiveness and diagnostic utility is its ability to change patient outcomes in a more beneficial or effective manner than currently possible. Good correlation with histology is not enough to prove clinical effectiveness. As in vivo imaging systems become available and human clinical trials are performed, studies must be designed to correctly assess the value of OCT from a large-scale perspective. As target applications are identified, investigators must keep in mind that alternative diagnostic techniques may be available. To justify the use of a new diagnostic technique, it must be cost-effective and offer greater sensitivity and specificity than alternative techniques. In addition, the diagnostic must have clinical utility, that is, the information must be relevant to clinical decision making regarding treatment options or management of the disease.

Optical coherence tomography is still in its infancy, but despite the current lack of extensive clinical studies, the possibility of application in the detection and management of early neoplasia and cancer remains very high and opens a new, exciting field of research. In the near future as OCT becomes more standardized and new, faster and portable systems emerge, we expect to see a surge in the amount of research in this area. This will spark not only new applications of OCT in the diagnosis of cancer but also innovations in technology that will move OCT toward clinical acceptance.

ACKNOWLEDGMENTS

We would like to express our appreciation to Dr. Stephen A. Boppart, Christine A. Jesser, Dr. Wolfgan Drexler, and Dr. Xingde Li for their support. We are also grateful to Dr. Bouma and Dr. Tearney for their contributions. This research is sponsored in part by the National Institutes of Health Contracts NIH-9-RO1-EY11289-13 (JGF), NIH-1-RO1-CA75289-02 (JGF&MEB), NIH-1-R29-HL55686-01A1 (MEB), NIH-1-RO1-AR44812-01 (MEB), the Medical Free Electron Laser Program, Office of Naval Research Contract N00014-94-1-0717 (JGF), the Air Force Office of Scientific Research Contract F4920-98-1-0139 (JGF), and the Whitaker Foundation Contract 96-0205 (MEB).

REFERENCES

1. Landis SH, Murray T, Bolden S, Wingo PA. Cancer Stat 1:6–30, 1998.
2. Osteen RT, ed. Cancer Manual. 9th ed. Framingham, MA: Am Cancer Soc, LoCCC 96-86232.
3. Huang D, Swanson EA, Lin CP, Schuman JS, Stinson WG, Chang W, et al. Optical coherence tomography. Science 254:1178–1781, 1991.
4. Tearney GJ, Brezinski ME, Bouma BE, Boppart SA, Pitris C, Southern JF, Fujimoto JG. In vivo endoscopic optical biopsy with optical coherence tomography. Science 276:2037–2039, 197.
5. Burchenal JH, Oettgen HF, eds. Cancer: Achievements, Challenges and Prospects for the 1980s, Vol 1. New York: Grune & Stratton, 1981.
6. Folkman J, Klagsbrum M. Angiogenic factors. Science 235:444, 1987.
7. Kramer BS. The screening editorial board of the physician query: NCI state-of-the-art statements on cancer screening. Washington, DC: Natl Cancer Inst 1995:719.
8. Doll R, Pet R. The causes of cancer: Quantitive estimates of avoidable risks of cancer in the United States today. J Natl Cancer Inst 66:1191, 1988.
9. DeVita VT, Hellman S, Rosenberg SA, eds. Cancer: Principles and Practice of Oncology. Philadelphia: Lippincott-Raven, 1997.
10. Rimer BK, Demark-Wahnefried W, Egert JR. Acceptance of cancer screening. In: Handbook of Health Behavior Research. Philadelphia: JB Lippincott.
11. Moosa AR, Schimpff SC, Robson MC, eds. Comprehensive Textbook of Oncology. Baltimore: Williams and Wilkins, 1991.
12. Cotran RS, Kumar V, Robbins SL. Robbins' Pathologic Basis of Disease. Philadelphia: WB Saunders, 1989.
13. Rabbani F, Stroumbakis N, Kava BR, Cookson MS, Fair WR. Incidence and clinical significance of false-negative sextant prostate biopsies. J Urol 159:1248–1250, 1998.
14. Adami B, Eckardt VF, Paulini K. Sampling error and observer variation in the interpretation of esophageal biopsies. Digestion 19:404–410, 1979.
15. Marshall JB, Diaz-Arias AA, Barthel JS, King PD, Butt JH. Prospective evaluation of optimal number of biopsy specimens and brush cytology in the diagnosis of cancer of the colorectum. Am J Gastroenterol 88:1352–1354, 1993.
16. Brenner RJ, Fajardo L, Fisher PR, Dershaw DD, Evans WP, Bassett L, Feig S, Mendelson E, Jackson V, Margolin FR. Percutaneous core biopsy of the breast: Effect of operator experience and number of samples on diagnostic accuracy. Am J Roentgenol 166:341–346, 1996.
17. Burns RP. Image-guided breast biopsy. Am J Surg 173:9–11, 1997.
18. Bonham CA, Dominguez EA, Fukui MB, Paterson DL, Pankey GA, Wagener MM, Fung JJ, Singh N. Central nervous system lesions in liver transplant recipients: Prospective assessment of indications of biopsy and implications for management. Transplantation 66:1596–1604, 1998.
19. Parrillo JE. Transvenous endomyocardial biopsy. Clinical indications, potential complications, and future applications. Chest 90:155–157, 1986.
20. American Joint Committee on Cancer. Manual for Staging of Cancer. 3rd ed. Philadelphia: JB Lippincott, 1988.
21. Oguro Y, Takagi K. Recent advances in endoscopic diagnosis of esophago-gastric cancer. In: Endoscopic Approaches to Cancer Diagnosis and Treatment. London: Taylor & Francis, 1990:19.
22. Graham DY, Schwartz JT, Gain GD, Gyorkey F. Prospective evaluation of biopsy number in the diagnosis of esophageal and gastric number. Gastroenterology 82:228–231, 1982.

23. Bond SH. Outcomes and effectiveness of endoscopic procedures. Gastrointest Endosc 38:725–725, 1992.
24. Milnes JP, Hine KR, Holmes GK, Cohen ME. Limitations of endoscopy in the diagnosis of carcinoma of the cardia of the stomach. Br J Radiol 55:593–595, 1982.
25. Winawer SJ, Posner G, Lightdale CJ, Sherlock P, Melamed M, Fortner JG. Endoscopic diagnosis of advanced gastric cancer. Factors influencing yield. Gastroenterology 96:1183–1187, 1975.
26. Yamaguchi K, Enjoji M, Kitamura K. Endoscopic biopsy has limited accuracy in the diagnosis of ampullary tumors.
27. Tanaka M, Kawanami O, Satoh M. Endoscopic observation of peripheral airway lesions. Chest 93:228, 1988.
28. Lightdale CJ. Diagnostic laparoscopy in gastroenterologic practice. Prog Gastroenterol, 4:461–475, 1983.
29. Botet JF, Lightdale CJ, Zauber AG, Gerdes H, Winawer SJ, Urmacher C, Brennan MNF. Preoperative staging of gastric cancer: Comparison of endoscopic US and dynamic CT. Radiology 1991:181–426.
30. Yanai H, Tada M, Karita M, Okita K. Diagnostic utility of 20-megahertz linear endoscopic ultrasonography in early gastric cancer. Gastrointest Endosc 44:29–33, 1996.
31. Schuder G, Isringhaus H, Kubale B, et al. Endoscopic ultrasonography of the mediastinum in the diagnosis of bronchial carcinoma. Thorac Cardiovasc Surg 39:299–303, 1991.
32. Rosh T. Endoscopic ultrasonography. Endoscopy 26:148–168, 1994.
33. Souquet JC, Napoleon B, Pujol B, Kerriven O, Ponchon T, Descos F, Lamber R. Endoscopic ultrasonography in the preoperative staging of esophageal cancer. Endoscopy 26:764–766, 1994.
34. Catalano MF, Sivak MV Jr, Bedford RA, Falk GW, van Stolk R, Presa F, Van Dam J. Observer variation and reproducibility of endoscopic ultrasonography. Gastrointest Endosc 41:115–120, 1995.
35. Templeton PA, Caskey CI, Zerhouni EA. Current uses of CT and MR imaging in the staging of lung cancer. Radiol Clin Am 28:631–646, 1990.
36. Kramer ED, Vezina LG, Packer RJ, Fitz CR, Zimmerman RA, Cohen MD. Staging and surveillance of children with central nervous system neoplasms: Recommendations of the Neurology and Tumor Imaging Committees of the Children's Cancer Group. Pediatr Neurosurg 20:254–262, 1994; discussion 262–263.
37. Adams S, Baum RP, Stuckensen T, Bitter K, Hor G. Prospective comparison of 18F-FDG PET with conventional imaging modalities (CT, MRI, US) in lymph node staging of head and neck cancer. Eur J Nucl Med 25:1255–1260, 1998.
38. Schmitt J, Yadlowsky M, Bonner R. Subsurface imaging of living skin with optical coherence microscopy. Dermatology 191:93–98, 1995.
39. Fujimoto JG, Brezinski ME, Tearney GJ, Boppart SA, Bouma BE, Hee MR, Southern JF, Swanson EA. Optical biopsy and imaging using optical coherence tomography. Nature Med 1:970–972, 1995.
40. Brezinski ME, Tearney GJ, Bouma BE, Izatt JA, Hee MR, Swanson EA, Southern JF, Fujimoto JG. Optical coherence tomography for optical biopsy. Properties and demonstration of vascular pathology. Circulation 93:1206–1213, 1996.
41. Brezinski ME, Tearney GJ, Boppart SA, Swanson EA, Southern JF, Fujimoto JG. Optical biopsy with optical coherence tomography: Feasibility for surgical diagnostics. J Surg Res 71:32–40, 1997.
42. Welzel J, Lankenau E, Birngruber R, Engelhardt R. Optical coherence tomography of the human skin. J Am Acad Dermatol 37:958–963, 1997.
43. Kobayashi K, Izatt JA, Kulkarni MD, Willis J, Sivak MV Jr. High-resolution cross-sectional imaging of the gastrointestinal tract using optical coherence tomography: Preliminary results. Gastrointest Endosc 47:515–523, 1998.

44. Tearney GJ, Brezinski ME, Southern JF, Buma BE, Boppart SA, Fujimoto JG. Optical biopsy in human gastrointestinal tissue using optical coherence tomography. Am J Gastroenterol 92:1800–1804, 1997.

45. Tearney GJ,Brezinski ME, Southern JF, Bouma BE, Boppart SA, Fujimoto JG. Optical biopsy in human urologic tissue using optical coherence tomography. J. Urol 157:1915–1919, 1997.

46. Tearney GJ, Brezinski ME, Southern JF, Bouma BE, Boppart SA, Fujimoto JG. Optical biopsy in human pancreatobiliary tissue using optical coherence tomography. Dig Dis Sci 43:1193–1199, 1998.

47. Drexler W, Morgner U, Kartner FX, Pitris C, Boppart SA, Li, XD, Ippen EP, Fujimoto JG. In vivo ultrahigh-resolution optical coherence tomography. Opt Lett 24:1999.

48. Boppart SA, Bouma BE, Pitris C, Southern JF, Brezinski ME, Fujimoto JG. In vivo cellular optical coherence tomography imaging. Nature Med 4:861–865, 1998.

49. Puliatifo CA, Hee MR, Schumann JS, Fujimoto JG. Optical Coherence Tomography of Ocular Diseases Thorofare, NJ: Slack, Inc 1995.

50. Hee MR, Izatt JA, Swanson EA, Huang D, Lin CP, Schuman JS, Puliafito CA, Fujimoto JG. Optical coherence tomography of the human retina. Arch Ophthalmol 113:325–332, 1995.

51. Puliafito CA, Hee MR, Lin CP, Reichel E, Schuman JS, Duker JS, Izatt JA, Swanson EA, Fujimoto JG. Imaging of macular disease with optical coherence tomography (OCT). Ophthalmology 1995:217–229.

52. Tearney GJ, Brezinski ME, Southern JF, Bouma BE, Boppart SA, Fujimoto JG. Optical biopsy in human gastrointestinal tissue using optical coherence tomography. Am J Gastroenterol 92:1800–1804, 1997.

53. Pitris C, Brezinski ME, Bouma BE, Tearney GJ, Southern JF, Fujimoto JG. High resolution imaging of the upper respiratory tract with optical coherence tomography: A feasibility study. Am J Respir Crit Care Med 157:1640–1644, 1998.

54. Tearney GJ, Brezinski ME, Southern JF, Bouma BE, Boppart SA, Fujimoto JG. Optical biopsy in human urologic tissue using optical coherence tomography. J Urol 157:1915–1919, 1997.

55. Cameron AJ, Ott BJ, Payne WS. The incidence of adenocarcinoma in columnar-lined (Barrett's) esophagus. N Engl J Med 313:857–859, 1985.

56. Pack GT. Unusual tumors of the stomach. Ann NY Acad Sci 114:985, 1964.

57. Mishima Y, Hirayama R. The role of lymph node surgery in gastric cancer. World J Surg 11:406, 1987.

58. Kaneko E, Nakamura T, Umeda N, et al. Outcome of gastric carcinoma detected by gastric mass survey in Japan. Gut 18:626, 1977.

59. Feczko PJ, Halpert RD. Reassessing the role of radiology and hemoccult screening. Am J Radiol 146:697, 1986.

60. Jass JR, Atkin WS, Cuzick I, et al. The grading of the rectal cancer: Histological perspectives and a multivariate analysis of 447 cases. Histopathology 10:437, 1986.

61. Lofberg R, Brostrom O, Karlen P, Tribukait B, Ost A. Colonoscopic surveillance in long-standing total ulcerative colitis: A 15-year follow-up study. Gastroenterology 99:1021, 1990.

62. Department of Health and Human Services. Guide to Clinical Preventive Services: Report of the US Preventive Services Task Force, 2nd ed. Washington, DC.

63. Lowenfels AB. Why are small-bowel tumours so rare: Lancet 1:24, 1973.

64. Staley CA, Lee JE, Cleary KA, et al. Preoperative chemoradiation, pancreaticoduodenectomy and intraoperative radiation therapy for adenocarcinoma of the pancreatic head. Am J Surg 171:118, 1996.

65. Pitt HA, Dooley WC, Yeo CJ, Cameron JL. Malignancies of the biliary tree. Curr Probl Surg 32:1, 1995.

66. Sergeev AM, Gelikonov VM, Gelikonov GV, Feldchtein FI, Kuranov RV, Gladkova ND, Shakhova NM, Snopova LB, Shakov AV, Kuznetzova IA, Denisenko AN, Pochinko VV, Chumakov YP, Streltzova OS. In vivo endoscopic OCT imaging of pre-cancer and cancer states of human mucosa. Opt Express 1:432–440, 1997.

67. Pitris C, Jesser C, Boppart SA, Stamper D, Brezinski ME, Fujimoto JG. Feasibility of optical coherence tomography for high resolution imaging of human gastrointestinal tract malignancies. Gastroenterol.

68. Hizawa K, Suekane H, Aoyasi K, et al. Use of endosonographic evaluation of colorectal tumor depth in determining the appropriateness of endoscopic mucosal resection. Am J Gastroenterol 91:768–771, 1996.

69. Regan JW, Ng ABP. The cellular manifestations of uterine carcinomas. In: JH Norris, AT Hertig, MR Abell, eds. The Uterus. Int Acad Pathology, Monographs in Pathology. Baltimore: Williams & Wilkins, 1973.

70. Richard RM. Natural history of cervical intraepithelial neoplasia. Clin Obstet Gynecol 110:748, 1967.

71. Fidler HK, Boyes DA, Worth AJ. Cervical cancer detection in British Columbia. A progress report. J Obstet Gynaecol Br Commonw 75:392–404, 1968.

72. American College of Obstetricians and Gynaecologists. Statement of Policy: Periodic Cancer Screening. ACOG, 1980.

73. Gore H, Hertig A. Premalignant lesions of the endometrium. Clin Obstet Gynecol 5:1148, 1962.

74. Malkasian GJ. Carcinoma of the endometrium: Effect of stage and grade on survival. Cancer 41:996–1001, 1978.

75. Roberts JA, Lifshitz S. Primary adenocarcinoma of the fallopian tube. Gynecol Oncol 13:301–308, 1982.

76. Scully RE. Pathology of ovarian cancer precursors. J Cell Biochem 23 (suppl):208–218, 1995.

77. Van Nagell JR, Higgins RV, Donaldson ES, et al. Transvaginal sonography as a screening method for ovarian cancer. A report of the first 1000 cases screened. Cancer 65:573, 1990.

78. Bjorkholm E, Petterson F, Einhorn N, et al. Long term follow-up and prognostic factors in ovarian carcinoma: The Radiumhemmtseries, 1953–1973. Acta Rad Oncol 21:413–419, 1982.

79. Pitris C, Goodman A, Boppart SA, Libus JJ, Fujimoto JG, Brezinski ME. High-resolution imaging of gynecologic neoplasms using optical coherence tomography. Obstet Gynecol 93:135–139, 1999.

80. Sergeev AM, Gelikonov VM, Gelikonov GV, Feldchtein FI, Kuranov RV, Gladkova ND, Shakhova NM, Snopova LB, Shakov AV, Kuznetzova IA, Denisenko AN, Pochinko VV, Chumakov YP, Streltzova OS. In vivo endoscopic OCT imaging of pre-cancer and cancer states of human mucosa. Opt Express 1:432–440, 1997.

81. Stearns V, Gelman EP. does tamoxifen cause cancer in humans? J Clin Oncol 16:779–792, 1998.

82. American College of Obstetricians and Gynecologists (ACOG) Committee on Gynecologic Practice. Committee opinion: Tamoxifen and endometrial cancer, number 169. Int J Gynecol Obstet 53:197–199, 1996.

83. Boppart SA, Goodman A, Libus JJ, Pitris C, Jesser CA, Brezinski ME, Fujimoto JG. High resolution imaging of endometriosis and ovarian carcinoma with optical coherence tomography: Feasibility for laparoscopic-based imaging. Br J Obstet Gynecol.

84. Pode D, Fair WR. The development of bladder cancer. AUA Update, Vol 7, lesson 40. Bellaire, TX: Am Urological Assoc Office of Education, 1987.

85. Jewett JH, Strong GH. Infiltrating carcinoma of the bladder: Relation of depth of penetration of the bladder wall to incidence of local extensions of metastases. J Urol 55:366, 1946.

86. Whitemore WF Jr. Management of invasive bladder neoplasms. Semin Urol 1:34, 1983.

87. Jesser CA, Boppart SA, Pitris C, Stamper DL, Nielsen GP, Brezinski ME. Fujimoto JG. High resolution imaging of transitional cell carcinoma with optical coherence tomography: Feasibility for the evaluation of bladder pathology. Br J Urol.

88. Taphoorn MJ, Heimans JJ, Kaiser MC, de Slegte RG, Crezee FC, Valk J. Imaging of brain metastases: Comparison of computerized tomography (CT) and magnetic resonance imaging (MRI). Neuroradiology 31:391–395, 1989.

89. Grimson WEL, Ettinger GJ, White SJ, Lozano-Perez T, Wells WM III, Kikinis R. An automatic registration method for frameless stereotaxy, image-guided surgery, and enhanced reality visualization. IEEE Trans Med Imaging 15:129–140, 1996.

90. Mizuno A, Hayashi T, Tashibu K, Maraishi S, Kawauchi K, Ozaki Y. Near-infrared FT-Raman spectra of the rat brain tissues. Neurosci Lett 141:47–52, 1992.

91. Poon WS, Schomacker KT, Deutsch F, Martuza RL. Laser-induced fluorescence: Experimental intraoperative delineation of tumor resection margins. J Neurosurg 76:679–686, 1992.

22

Optical Coherence Tomography in Dentistry

BILL W. COLSTON, JR., MATTHEW J. EVERETT, UJWAL S. SATHYAM, and LUIZ B. DA SILVA

Lawrence Livermore National Laboratory, Livermore, California

22.1 INTRODUCTION

Optical coherence tomography (OCT) has the potential of offering a safe, novel method for imaging dental microstructure for the evaluation of dental health. Potential dental applications of OCT include, among others, diagnosis of periodontal diseases, detection of caries, and evaluation of dental restoration integrity. This technique can potentially benefit any accessible region of the oral cavity that contains useful information within the first 2–3 mm of tissue.

This chapter is intended to provide an overview of dental OCT technology, highlighting those system characteristics or design constraints that are specific to dentistry. In addition, we will touch on some of the most important challenges currently facing dental clinicians and describe how OCT imaging could be applied to these problems. Finally, a perspective on future directions for OCT in dentistry will be provided, including an outline of the most promising clinical applications and prospects for future development.

22.2 HISTORY OF DENTAL OCT

Dental OCT imaging was pioneered by a collaboration between physicists at Lawrence Livermore National Laboratory (LLNL) and clinicians at the University of Connecticut Health Center [1,2]. Preliminary work with an animal model focused on correlating optical scattering signatures with tissue structures in the periodontium region of the oral cavity [3]. The subsequent construction of an intraoral handpiece then allowed us to produce a prototype system capable of operating in a dental clinic. This system was used to produce the first in vivo OCT images of the oral cavity, focusing on the periodontium region [4]. Recently, other researchers expanded this work to include OCT imaging of other tissue structures in the oral cavity [5]. Detection of caries based on birefringence changes visible in polarization-sensitive OCT (PS-OCT) phase images was initially suggested by an Austrian group of researchers [6]. Researchers at LLNL and the University of California at San Francisco later determined that PS-OCT is capable of caries detection, but based on depolarization of light associated with changes in optical scattering rather than birefringence changes [7].

22.3 OPTICAL PROPERTIES OF DENTAL TISSUES

A cartoon highlighting the cross-sectional anatomy of a tooth and connected soft tissue is shown in Fig. 1. The upper part of the drawing corresponds to the crown or top of the tooth. The enamel layer consists of prisms that run like the spokes of a wheel from the dento-enamel junction (DEJ) to the outer enamel surface. These prisms, made up of hydroxyapatite crystals, can be as long as 3–4 mm near the cervix of the tooth and average 6 μm in diameter, with neighboring prisms separated by glycoprotein prism sheaths 0.1–0.2 μm wide (Fig. 2). Inside the enamel shell, dentin is a complex structure composed of dentinal tubules honeycombed in a collagen matrix. The tubules are composed of long cell processes (ondontoblasts) and are surrounded by small needle-like hydroxyapatite crystals (1–3 μm in diameter) in a fibrous matrix (type I collagen fibers).

The gingival margin marks the beginning of the gingival tissue. The gingiva consists of two basic tissue types—a superficial layer of epithelium and an underlying, supportive connective tissue layer. The epithelium provides a mechanical barrier that protects the underlying tissues. The connective tissue, or lamina propria, adds mechanical support and contains essential entities such as blood vessels and nerves. The epithelium folds over the crest of the free gingiva and then faces the

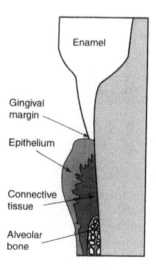

Figure 1 Cartoon showing soft and hard tissue interfaces in the oral cavity.

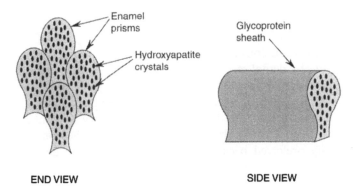

END VIEW · SIDE VIEW

Figure 2 Illustration showing structure of enamel prisms.

tooth surface. The sulcus is defined as the shallow groove between the epithelium and the tooth and is an important feature of the diagnosing periodontal disease.

Because dental hard tissues are anisotropic, the scattering distribution is highly orientation-dependent. Average scattering and absorption properties, however, have been recorded for both enamel and dentin [8]. The average scattering coefficient for enamel is significantly affected by wavelength [μ_S (632 nm) = 60 cm^{-1}, μ_S (1053 nm) = 15 cm^{-1}] compared to dentin [μ_S (620 nm) = 280 cm^{-1}, μ_S (1053 nm) = 260 cm^{-1}], with the absorption coefficients in both cases being negligible. The indices of refraction for enamel and dentin are approximately 1.63 and 1.45 (λ = 633 nm), respectively. No study, to the best of our knowledge, has been performed for measuring the optical properties of dental soft tissues.

Two conclusions can be drawn from these optical property data with respect to dental OCT imaging: Longer wavelength sources should penetrate much further in enamel than shorter wavelengths, and visible to near-infrared light should propagate much further through enamel than through dentin. These findings are consistent with OCT image features, where penetration depths of more than 3 mm are not unusual in enamel. Although the optical scattering properties of gingival tissue are unknown, OCT images demonstrate a much larger scattering coefficient for gingiva (1–2 mm maximum penetration depth) than for enamel.

22.4 DENTAL OCT SYSTEM DESIGN

Optical coherence tomographic systems designed for use in dental clinics contain the basic elements essential to any OCT imaging system, including an optical source, a white light fiber-optic interferometer, detector and demodulation electronics, and a user display/interface. The design and function of these components are covered in some depth elsewhere in this textbook. In this section, therefore, we will focus on how various OCT system characteristics are applicable to dental imaging.

22.4.1 Optical Source Characteristics

The light sources currently used in dental OCT studies have relatively broad spectral bandwidths, on the order of 30–60 nm, with corresponding free-space axial resolutions of 10–25 μm. In detection of periodontal diseases, this high resolution is necessary for detecting important tissue interfaces such as the cemento-enamel junction and sulcus. This resolution is also a factor in determining the sensitivity of OCT systems for detecting small pre-carious lesions in dental hard tissue or evaluating the marginal and structural integrity of a dental restoration. Selection of a source wavelength for dental OCT systems is largely dictated by the availability of clinically portable sources such as superluminescent diodes and fiber-doped amplified spontaneous emission (ASE) sources. Because of this limitation, the majority of dental OCT systems operate at a wavelength of either 850 or 1310 nm. The longer 1310 nm, wavelength is generally preferred because it penetrates further in dental tissues.

22.4.2 Intraoral Handpieces

A variety of intraoral handpieces have been designed for use in the oral cavity. These handpieces, in general, are small enough to comfortably access most of the clinically relevant tissue in the oral cavity. This access is usually accomplished by coupling a single-mode optical fiber to some type of miniaturized sample arm collection optics. A transverse scanning mechanism, such as a pneumatic or dc motor-driven screw, is then employed to generate two- or three-dimensional OCT images. The primary limitation to transverse scanning dimensions is the size of the handpiece, because the end of the device that goes to the mouth must be large enough to accommodate the maximum distance of travel for all transverse scanning directions. A final consideration, besides access and scanning, is how the OCT image is registered against its physical location on the tissue. This is particularly challenging in posterior regions of the oral cavity where visual confirmation is limited. The type of intraoral handpiece used is largely driven by the clinical application (i.e., periodontal disease diagnosis, caries detection, etc.). Some examples of these devices are given below, along with a brief synopsis of their relative strengths and weaknesses.

One-Dimensional Imaging—OCT Dental Explorer

One very simple design for an intraoral handpiece incorporates the sample arm collection optics inside a dental explorer or mechanical periodontal probe (Fig. 3).

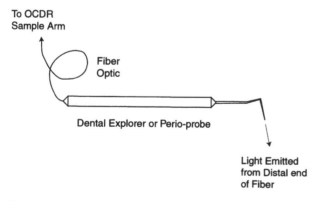

Figure 3   Schematic of dental explorer or mechanical periodontal probe containing a single-mode optical fiber from the OCT sample arm.

The addition of OCT imaging capabilities to the dental explorer provides the dentist with a profile of optical scattering versus depth in the tooth at the point where the tip of the dental explorer touches the tissue. The light from the probe tip can be angled to provide better access to the target tissue. For example, if it is desirable to create images of the loos gingiva in the periodontal pocket, the light can be angled perpendicular to the probe tip. Dragging the explorer across the tissue surface generates a series of one-dimensional scattering profiles. These profiles can then be combined to form a cross-sectional optical coherence tomographic (OCT) image of the internal structure of the tissue in the region of interest. The simple design of the OCT dental explorer compromises registration capabilities and lateral resolution for accessibility. This design is probably most useful for caries detection, because the explorer can be used on the contoured occlusal (top) and interproximal (between-teeth) surfaces of the tooth with relative ease. Because this device is a modification to an existing tool already widely used by dentists, it may gain acceptance more easily than handpieces that incorporate lateral scanning mechanisms and is likely to be more inexpensive to produce. The entire explorer, including a detachable optical fiber, would necessarily be sterilizable for infection control reasons.

Two-Dimensional Imaging—Side-Firing Intraoral Handpiece

There are, of course, a large number of possible designs for a two-dimensional intraoral handpiece. The anatomy of the oral cavity, however, makes a "side-firing" device particularly attractive [4]. In this configuration, the portion of the handpiece that enters the oral cavity is relatively long and thin,allowing it to fit comfortably between the cheek or lip and the gingival tissue. The desired transverse range of the OCT scan is used to determine the height of the handpiece device,. The end of the device shown in Fig. 4, for example, is approximately 13 mm in height and about 2 mm in width. The collection optics consist of a combination of a gradient refractive index (GRIN) lens with an angle prism mounted on the end of the sample arm single-mode optical fiber. Light emerging from the fiber is focused by the GRIN lens onto the tissue and reflected 90° by internal reflection off the prism. The fiber-optic–GRIN lens assembly is linearly scanned parallel to the surface of the target tissue

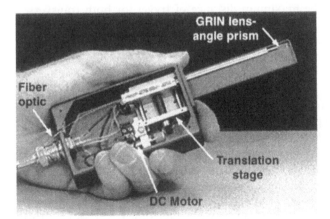

Figure 4 Intraoral OCT handpiece (one dimension of lateral scanning).

and perpendicular to the fiber axis, through translation of a traveling stage via a dc motor-driven screw. Scan activation is accomplished via a foot pedal. The foot pedal, when depressed, creates a digital signal (generated from the dc motor power supply) that is fed to the computer and used to apply an appropriate bias to the motor. Limit switches constrain lateral motion of the fiber assembly to the desired transverse scan dimension. The average B-scan image acquisition is approximately 42 s based on a Doppler shift modulation of 82 kHz, an axial scan range of 4 mm, a transverse scan range of about 7 mm, and a transverse resolution of 25 μm. The waist size of the 1.8 mm diameter GRIN lens was measured to be 20 μm at the focus, with a Rayleigh range of 1.9 mm. The probe light passes through a slot in the tip of the handpiece that is parallel to the transverse scanning direction. A disposable plastic sleeve is used to cover this slot for infection control purposes.

   Most tissues in the oral cavity can be accessed using this handpiece, although stabilization on the lingual aspects of the tooth is still difficult. A slot cut in the back of the handpiece allows visual registration of the OCT scan against the tissue. When visual registration is difficult, however, such as in the posterior portion of the mouth or occlusal tooth surfaces, it remains challenging to accurately position the handpiece against the tissue. This is an important concern when trying to monitor disease progression, where it is desirable to make multiple measurements at the same location over a given period of time. Some type of conventional imaging modality (such as a charge-coupled device coupled to an imaging fiber) could conceivably be used to improve registration.

Three-Dimensional Imaging

A third type of intraoral handpiece incorporates three-dimensional scanning capabilities [5]. Here the distance between adjacent B-scans is precisely controlled. This type of scanning is particularly useful when volumetric estimates of tissue density (such as the extent of a carious lesion) are desirable. As an example of a three-dimensional data set, an image of a rat's jaw collected using a table-mounted X-Y galvanometer is shown in Fig. 5. Here multiple cross-sectional tomograms have been stacked to create a three-dimensional image. Internal tissue information can be analyzed by taking a slice through any portion of this figure. The primary limitations of intraoral handpieces of this type is their size; the end of the handpiece must be large enough to accommodate the maximum distance of travel for both transverse scanning directions. This makes posterior tissue difficult to access but may be desirable for imaging the occlusal surfaces of teeth.

22.4.3   OCT Image Artifacts

Three primary types of image artifacts can occur in any OCT image: motion, echo, and birefringence. The first type, motion artifacts, can lead to a loss of spatial resolution in both the axial and transverse directions. Because the B-scan intensity image is formed from a series of longitudinal A-scans, axial motion can lead to misalignment of subsequent transverse scans with a resulting loss of the surface contour profile (Fig. 6). This is obvious here, because the enamel surface (E) follows the same contour as the interface between the enamel and dentin (D). Transverse motion error can occur during relatively long image acquisition times and lead to inaccuracies in the transverse resolution and nonlinear longitudinal information.

1 mm

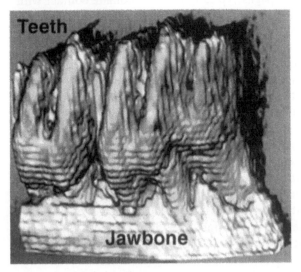

Figure 5 Three-dimensional image of stacked OCT cross-sectional scans taken of a rat's jaw.

1 mm

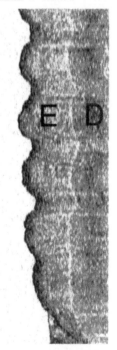

Figure 6 Optical coherence tomographic image of tooth surface (in vivo) showing motion artifacts.

Because current intraoral handpiece designs typically involve intimate contact with the tissue, however, these types of motion artifacts are greatly reduced. Based on our experience, total B-scan image acquisition times on the order of a few seconds are fast enough to minimize motion artifacts.

A second, and potentially more serious, type of artifact are reflection echoes crated by multiple reflection paths in the OCT interferometer. The strength of these echoes is proportional to the magnitude of the interface creating a specular reflection and is a function of the source output power. The interface that typically creates problems in dental OCT applications is found between the infection control plastic sleeve and the tissue surface. Angling the light incident on the plastic sleeve from the handpiece tip or adjusting the focus of the collection optics can minimize this reflection. Fogging of the infection control sleeve that leads to regional changes in OCT image brightness (Fig. 7, left) further complicates this situation One solution to this problem is to use an imaging gel at the plastic/tissue interface. The gel provides an index-matching medium that prevents overly bright specular reflections and eliminates fogging artifacts (Fig. 7, right). In the example shown, much more structure is evident in the enamel and gingival tissue when the imaging gel is used.

Tissue birefringence can also lead to artifacts in conventional OCT systems. This is of particular concern in enamel, owing to its high birefringence. This birefringence is created by the different between the index of refraction for light polarized along the hydroxyapatite crystal axis and that of the light polarized perpendicular to the axis. When the enamel surface is perpendicular to the incident light form the optical handpiece, the two axes of polarization of the incident light are both perpendicular to the axes of the prisms, and minimal birefringence effects

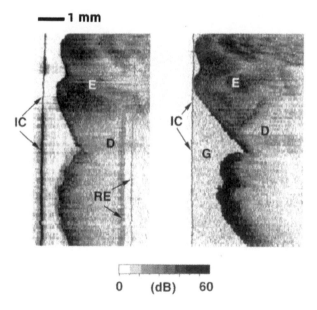

Figure 7 Comparison of in vivo OCT image taken without (right) and with (left) imaging gel (G) between the infection control plastic (IC) and tooth surface. Reflection echoes (RE) result in artifacts inside the dentin (D) structure.

occur. As the contour of the tooth changes, however, the prisms become more perpendicular to the probe light and birefringence-induced artifacts appear in the OCT images. The effect of these artifacts, unfortunately, is to obscure structural features in the enamel that might otherwise be visible, such as pre-carious or carious lesions (Fig. 8). One method for eliminating these artifacts is to use a polarization-sensitive OCT (PS-OCT) system.

22.5 APPLICATIONS

The information available to dental clinicians for evaluating diseases in the oral cavity is currently inadequate, relying on methods that are, by nature, either qualitative or inaccurate. The goal of dental optical coherence tomography is to produce in vivo images of dental microstructure that can be used to make both qualitative and quantitative assessments of oral tissue health. In particular, we hope to derive from these images clinically important anatomical features such as the location of the soft tissue attachment, morphological changes in gingival tissue, tooth decay, and structural integrity of dental restorations.

22.5.1 Diagnosing Periodontal Diseases

Periodontal diseases are plaque-induced disorders that result in loss of connective tissue attachment and resorption of alveolar bone. An important aspect of periodontal disease assessment is determination of the location of the soft tissue attachment to the tooth surface [9]. Currently, mechanical or pressure-sensitive probes are used to assess periodontal conditions [10]. The periodontal probe is placed between the soft tissue and the tooth. The depth of probe penetration (probable pocket depth) is measured, and the attachment level is estimated from a fixed reference point on the tooth, the cemento-enamel junction (CEJ).

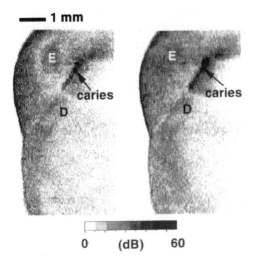

Figure 8 Extracted tooth with caries occurring along the dentin/enamel interface. Unlike demineralization in the enamel layer, caries that occurs in dentin is much easier to visualize in the OCT total intensity plot (right) than in the OCT single-detector plot (left).

Unfortunately, periodontal probing is not a precise diagnostic. These probes have several sources of error resulting from variations in insertion force [11], inflammatory status of tissue [12], diameter of probe tips [13], and anatomical tooth contours [14] in addition to being painful for the patient. These errors limit the ability of clinicians to evaluate subtle differences in clinical values that may be important in early disease detection and intervention [14].

Radiographs can be used as a supplementary tool in periodontal disease diagnosis to reveal morphological characteristics of alveolar bone. Although radiographs are highly sensitive to detecting regions of alveolar bone loss, they are incapable of identifying active disease. Periodontal disease is therefore not identified until significant bone loss has occurred. Moreover, radiographs provide no information on the state of the soft tissue. Because OCT records soft tissue contour and microstructure, it offers the potential to quantify the soft tissue changes that occur in gingivitis and periodontal diseases.

OCT Imaging in an Animal Model

An animal model was used to conduct the first OCT imaging studies of dental structures [3]. A bench-top dental OCT system was used to image selected regions from the oral cavity of two young pigs shortly after sacrifice. The source used in this experiment was relatively low powered ($\sim 70\,\mu$W) with a net system signal-to-noise ratio of 90 dB. The axial and lateral resolution of the system were 17 μm and 20 μm, respectively. Histological confirmation of the OCT images was made by freezing the specimens and then slicing them axially using a diamond-tipped rotating disk. The internal tooth and soft tissue microstructure was thus exposed and the critical tooth/gingiva interface maintained. A digital camera mounted on a microscope was used to obtain photomicrographs of the sectioned teeth.

This in vitro approach had the benefit of allowing direct comparisons of the acquired OCT cross-sectional images (Fig. 9, left) to histology (Fig. 9, right). The axial scale for the OCT image is given in terms of optical pathlength and needs to be divided by the refractive index of the relevant tissue to obtain true physical dimensions, resulting in an axial compression of the image. The refractive indices for gingiva, enamel, and dentin are ~ 1.33, ~ 1.63, and ~ 1.45 ($\lambda = 633$ nm), respectively. An important reference point for determining attachment level in elevation of periodontal diseases, the sulcus (S), is clearly visible in these early in vitro OCT images. In addition, the dento-enamel junction, whose integrity is important in caries diagnosis, is also discernible. Although the periodontal tissues of the porcine specimens used in this study were healthy, the images demonstrated the ability of OCT to locate the tooth surface and contour beneath the gingival tissue. The first study was an important milestone in establishing the validity of this technique for dental medicine.

OCT Imaging in the Clinic

Preliminary clinical data are currently being collected using in vivo dental OCT systems. These imaging devices are relatively compact and incorporate intraoral handpieces for accessing most parts of the oral cavity. The images created using these systems contain structural details of hard and soft tissue anatomy (Fig. 10). The image shown in Fig. 10, for example, was collected from a healthy volunteer and represents a cross section of the tooth at the midbuccal region. No postprocessing

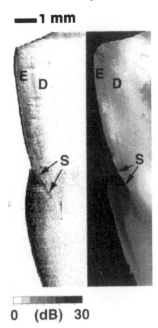

Figure 9 In vivo B-scan image of pig's jaw (left) matched against histology (right). Visible structures include the enamel (E), dentin (D), and sulcus (S).

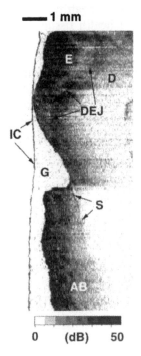

Figure 10 In vitro B-scan image of a human healthy mandibular premolar taken perpendicular to the gingival margin. E, enamel; D, dentin; DEJ, dento-enamel junction; IC, infection control, G, imaging gel, S, sulcus; AB, alveolar bone.

was used in creating this image. The surface contour of this tissue is well represented, although a small amount of motion artifact can be seen as modulations of the facial surface. The plastic infection control sleeve (IC) is visible as a thin black line at the air/imaging gel (*G*) interface. The imaging gel reduces the backreflection from the infection control sleeve and prevents artifacts due to fogging. At the crown of the tooth, the dento-enamel function (DEJ), or interface between the outer enamel layer (*E*) and the inner dentin microtubules (*D*), is clearly visible. The interface between the gingiva and tooth, the sulcus (*S*), is also easily distinguished in this image. The checkered region underlying the dark epithelial layer at the base of the image has been presumptively identified as alveolar bone (AB).

Because progression of periodontal disease results in alterations of the connective tissue architecture, the identification of these anatomical features by the use of dental OCT is promising. More expansive clinical studies correlating OCT image characteristics with standard assessments of oral health, however, must be performed before this technique will be useful for diagnosis of gingivitis or periodontal diseases

22.5.2 Detecting Caries

Although the number of cases of dental caries diagnosed in the United States has decreased over the past few decades, dental decay is still the leading cause of tooth loss [15]. Caries lesions are difficult to detect in the early stages of development and as a result are usually found after they have progressed to the point at which surgical intervention and restoration are necessary, resulting in the loss of healthy tissue structure and weakening of the tooth. To minimize their loss of health tissue and the need for surgical intervention, new, more sophisticated diagnostic tools are needed.

Dental caries is currently diagnosed by using radiography in conjunction with visual and tactile exploration. The traditional method of caries detection, probing the teeth with a sharp dental explorer, has fallen into disfavor because it causes damage to the tooth by penetrating into the enamel and may also cause microbiological cross-contamination between teeth. Although radiography uses ionizing radiation that carries the potential for detrimental biological effects, it remains an essential component of caries diagnosis. Radiography has high predictive value for detecting interproximal lesions involving the dentin. Radiography also shows a high sensitivity for detecting occlusal caries that involves dentin, although the false positive fraction is high. The predictive value of radiography for lesions confined to the enamel is poor [16,17]. OCT holds promise as a supplement to radiographic diagnosis for detecting early occlusal lesions and for quantifying enamel demineralization. OCT may also prove to be more sensitive for detecting recurrent caries because the margins of restorations are imaged in tomographic sections with a higher resolution that can be obtained using current radiographic methods.

Overview of Dental PS-OCT Imaging

The imaging depth of OCT systems in dental hard structures is superior to that in soft tissue, particularly in enamel, where imaging depths of up to 4 mm have been demonstrated. Conventional OCT images, however, often contain birefringence artifacts (as described above) that can obscure important structural features such as small demineralized regions of the tooth. These artifacts are particularly prevalent when imaging highly contoured tooth surfaces, because the tooth birefringence is dependent on the relative orientation between the incident probe light and the tooth structure. PS-OCT systems can potentially be used to eliminate these artifacts and measure the polarization state of the light backscattered from the tooth, allowing sensitive detection of demineralized or carious regions.

The first polarization-sensitive OCDR system was developed by Hee et al. [18], who used a pair of detectors to measure the two orthogonal polarization states of light backscattered from the tissue. An alternative technique using a single detector and a rotating waveplate in conjunction with a transverse scanning capability was then developed by de Boer et al. [19] and used to demonstrate the first two-dimensional PS-OCT images of tissue. The Stokes parameters were determined using multiple PS-OCT scans in rodent muscle and skin by de Boer et al. 20]. Other investigators attempted to measure changes in tooth birefringence using PS-OCT as a caries diagnostic [6]. Their system, however, had limited sensitivity and penetration depth, making it difficult to discriminate between birefringence and depolarization of light. We recently demonstrated, in collaboration with investigators at the University of California at San Francisco, that demineralization of enamel increases optical scattering and causes depolarization of light rather than changes in birefringence [7]. The PS-OCT system used in these trials was a bulk optic system that combines the initial two-detector design of Hee et al. [18] with transverse scanning and is described in detail elsewhere [21]. Circularly polarized low coherence light is focused on biological tissue in the sample arm. High resolution cross-sectional imaging and birefringence characterization of the tissue are then obtained by measuring the backscattered light intensity and polarization as a function of axial depth and transverse location in the tissue. A scanning retroreflector varies the pathlength of the reference arm for each transverse location on the sample. An interferometric signal is detected when the distances to the reference and sample arm reflections are matched to within the source coherence length. The return light is spilt into orthogonal polarizations (horizontal and vertical) before being detected.

The resulting signals are squared to determine the power $P_H(z)$ and $P_V(z)$ in the two detectors scattered from the tissue as a function of depth z. The total backscattered light versus penetration depth in the tissue is given by

$$P_T(z) = P_V(z) + P_H(z)$$

and the degree of polarization of this light by

$$\rho(z) = \frac{P_V(z) - P_H(z)}{P_V(z) + P_H(z)}$$

When there is no birefringence or depolarization in the tissue, $P_H(z) = 0$ and the degree of polarization $\rho(z)$ is equal to 1. Depolarization of the light spreads the light equally between the detectors, causing $\rho(z)$ to approach zero. Birefringence in the tissue can also affect this measurement of the degree of polarization, causing the light to swing back and forth between the two detectors and leading to an oscillation in the value of $\rho(z)$ between 1 and -1 with tissue depth z.

PS-OCT Imaging of Bovine Blocks

The ability of PS-OCT to detect demineralized regions was initially evaluated using tissue phantoms (Fig. 11). A surface zone of demineralization approximately 50 μm thick was produced on the polished surface of half of 5 mm × 5 mm bovine enamel block by soaking it in an acidic solution while half of the block was covered by an acid-resistant varnish. Cross-sectional PS-OCT backscattering intensity and polarization state images of these bovine enamel blocks were taken such that half of each image was of normal enamel and half of demineralized enamel. Backscattering and degree of polarization state images for a typical bovine enamel block are shown in Fig. 11. The backscattering intensity was only slightly affected by the demineralization (Fig. 11, left). The polarization state image, however, shows clear contrast between the normal and carious enamel microstructure (Fig. 11, right).

PS-OCT Imaging of Extracted Human Teeth

Having demonstrated the efficacy of PS-OCT for detection of caries in tissue models, we next applied it to in vitro detection of naturally occurring caries in extracted human teeth [7]. Histological thin sections examined under polarized light were used to verify the discrimination between normal and carious enamel in the PS-OCT images. The histology confirmed the high sensitivity and specificity of the PS-OCT system for detection of caries both on and just below the facial surface of the tooth (Fig. 12). The white spot lesion, visible in the histology as a darkened region near the enamel surface, is clearly detected in the polarization image, as indicated by the depolarization of the light between the two horizontal lines. The health enamel above the lines is highly birefringent, as indicated by the black and white stripes caused by $\rho(z)$ varying from 1 to -1, while below the lines there is little birefringence, as indicated by the maintenance of polarization state with depth. The capability of PS-OPCT to pinpoint the location of caries based on the depolarization, which is localized to the regions of demineralization, is well illustrated in this example.

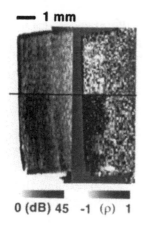

0 (dB) 45   -1 (ρ) 1

Figure 11 Bovine block with top half of enamel demineralized. Contrast between the demineralized and normal regions is much better in the OCT polarization state plot (right) than in the OCT intensity plot (left).

1 mm

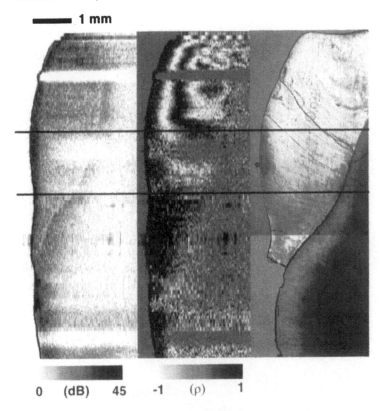

0 (dB) 45   -1 (ρ) 1

Figure 12 Extracted tooth with a large demineralized section in the center of the enamel layer. Contrast between the demineralized and normal regions is much better in the OCT phase plot (center) than in the OCT intensity plot (left). Histology is shown in the right-hand image, with the dark layer on the tooth surface corresponding to demineralized structure.

We also explored the use of PS-OCT caries detection on the occlusal (biting) surface of teeth, where many cavities occur that are difficult to detect using standard methods. The PS-OCT images were more difficult to interpret than those collected on the facial (front) surface of teeth. The highly contoured occlusal surface produced large variations in tooth birefringence along the tooth surface (Fig. 13). The extracted tooth, as demonstrated in the histological section, has a large carious section in the center with less extensive decay extending to the edges of the tooth (Fig. 13, left). There is a good correspondence between the histology (Fig. 13, right) and phase image (Fig. 13, center). Although demineralization-induced depolarization is visible across the majority of the PS-OCT image, depolarization of the incident light occurs most rapidly in the center of the tooth, which marks where the histology shows the greatest amount of decay. This rapid depolarization is visible as a reduction in the depth to which the light remains polarized, leading to a narrowing of the black band at the surface of the tooth in the PS-OCT polarization image. This particular figure demonstrates the capability of PS-OCT to provide some measure of the degree of demineralization.

Optical coherence tomographic backscatter images, however, are useful for the detection of carious lesions in dentin [22]. Unlike the carious enamel, the carious

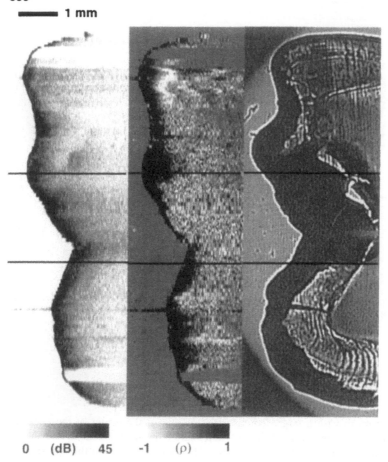

Figure 13 Caries detection on occlusal surface of extracted human teeth demonstrates complications associated with variable birefringence. Demineralized regions of enamel are between the black lines. The figure consists of three images of the same cross section of a tooth, with a PS-OCT intensity image on the left, a PS-OCT polarization image in the center, and histology on the right. Greatest depolarization of light occurs in area contained within the lines, where histology shows the greatest damage associated with caries.

dentin below the composite restoration is easily imaged in the backscattering intensity image (Fig. 14). This result could have been predicted by the relatively low birefringence of dentin compared to that of enamel. Because both intensity and polarization OCT provide useful information for caries detection, future dental OCT systems will likely incorporate PS-OCT capabilities in a fiber-based system.

22.5.3 Evaluating Dental Restorations

Dental restorations, such as fillings and crowns, provide a barrier restricting oral fluid and bacteria from entering the tooth. An inadequate marginal seal between the restoration and the native tooth can result in further loss of tooth structure and dissemination of bacteria [23]. The most commonly used methods for evaluating the margins and structural integrity of restorations are visual, radiographic, and tactile

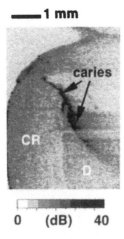

1 mm

0 (dB) 40

Figure 14 Intensity OCT image showing carious lesion along the dentin/composite interface, as imaged from the occlusal surface. (Image provided by Felix I. Feldchtein, Institute of Applied Physics of Russian Academy of Science.)

examination [24]. OCT has the potential advantage over these methods of visualizing structural and marginal restoration defects before significant leakage occurs, minimizing tooth loss and decreasing the number of unnecessary replacement restorations.

In Vivo Imaging of the Tooth/Restoration Margin

A variety of restoration materials have been imaged using dental OCT systems [4,5]. The most serious challenges to this effort are the limited imaging depths of existing OCT systems and their inability to penetrate the supportive metal coping beneath a crown. Prosthetics such as porcelain crowns have scattering characteristics similar to enamel, but other restorations such as metal fillings and composites are either impenetrable or much more highly scattering than the tooth itself. We imaged, for example, a composite restoration (CR) from the occlusal surface of the tooth using the in vivo dental OCT system (Fig. 15). The scattering coefficient of the composite material is relatively homogeneous and much higher than that of the surrounding enamel microstructure (E). In this particular case, the restoration is shallow enough that the restoration margin is clearly visible. The birefringence artifacts present in the enamel layer provide an excellent contrast that aids in identifying this interface.

Imaging Structural Defects in Restorations

The ability of OCT to evaluate the structural quality of a restoration has been nicely demonstrated by Feldschtein and coworkers at the Russian Academy of Science. The OCT image in Fig. 16, for example, shows bubble (left image) and gap (right image)_ filling defects in a composite resin restoration. The bubble defect is present just above the tooth/restoration margin. The restoration in this case was deep enough that only the left edge of the margin is visible. The gap defect image, on the other hand, had a shallow enough restoration that the entire tooth/resin interface is visible. It is unclear whether this gap is filled with some type of transparent glue or is an

— 1 mm

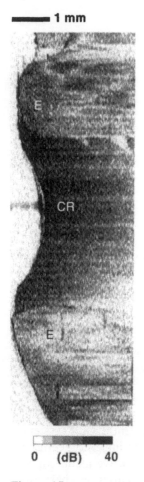

0   (dB)   40

Figure 15   In vivo OCT image, taken from the occlusal surface, of a composite restoration (middle). Birefringence artifacts (banding) is obvious in the surrounding enamel.

—1 mm

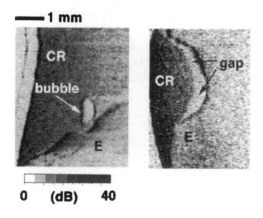

0   (dB)   40

Figure 16   Optical coherence tomographic image of bubble (left) and gap (right) filling defects. (Image provided by Felix I. Feldchtein, Institute of Applied Physics of Russian Academy of Science.)

actual air gap. The presence of either of these defects could require replacement of the restorative material.

Monitoring Restoration Placement and Quality Control

Another exciting prospect for this application is the ability to dynamically assess the quality of a new restoration. An example of this process is shown in Fig. 17. The image on the left shows a carious lesion in the cervical region of the root before any type of operative procedure has been applied. Demineralization is likely the cause of the bright image region that extends about 300 μm below the surface of the crater. The lesion after diamond burr drilling and acid etching of this region is then shown in the center image. Finally, the right image shows the tooth after a filling (composite resin) has been placed. The restoration covers over the enamel layer, with the entire margin of the restoration being clearly visible. No structural defects are apparent in this image.

22.6 THE FUTURE OF DENTAL OCT

The optical accessibility of clinically relevant structures in the oral cavity makes it a particularly attractive location for the application of OCT imaging techniques. Despite the promise of the early imaging studies provided in this chapter, however, at least two series of events must occur for OCT to become a widely available diagnostic in dental clinics. First, extensive clinical evaluations must be performed correlating OCT imaging and currently accepted diagnostic markers of disease state. Second, the cost and complexity of dental OCT systems must be reduced to the level of current radiographic devices. The areas in which OCT is most likely to be useful in dentistry include diagnosis of soft tissue diseases, detection of caries, and evaluation and monitoring of tooth restorations.

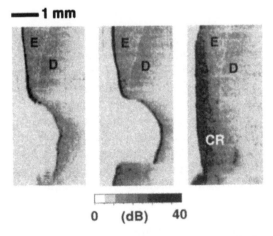

Figure 17 Optical coherence tomographic images showing placement of new composite restoration: preoperative lesion (left), lesion after diamond burr drilling and acid etching (center), and tooth after filling has been placed (right). (Image provided by Felix I. Feldchtein, Institute of Applied Physics of Russian Academy of Science.)

22.6.1 Diagnosis Gingivitis and Periodontal Disease

Soft tissue health is one area where OCT imaging could make a significant impact. There are no cross-sectional imaging modalities that can be used intraorally for visualizing oral soft tissue structures such as the soft and hard palate. gingiva, buccal mucosa, mucogingival folds, tongue, sublingual areas, pharyngeal areas, and peri-oral area. One focus of our group is to evaluate the use of OCT for the diagnosis of gingivitis and periodontal diseases. Because gingivitis leads to swelling of the tissue and an increase in blood flow, OCT may be capable of resolving subtle scattering and/or absorption differences in diseased tissues. These image features could range from a change in image brightness relative to surrounding structures to the appearance or disappearance of clinically relevant interfaces such as the sulcus. Alternative OCT imaging systems may need to be employed to provide sufficient contrast for making these determinations. One example of such a system would be use of a Doppler OCT system for imaging blood movement in the gingiva. Another might be the application of color or multiple-wavelength OCT systems for selective image enhancement of tissue absorbers such as hemoglobin or water.

Diagnosis of periodontal diseases using OCT imaging should, in theory, be a much more straightforward task, because the physical changes in tissue microstructure (i.e., bone loss, gingival detachment, etc.) are more extreme than those that occur due to gingivitis. The primary limitation of this application, however, is likely to be the useful imaging depth of OCT through soft tissue. Loss of resolution due to multiple scattering or poor image brightness caused by insufficient light penetration may combine to hide important structural interfaces. The clinician would then be in the position of relying on subtle changes in the tissue optical properties, such as those described above for diagnosis of gingivitis, for determining periodontal disease activity. The early studies discussed in this chapter provide a promising base for future work, although more extensive clinical studies aimed at correlating OCT image features with disease biomarkers will be necessary before dental OCT can be adequately validated as a tool for evaluating soft tissue health.

22.6.2 Detecting Caries

Optical coherence tomographic systems may provide a valuable tool for early detection of carious and pre-carious lesions. The imaging depths of OCT systems in teeth are relatively large compared to those attainable in the oral soft tissue. The image contrast between healthy and carious tooth structures attainable from PS-OCT polarization state images is also a very promising prognosis for OCT detection of caries. The primary hurdles to be overcome in this area concern the inability to adequately define and access decayed tooth structures. Studies targeted at correlating PS-OCT and OCT images of carious teeth with histological sectioning, followed by patient-oriented clinical trials, are the next step toward validating this technique for caries detection.

22.6.3 Evaluating the Structural Integrity of Restorations

Finally, OCT could be used to evaluate the structural and marginal integrity of dental restorations. The preliminary research indicates that OCT is capable of imaging and quantifying marginal discrepancies with very high resolution. The tomographic nature of the images should provide important information regarding the degree of mineralization of enamel or dental tissue that is contiguous to the restoration margin. Obviously, this application of OCT will be limited by the scattering properties and filling depth of the restoration material. Further studies using extracted teeth are necessary to obtain a clearer understanding of the limitations of OCT for this application.

REFERENCES

1. Nathel H, Colston B, Armitage G, Otis L. Specular reflectivity of dental hard tissues as determined by time-domain reflectometry. OSA Annul Meeting, Rochester, NY, 1994, Abstract 32.
2. Otis L, Colston B, Armitage G, Nathel H. Specular reflectivity of dental hard tissues. J Dental Res 74(SI):67, 1995.
3. Colston BW, Everett MJ, Da Silva LB, Otis LL, Stroeve P, Nathel H. Imaging of hard and soft tissue structure in the oral cavity by optical coherence tomography. Appl Opt 37(19):3582–3585, 1998.
4. Colston BW, Sathyam US, Da Silva LB, Everett MJ, Stroeve P, Otis LL. Dental OCT. Opt Express 3:230–328, 1998.
5. Feldchtein FI, Gelikonov GV, Gelikonov VM, Iksanov RR, Kuranov RV, Sergeev AM, Gladkova ND, Ourutina MN, Warren JA, Reitze DH. In vivo OCT imaging of hard and soft tissue of the oral cavity. Opt Express 3:239–250, 1998.
6. Baumgartner A, Hitzenberger CK, Dichtl S, Sattmann H, Moritz A, Sperr W, Fercher AF. Optical coherence tomography of dental structures. SPIE 3248:130–136, 1998.
7. Everett MJ, Colston BW Jr, Sathyam US, Da Silva LB, Fried D, Featherstone JD. Noninvasive diagnosis of early caries with polarization sensitive optical coherence tomography (PS-OCT). SPIE Proc Lasers in Dentistry V, 1999:3593.
8. Fried D, Glena RE, Featherstone JDB, Seka W. Nature of light scattering in dental enamel and dentin at visible and near-infrared wavelengths. Appl Opt 34(7):1278–1285, 1995.
9. Machtei EE, Christersson LA, et al. Alternative methods for screening periodontal disease in adults. J Clin Periodontol 20:81–87, 1993.
10. Pihlstrom BL. Measurement of attachment level in clinical trials. Probing methods. J Periodontol 63:1072–1077, 1992.
11. Mayfield L, Bratthall G, Attstrom R. Periodontal probe precision using four different periodontal probes. J Clin Periodontol 23:76–82, 1996.
12. Aguero A, Garnick JJ, et al. Histological location of a standardized periodontal probe in man. J Periodontol 66:184–190, 1995.
13. Keagle JG, Garnick JJ, et al. Gingival resistance to probing forces: Determination of optimal probe diameter. J Periodontol 60:167–171, 1989.
14. Van der Welden U. Errors in the assessment of pocket depth in vitro. J .Clin periodontol 5:182–187, 1978.
15. Chauncey HH, Glass RL, Alman JE. Dental caries, principal cause of tooth extraction in a sample of US male adults. Caries Res 23:200–205, 1989.
16. Hintze H, Wenzel A, Larsen MJ. Stereomicroscopy, film radiography, microradiography and naked-eye inspection of tooth sections as validation for occlusal caries diagnosis. Caries Res 29:359–363, 1995.
17. Wenzel A. Digital radiography and caries diagnosis. Dentomaxillofac Radiol 1:3–11, 1998.
18. Hee MR, et al. Polarization-sensitive low-coherence reflectometer for birefringence characterization and ranging. J Opt Soc Am B 9(6):903–908, 1992.

19. de Boer JF, Milner TE, vanGemert MJC, Nelson JS. Two-dimensional birefringence imaging in biological tissue by polarization-sensitive optical coherence tomography. Opt Lett 22(12):934–936, 1997.
20. de Boer JF, Milner TE, Nelson JS. Determination of the depth-resolved Stokes parameters of light backscattered from turbid media by use of polarization-sensitive optical coherence tomography. Opt Lett 24(5):300–302, 1999.
21. Everett MJ, Schoenenberger K, Colston BW Jr, DaSilva LB. Birefringence characterization of biological tissue using optical coherence tomography. Opt Lett 23:228–230, 1998.
22. Warren JA, Gelikonov GV, Gelikonov VM, Feldchtein FI, Sergeev AM, Beach NM, Moores MD, Reitze DH. Imaging and characterization of dental structure using optical coherence tomography. Opt Soc Am Tech Dig 6:128, 1998.
23. Leinfelder KF, Lemons JE. Clinical Restoration materials and Techniques. Philadelphia: Lea & Febiger, 1988.
24. Cvar JF, Ryge G. Criteria for the Clinical Evaluation of Dental Restoration Materials. San Francisco: US Dept HEW PHS, Dental Health Center, 1971.

23

Surgical Guidance and Intervention

STEPHEN A. BOPPART and JAMES G. FUJIMOTO

Massachusetts Institute of Technology, Cambridge, Massachusetts

MARK E. BREZINSKI

Harvard Medical School, Massachusetts General Hospital, Boston, Massachusetts

23.1 IMAGE-GUIDED SURGERY

The use of imaging modalities for surgical guidance has the potential to improve patient outcome and reduce patient morbidity. If the surgeon is provided with enhanced abilities to view or image tissue intraoperatively, then collateral damage to normal tissue can be minimized. Imaging techniques may also enhance discrimination between normal and abnormal tissues by exploiting differences in tissue properties that cannot be recognized with standard visual cues. Integrating imaging modalities with surgical techniques requires solutions to a number of technical problems. Resolution and contrast must be sufficient to discriminate microstructural tissue morphology. Fast image acquisition is necessary to eliminate motion artifacts from either the patient's physiological processes or the surgeon's repositioning of instruments. An accurate system of registration between acquired images and the tissue is necessary to enable guidance of the surgical procedure. Overcoming these technical challenges of introducing imaging modalities into the surgical suite will no doubt improve patient care.

The surgical suite is a demanding environment that presents challenges for optical coherence tomographic (OCT) imaging. The sterile surgical field requires that all instruments be frequently sterilized with high temperatures and pressures. Often the surgical field is small, making it difficult to integrate additional surgical instruments into the field. The number of instruments available and the frequency with which the surgeon must switch between instruments must be kept to a minimum. Finally, the presence of blood and other body fluids can quickly obscure the viewing and imaging capabilities of optical instruments. Still, it is essential for the surgeon to visualize the tissue he or she is operating on, and imaging modalities that enable better visualization will be of interest to the surgical community. Imaging modalities such as computed tomography (CT), magnetic resonance imaging (MRI), ultrasound (US), and microscopy are techniques that play a role in surgery both in and out of the operating room. Minimally invasive surgery (MIS) uses multiple small incisions through which imaging and mechanical instruments are passed. These MIS instruments can be flexible, such as the endoscope for examining the upper and lower gastrointestinal tract, or rigid, such as the laparoscope for transabdominal access. In MIS, the surgeon does not have full visualization as in the open surgical field; therefore, imaging instruments play a critical role.

Principles for image-guided interventions and surgery have been established [1]. One precedent for image-guided surgery is the open-magnet MRI, which permits the surgeon to obtain three-dimensional (3-D) MRI volumes of the surgical field intraoperatively [2,3]. These instruments, few in number, are extremely expensive and complex systems. Studies have yet to show a positive patient outcome compared to standard surgical procedures, partly because of the relatively small numbers of patients undergoing these procedures. Ultrasound has been used to guide placement of needles for biopsies with good success due to imaging penetrations of 10–30 cm. However, 100 μm resolutions limit ultrasound to imaging larger tissue morphology. Optical coherence tomography can produce high resolution cross-sectional images of biological tissue [4–8]. Advances in OCT technology have permitted in vivo biological imaging in real time [9,10]. The high resolution of OCT may enable image-guided surgery to approach another level of investigation. OCT has already been demonstrated for imaging surgically relevant tissue [11–14], and imaging may be performed at near-histological or cellular resolutions [15]. The localization of small vessels and nerves may be possible, as may the discrimination of abnormal neoplastic tissue. The use of OCT for surgical diagnostics, guidance, and intervention could enhance the precision of existing procedures as well as make new ones possible [16]. In this chapter, applications in surgical guidance and intervention are demonstrated with examples of OCT for guiding microsurgical anastomosis of arteries and nerves, avoiding sensitive structures, identifying pathological tissue, determining tumor margins, and guiding laser intervention. Taken together, the high resolution, high speed imaging capabilities of OCT offer a new methodological approach to intraoperative surgical guidance and intervention.

23.1.1 Current Modalities

The integration of imaging modalities into the surgical suite has been fueled by improvements in visualization and the additional information that can be obtained from the tissue. Light microscopy has been well established in the surgical suite, particularly for microsurgery of vessels [17] and nerves [18] and for delicate procedures involving the central nervous system [19]. Surgical microscopes and loupes magnify the tissue under examination to recognize and avoid injury, visualize abnormal changes, and practice delicate surgical techniques using fine microsurgical instruments and suture materials. Resolutions as high as 1 μm can be achieved with high magnification surgical microscopes. The disadvantages of light microscopy in surgery, however, include the limited field of view and the inability to visualize subsurface tissue morphology.

Computed tomography has been primarily used to plan surgical procedures and guide placement of needle biopsies. Within a single plane, resolutions of 0.5–1.0 mm are possible [20]; multiple planes are acquired by stepping the patient through the source–detector plane in increments of 5–10 mm. X-rays have been applied to microscopy for research applications. The shorter wavelengths of X-ray ($\approx$ 1 nm) compared to those of visible wavelengths (300–700 nm) allow higher resolutions. Using a configuration with a single source and detector that is scanned over specimens, X-rays have been used to image in vitro insects [21] and more recently individual live bacteria with 200 nm resolutions—high enough to resolve bacterial DNA [22].

Magnetic resonance imaging is ideally suited for whole-body or organ imaging. The resolution of MRI is dependent on the magnetic field strength that can be generated within the tissue. Most clinical MRI machines have a 1.5 T magnet and provide 0.5–1 mm resolution within an imaging plane [23]. Image acquisition times have been reduced to 50 ms. The instrument size is equivalent to that of a CT scanner. However, extra precautions are necessary surrounding the magnet to prevent the introduction of metal instruments, which are attracted to the strong magnetic field. Engineering improvements in the MRI technology have enabled high resolution research systems for MRI microscopy. Resolutions as high as 12 μm have been demonstrated on in vivo *Xenopus laevis* (African frog) tadpoles during development [24,25]. However, to attain these resolutions, 7 T field strengths are needed across small ($\approx$ 1 cm) magnet bores. Acquisition times are prohibitively slow, with three-dimensional volumes of developing tadpoles requiring 2 h. Gadolinium contrast agents can be used to label blood flow within mouse embryos, and striking image sequences of vascular development in the mouse have been demonstrated [26].

Ultrasound is routinely used in an outpatient setting with image guidance used for the placement of needles for biopsy. Ultrasound transducers have been placed on the tips of endoscopes and laparoscopes to develop multimodality instruments for imaging subsurface tissue structures [27]. Transducers less than 1 mm in size have been placed within rotating catheters for intravascular ultrasound (IVUS) imaging of atherosclerosis and stenosis in human coronary arteries [28]. Most clinically available instruments today operate at 10–20 MHz, with high frequency ultrasound considered to be 30 MHz and higher. These acoustic frequencies provide 100–200 μm resolutions with imaging depths up to tens of centimeters [29]. Ultrasound backscatter microscopy is a research field employing extremely high frequency transducers (> 100 MHz) to image microstructure [30]. High frequency ultrasound, however, is more highly attenuated in biological tissue, limiting the imaging penetration depth. Human myocardial cells have been imaged with 1.7 μm resolutions using a 600 MHz transducer [31]. However, a fixed 5 μm thick tissue section was used as the sample because image penetration was poor. Currently, these ultrahigh resolutions are not available in any clinical instrument. Ultrasound backscatter microscopy using 40–100 MHz transducers providing 17–30 μm axial and 33–94 μm lateral resolution has been applied clinically for imaging skin in humans and the progression of melanoma in the mouse animal model [32,33].

23.1.2 Minimally Invasive Surgery

Minimally invasive surgery (MIS) is a relatively new methodology that has contributed significantly to patient care by reducing the morbidity associated with more invasive procedures. By reducing the size of the surgical access site, patient recovery time and risk of infection are likewise reduced. Because of this, MIS procedures are becoming the standard for many surgical procedures. The increase in MIS procedures has, in turn, resulted in advancements in instrument design. Optical as well as nonoptical imaging technologies have been developed for specific tissue or organ system access [34]. Examples include the rigid laparoscope for abdominal or pelvic access, the flexible bronchoscope or endoscope for respiratory or gastrointestinal systems, and the small rigid arthroscope for access into joint spaces. Recent advancements have begun to take advantage of synergistic benefits from multiple imaging modalities integrated into a single MIS instrument [27,35,36]. Common to all instruments, both mechanically and optically, are design features that permit entry via narrow incisions or natural body openings.

Endoscopy is a well-established technique used primarily for visualizing tortuous internal body lumens and cavities. Although specific names have been given to endoscopic procedures in each organ system, the general technique involves the insertion of a long, thin, and flexible device for video-based imaging of surface features at remote internal sites. The use of endoscopes include the investigation and biopsy of sites throughout the gastrointestinal tract ranging from the esophagus and stomach to the small intestine and colon [37]. Using bronchoscopes, the respiratory tract is visualized and biopsied. Tumors of the lung are imaged during video-assisted thoracic surgical (VATS) procedures [38]. The urinary tract is examined for polyps or masses using cystoscopy. Endoscopes can be made extremely small in diameter, permitting the passage into individual vessels (angioscopy) for the repair of valves [39].

Laparoscopy is becoming the standard for cholecystectomy, tubal sterilization, and aspiration of ovarian cysts. Laparoscopy is increasingly being used for diagnosing abdominal disorders [40] and for staging intra-abdominal malignancies [41]. In fact, laparoscopy has even been found to be significantly more sensitive and more accurate than either US or CT for detecting intra-abdominal metastases [42]. Unlike the flexible endoscope, the laparoscope is a rigid instrument approximately 2–10 mm in diameter and 10–40 cm in length. The rigid design permits the use of glass optical relay elements to relay the image from the distal end to the proximal end [43], where it is either observed with the human eye or digitized with a charge-coupled device (CCD) camera and displayed on a monitor. The hallmark MIS procedure is laparoscopic cholecystectomy, which is now a gold standard because of its high success rate, the efficiency with which the procedure can be performed, and the low level of postoperative morbidity [44,45].

23.2 SURGICAL GUIDANCE WITH OPTICAL COHERENCE TOMOGRAPHY

Optical coherence tomography is a new modality for surgical guidance. The high resolution (2–10 μm) of OCT imaging is unique compared to many of the other surgical guidance modalities. Because of this, OCT has the potential to explore tissue morphology from a previously unrealized perspective. Performing surgical procedures under guidance at near-histological resolutions is a new methodological approach. In addition to its high resolution, several features of OCT suggest that it will be useful for guiding surgical procedures. First, unlike MRI, the OCT instrument is compact and portable, approximately the size of a personal computer. Second, unlike ultrasound, OCT is noncontact, with no requirement for a transducing medium. Third, the fiber-based design allows straightforward integration with scalpels, microscopes, or pencil-sized hand held probes, which are well suited for the tight confines of the operative suite [46,47]. Developments in high speed OCT imaging and beam delivery systems have provided the necessary advancements for the use of OCT in surgical guidance. Mechanisms for rapid axial scanning have enabled real-time OCT imaging at up to several frames per second. Image acquisition at these rates eliminates the majority of motion artifacts induced by either patient or surgeon movement. More important, real-time acquisition yields high speed visual data for the surgeon, providing him or her with feedback during exploration or intervention. Used alone or as an adjunct imaging modality with CCD-based imaging, OCT has the potential to improve visualization during surgical procedures.

In this chapter we will outline several scenarios where OCT imaging can be applied to surgical guidance and cite examples of each. OCT imaging for surgical guidance is demonstrated with examples of three-dimensional imaging for improved visualization of spatially complex structures. Because microsurgical procedures are often limited by visualization of small structures, OCT is used to monitor the microsurgical repair of small vessels and nerves. By intraoperatively identifying sensitive structures such as vessels and nerves, OCT may help reduce iatrogenic injury. OCT is used to identify and localize pathological tissue such as tumors. Biopsy sampling rates maybe improved if OCT can intraoperatively identify abnormal tissue. Complete tumor resection is crucial. Because OCT can image at near-histological resolutions, OCT may have the potential to more precisely identify tumor margins. Imaging of lymph nodes suggests that OCT may be effective at recognizing changes in node morphology that reflect tumor involvements.

23.2.1 Three-Dimensional OCT Imaging

Three-dimensional OCT imaging provides a surgical diagnostic tool for improved visualization of tissue structure. Improved visualization is critical for assessing proper approaches for surgical resection of tumors, particularly when vessels and nerves are in close proximity or intertwined. Understanding the network of vessels and nerves is extremely difficult on the basis of a series of 2-D images because of the unpredictable 3-D spatial orientations that these structures may have. The importance of binocular viewing and 3-D imaging is most appreciated when it is absent, as in current MIS endoscopes and laparoscopes. The 2-D image of distant tissue visualized through endoscopes and laparoscopes makes surgical manipulation extremely difficult.

The acquisition of 3-D data has three primary advantages: (1) The entire volume representing the 3-D configuration of the tissue is available for analysis, (2) the 3-D volume can be rotated about arbitrary axes and visualized at arbitrary angles, and (3) the 3-D volume of data can be resectioned postacquisition to extract 2-D planes along axes different from the axes in which the data were collected. A 3-D OCT data set allows repeatable resectioning at arbitrary planes, particularly at cross-sectional planes that can be correlated with histological findings. The user is not confined to the imaging plane established at the time of data collection. This is an advantage over histology, where a single sectioning plane is identified and maintained.

Several algorithms exist for representing data in three dimensions. The reconstruction can be performed on the volume as a whole using voxels or only on the surface using sheets of polygons. Three-dimensional projections project the 3-D data volume onto a 2-D screen positioned at arbitrary angles. When sectioning 3-D OCT data sets, only the selected planes are seen, and much of the information in the data set is not used. The volumetric display of 3-D reconstructions incorporates all of the 3-D voxel information. The imaged tissue represents an object that has both surface and volume features. Generating an image of an object's surface that approximates the appearance of a real physical surface is a process called surface rendering. Smooth surface rendering of 3-D objects requires the use of triangles or polygons to connect adjacent discrete-height pixels [48,49]. Creating realistic-looking objects is computationally difficult because of the number of polygons that must be calculated and drawn. Surface rendering can be combined with transparency factors to permit visualization of structures within the 3-D volume. In this case, volume rendering must be performed, increasing the level of computation.

Examples of three-dimensional OCT reconstructions using surface and volume rendering are shown in Fig. 1. These renderings were generated from a series of 60

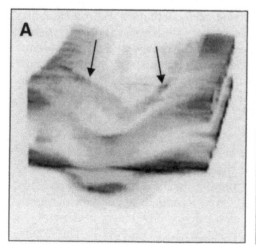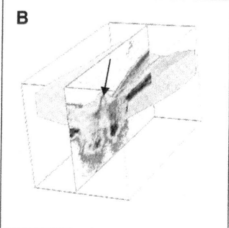

Figure 1 Three-dimensional surface and volume rendering of in vivo optic disk. (A) Arrows indicate retinal vessels exiting optic disk. (B) Cross section through volume-rendered data set illustrates retinal vessel lumen (arrow). (From Ref. 16.)

cross-sectional OCT images of the in vivo rhesus optic disk as part of an OCT imaging study investigating retinal injury [50]. OCT images were imported and processed on a computer workstation (Silicon Graphics, Inc., Mountain View, CA) using SegmentView software [51]. The surface rendering of the 3-D data set is shown in Fig 1A. From this 3-D surface image, the spatial orientation of the retinal vessels can be observed as they exit the optic disk (arrows). Volume rendering was performed on the same data set and shown in Fig. 1B. A highlighted slice through the volume-rendered data shows a retinal artery lumen (arrow). Three-dimensional images of the optic disk may be useful for the assessment of early stages of glaucoma when changes in cup-to-disk ratio occur.

Three-dimensional projections are obtained from less computationally taxing algorithms. A series of 2-D images represent a stack or 3-D volume. Projections of this 3-D volume are made onto a 2-D screen located at arbitrary positions. The projection onto the 2-D screen can be the maximum value, mean value, or sum of values through the 3-D volume. Variations in surface and interior depth cuing as well as surface and depth opacity permit the highlighting of particular features. Three-dimensional OCT projections of the developing *Xenopus laevis* (African frog) heart [52] are shown in Chapter 19, Fig. 6. Four projections of the 3-D data set illustrate the 3-D morphological arrangement of developing cardiac structure, which is often difficult to envision from a series of 2-D images. Additional examples of 3-D OCT projections will be illustrated in later sections of this chapter.

Current limitations for 3-D OCT imaging in surgery include the lack of high speed, multiaxis beam delivery systems, fast image acquisition rates, and maintenance of image registration. Surgical microscopes, handheld surgical probes, and laparoscopes can be readily modified for 3-D OCT imaging by the addition of orthogonal scanning mirrors to direct and scan the OCT beam in the operating field. Three-dimensional OCT imaging with endoscopes requires the implementation of an additional translation mechanism similar to that used in 3-D intravascular ultrasound imaging [53,54]. For example, radial-imaging OCT catheters [47] used in biological lumens would require a computer-controlled motorized pullback system to translate the rotating beam along the axis of the catheter, thereby collecting a 3-D data set in the form of a cylinder. OCT image acquisition times are primarily limited by the axial scanning mechanism. High speed phase-controlled optical delay lines have demonstrated axial scanning at 2000 Hz [55]. Faster scanning rates are possible using a resonant galvanometer in the optical delay line. However, for moderate 3-D volumes sizes ($256 \times 256 \times 256$ pixels), no current mechanism is capable of acquisition rates sufficient for real-time 3-D intraoperative guidance. Difficulties with image registration during 3-D OCT data acquisition are due to the limitation in 3-D volume acquisition rates. Patient and surgeon movement during 3-D volume acquisitions result in motion artifacts in OCT images. Although computer algorithms can correct for small positional changes, technological advancements for faster acquisition rates will likely improve on this limitation as well.

23.2.2 OCT Image-Guided Microsurgery

"Microsurgery" refers to microscopic techniques used to repair injured or severed vessels and nerves. The repair of vessels and nerves is necessary to restore function following traumatic injury [56]. Although the repair of these sensitive structures is performed with the aid of surgical microscopes and loupes to magnify the surgical field [17], surgeons are limited to the *en face* view that they provide. A technique capable of subsurface, three-dimensional, micrometer scale imaging in real time would permit the intraoperative monitoring of microsurgical procedures, offering immediate feedback to the surgeon and likely an improvement in patient outcome. The capabilities of OCT for the intraoperative assessment of microsurgical procedures has been demonstrated [13]. High speed OCT imaging was integrated with a surgical microscope to performed micrometer scale three-dimensional imaging on microsurgical specimens.

The ability of OCT to assess internal structure and luminal patency within an arterial anastomosis was demonstrated by acquiring the cross-sectional OCT image (2.2 mm × 2.2 mm, 250 × 600 pixels) and 3-D projections of a 1 mm diameter in vitro rabbit inguinal artery shown in Fig. 2A. The arterial segment was bisected cross

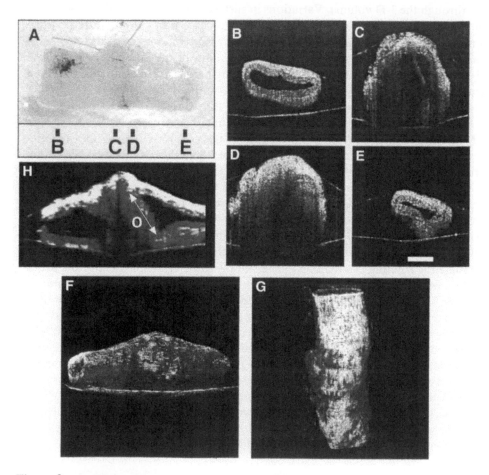

Figure 2 Arterial anastomosis. Labeled vertical lines in (A) refer to cross sectional imaging locations (B–E) from an anastomosis of an in vitro rabbit artery. An obstructive flap is identified in (C). By resectioning the 3-D data set, a complete obstruction is observed in (H). Horizontally and vertically rotated 3-D projections are shown in (F) and (G), respectively. f, flap; o, occlusion. Bar represents 1 mm. (From Ref. 13.)

sectionally with a scalpel and then reanastomosed. A No. 10-0 nylon suture with a 50 μm diameter needle was used to place a continuous suture and perform and end-to-end anastomosis. For precise registration of 3-D images, the anastomosed segment was positioned on micrometer step, computer-controlled, motorized translational stages for OCT imaging A series of 40 cross-sectional images were acquired perpendicular to the long axis at 100 μm interval spacing. Imaging was performed through the anastomosis site and several milimeters on either side of it. Following imaging, the specimen was digitally imaged with a CCD camera.

Two-dimensional cross-sectional images in Figs 2B–2E were acquired from the locations labeled in Fig. 2A. Figures 2B and 2E were acquired from each end of the anastomosis. These images clearly show arterial morphology corresponding to the intimal, medial, and adventitial layers of the elastic artery. The muscular media appears less backscattering than the adventitia, which merges with the surrounding collagenous tissue. The patent lumen is readily apparent. This is in contrast to what is observed in Fig. 2D, where at the site of anastomosis the lumen has been obstructed by tissue. The image in Fig. 2C reveals the obstructing tissue in cross section. Note that the presence of additional tissue has attenuated the signal from the lower wall and hence reduces the resolution of individual layers. by assembling a series of cross-sectional 2-D images, a 3-D data set was produced. From this data set, arbitrary planes can be selected and corresponding sections displayed. For an arterial anastomosis, often it is more informative to image longitudinally along the axis of the artery and through the anastomosis site. Figure 2H is a longitudinal section from the 3-D data set that confirms the occlusion within the anastomosis site.

Three-dimensional projections of the arterial anastomosis are shown in Figs. 2F and 2G. These horizontally and vertically rotated projections each comprise 80 slices at 50 μm spacing. At this high slice density, the internal structure shown in Figs. 2B–2E is difficult to visualize. However, high slice densities are necessary if the 3-D data set is to be sectioned at arbitrary planes as shown in Fig. 2H. Additionally, micrometer scale surface features that were not readily apparent from the 2-D slices are more prominent.

During microsurgical procedures, patient outcome can be substantially influenced by the ability of the surgeon to assess tissue microstructure [57]. The use of a surgical microscope serves to magnify the tissue but only provides a surface, or *en face*, view. OCT should improve intraoperative diagnostics by providing high resolution, subsurface, cross-sectional imaging of vessels in real time. The in vitro arterial anastomosis imaged in Fig. 2 demonstrates the ability to assess internal structure within an anastomosis site and evaluate patency. Intraoperative assessment of luminal obstructions is critical if a successful procedure is to be performed. OCT can be used to identify the location of the obstruction and its longitudinal extent. This would include the presence of a thrombogenic adventitial flap or intimal inversion, which predisposes the site to postoperative subacute occlusion.

The peripheral nervous system encompasses distal nerves that relay sensory and motor signals to and from the central nervous system. Peripheral nerves are frequently injured during complex surgical procedures and trauma, often requiring the microsurgical anastomosis or reconnection of the two severed ends [18]. The incidence of neurosensory changes in the oral cavity and lip ranges from 0.4% to 11.5% following mandibular third molar removal because of the proximity to the lingual and inferior alveolar nerves [57]. Trauma seen at military medical units during troop engagements are predominantly of the limbs, requiring microsurgical repair of small vessels and nerves [59]. A peripheral nerve is actually a bundle of fascicles contained within an outer sheath called the epineurium. Microsurgical anastomosis can be performed either epineurally or perineurally [60]. Epineural anastomosis involves suturing only the outer neural sheath. Greater neural function is restored if the corresponding fascicles can be aligned during perineural attachment. This, however, requires the identification of fascicles based on their longitudinal orientation and their relative diameter. Currently, no technique exists for obtaining this information without physical dissection of the nerve ex vivo.

Optical coherence tomography has been used to image in vitro peripheral nerves and identify individual fascicles [13]. Longitudinal tracking of the spatial orientation of rabbit peripheral nerve fascicles is demonstrated in Fig. 3 using OCT. Representative cross-sectional images (3 mm × 2.2, 300 × 600 pixels) of the peripheral nerve are shown in Figs. 3A–3D. For each slice, one fascicle was manually segmented, colored white, and tracked through the acquired volume of data. Forty

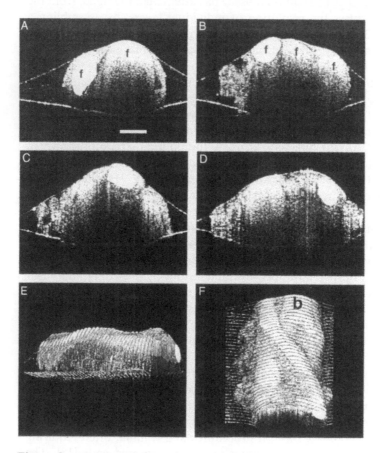

Figure 3 (A–D) Longitudinal tracking of rabbit peripheral nerve fascicles. A single fascicle was segmented and followed longitudinally along the length of the in vitro nerve. (E,F) Three-dimensional projections rotated in the horizontal and vertical directions. b, bifurcation; f, fascicle. Bar represents 1 mm. (From Ref. 13.)

images at $100\,\mu$m spacing were assembled for the 3-D projections shown in Figs 3E and 3F. The horizontally and vertically rotated projections of the peripheral nerve dramatically reveal the twisted path of the segmented fascicle along the longitudinal axis of the nerve. In addition, a branch in another, unsegmented fascicle is observed in Fig. 3F. Previously, this feature had not been recognized from examining the 2-D images.

Precision realignment of individual nerve fascicles increases the likelihood that end-organ function will be restored after peripheral nerve reconstruction [61]. These results show that OCT can image peripheral nerves in cross section and that individual fascicles can be identified and segmented. The use of OCT to acquire multiple cross-sectional images and three-dimensionally reconstruct the peripheral nerve offers the opportunity to determine the relative diameters of individual fascicles and to longitudinally track their spatial orientation. The 3-D projection of the segmented peripheral nerve in Fig. 3F not only revealed the twisted course of one fascicle but also revealed a bifurcation of a second fascicle, a feature not previously appreciated from the 2-D images.

A surgical microscope-based OCT system was used to demonstrate the potential of OCT for guiding microsurgical procedures. Performance of many fine surgical procedures in vulnerable tissue would likely benefit from high resolution subsurface imaging. By imaging and recognizing vessels, nerves, and other sensitive tissues intraoperatively, iatrogenic injury is likely to be reduced. In an analogous manner to Doppler ultrasound, OCT may be configured to perform laser-Doppler velocimetry. This technique has been used to measure blood flow velocities through in vivo animal model vessels [62] and may be useful for assessing perfusion following vascular anastomosis. Potential limitations of OCT include the imaging penetration and the effect of blood within the surgical field. Utilizing longer wavelengths in the near-infrared, imaging depths have been increased from 1 mm (using 800 nm wavelengths) up to 2–3 mm (using 1300 nm wavelengths) due to decreased optical absorption and scattering in tissue. These depths may still appear somewhat limiting. However, the majority of microsurgical complications occur in vessels less than 2 mm in diameter and are suitable for OCT imaging. The presence of blood in the surgical field may influence the quality of OCT images.

These results have shown how 2-D OCT images and 3-D OCT projections can provide diagnostic feedback to assess microsurgical anastomoses. This previously unavailable diagnostic ability offers the potential to directly impact and improve patient outcome by incorporating high speed, high resolution intraoperative image guidance during microsurgical procedures.

23.2.3 Reducing Iatrogenic Injury

Iatrogenic injury is defined as an adverse physical condition induced in a patient by the effects of treatment by a surgeon. Examples in surgery include making incisions at improper locations, extending incisions larger than necessary, and inadvertently incising sensitive tissue structures such as vessels and nerves. One study predicted that advancements in technology and complexity in surgery would increase the rate of iatrogenic injury, but the advancements would outweigh the adverse events, resulting in improved surgical outcomes [63]. As a high resolution subsurface imaging modality for surgical guidance, OCT has the potential to reduce iatrogenic injury during surgical procedures. OCT must provide real-time imaging that differentiates tissue morphology, enabling the surgeon to rapidly and accurately identify sensitive tissue structures and discriminate between normal and pathological tissue. Identifying and avoiding vessels and nerves as well as sensitive tissue of the central nervous and cardiovascular systems will likely reduce iatrogenic injury. Two examples in this section demonstrate the use of OCT for identifying and avoiding sensitive structures.

A surgical microscope was modified to perform high speed OCT imaging. A pair of orthogonal galvanometer scanners and a dichroic mirror directed the OCT imaging beam in the optical axis of the surgical microscope. To demonstrate the ability of OCT to locate vessels and sensitive structures embedded in highly scattering tissue in real time, a 1 cm^3 block of in vitro human tissue was removed from the left lateral ankle of an amputated foot. The foot had been amputated as a result of complications associated with vascular insufficiency secondary to diabetes mellitus. The surgical microscope was used to obtain the images shown in Fig. 4. Because the OCT imaging beam and visible aiming beam were coaligned with the optical axis of the microscope, the scan location on the specimen could be directly viewed through the microscope. The magnified view enabled visualization of small surface structures and the precise alignment of the OCT scan location on the tissue. The block of tissue was manually manipulated under the microscope while images (3 mm × 2.75 mm 25 6 × 256 pixels) were acquired at 8 frames per second. Subsurface microsurgical structures were immediately identified, including numerous small arteries, veins, and nerves and even a vascular clip from a previous surgical repair. All structures were embedded in adipose and connective tissue. Figure 4A illustrates a cross section of an artery located 500 μm below the surface and surrounded by adipose tissue. This artery could not be visualized through the microscope alone but was readily apparent in the OCT image display. The image clearly shows the characteristically thick wall and multiple layers of the artery. To the right of the artery is a portion of dense connective tissue that does not have the clear, low-backscattering regions present in adipose tissue. Figure 4b is a longitudinal section of the same artery after the tissue

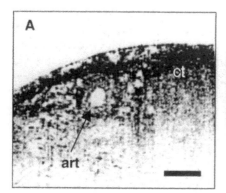 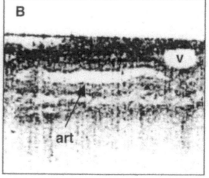

Figure 4 High-speed (8 fps) imaging of embedded in vitro human vessels. (A) Cross sectional image of artery adjacent to connective tissue. (B) The same artery was rotated and viewed in longitudinal cross section. An oblique cross section of a vein is also observed. art, artery; ct, connective tissue; v, vein. Bar represents 500 μm. (From Ref. 13.)

block had been rotated by 90°. The thick arterial wall is readily identified. The right edge of Fig. 4b shows an oblique cross section of a vein with its characteristic thin wall. The tissue block was stored in saline prior to imaging. Hence, the lumens of the artery and the vein were filled with saline rather than blood. The saline-filled lumens have low optical backscatter compared to the surrounding tissue.

Iatrogenic injury to vessels and nerves has the potential to increase patient morbidity and mortality. The repair of these structures following iatrogenic injury results in increased operation times, which can substantially delay the progress of the surgical procedure. Therefore, avoiding such injury will be extremely beneficial to both the patient and the surgeon. To prevent iatrogenic injury, high speed subsurface OCT imaging may provide forewarning to the surgeon as to the proximity of vulnerable tissue structures.

23.2.4 Guiding Biopsies

The ability of OCT to discriminate between tissue morphologies has practical application for guiding surgical biopsies. A biopsy is a procedure in which a portion of tissue is physically removed for ex vivo histological processing and light microscopic examination. The placement of the biopsy instrument is usually guided with some imaging technique as in ultrasound-guided needle biopsies of breast masses or endoscope-guided resection of colonic polyps and lesions. For screening procedures, as in the endoscopic examination of Barrett's esophagus patients for disease progression to adenocarcinoma, random biopsies are obtained every several centimeters throughout the distal esophagus in search of small foci of neoplastic tissue. This screening and sampling procedure is time-consuming and costly. It is recommended that patients undergo endoscopy every 6 months, and the repeated biopsies result in significant morbidity for the patient. In this and other similar screening scenarios, sampling errors are high, thereby giving unacceptably high false-negative rates. The high resolutions of OCT may improve sampling error rates by intraoperatively directing the placement of biopsy instruments to suspect regions of tissue. In addition, by reducing the number of biopsy specimens that are required, processing time, costs, and patient discomfort are all minimized. Examples of OCT imaging applications for guiding biopsies in the gastrointestinal tract, in the female reproductive tract, and in lymph nodes are demonstrated.

The upper and lower gastrointestinal tracts are readily accessed with catheters and flexible endoscopes [64]. Diagnostic procedures provide *en face* visualization of the epithelial lining to evaluate colonic polyps or esophageal disorders. Barrett's esophagus is a condition where the stratified squamous epithelial lining of the lower esophagus is replaced by columnar epithelium of the stomach [65]. This metaplastic change is likely a result of acid reflux from the stomach and is found in up to 20% of patients who undergo endoscopic examination for evaluation of gastroesophageal reflux disease [66]. Patients with Barrett's esophagus are 30–40 times more likely to develop adenocarcinoma than the general population [67]. Therefore, these patients must be routinely examined endoscopically and biopsied. High resolution imaging with OCT may be useful to sample large areas of the esophagus and to guide surgical biopsy for diagnosis. Imaging of the in vitro human gastrointestinal tract has been performed with OCT [68,69], including some of the common neoplasms [70]. Depths of penetration are sufficient to image through the esophageal mucosa and submucosa. Resolutions are sufficient to identify morphological changes of colonic inflammation and pseudomembranes. To demonstrate high speed catheter-based OCT imaging of in vivo esophageal mucosa, a rabbit animal model was used. Representative catheter-acquired images are shown in Fig. 5. The upper esophagus, shown in Fig. 5A, reveals a lumen with fewer folds. The OCT image in Fig. 5A demonstrates full-thickness imaging through the esophageal wall. The OCT image in Fig. 5B shows increasing numbers of folds. The lower esophageal sphincter is shown in Fig. 5C. The esophageal wall is surrounded by smooth muscle. OCT imaging penetration falls off rapidly in the outer muscle layers.

The in vivo images of the rabbit esophageal epithelium suggest a feasibility for staging and following conditions such as Barrett's esophagus. Because early dysplastic changes result in an increase in numbers and sizes of epithelial nuclei, changes in optical backscatter may be able to identify suspect regions. Larger scale structural epithelial changes occurring in later stages of Barrett's esophagus will be even more evident.

The use of minimally invasive surgical and diagnostic optical techniques is frequently applied to imaging the organs of the female reproductive tract. OCT has shown feasibility for imaging the microstructural features of the fallopian tubes [71]. Laparoscopic imaging is becoming the gold standard for diagnostic and surgical gynecological procedures such as tubal ligation, management of benign

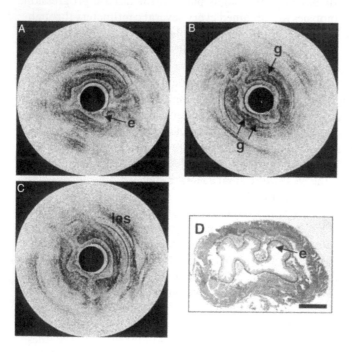

Figure 5 In vivo rabbit esophagus at three longitudinal positions. Images were acquired at 4 frames per second using a radial imaging OCT catheter. OCT images of the (A) proximal, (B) middle, and (C) distal esophagus with (D) corresponding histology show varying morphological features including muscular layers, secretory glands (g), stratified squamous epithelium (e), and the lower esophageal sphincter (les). Bar represents 1 mm.

ovarian cysts, and oophrectomy. Laparoscopy is used as a second-look procedure when ultrasound resolutions fail to diagnose ovarian pathology and has been suggested as a surgical screening tool for the early detection of ovarian cancer [72]. Although laparoscopy provides a closer look at tissue structure, only surface features are visible and subsurface microstructural abnormalities are undetectable. A nonexcisional means of imaging tissue at near-histological resolutions has the potential to improve diagnostic capability without the need to physically respect suspect samples of sensitive tissue.

Optical coherence tomography was used to image over 80 in vitro sites on laparoscopically accessible gynecological pathology to demonstrate its feasibility for imaging and assessing normal and abnormal microstructure [73]. Images were correlated with histology. High speed nonexcisional OCT imaging through laparoscopes has the potential to guide biopsies or even increase and improve sampling without the need for physical resection. Intraoperative OCT imaging has the potential for in situ diagnoses of early-stage gynecological neoplasms [74].

The laparoscopic approach to the uterus is transabdominal. The peritoneal surface of the uterus is often the site of endometrial foci. Endometriosis is the transplantation of endometrial cells from the interior uterine wall to sites on the peritoneal abdominal wall, peritoneal surface of the uterus, ovaries, or fallopian tubes. Studies suggest that this occurs as a result of cells passing through the fallopian tubes following endometrial wall shedding [75]. The growth of endometrial sites results in extreme abdominal pain. In a recent U.S. Health Interview Survey, 50% of those reporting having endometriosis had stayed in bed all day because of their condition at some time during the previous year, with the average of 17.8 bed-days [76], Thus, this disease is costly in terms of a woman's quality of life, medical expenses, and impact in the workplace. Because endometriosis can be definitively diagnosed only during a course of pelvic surgery or laparoscopic exam, prevalence estimates are based on surgical populations. Endometriosis was diagnosed in approximately 25% of women (range is 4.5–82% across all studies) who had laparoscopy because of pelvic pain [77]. Surgical treatment is by laparoscope-guided ablation of foci with either electrosurgery, radio-frequency electrodes, or a laser. Visual determination of endometrial sites is difficult, relying solely on surface color cues. Foci can also be located below the peritoneal surface, making *en face* visualization and diagnosis uncertain. OCT was used to image subsurface endometrial foci to demonstrate its feasibility for improved discrimination.

Cross-sectional OCT images (6 mm × 3 mm, 600 × 400 pixels) were obtained in vitro from the peritoneal surface of each specimen, with the orientation consistent with that encountered during a laparoscopic examination. Figure 6 compares and contrasts normal human uterus with a site of endometriosis. Both images were acquired from the peritoneal surface that would be imaged laparoscopically. The normal peritoneal uterine surface in Fig. 6A shows a relatively smooth peritoneal surface with occasional invaginations. Small regions of adipose cells surrounded by normal myometrium are observed in the OCT image. This is in contrast to the endometriosis observed in Fig. 6B. The elevated peritoneal surface with irregular boundaries and glandular spaces is indicative of secretory endometrium. It is this tissue morphology that is believed to result in extreme abdominal pain.

Ovarian cancer has a high mortality rate largely due to poor techniques for early detection. In 1998, ovarian cancer was responsible for over half of the deaths

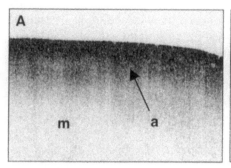
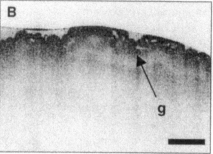

Figure 6   Endometriosis. (A) Normal peritoneal surface of in vitro human uterus and (B) endometriosis. a, adipose cells, g, glandular tissue; m, myometrium. Bar represents 1 mm.

from neoplasms of the female reproductive system [78]. High resolution in vitro OCT imaging from the external surface of the ovary can identify morphological differences as shown in Fig. 7. Normal ovary in Fig. 7A is relatively homogeneous compared to the cystic and papillary structures observed in the ovarian tumor shown in Fig. 7B. The ability to image and diagnose early precursors of ovarian cancer [79,80] would enable more effective treatment options and improve patient outcomes. Laparoscopy is one minimally invasive technique that enables diagnostics and surgery to be performed with decreased morbidity. Although laparoscopy offers exceptional visualization of remote, internal tissue, imaging is limited to surface features. OCT enables cross-sectional, subsurface imaging of biological

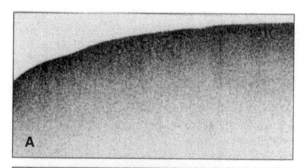
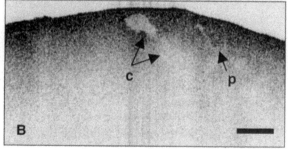

Figure 7   Ovarian cancer. (A) Normal in vitro human ovary and (B) ovarian cancer. c, cystic cavities; p, papillary structures. Bar represents 500 μm.

structure. The combination of these two techniques has the potential for significantly improving the ability to nonexcisionally sample suspect gynecological tissue at high resolutions.

Optical coherence tomography imaging studies of in vitro laparoscopically accessible gynecological tissue suggest the feasibility for integrating this technology into a clinically useful device. Demonstrated performance of current laparoscopic imaging may be improved by OCT imaging of subsurface morphology in real time at near-histological resolutions. The use of OCT to identify subtle morphological changes, as seen here, is a powerful diagnostic tool. In addition, the use of OCT laparoscopy can guide the surgical ablation of suspect tissue sites or the placement of biopsy forceps when tissue specimens are physically resected for histopathological examination. The use of OCT for the early detection of neoplasms without having to physically resect sensitive tissue has the potential to improve treatment protocols and reduce patient morbidity and mortality.

Advances in minimally invasive surgery have been applied to the oncology patient for tumor staging, assessment of resectability, and evaluation of recurrent and metastatic disease. Staging of tumors is often performed laparoscopically [81] with subsequent lymph node biopsy. Staging requires sampling of numerous lymph nodes, only a few of which can be physically resected for histopathological examination. Ultrasonography has been used to image relative sizes of normal and abnormal lymph nodes in vitro, but resolutions were not sufficient to resolve internal architecture [82]. A means of optically imaging the architectural morphology of lymph nodes in real time with high resolution and without having to physically resect and histologically prepare specimens would permit the rapid intraoperative staging of tumor extent. The ability to image subsurface lymph node microstructure offers the potential for reducing the number of biopsies necessary to stage tumors. Integration of OCT imaging with current laparoscope designs will permit simultaneous subsurface OCT imaging with existing *en face* visualization. By sampling greater numbers of lymph nodes, a potential exists for more accurate tumor staging and more precise treatment protocols.

Thirty-five cross-sectional OCT images (2 mm × 1 mm, 500 × 500 pixels) were obtained in vitro from the outer surface of two human lymph node specimens. The orientation was consistent with that encountered during a laparoscopic examination. Two OCT images are shown with corresponding histology in Fig. 8. The OCT image shows characteristic follicular morphology. A cross section of a lymphatic vessel surrounded by adipose tissue is identified in Fig. 8A. The vessel and adipose tissue have been displaced in the histological section (Fig. 8B) due to processing artifact. An outer capsule is noted in Figs 8C and 8D. Correspondence between OCT images and histology is strong. Much of the internal cortex is relatively homogeneous at these image resolutions.

The ability to accurately guide biopsies, assess tumor stage, and evaluate recurrent or metastatic disease allows more effective treatment options and improved patient outcomes. Laparoscopy is one minimally invasive technique that enables more sensitive tumor staging by lymph node involvement with deceased surgical morbidity. Although laparoscopic and endoscopic techniques offer exceptional visualization of remote, internal tissue, imaging is limited to surface features. OCT enables cross-sectional, subsurface imaging of biological structure. The combination of OCT with laparoscopic and endoscopic techniques has the potential to rapidly

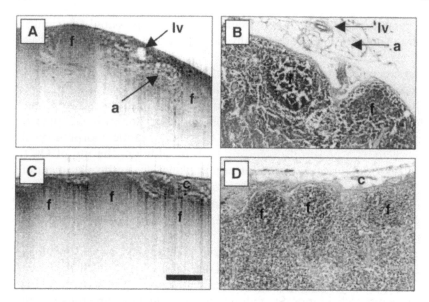

Figure 8 Pediatric lymph nodes with corresponding histology. In vitro images of pediatric lymph nodes show characteristic follicular structures. a, adipose tissue; c, capsule; lv, lymphatic vessel; f, fascicle. Bar represents 1 mm. (From Ref. 16.)

scan larger areas of tissue for suspect pathological regions, to guide biopsies in real time, and to reduce biopsy sampling error rates.

23.2.5 Identifying Tumors and Tumor Margins

The ability of OCT to identify tumors and tumor margins in situ represents a significant advancement in image-guided surgery. Identification of tumor margins remains a central problem in surgery. To ensure that the entire tumor has been removed, wide resections of surrounding tissue are performed. The surgical specimen is immediately sent for histopathological evaluation using staining techniques and light microscopy to determine if any tumor is present on the outer surfaces of the resected tissue block. If the result is positive, further resections of tissue are performed. This process, which can be iterative, can result in significant delays in the operating room during which the patient remains under anesthesia. To demonstrate the use of OCT for the identification of tumors and tumor margins, a human brain melanoma was investigated.

Tumors of the central nervous system have several unique characteristics that are not common to neoplastic processes in other parts of the body. The distinction between benign and malignant lesions is less evident. In certain locations, benign lesions can have equally lethal consequences. In addition, the ability to surgically remove neoplasms is restricted by functional anatomical considerations. The incidence of intracranial tumors ranges from 10 to 17 per 100,000, and they account for as many as 20% of all cancers in childhood [67]. Although the five-year survival rate has shown a statistically significant improvement ($p < 0.05$) since 1974, it still remains around 29% [78]. The sensitivity of these tissues limits the amount that can be physically biopsied for histopathological examination. The use of OCT to optically biopsy and identify tumors and tumor margins may offer the potential to reduce patient morbidity.

During the resection of central nervous system neoplasms, precise intraoperative identification of the tumor margin is vital both for the complete resection of the neoplasm and the prevention of iatrogenic injury. Because of this, various imaging modalities including ultrasound, CT, and MRI have been used in an attempt to improve patient morbidity [19,83–86]. Unfortunately, the resolutions of such modalities are often hundreds of micrometers, thereby poorly resolving small tumors and reducing the sharp definition of the tumor margin. Optical techniques including fluorescence and Raman spectroscopy have enabled quantitative identification of brain tumor cells and tumor margins based on native spectroscopic characteristics of the tissue [87–89]. However, imaging tumors based on these techniques is limited to surface features without cross-sectional imaging or optical ranging into the tissue. High resolution video imaging for discrimination of brain tissues has been effective but requires the administration of topical or systemic fluorescent dyes [19,90].

The optical properties of brain and nervous system tissue have been previously characterized [91,92]. A technology, such as OCT, capable of performing intraoperative optical biopsy may provide high resolution discrimination between normal and pathological tissue. If this optical biopsy could be performed in real time, it could be a powerful tool for the surgeon resecting central nervous system neoplasms, allowing tumor margins to be rapidly defined as the intervention progresses.

Optical coherence tomography has been demonstrated for the detention of brain tumors and their margins with normal brain parenchyma, suggesting a role for guiding surgical resection [14]. A handheld surgical imaging probe and modified surgical microscope were constructed for 2-D and 3-D imaging, respectively. The compact and portable probe will enable OCT imaging within the surgical field, whereas the OCT instrument can be remotely located in the surgical suite. An in vitro specimen of outer human cerebral cortex with metastatic melanoma was imaged. The OCT images in Figs. 9A and 9B were acquired through the tumor as indicated by the lines on the digital *en face* view of the cortex (Fig. 9G). These original images were threshold segmented to identify regions of high backscatter within the tumor. The original images were then overlaid with the segmented data, as shown in Figs. 9C and 9D. The OCT images show increased optical backscattering in the region of the larger tumor (white arrows). Small tumor lesions also appear within the image (black arrows). A shadowing effect is observed below each tumor site due to the increased optical backscatter and the subsequent loss of optical power penetrating beneath the tumor. In Figs. 9A and 9C, the boundary of the tumor can be identified. In Figs. 9B and 9D, the tumor is identified below the surface of normal cortex. The histology in Figs 9E and 9F confirms the presence and relative size of the tumor. The digital image shown in Fig. 9G illustrates the characteristics of this particular metastatic melanoma. Multiple small ($< 500 \, \mu$m) metastases are shown surrounding the larger lesion. It is likely that the primary tumor had seeded a large number of tumor cells that were widely distributed across the gray matter of the cortex.

Subsurface visualization of the tumor and its margins was demonstrated by sectioning the three-dimensional data set at planes parallel to the cortical surface as shown in Fig. 10. The top image in Fig. 10 illustrates the section plane orientation through the tumor. Sections 100–1200 μm below the cortical surface are shown in

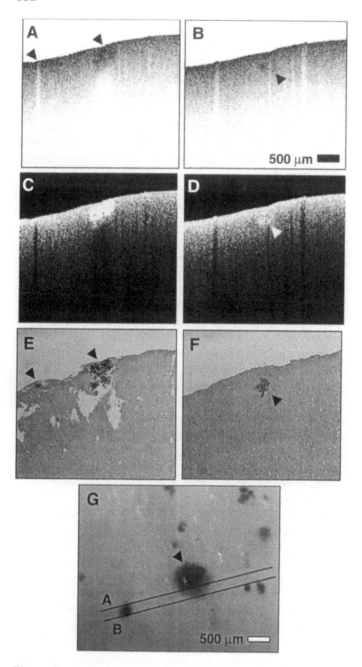

Figure 9 Malignant melanoma in human cortical brain tissue. Original in vitro images (A, B) were threshold segmented (C, D) to highlight backscattering tumor. Comparison with histology (E, F) is strong. Scan locations are shown in the digitized image of the cortex surface (G). Bar represents 500 μm. (From Ref. 14.)

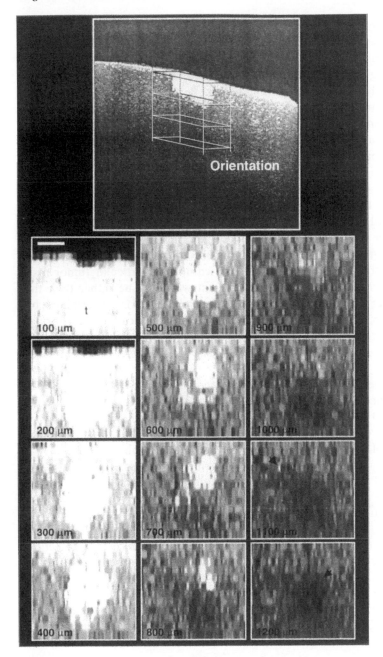

Figure 10 Resectioning of 3-D brain tumor data set. Resectioning produces planar sections from data sets acquired in cross section. Arrow at $1100\,\mu$m indicates deepest tumor (t) extent. Arrow at $1200\,\mu$m indicates shadowing from tumor above. Bar represents $500\,\mu$m. (From Ref. 14.)

the lower part of the figure. The tumor distribution, which appears white is shown at varying depths. The section at $1100\,\mu$m depth indicates a small region of tumor (arrow) that had penetrated beyond the central lesion. The gray-scale transition of normal cortex from light gray (at $100\,\mu$m) to dark gray (at $1200\,\mu$m) is a result of signal attenuation with increasing depth. The darkest region (arrow) shown most prominently at $1200\,\mu$m depth is the result of shadowing form the tumor above.

These results demonstrate micrometer scale optical coherence tomographic imaging of in vitro metastatic melanoma in the human brain. The OCT images acquired with the probe in Fig. 9 show excellent correlation with the corresponding histology despite the histological sectioning artifact in Fig. 9e. This artifact is likely due to the differences in mechanical tissue properties between normal cortex and tumor, which resulted in different tensions across the microtome blade. The tumor shows increased optical backscatter compared to normal cortex. The difference likely results from the higher concentration of subcellular organelles (i.e., nuclei and mito-chondria) in the tumor compared with the high concentration of loose supportive tissue in the gray matter [93]. However, melanin within the particular tumor may also contribute. OCT relies on the inherent contrast within tissue rather than the addition of exogenous dyes. Contrast within images is therefore determined by variations in the index of refraction, as would occur between tumor and normal cortex. Future studies are needed to examine other tumor morphologies that do not contain melanin, such as astrocytomas and glioblastomas, to determine their ima-ging properties.

The depth of penetration for OCT imaging in cortical brain tissue is somewhat limiting. However, once a tumor is identified and resection begins, OCT can con-tinually image ahead of the resection plane to search for the tumor margin or subsur-face vessels. The use of OCT for optical biopsy may permit the nonexcisional imaging of thc walls of the brain cavity to ensure that all tumor has been removed.

The resolutions achieved in this study were as high as $16\,\mu$m, higher than any current ultrasound, CT, or MRI intraoperative imaging technique. This allowed the tumor/cortex interface and the extent of tumor below the surface to be defined with high resolution. Resolutions as high as 2–$3\,\mu$m have been achieved using solid-state ultrafast laser sources [94,95]. At these resolutions, it may be possible to image individual tumor cells that have migrated away from the central tumor. Resection must include these cells to prevent recurrence of tumor. OCT represents a new high resolution optical imaging technology that has the potential for identifying tumors and tumor margins on the micrometer scale and in real time. OCT offers imaging performance not achievable with current imaging modalities and may contribute significantly to the surgical resection of neoplasms.

23.3 INTERVENTION WITH OPTICAL COHERENCE TOMOGRAPHY

Surgical intervention is the process of interfering with disease pathogenesis by sur-gically modifying its course. Because surgical intervention requires visualization to identify tissue morphology, precision to avoid sensitive tissue structures, and con-tinuous feedback to monitor the extent of the intervention, OCT may provide the technology advancements to improve the operative procedure. Scalpels, catheters, radio-frequency ablation electrodes, and lasers are examples of instruments used for surgical intervention. Lasers have been used extensively in interventional procedures to thermally coagulate tissue, control bleeding, and remove unwanted or diseased tissue through ablation. The feasibility of OCT to perform image-guided surgical intervention is investigated in this section. The imaging capabilities of OCT can be used to guide and assess the progress of the surgical intervention. High-power argon laser ablation will be used as the representative interventional technique. Emphasis should be given to the fact that thermal argon laser ablation is representative of a wide array of interventional devices and techniques that OCT can potentially guide. The tissue response to thermal injury has been well characterized over the last several decades, and this research does not attempt to verify previous results. Instead, this research using high speed OCT demonstrates dynamic changes that occur in a variety of clinically relevant tissues. These results will demonstrate the concept and limitations of OCT image guidance during representative surgical interventions.

The use of OCT in an interventional procedure was first demonstrated by the OCT image-guided placement and assessment of retinal laser lesions in the in vivo primate eye [50]. This study examined the dynamic evolution of retinal lesions from continuous wave and nanosecond, picosecond, and femtosecond pulses at visible wavelengths (514–580 nm). Although images were acquired every 5 s, the time evolution of lesion morphology enabled a better understanding of the mechanisms of damage. Faster OCT image acquisition rates now enable rapid microstructural changes to be observed sequentially over time, making it possible to intraoperatively monitor the interventional process and observe the dynamic changes taking place within the tissue.

The pathological effects in tissue that result from increasing temperatures have been well described [96]. The thermal and mechanical effects of laser tissue ablation have also been previously analyzed [97]. The majority of studies have used static histological preparations to document the tissue changes that occur. Dynamic changes in tissue optical properties have been characterized previously [98,99] but without the use of imaging techniques. High speed OCT has been used to image changes in optical backscatter in highly scattering tissues [12]. To image the dynamic effects of thermal injury, an OCT setup using a modified surgical microscope was constructed. An argon beam was incorporated and aligned within the OCT imaging plane, centered within the transverse OCT scan length. A mechanical shutter was used for timed argon laser (514 nm) exposures on the sample. The 1–3 W argon beam was focused to a 0.8 mm diameter spot on the tissue surface. This setup permitted image acquisition immediately prior to and after exposure to track the optical changes occurring within the tissue due to the thermal damage.

Before performing dynamic imaging studies, a single thermal lesion was thoroughly investigated to determine what optical changes were detactable with OCT. A 10 s, 3 W exposure on in vitro rat rectus abdominis muscle was used to form an ablation crater. The specimen was then placed on a multiaxis translational stage to perform 3-D imaging of the crater. Sixty cross-sectional images (400 × 600 pixels, 4 mm × 6 mm) were acquired at 100 μm intervals to produce a 3-D data set. Two projections of this data set are shown in Fig. 11. The deep crater can be seen in the center of the projection. Surrounding the crater is an elevated region of damage that decreases radially outward from the center. The projection in Fig. 11B shows the crater viewed from below the tissue surface, illustrating the deep penetration of the lesion into the tissue.

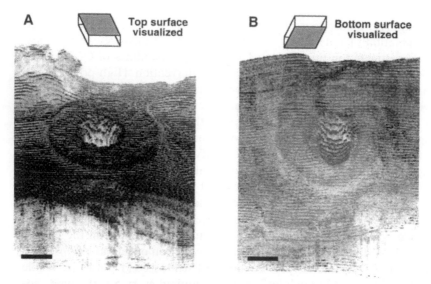

Figure 11 Three-dimensional projections of laser ablation crater in in vitro rat rectus abdominis muscle. Crater was formed by 3 W of argon power during a 10 s exposure. Argon beam was focused to a 0.8 mm diameter spot. Crater and concentric zone of thermal injury are viewed from (A) above and (B) below the tissue surface. Bar represents 1 mm. (From Ref. 12.)

A sequence of cross-sectional images from this data set is shown in Fig. 12. These provide information on the depth-dependent distribution of the thermal energy. The number in each image refers to the distance from the center of the crater at which the cross-sectional image was acquired. At a distance of 3.75 mm from the center, small distortions in the muscle layers (arrow) are observed, although little change has occured at the tissue surface. At 3.0 mm, thermal injury has elevated the tissue surface and distorted an internal low-backscattering layer. At 2.25 mm, a region of increased optical backscatter has appeared. This region appears deeper in the 1.5 mm section. At 0.75 mm from the center, carbonization of the tissue results in significant shadowing of underlying structures. A cross section through the center of the crater is shown in the last image. The vertical bands of low backscatter adjacent to the crater are due to shadowing by the vertical crater walls, which are lined with carbonized tissue. Carbonized tissue scatters and absorbs the incident light, decreasing imaging penetration.

Figure 11A shows concentric rings of birefringent effects and tissue damage that surround the deep crater. These are the result of a radial thermal distribution outward from the site of the incident beam. To optimally assess these radial distributions, the 3-D data set is resectioned in the *en face* plane, as would be viewed from the surface and with increasing depth into the tissue. Resectioned slices are shown in Fig. 13. The number in each figure refers to the depth from the surface at which the plane was sectioned. The shallow planes (150–600 μm) lack regions of tissue (lower white regions) because the axes of the tissue block were not precisely aligned with the translation stage axes. The image at 150 μm shows a relatively uniform ring consistent with the elevated region appearing in the 3-D projection of Fig. 11A. At greater depths (450–900 μm), however, a multiple-ring pattern is evident, possibly explained by a concentric elevation of birefringent tissue layers

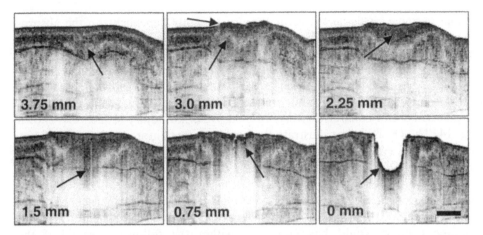

Figure 12 Cross sectional images of laser ablation crater shown in Fig. 11. Numbers refer to distance from crater center at which the image was acquired. At 3.75 mm, arrow indicates early subsurface changes of layered structure. Arrows at 3.0 mm show elevated tissue surface and irregular subsurface layers. Arrow at 0 mm illustrates deep crater with crabonized wall. Bar represents 1 mm. (From Ref. 12.)

presenting as regions of low and high optical backscatter. At a depth of 1350 μm, the crater bottom is approached and the concentric rings have diminished At 1500 μm, the region of high backscatter in the center represents tissue immediately below the crater bottom, and the white ring of reduced optical backscatter is due to the attenuation of the incident beam by the carbonized tissue lining the nearly vertical crater walls.

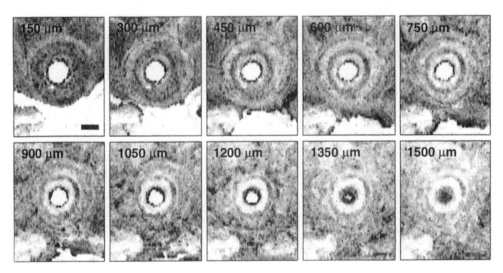

Figure 13 Resectioning of 3-D crater data set to illustrate *en face* plane. Three-dimensional data set was shown in Fig. 11. Numbers refer to depth below tissue surface. Concentric rings of birefringent effects and thermal injury are observed at all depths. Bar represents 1 mm. (From Ref. 12.)

The response of tissue to thermal injury is highly dependent on the absorption and scattering properties. To demonstrate the variability encountered between tissue types, sequences of thermal injury and ablation are shown for two strikingly different in vitro tissue types: rat kidney and brain. Laser therapy is used clinically to ablate regions of neoplastic tissue in the brain, liver, lung, and kidney, among others. The use of OCT to monitor this ablative therapy in real time may enable more precise control of laser delivery. A kidney thermal injury sequence is shown in Fig. 14. The OCT images illustrate the homogeneous nature of the outer cortex of the kidney ($\mu_a = 1.21\,\mathrm{cm}^{-1}$) [100]. Imaging penetration in this tissue is limited to $\approx 1\,\mathrm{mm}$. This 1 W, 3 s exposure was below the threshold for surface membrane rupture, tissue ablation, and crater formation. An outward front of increased backscatter is observed (0.6 s) followed by a region of low backscatter at the center of the lesion (1.6 s). Backscatter from this region increases over time (2.0–3.0 s). Membrane rupture would have occurred within the following second if the exposure had continued. The corresponding histology is also shown, indicating a region of coagulated tissue (arrows) with no tissue fragmentation. Contrasted with this tissue is the ablation of rat brain tissue ($\mu_a = 0.19\,\mathrm{cm}^{-1}$) [100] in Fig. 15. The

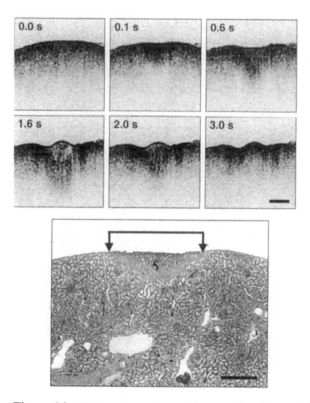

Figure 14   Kidney laser thermal damage. In vitro rat kidney was exposed to 1 W of argon power for 3.0 s. Exposure was stopped prior to membrane rupture of rat kidney. Arrows in the corresponding histology indicate zone of thermal damage. Bar represents 1 mm. (From Ref. 12.)

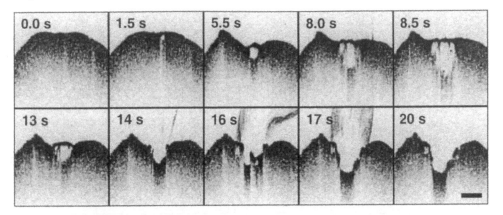

Figure 15 Brain laser ablation. In vitro rat brain was exposed to 1 W of argon power for 20 s. Bar represents 1 mm. (From Ref. 12.)

lower absorption coefficient implies that longer exposure durations are required for the same incident power to produce similar effects. This was observed for 1 W incident on brain tissue for 20 s. In this sequence, significant vacuolization and tissue heating occur (5.5–13 s) before the surface membrane is ruptured at 14 s. Membrane rupture is followed by ejection of tissue from the lesion, evolution of a smoke plume (16–17 s), and crater formation (20 s).

Observations from high speed OCT imaging of thermal laser injury suggest that prior to crater formation the outer membrane of the tissue must first be ruptured. Considerable thermally induced cell injury and death occurs before membrane rupture and crater formation. Membrane rupture represents a catastrophic event that results in ejection of tissue from the lesion site. In particular surgical applications, rupturing the outer membrane is undesirable and can lead to significant bleeding. OCT image guidance can be used to monitor the progress of thermal ablation and prevent membrane rupture.

The membrane rupture threshold is documented by a comparison of thermal injury in in vitro rat liver ($\mu_a = 12\,\text{cm}^{-1}$) [100] for thermal energy doses below and above the membrane rupture threshold. Two sequences are shown in Fig. 16. The first exposure at 1 W is halted after 1 s, prior to the membrane rupture. The second exposure is allowed to continue for 7 s, resulting in membrane rupture, ejection of tissue, and crater formation. The corresponding histology for the subthreshold lesion indicated a region of coagulated tissue. In contrast, the above-threshold lesion histology showed marked tissue ablation and fragmentation within the lesion crater. Below the crater extended a zone of coagulated tissue that was not observed in the OCT image due to the poor penetration through the carbonized crater wall.

These examples demonstrate the use of OCT for guiding and monitoring surgical intervention. Although a continuous wave argon laser was used as an interventional device, the laser is only a representative technique for a wide range of instruments and techniques including scalpels, electrosurgery, radio frequency, microwaves, and ultrasound ablation. OCT imaging was performed at 8 frames per second, fast enough to capture dynamic changes in the optical properties of

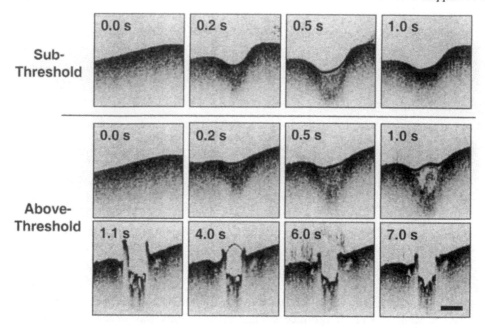

Figure 16 Subthreshold and above-threshold ablation of liver. In vitro rat liver was exposed to 1 W argon power for 1 s and 7 s. Bar represents 1 mm. (From Ref. 16.)

the tissue during thermal ablation. these image sequences provided interesting insight into ablation mechanism for a variety of tissue types. Although high speed ablation techniques such as pulsed laser ablation may occur on faster time scales, OCT is still effective at imaging the integrated effects of the ablation process. OCT can monitor the extent of thermal injury below the surface of the tissue by imaging the changes in optical backscatter. OCT imaging can therefore provide empirical information for dosimetry to minimize the extent of collateral injury. The use of OCT for guiding surgical interventions has the potential to improve intraoperative monitoring and more effectively control interventional procedures.

23.4 CONCLUSIONS

Optical coherence tomography has unique characteristics that are advantageous for surgical guidance and intervention. First, OCT can acquire cross-sectional images of surgical tissue at resolutions that are unprecedented in the surgical community. Second, imaging can be performed in situ without having to physically resect and histologically prepare tissue, which are both costly and time-consuming. Third, imaging can be performed in real time, enabling immediate feedback to the surgeon to guide procedures. Fourth, the fiber-optic OCT technology can be readily integrated into existing instruments, including hand held probes, catheters, endoscopes, laparoscopes, and surgical microscopes. Finally, OCT can be integrated with interventional techniques such as laser ablation.

The capabilities of OCT for surgical guidance and intervention has been demonstrated in five major areas of application.

OCT was first demonstrated for guiding microsurgical procedures. It was used to assess the quality of a microsurgical arterial anastomosis and was able to identify occlusions transmurally that would lead to postoperative complications. The use of OCT to longitudinally track peripheral nerve fascicles and estimate fascicle diameters provides previously unavailable information to the microsurgeon to successfully anastomose corresponding ends of a severed peripheral nerve.

Second, the potential of OCT for reducing iatrogenic injury during surgical procedures was demonstrated. High speed OCT imaging provided real-time feedback and identified subsurface vessels. Avoiding vulnerable vessels, nerves, and other sensitive tissues will help reduce iatrogenic injury.

Third, the use of OCT for guiding biopsies of suspect regions of tissue was demonstrated. Examples in the gastrointestinal tract, the female reproductive tract, and lymph nodes were shown. In these areas, a reduction in biopsy sampling error rates would be beneficial.

Fourth, OCT has the potential to identify tumors and tumor margins. Imaging of metastatic melanoma of the brain is one case where accurate tumor margin localization is necessary. Complete resection of tumor is required while minimizing the resection of surrounding normal brain tissue to preserve function.

Finally, OCT was demonstrated for intraoperatively guiding and monitoring surgical interventions. A representative surgical interventional technique using an argon laser to thermally ablate tissue was shown. Thermal and mechanical damage mechanisms were observed with OCT and confirmed with histology.

The use of OCT shows promise for rapid feedback, visualization, and control of surgical intervention.

Studies have explored the feasibility of using OCT in surgical guidance and intervention. However, more detailed investigation is needed and must focus on specific surgical procedures associated with given clinical conditions in order to evaluate the ultimate applicability of OCT for that clinical situation. Outcomes as well as efficiency and economic measures must also be considered. However, the unique abilities of OCT to visualize tissue and tissue pathology in ways that were previously impossible suggest that it has the potential to create entirely new methodologies in surgery. The incorporation of OCT imaging into surgery promises to both improve the outcomes of many existing procedures and enable new ones.

STATEMENT OF ANIMAL CARE AND TISSUE USE

The animals used in this research were cared for and maintained under the established and approved protocols of the Committee on Animal Care, Massachusetts Institute of Technology, Cambridge, MA.

The protocol for the use of discarded human tissue has been approved by the Committee on the Use of Human Subjects, Massachusetts General Hospital, Boston, MA.

ACKNOWLEDGMENTS

The material in this chapter is excerpted in part from the doctoral dissertation of Stephen A. Boppart, entitled "Surgical Diagnostics, Guidance, and Intervention Using Optical Coherence Tomography," which was submitted to the Harvard-MIT Division of Health Sciences and Technology and the Massachusetts Institute of Technology in May 1998. These studies were performed in the Department of Electrical Engineering and Computer Science and the Research Laboratory of Electronics at the Massachusetts Institute of Technology. We wish to thank Drs. Gary Tearney, Brett Bouma, Juergen Herrmann, and James Southern for their invaluable scientific contributions. We also thank Costas Pitris and Christine Jesser for their contributions. This research is sponsored in part by the National Institutes of Health Contracts NIH-9-RO1-EY11289-12 (JGF), NIH-1-RO1-CA75289-02 (JGF and MEB), NIH-1-R29-HL55686-01A1 (MEB), NIH-1-RO1-AR44812-01 (MEB), the Medical Free Electron Laser Program, Office of Naval Research Contract N00014-94-1-0717 (JGF), the Air Force Office of Scientific Research Contract F4920-98-1-0139 (JGF), and the Whitaker Foundation Contract 96-0205 (MEB). Dr. Stephen Boppart gratefully acknowledges the support of the Air Force Palace Knight Program.

REFERENCES

1. Melzer A, Schmidt A, Kipfmuller K, Gronemeyer D, Seibel R. Technology and principles of tomographic image-guided interventions and surgery. Surg Endosc 11:946–956, 1997.
2. Black MP, Moriarty T, Alexander E, Stieg P, Woodward EJ, Gleason PL, Martin CH, Kikinis R, Schwartz RB, Jolesz FA. Development and implementation of intraoperative magnetic resonance imaging and its neurosurgical applications. Neurosurgery 41:831–845, 1997.
3. Grimson WEL, Ettinger GJ, White SJ, Lozano-Perez T, Wells WM III, Kikinis R. An automatic registration method for frameless stereotaxy, image-guided surgery, and enhanced reality visualization. IEEE Trans Med Imaging 15:129–140, 1996.
4. Huang D, Swanson EA, Lin CP, Schuman JS, Stinson WG, Chang W, Hee MR, Flotte T, Gregory K, Puliafito CA, Fujimoto JG. Optical coherence tomography. Science 254:1178–1181, 1991.
5. Hee MR, Izatt JA, Swanson EA, Huang D, Lin CP, Schuman JS, Puliafito CA, Fujimoto JG. Optical coherence tomography of the human retina. Arch Ophthalmol 113:325–332, 1995.
6. Fujimoto JG, Brezinski ME, Tearney GJ, Boppart SA, Bouma B, Hee MR, Southern JF, Swanson EA. Optical biopsy and imaging using optical coherence tomography. Nature Med 1:970–972, 1995.
7. Schmitt JM, Yadlowsky MJ, Bonner RF. Subsurface imaging of living skin with optical coherence microscopy. Dermatology 191:93–98, 1995.

8. Brezinski ME, Tearney GJ, Bouma BE, Izatt JA, Hee MR, Swanson EA, Southern JF, Fujimoto JG. Optical coherence tomography for optical biopsy: Properties and demonstration of vascular pathology. Circulation 93:1206–1213, 1996.

9. Tearney GJ, Brezinski ME, Bouma BE, Boppart SA, Pitris C, Southern JF, Fujimoto JG. In vivo endoscopic optical biopsy with optical coherence tomography. Science 276:2037–2039, 1997.

10. Feldchtein FI, Gelikonov GV, Gelikonov VM, Kuranov RV, Sergeev AM, Gladkova ND, Shakhov AV, Shakhova NM, Snopova LB, Terent'eva AB, Zagainova EV, Chumakov YuP, Kuznetzova IA. Endoscopic applications of optical coherence tomography. Opt Express 3:257–270, 1998.

11. Breazinski ME, Tearney GJ, Boppart SA, Swanson EA, Southern JF, Fujimoto JG. Optical biopsy with optical coherence tomography, feasibility for surgical diagnostics. J Surg Res 71:32–40, 1997.

12. Boppart SA, Herrman JM, Pitris C, Stamper DL, Breazinski ME, Fujimoto JG. High-resolution optical coherence tomography guided laser ablation of surgical tissue. J Surg Res 82:275–284, 1999.

13. Boppart SA, Bouma BE, Pitris C, Tearney GJ, Southern JF, Brezinski ME, Fujimoto JG. Intraoperative assessment of microsurgery with three-dimensional optical coherence tomography. Radiology 208:81–86, 1998.

14. Boppart SA, Brezinski ME, Pitris C, Fujimoto JG. Optical coherence tomography for neurosurgical imaging of intracortical melanoma. Neurosurgery 43:834–841, 1998.

15. Boppart SA, Bouma BE, Pitris C, Southern JF, Brezinski ME, Fujimoto JG. In vivo cellular optical coherence tomography imaging. Nature Med 4(7):861–864, 1998.

16. Boppart SA. Surgical diagnostics, guidance, and intervention using optical coherence tomography. Doctoral Thesis, Harvard-MIT Division of Health Sciences and Technology, Massachusetts Institute of Technology, Cambridge, MA, 1998.

17. Rooks MD, Slappey J, Zusmanis K. Precision of suture placement with microscope- and loupe-assisted anastomoses. Microsurgery 14:547–550, 1993.

18. Merle M, De Mcdinaceli L. Primary nerve repair in the upper limb. Our preferred methods: Theory and practical applications. Microsurgery 8:575–586, 1992.

19. Haglund MM, Berger MS, Hochman DW. Enhanced optical imaging of human gliomas and tumor margins. Neurosurgery 38:308–317, 1996.

20. Allemond R. Basic technical aspects and optimization problems in x-ray computed tomography. In: R Guzzardi, ed. Physics and Engineering of Medical Imaging. Boston, MA: Martinus Nijhoff, 1987:207–217.

21. Morton EJ, Webb S, Bateman JE, Clarke LJ, Shelton CG. Three-dimensional x-ray microtomography for medical and biological applications. Phys Med Biol 35:805–820, 1990.

22. Rajyaguru JM, Kado M, Nekula K, Richardson MC, Muszynski MJ. High resolution x-ray micrography of live *Candida albicans* using laser plasma pulsed point x-ray sources. Microbiology 143:733–738, 1997.

23. Markisz JA, Aquilia MG. Technical Magnetic Resonance Imaging. Stamford, CT: Appleton & Lange, 1996.

24. Jacobs RE, Fraser SE. Magnetic resonance microscopy of embryonic cell lineages and movements. Science 263:681–684, 1994.

25. Jacobs RE, Fraser SE. Imaging neuronal development with magnetic resonance imaging (MRI) microscopy. J Neurosci Meth 54:189–196, 1994.

26. Smith BR, Johnson GA, Groman EV, Linney E. Magnetic resonance microscopy of mouse embryos. Proc Natl Acad Sci USA 91:3530–3533, 1994.

27. Goldberg BB, Liu J-B, Merton DA, Feld RI, Miller LS, Cohn HE, Barbot D, Gillum DR, Vernick JJ, Winkel CA. Sonographically guided laparoscopy and mediastinoscopy using miniature catheter-based transducers. J Ultrasound Med 12:49–54, 1993.

28. Hibberd MG, Vuille C, Weyman AE. Intravascular ultrasound: Basic principles and role in assessing arterial morphology and function. Am J Cardiol Imag 6:302–324, 1992.

29. Masotti L. Basic principles and advanced technical aspects of ultrasound imaging. In R Guzzardi, ed. Physics and Engineering of Medical Imaging. Boston, MA: Martinus Nijhoff, 1987:263–317.

30. Foster FS, Pavlin CJ, Lockwood GR, Ryan LK, Harasiewicz KA, Berube LR, Rauth AM. Principles and applications of ultrasound backscatter microscopy. IEEE Trans Ultrason Ferroelec Freq Contr 40:608–617, 1993.

31. Chandraratna PAN, Award MI, Chandrasoma P, Khan M. High-frequency ultrasound: Determination of the lowest frequency required for cellular imaging and detection of myocardial disease. Am Heart J 129:15–19, 1995.

32. Turnbull DH, Starkoski BG, Harasiewicz KA, Semple JL, From L, Gupta AK, Sauder DN, Foster FS. A 40–100 MHz B-scan ultrasound backscatter microscope for skin imaging. Ultrasound Med Biol 21:79–88, 1995.

33. Turnbull DH, Ramsay JA, Shivji GS, Blomfield TS, From L, Sauder DN, Foster FS. Ultrasound backscatter microscope analysis of mouse melanoma progression. Ultrasound Med Biol 22:845–853, 1996.

34. Boppart SA, Deutsch TF, Rattner DW. Optical imaging technology in minimally invasive surgery. Surg Endosc 13:718–722, 1999.

35. Geis WP, Kim HC, McAfee PC, Kang JG, Brennan EJJ. Synergistic benefits of combined technology in complex minimally invasive surgical procedures: Clinical experience and educational processes. Surg Endosc 10:1025–1028, 1996.

36. Grimm H. Endoscopic ultrasonography with the ultrasonic esophagoprobe. Endoscopy 26:818–821, 1994.

37. Walsh RM, Ackroyd FW, Shelito PC. Endoscopic resection of large sessile colorectal polyps. Gastrointest Endosc 38:303–309, 1992.

38. Asamura H, Nakayama H, Kondo H, Tsuchiya R, Naruke T. Thoracoscopic evaluation of histologically/cytologically proven or suspected lung cancer: A VATS exploration. Lung Cancer 16:183–190, 1997.

39. Miller A, Stonebridge PA, Tsoukas AI, Kwolek CJ, Brophy CM, Gibbons GW, Freeman DV, Pomposelli FB, Campbell DR, LoGerfo FW. Angioscopically directed valvulotomy: A new valvuotome and technique. J Vasc Surg 13(6):813–820, 1991.

40. Easter DW, Cuschieri A, Nathanson LK, Jones ML. The utility of diagnostic laparoscopy for abdominal disorders. Diag Laparos 127:379–383, 1992.

41. Hemming AW, Nagy AG, Scudamore CH, Edelmann K. Laparoscopic staging of intraabdominal malignancy. Surg endosc 9:325–328, 1995.

42. Watt I, Stewart I, Anderson D, Bell G, Anderson JR. Laparoscopy, ultrasound and computed tomography in cancer of the oesophagus and gastric cardia: A prospective comparison for detecting intra-abdominal metastases. Br J Surg 76:1036–1039, 1989.

43. Tomkinson TH, Bentley JL, Crawford MK, Harkrider CH, Moore DT, Rouke JL. Rigid endoscopic relay systems: A comparative study. Appl Opt 35:6674–6683, 1996.

44. Reddick EJ, Olsen DO. Laparoscopic laser cholecystectomy: A comparison with minilap cholecystectomy. Surg endosc 3:131, 1989.

45. Escarce JJ, Bloom BS, Hillman AL, Shea JA, Schwartz JS. Diffusion of laparoscopic cholecystectomy among general surgeons in the United States. Med Care 33:256–271, 1995.

46. Boppart SA, Bouma BE, Pitris C, Tearney GJ, Fujimoto JG. Forward-imaging instruments for optical coherence tomography. Opt Lett 22:1618–1620, 1997.

47. Tearney GJ, Boppart SA, Bouma BE, Brezinski ME, Weissman NJ, Southern JF, Fujimoto JG. Scanning single-mode fiber optica catheter-endoscope for optical coherence tomography. Opt Lett 21:543–545, 1996.

48. Bolle RM, Vemuri BC. On three-dimensional surface reconstruction methods. IEEE Trans Pattern Anal Mach Intell 13:1–13, 1991.

49. Lorensen WE, Cline HE. Marching cubes: A high resolution 3D surface reconstruction algorithm. Comput Graphics 21:163–163, 1987.

50. Toth CA, Birngruber R, Boppart SA, Hee MR, Fujimoto JG, DiCarlo CD, Swanson EA, Cain CP, Narayan DG, Noojin GD, Roach WP. Argon laser retinal lesions evaluated in vivo by optical coherence tomography. Am J Ophthalmol 133:188–198, 1997.

51. Dobrezyneki A. Personal communication, 1995.

52. Boppart SA, Tearney GJ, Bouma BE, Southern JF, Brezinski ME, Fujimoto JG. Noninvasive assessment of the developing *Xenopus* cardiovascular system using optical coherence tomography. Proc Natl Acad Sci USA 94:4256–4261, 1997.

53. von Birgelen C, de Very EA, Mintz GS, Nicosia A, Bruining N, Li W, Slager CJ, Roelandt JR, Serruys PW, de Feyter PJ. ECG-gated three-dimensional intravascular ultrasound: Feasibility and reproducibility of the automated analysis of coronary lumen and atherosclerotic plaque dimensions in humans. Circulation 96:2944–2952, 1997.

54. Ng K-H, Evans JL, Vonesh MJ, Meyers SN, Mills TA, Kane BJ, Aldrich WN, Jang Y-T, Yock PG, Rold MD, Roth SI, McPherson DD. Arterial imaging with a new forward-viewing intravascular ultrasound catheter, II: Three-dimensional reconstruction and display of data. Circulation 89:718–723, 1994.

55. Tearney GJ, Bouma BE, Fujimoto JG. High-speed phase- and group-delay scanning with a grating-based phase control delay line. Opt Lett 22:1811–1813, 1997.

56. Zhong-wei C, Dong-yue Y, Di-Sheng C, eds. Microsurgery. New York: Springer-Verlag, 1982.

57. Culbertson JH, Rand RP, Jurkiwicz MJ. Advances in microsurgery. Adv Surg 23:57–88, 1990.

58. Zuniga JR, Labanc JP. Advances in microsurgical nerve repair. J Oral Maxillofac Surg 51(suppl 1):62–68, 1993.

59. Ryan JM, Milner SM, Cooper GJ, Haywood IR. Field surgery on a future conventional battlefield: Strategy and wound management. Ann Roy Coll Surg Engl 73:13–20, 1991.

60. Terris DJ, Fee WE. Current issues in nerve repair. Arch Otolaryngol Head Neck Surg 119:725–731, 1993.

61. Wyrick JD, Stern PJ. Secondary nerve reconstruction. Microsurgery 8:587–598, 1992.

62. Yazdanfar S, Kulkarni MD, Izatt JA. High resolution imaging of in vivo cardiac dynamics using color Doppler optical coherence tomography. Opt Express 1:424–431, 1997.

63. Adar R, Bass A, Walden R. Iatrogenic complications in surgery. Five years' experience in general and vascular surgery in a university hospital. Ann Surg 196:725–729, 1982.

64. Botet JF, Lightdale C. Endoscopic ultrasonography of the upper gastrointestinal tract. Radiol Clin N Am 30:1067–1083, 1992.

65. Phillips RW, Wong RKH. Barrett's esophagus. Gastroenterol Clin N Am 20:791–815, 1991.

66. Spechler SJ. Gastroesophageal reflux disease and other disorders of the esophagus. In S Chopra, RJ May, eds. Pathophysiology of Gastrointestinal Diseases. Boston, MA: Little, Brown, 1989:37–70.

67. Cotran RS, Kumar V, Robbins SL. *Robbins Pathogenic Basis of Disease*. 5th ed. FJ Schoen, Philadelphia: WB Saunders, 1994.

68. Tearney GJ, Brezinski ME, Southern JF, Bouma BE, Boppart SA, Fujimoto JG. Optical biopsy in human gastrointestinal tissue using optical coherence tomography. Am J Gastroenterol 92:1800–1804, 1997.

69. Izatt JA, Kulkarni MD, Wang H-W, Kobayashi K, Sivak MV. Optical coherence tomography and microscopy in gastrointestinal tissues. IEEE J Selected Topics Quant Electron 2:1017–1028, 1996.

70. Pitris C, Jesser CA, Boppart SA, Stamper DL, Brezinski ME, Fujimoto JG. Feasibility of optical coherence tomography for high-resolution imaging of human gastrointestinal tract malignancies. J Gastroenterol, 35:87–92, 2000.

71. Herrmann JM, Brezinski ME, Bouma BE, Boppart SA, Pitris C, Southern JF, Fujimoto JG. Two- and three-dimensional high-resolution imaging of the human oviduct with optical coherence tomography. Fertil Steril 70:155–158, 1998.

72. Runowicz CD. Office laparoscopy as a screening tool for early detection of ovarian cancer. J Cell Biochem 23(suppl):238–242, 1995.

73. Boppart SA, Goodman AK, Pitris C, Jesser C, Libis JJ, Brezinski ME, Fujimoto JG. High-resolution imaging of endometriosis and ovarian carcinoma with optical coherence tomography: Feasibility for laparoscopic-based imaging. Br J Obstet Gyn 106:1071–1077, 1999.

74. Pitris C, Goodman AK, Boppart SA, Libus JJ, Fujimoto JG, Brezinski ME. High resolution imaging of gynecological neoplasms using optical coherence tomography. Obstet Gynecol 93:135–139, 1999.

75. Nisolle M, Donnez J. Peritoneal endometriosis, ovarian endometriosis, and adenomyotic nodules of the rectovaginal septum are three different entities. Fertil Steril 68:585–596, 1997.

76. Kjerulff KH, Erickson BA, Langenberg PW. Chronic gynecological conditions reported by US women: Findings from the National Health Information Survey, 1984 to 1992. Am J Public Health 86:195–199, 1996.

77. Eskenazi B, Warner ML. Epidemiology of endometriosis. Obstet Gyn Clin N Am 24:235–258, 1997.

78. American Cancer Society. Cancer Statistics 1998. CA Cancer J Clin 48:6–29, 1998.

79. Scully RE. Pathology of ovarian cancer precursors. J Cell Biochem 23(suppl):208–218, 1995.

80. Tortolero-Luna G, Mitchell MF. The epidemiology of ovarian cancer. J Cell Biochem 23(suppl):200–207, 1995.

81. Childers JM, Balserak JC, Kent T, Surwit EA. Laparoscopic staging of Hodgkin's lymphoma. J Laparoendosc Surg 3:495–499, 1993.

82. Vassallo P, Edel G, Roos N, Naguib A, Peters PE. In-vitro high-resolution ultrasonography of benign and malignant lymph nodes. Invest Radiol 28:698–705, 1993.

83. Chandler WF, Knake JE, McGillicuddy JE, Lillehei KO, Silver TM. Intraoperative use of real-time ultrasonography in neurosurgery. J Neurosurg 57:157–163, 1982.

84. Gooding GAW, Boggan JE, Weinstein PR. Characterization of intracranial neoplasms by CT and intraoperative sonography. Am J Neuroradiol 5:517–520, 1984.

85. Kaye AH, Morstyn G, Apuzzo MLJ. Photoradiation therapy and its potential in the management of neurological tumors. J Neurosurg 69:1–14, 1988.

86. Taphoorn MJ, Heimans JJ, Kaiser MC, de Slegte RG, Crezee FC, Valk J. Imaging of brain metastases: Comparison of computerized tomography (CT) and magnetic resonance imaging (MRI). Neuroradiology 31:391–395, 1989.

87. Jeannesson P, Manfait M, Jardillier JC. A technique for laser Raman spectroscopic studies of isolated cell populations. Anal Biochem 129:305–309, 1983.

88. Mizuno A, Hayashi T, Tashibu K, Maraishi S, Kawauchi K, Ozaki Y. Near-infrared FT-Raman spectra of the rat brain tissues. Neurosci Lett 141:47–52, 1992.

89. Poon WS, Schomacker KT, Deutsch TF, Martuza RL. Laser-induced fluorescence: Experimental intraoperative delineation of tumor resection margins. J Neurosurg 76:679–686, 1992.

90. Hansen DA, Spence AM, Carksi T, Berger MS. Indocyanine green (ICG) staining and demarcation of tumor margins in a rat glioma model. Surg Neurol 40:451–456, 1993.

91. Svaasand LO, Ellingsen R. Optical properties of human brain. Photochem Photobiol 38:293–299, 1983.

92. Eggert HR, Blazek V. Optical properties of human brain tissue, meninges, and brain tumors in the spectral range of 200 to 900 nm. Neurosurgery 21:459–464, 1987.
93. Dunn A, Richards-Kortum R. Three-dimensional computation of light scattering from cells. IEEE J Selected Topics Quant Electron 2:898–905, 1996.
94. Clivaz X, Marquis-Weible F, Salathe RP. Optical low coherence reflectometry with 1. 9 μm spatial resolution. Electronics Lett 28:1553–1555, 1992.
95. Bouma BE, Tearney GJ, Boppart SA, Hee MR, Brezinski ME, Fujimoto JG. High resolution optical coherence tomographic imaging using a modelocked Ti : Al$_2$O$_3$ laser. Opt Lett 20:1486–1488, 1995.
96. Thomsen S. Pathologic analysis of photothermal and photomechanical effects of laser-tissue interactions. Photochem Photobiol 53:825–835, 1991.
97. LeCarpentier GL, Motamedi M, McMath LP, Rastegar S, Welch AJ. Continuous wave laser ablation of tissue: Analysis of thermal and mechanical events. IEEE Trans Biomed Eng 40:188-200, 1993.
98. Lin W-C, Motamedi M, Welch AJ. Dynamics of tissue optics during laser heating of turbid media. Appl Opt 35:3413–3420, 1996.
99. Pettit GH, Ediger MN, Weiblinger RP. Dynamic optical properties of collagen-based tissue during ArF excimer laser ablation. Appl Opt 32:488–493, 1993.
100. Welch AJ, van Gemert MJC. Optical-Thermal Response of Laser-Irradiated Tissue. New York: Plenum Press, 1995.

24

Applications of Optical Coherence Tomography in Gynecology

N. M. SHAKHOVA

Nizhny Novgorod Medical Academy, Nizhny Novgorod, Russia

FELIX I. FELDCHTEIN and A. M. SERGEEV

Institute of Applied Physics, Nizhny Novgorod, Russia

24.1 BACKGROUND OF OCT APPLICATIONS IN GYNECOLOGY

Modern gynecology tends to treatment approaches that provide termination of pathological processes along with preservation of the patient's quality of life. This implies the performance of corrective hormonal therapy, organ-preserving operations for removal of tumors, and so on. There is, therefore, a need for earlier and more accurate diagnosis of pathological states, objective assessment of physiological processes, and adequate monitoring of the course of treatment.

Various high-technology methods are currently in use to diagnose gynecological pathologies. These include ultrasound, magnetic resonance imaging, and computed tomography, among others. Nevertheless, the problem of reducing the number of false diagnoses retains its importance. One of the possible trends here is the use of optical technologies for medical diagnostics. Spectroscopy, for example, has already found a place in clinical practice [1]. The advent of OCT [2] capable of imaging subsurface microstructure of biological objects as well as further development of this technique toward the creation of portable, easy-to-use clinical devices offers new diagnostic opportunities for the gynecologist [3–5].

The attractiveness of the OCT technique in gynecology is due to its capability to obtain unique in vivo information on epithelial structures of female genital organs. Clearly, the mucosa of different organs is not equally amenable to OCT

649

imaging. Our experience shows [4] that OCT is more informative in the case of internal organs with a stratified (horizontally layered) architecture of the normal mucosa. An example is a tissue covered with stratified squamous epithelium that is separated from underlying stroma by a smooth basement membrane, such as in the vagina and uterine cervix. Due to different light-scattering properties of the epithelium and stroma, the position of the basement membrane is distinctly seen in those OCT images. For organs covered with thin transitional or columnar epithelium on the smooth basement membrane, such as the endocervix, its position may not be easily observed; however, a stratified architecture of images is also typical. OCT is also sensitive to the presence of subsurface structural inhomogeneities such as blood vessels and glands, which is characteristic of mucosa in most female genital organs. In general, the architecture and optical properties of superficial tissue in the female genital tract are favorable for OCT to extract novel biomedical information.

This information is important, particularly for monitoring physiological processes in the human body (i.e., functional imaging). For instance, the mucous membranes of female genital organs are "targets" that undergo dynamic alterations in different periods of a woman's life and reflect the operation of control systems such as the hypothalamic-hypophysial-ovarian system [6]. Changes in the architecture of mucosa are caused not only by endogenic but also by exogenic hormones and, if monitored by OCT, may be a sign indicating whether or not the hormonal therapy is adequate.

Due to the capability to image structural violations in normal tissue, the technique can be successfully used in diagnostics of pathological processes, especially at their early stages. Most pronounced morphological alterations in biological tissue are related to the development of tumors. Upon detection of a tumor the physician also needs to precisely determine its characteristics that are indicative of the stage and dissemination of the disease. This, in turn, is important to adoption of a treatment strategy [7].

In modern gynecology, minimally invasive and organ-preserving methods are being extensively used in the treatment of both benign and malignant tumors. When minimizing the volume of an excised tissue, however, a surgeon should be confident of the complete removal of the lesion. It is obvious that the capability of OCT to precisely detect the margins of a pathological area makes this imaging technique promising for intraoperative control in minimally invasive surgery.

The ease of the OCT device application and the noninvasiveness of the probing light allow frequent and multiple use of OCT for dynamical observation of a patient over time. This is important for postoperative control and especially for long-term follow-up, keeping in mind that the criterion of recovery is nonrecurrence of the disease during a control period after treatment.

To demonstrate OCT imaging in gynecological practice, we used an endoscopic OCT device described in previous work [3]. The probing low coherent light was generated by a superluminescent semiconductor diode operating at a center wavelength of 830 nm full width at half-maximum (FWHM) spectral bandwidth 25 nm, and an output power of 1.5 mW. The in-depth resolution was $\sim 15\,\mu$m in free-space units; the lateral resolution 20 μm. The in-depth scanning was performed with a piezofiber modulator [8] with a scanning range of 1–2 mm (free space units) and a scan rate of 70–150 Hz, resulting in the typical acquisition time for a 200 × 200 pixel image of 1.5–3 s. All acquired OCT images are represented in the negative gray-scale "palette," in which a darker gradation corresponds to a higher intensity of back-scattered light (analogous to echo-positive regions in ultrasonography). The scale in these images is given by the 1 mm bar, and the vertical scale is normalized with the assumption that the average group refractive index of mucosa is 1.4. The galvanometer-type probe with outer diameter 2.7 mm (Fig. 2) delivered ∼ 0.5 mW of the optical power to the tissue and provided lateral scanning over 1.6 mm. Our two-year experience in exploitation of endoscopic OCT devices has shown that OCT imaging is an attractive technique for clinical use, because it is noninvasive, its wavelength and power cause no side effects, and information is acquired at a high rate and displayed in real time. Besides, the device is compatible with a standard personal computer and allows a doctor to record an OCT database for further processing and storage of information. The design of optical microprobes [3] used in endoscopic OCT devices permits sterilization by traditional procedures and integration with standard endoscopic equipment, thus making it possible to perform imaging of all organs of the female genital system.

To evaluate the state of the female external genital organs, vagina, and uterine cervix, OCT vulvocolposcopy was performed (Fig. 1). In this procedure, an OCT probe was introduced to the area of interest under the control of a colposcope. As additional information, data of hormonal examination and cytological analyses were used. When indicated, histological verification of biopsy material was carried out.

To diagnose intrauterine pathologies, OCT hysteroscopy was performed (Figs. 2a and 2b). In this case, a microprobe of the OCT device was inserted through a biopsy channel of a standard rigid hysteroscope. Information obtained was then analyzed in parallel with clinical, endoscopic, and morphological data.

Optical coherence tomographic information of the state of the ovaries, fallopian tubes, and pelvic peritoneum was acquired during laparoscopy (Fig. 3). The OCT probe was introduced into the peritoneum through an additional trocar using a specially designed guide.

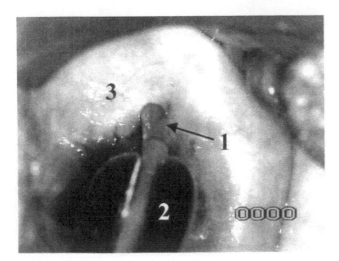

Figure 1   Optical coherence tomographic colposcopic examination of the uterine cervix. *1*, Tip of OCT probe; *2*, holder; *3*, surface of exocervix.

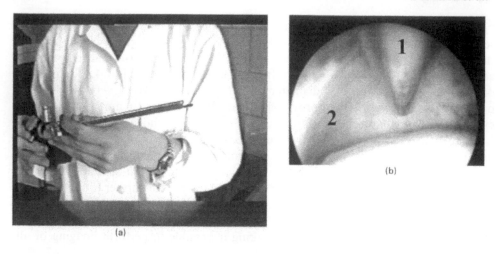

Figure 2 (a) Hysteroscope with inserted OCT probe and (b) view of OCT probe in the uterine cavity. *1*, Tip of OCT probe; *2*, uterine cavity.

To date, we have examined over 150 female patients. Clinical approbation of the OCT technique has been carried out in the gynecological clinic of the Nizhny Novgorod State Medical Academy, Nizhny Novgorod, Russia (head of clinic, Prof. T. S. Kachalina), in the gynecological department of the Municipal Hospital, Chartres, France (head of department, Prof. G. Pennehouat), and in the clinics of Prof. J. E. Hamou in Paris and Prof. M. Bruhat in Clermont-Ferrand, France.

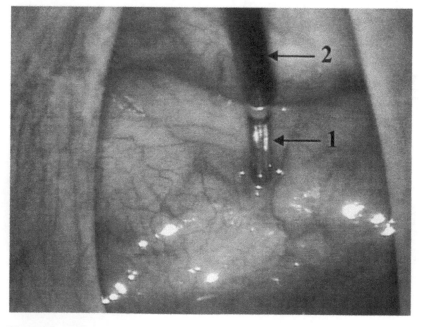

Figure 3 View of OCT probe in abdominal cavity (cul-de-sac of Douglas). *1*, Tip of OCT probe; *2*, holder.

24.2 OCT IMAGING OF NORMAL TISSUE AND FUNCTIONAL IMAGING

To realize the diagnostic potential of OCT in gynecology, a comparative analysis of tomographic data obtained from the same tissue in different physiological states should be performed. It is natural to begin with a discussion of normal tissue images. First, tomograms of the female genital tract were obtained ex vivo and interpreted using results of parallel examination of the material at the macroscopic and microscopic levels by means of standard morphometry and histology. Figure 4a is a histological view of the uterine cervix in the zone of transition of stratified squamous epithelium (SSE) of the vaginal portion (exocervix) into the simple columnar epithelium (SCE) of the cervical canal (endocervix). In the tomogram of this zone (Fig. 4b), a light stripe to the left corresponds to stratified squamous epithelium; the boundary between the light stripe and a darker area below indicates the position of the basement membrane (BM). The BM itself apparently cannot be resolved by OCT due to its extremely small thickness. However, because the basement membrane separates tissue with different light-scattering properties, i.e., epithelium from stroma (S), its topography can be defined in optical images of mucosa with a rather thick epithelial layers. A light, rounded formation in the center represents a cervical gland (G) with mucus. The area covered with columnar epithelium has no tomographically differentiable position of the basement membrane due to the presence of only a single row of epithelial cells that are too small to be resolved by the OCT device.

When imaging in vivo, we obtained tomograms of unaltered epithelium of the vaginal portion of the uterine cervix, which showed some regular features (Fig. 5). In all tomograms, epithelium appears as a light stripe clearly delineated from the underlying tissue. The stripe width varies in the range of 50–600 μm, depending on the functional state of the body. These measurements are in accord with well-known morphological data on the thickness of squamous epithelium in the uterine cervix [9]. In the underlying tissue, vessels of different sizes can sometimes be seen, appearing in tomograms as light rounded or elongated formations. When examining the vagina,

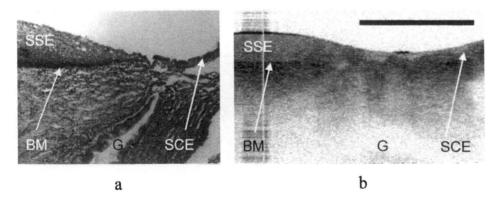

a   b

Figure 4   (a) Histological sample of squamocolumnar junction and (b) in vitro OCT image of the same area, showing stratified squamous epithelium (SSE), basement membrane (BM), transition of stratified squamous epithelium into simple columnar epithelium (SCE), cervical gland (G).

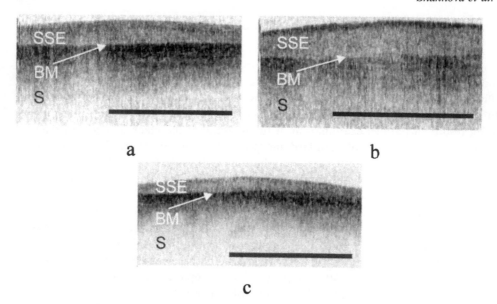

a   b

c

Figure 5 Optical coherence tomographic images of normal cervix in different female patients. Less scattering stripe of epithelium (SSE) is delineated from more scattering stromal tissue (S) by basement membrane (BM). Image (c) is averaged over three frames.

whose morphology is quite similar to that of the uterine cervix, we obtained OCT patterns resembling those of the uterine cervix, except that the subepithelial area looks more inhomogeneous, which corresponds to the less compact structure of subepithelial tissue of the vaginal wall with a higher degree of vascularization of the lamina propria (LP) (Fig. 6). Thus, a well-organized layer architecture can be clearly seen in all tomograms of female genital organs covered with stratified squamous epithelium. This fact allows us to draw preliminary conclusions about OCT criteria of unaltered tissue in gynecology.

It is known that the mucosa of the uterine cervix and vagina is hormone-dependent, i.e., its structure is determined by the hormonal status of the woman.

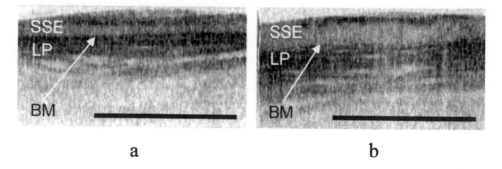

a   b

Figure 6 Optical coherence tomographic images of vaginal wall in different female patients, demonstrating less compact structure of subepithelial tissue of the vaginal wall compared to the normal cervical mucosa in Fig. 5. LP, lamina propria.

In hypoestrogenia, the exocervix is atrophied, the epithelium is represented by basal and parabasal cells, and the superficial cell layers are practically absent. In contrast, in hyperestrogenia, the amount and size of epithelial cells are increased, and glycogen is accumulated in the cells, which leads to thickening of the epithelium. The capability of OCT to evaluate the tissue structure in vivo and to measure exactly the size of different components may be used in monitoring hormone-dependent functional states. OCT images in Figs. 7a and 7b demonstrate the difference in epithelium of an older woman with age-related hypoestrogeny and a young woman with clinically pronounced hyperstrogenia. The functional epithelial difference can be seen even more clearly in OCT images of the cervix of pregnant women. It is known that, during pregnancy, hypervasculation of the cervix, extracellulation of fluid, and disintegration of collagen fibers occur [10]. All these factors are evidenced in tomograms by the occurrence of weakly scattering stripes and dots in the subepithelial layer (Figs. 8a and 8b).

Changes in the hormonal status influence not only the exocervix but also, first of all, the endometrium. By means of OCT hysteroscopy we obtained tomograms of the endometrium of females of different ages that demonstrate the functional specificity of mucosa of the uterine cavity. The endometrium of women of reproductive age exhibits cyclical changes, with each phase of these changes being characterized by its own specific features. Histological and OCT data of the secretory endometrium are presented in Figs 9a and 9b that demonstrate some morphological parallels. The compact layer (CL) appears as a highly backscattering stripe on the surface; the underlying spongy layer (SL) containing glands and blood vessels (BV) is imaged with a number of low backscattering rounded structures of different diameters. In older women, during menopause the endometrium becomes atrophied and is characterized by the sclerosed functional layer, the presence of rare nonfunctioning glands, and a low degree of vascularization (Figs 10a and 10b).

As indicated earlier, dynamical alternations in female genital organs, in particular, the ovaries, are determined by the operation of control systems. OCT images of the ovaries obtained during laparoscopy reflect some characteristic mor-

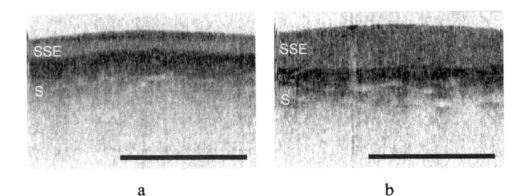

a   b

Figure 7 Optical coherence tomographic images demonstrating the difference between the epithelium of (a) an older woman with age-related hypoestrogeny and (b) a young woman with clinically pronounced hyperestrogenia.

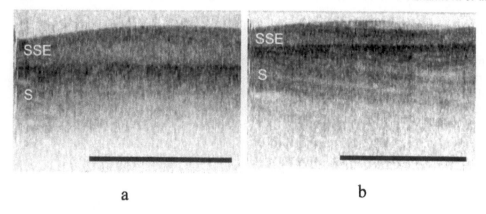

a   b

Figure 8   Optical coherence tomographic images of normal cervix in (a) nonpregnant and
(b) pregnant women.

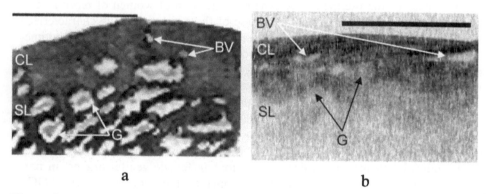

a   b

Figure 9   (a) Histological sample and (b) OCT image of secretory endometrium with compact layer (CL) and underlying spongy layer (SL) containing glands (G) and blood vessels
(BV).

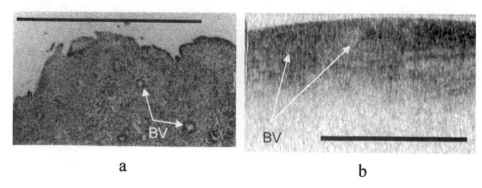

a   b

Figure 10   (a) Histology and (b) OCT data of atrophied endometrium.

phological features of these organs. Tunica albuginea of the ovaries is quite homo-geneous and compact. In the OCT image (Fig. 11b) it appears as a highly back-scattering medium without any optical structure. At the same time, an OCT image taken from the region of a growing follicle (Fig. 11d) shows the presence of a volume formation with a low scattering content. Thus, OCT not only can detect bulk formations but can also measure with high accuracy the thickness of their walls—in the case discussed above, the thickness of the follicle wall (FW). This capability may be important for differential diagnosis between functional cysts and ovarian cystadenoma.

By means of OCT laparoscopy we were able to record tomograms of other pelvic organs of the female genital system, in particular, the fallopian tubes. From the side of the abdomen cavity the fallopian tubes are covered by a very thin serous membrane that is transparent to the probing light and permits monitoring of a variety of subserous structures (Fig. 12). We believe that this information may be useful, for instance, for prognosis of the efficacy of oviduct reconstructive micro-surgery.

Of practical importance are tomograms recorded in parallel with laparoscopy from the pelvic peritoneum. Many gynecological diseases affect the peritoneum structure, altering it in different ways. These include endometriosis, disseminated

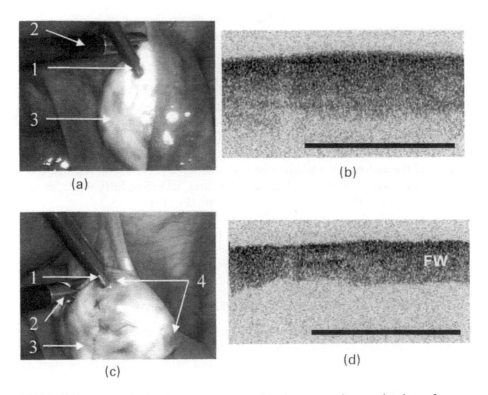

Figure 11 (a) Optical coherence tomographic laparoscopic examination of ovary and (b) corresponding OCT image of tunica albuginea; (c) OCT laparoscopic examination of a growing follicle; (d) corresponding OCT image. *1*, Tip of OCT probe; *2*, forceps; *3*, ovary; *4*, growing follicle. FW, follicle wall.

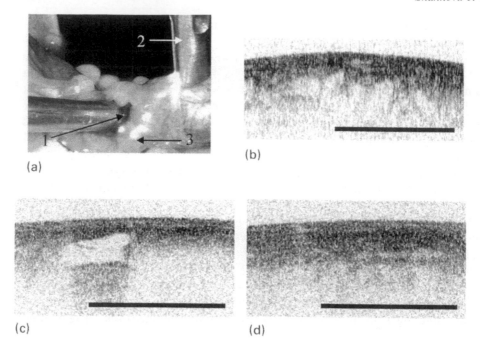

Figure 12 (a) Optical coherence tomographic laparoscopic examination of fallopian tubes and (b,c,d) corresponding OCT images demonstrating a variety of subserous structures. *1*, Tip of OCT probe; *2*, forceps, *3*, fallopian tube.

ovarian cancer, and trophoblastic disease. Timely determination of early and small forms of such diseases and the possibility of monitoring the reverse development of these processes in the course of therapy remain a problem in clinical practice. To our mind, OCT imaging is able to provide additional diagnostic information on the state of the peritoneum. To obtain such information, we examined different parts of the small pelvis and the abdominal wall covered with unaltered peritoneum. Because the serous membrane is very thin, the underlying structures, including fatty tissue, muscles, and vessels, are clearly seen in OCT tomograms (Fig.13).

Thus, the results of our OCT study demonstrate the applicability of OCT imaging in gynecological practice and allow us to draw initial conclusions about OCT criteria of normal states based on optical properties of the subsurface tissue architecture in female genital organs.

24.3 OCT IMAGING OF PATHOLOGICAL STATES

The potential of OCT for diagnosing pathological states of female genital organs were studied on the basis of preliminary information on unaltered tissue, therefore allowing us to set up comparative criteria of norm and pathology. Before we start a discussion of these results it should be noted that although OCT is very informative with regard to structural alterations, at today's stage of technological development it does not allow us to determine the origin of these alterations. Strictly speaking, at present OCT information lacks specificity. The technique can therefore be used in clinical practice to make a diagnosis only in combination with other methods. At the

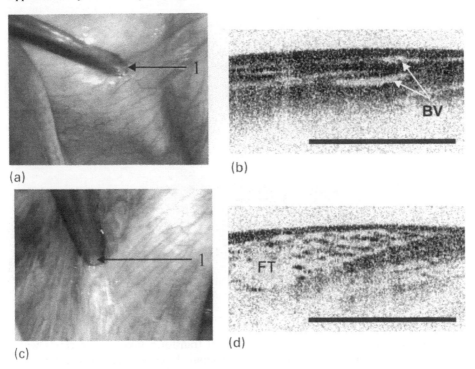

(a)

(b)

(c)

(d)

Figure 13 (a,c) Optical coherence tomographic laparoscopic examination of normal peritoneum. Under the serous membrane, (b) areas with numerous blood vessels and (d) fatty tissue are seen in corresponding OCT images. *1*, Tip of OCT probe. FT, fatty tissue.

same time, the unique capability of OCT to obtain in vivo information on structural alterations in tissue and to measure the dimensions of pathological areas with high accuracy opens up new opportunities for the physician. To demonstrate OCT prospects in this field, numerous tomograms of different pathological states were analyzed.

In our study, pathologies in the uterine cervix were presented most widely. As previously described, the OCT criterion of unaltered exocervix is a well-organized layer architecture. In contrast, in tomograms of the transformation zone (Fig. 14), characteristic morphological alterations [11] can be distinctly seen, evidencing overlapping layers of metaplastic epithelium (ME) and stratified squamous epithelium with ducts of open glands (OG) and formation of closed glands (CG).

Most pronounced structural alterations are indicative of precancer and cancer of the uterine cervix. One variant of loss of normal structure in uterine cervical precancer (a morphological analog of which is cervical intraepithelial neoplasia, CIN) is a specific response of subepithelial layers when stroma attempts to push its way toward the surface as vertical columns while epithelium sinks into underlying layers forming so-called "pillars" and blocks" [11]. OCT information (Fig. 15b) correlates well with histological findings taken from the same region (Fig. 15a) and with data known from the literature. In uterine cervical cancer, these alterations are even more profound. Whereas in the case of microcarcinoma there is only local destruction of the basement membrane,

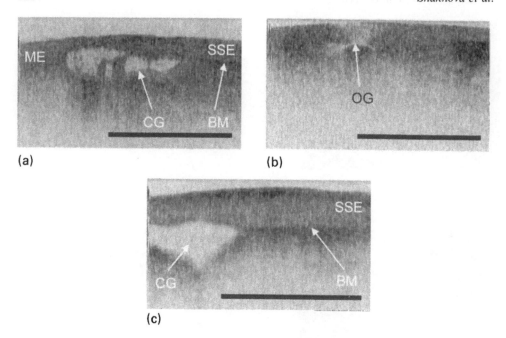

(a)   (b)

(c)

Figure 14 Optical coherence tomographic images of transformation zone in cervix with morphological alterations of mucosa containing overlapping layers of metaplastic epithelium (ME), stratified squamous epithelium (SSE), and open (OG) and closed (CG) glands.

invasive cancer completely "erases" the boundaries between layers, leading to the complete lack of optical structure (Fig. 16).

The foregoing examples demonstrate that OCT can detect zones where pathological alterations occur. However, as stated earlier, the final diagnosis on the origin of these alterations requires histological verification, especially when malignant processes are suspected. Accurate and timely diagnosis in such situations depends on an adequate choice of biopsy site. This is another field where OCT can help tremendously by indicating suspicious areas with an altered architecture from which a biopsy would be most informative.

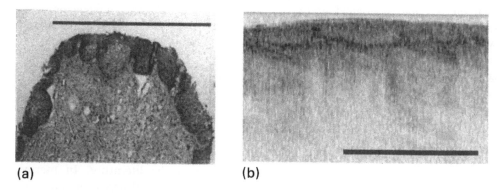

(a)   (b)

Figure 15 (a) Histology and (b) OCT image of cervical intraepithelial neoplasia (CIN II).

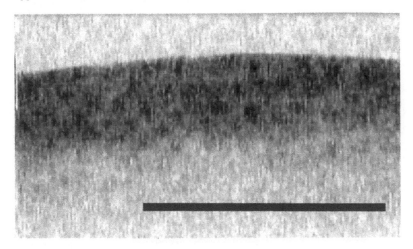

Figure 16   Optical coherence tomographic image of invasive cervical cancer with complete lack of optical structure.

Owing to this property, OCT could be one of the complementary components in a new scheme of early cervical cancer diagnosis, bridging smear analysis and biopsy. After discovering abnormal cells in a PAP smear from a visually unaltered cervix, OCT screening of the cervix can be performed to find areas with subsurface epithelial alterations and by localizing them target the excisional biopsy.

There is one more aspect that demonstrates the clinical significance of OCT in oncogynecology. It is well known that two criteria for staging cancer are the depth of invasion and the linear dimensions of a tumor. At early stages of cancer, the integrity of the basement membrane is preserved. According to our observations, OCT data are quite sensitive to the state of the basement membrane and hence can be used for diagnosing the stage of intraepithelial cancer. In the case of invasive cancer, OCT can play a role in the exact determination of the linear dimensions of a tumor. According to the 1995 FIGO classification of uterine cervical cancer, at an invasion depth of 3–5 mm, a linear tumor dimension of 7 mm is critical in making a decision concerning performance of an organ-preserving operation [12]. Current techniques are not 100% effective in determining the exact boundaries of a lesion. Endophytic tumors are most difficult in this regard, because their borders are not well differentiated visually. This is exactly a field where OCT may prove its usefulness. If a biopsy indicates that the depth of invasion is 3–5 mm, OCT can be engaged to trace the boundaries of the lesion and to determine its exact lateral dimensions. Figure 17 is a tomogram of invasive cancer of the uterine cervix. The transition from unaltered (left) to pathologically altered (right) epithelium can be clearly seen in this image, thus making it possible to exactly indicate the boundaries of the pathological zone. It is very important to note that this tomogram was recorded in the area where epithelium, according to colposcopic examination, had been found visually unaltered. Consequently, the visual and OCT-given borders of a tumor do not coincide. Further examinations confirmed the existence of a typical mismatch in the border position, which can amount to 2–3 mm. This fact can alter the treatment strategy

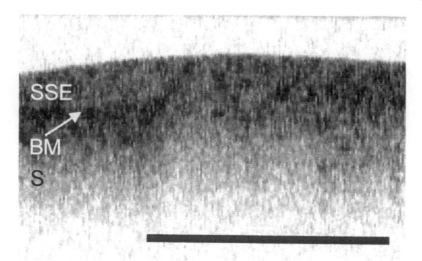

Figure 17 Optical coherence tomographic image of cervical mucosa with disappearing basement membrane at the border of invasive cancer (to the right). This tomogram was recorded in an area where epithelium according to colposcopic examination, was visually unaltered.

in minimally invasive surgery. Based on these results we can draw the conclusion that OCT is capable of detecting, most objectively and accurately among existing diagnostic methods, the boundaries of pathological regions and hence determining the real sizes of lesions.

Optical coherence tomographic data on pathologies in other organs of the female genital system are, to our mind, also interesting. In the previous section, tomograms of normal endometrium in various functional states were presented. Figure 18 demonstrates an image of the endometrium of an older woman (52 years old, postmenopause) suffering from abnormal uterine bleeding. In this tomogram, tissue appears as an inhomogeneous structure with alternation of moderately scattering components and nonscattering rounded formations. Morphologically, this state was determined to be cystic hyperplasia.

In patients with intrauterine tumorous formations, it is sometimes difficult to differentiate between submucosal myoma and an endometrical polyp. Tomographically (see Fig. 19), the presence of poorly backscattering formations with distinct and even borders, corresponding to cavities, speaks for polyp. The OCT image of polyps undoubtedly correlates with histological data. The following is a clinical example.

A 60-year-old female patient A.V. complained of vaginal bleeding, dizziness, and weakness. Examination showed low concentration of hemoglobin, corresponding to moderate anemia. Gynecological examination revealed an insignificant enlargement of the uterus. Ultrasound indicated an enlarged uterus due to an intramural myoma 18 mm in diameter and dilation of the uterine cavity due to a rounded echo-positive formation 23 mm in diameter. Hysteroscopy confirmed the presence of an intrauterine formation, visually resembling submucosal myoma of the uterus. OCT imaging related that this formation had an inhomogeneous structure (Fig. 20b). This finding allowed us to diagnose glandular polyp of the endometrium and to excise it without additional hormonal treatment. The diagnosis was further confirmed histologically (Fig. 20a).

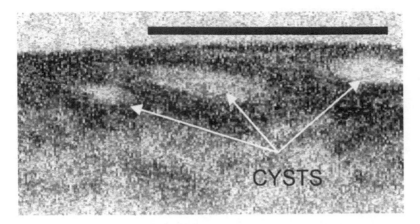

Figure 18 Optical coherence tomographic image of endometrical cystic hyperplasia.

Examination of the peritoneum in gynecology is well known to be of much diagnostic importance. We have attempted to find OCT signs of some pathological states of the peritoneum (Fig. 21a). As indicated earlier, unaltered peritoneum is seen in tomograms as a moderately scattering well-organized structure with a gradual attenuation of the signal with depth (Fig. 21b). When the serous membrane of the small pelvis is sclerosed because of inflammation or postoperative trauma, tomograms reveal increased backscattering from superficial layers with the preservation of

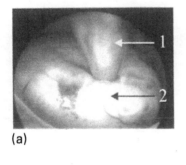

(a)

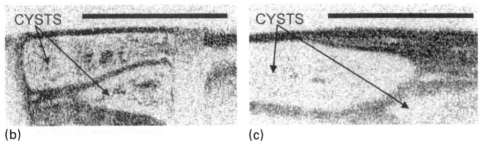

(b)　　　　　　　　　　　　　　(c)

Figure 19 (a) Optical coherence tomographic hysteroscopic examination of lesion in uterine body and (b,c) corresponding tomograms of endometrial polyp. *1*, Tip of OCT probe; *2*, polyp.

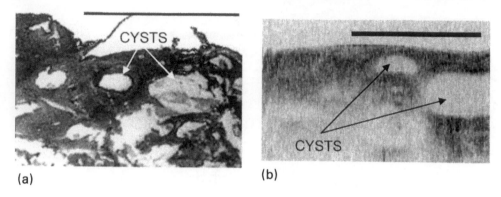

(a)   (b)

Figure 20   (a) Histology and (b) OCT image of endometrial polyp (female patient A.V.).

the optical structure (Fig. 21c). In endometriosis, the OCT signal is chaotic, and regions of low backscattering do not have distinct borders (Fig. 21d).

It is interesting to compare OCT data on alterations in different types of epithelium as a response to inflammation. To obtain these data, OCT colposcopy, OCT hysteroscopy, and OCT laparoscopy were performed in a patient with pelvic inflammatory disease caused by the use of an intrauterine device. In such patients, inflammation usually has a latent character and clinical signs are not pronounced. However, there was a sign repeated in all OCT images of the genital organs of this

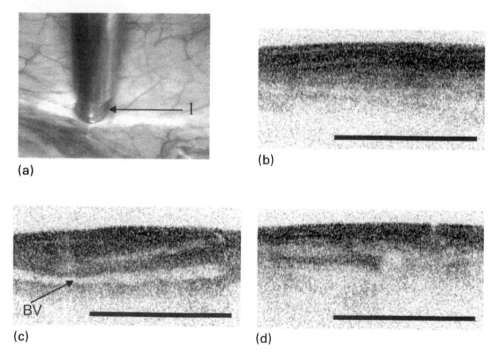

(a)   (b)

(c)   (d)

Figure 21   (a) Photo and (b,c,d) OCT images of peritoneum, (b) normal, (c) in postoperative sclerosis, and (d) in endometriosis. *1*, Tip of OCT probe.

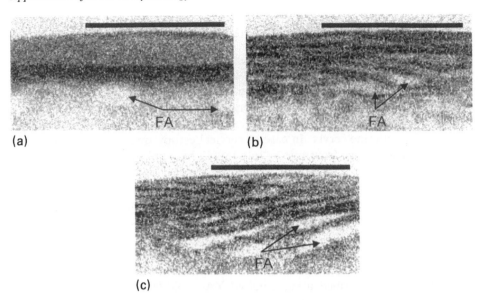

Figure 22 Optical coherence tomographic images of inflammation, recorded from (a) cervix, (b) endometrium and (c) fallopian tube with signs of fluid accumulation (FA) in the same female patient.

patient (Fig. 22)—the accumulation of fluid in tissue, which is indicative of the development of edema, a characteristic sign of inflammation. Mucosa of the uterine cervix covered with stratified squamous epithelium (Fig. 22a) preserves a stratified structure with signs of edematous formation in stroma and changed characteristics in the region of the basement membrane. This may be related to leukocytic infiltration of the latter zone. Regions covered with columnar epithelium (Figs. 22b and 22c) demonstrate the lack of organ specificity at inflammation: Tomograms are quite similar in the uterine cavity and in the wall of the fallopian tube, having a common "tiger skin" pattern.

Summarizing, it should be emphasized that OCT data in gynecology are informative as regards structural alterations that accompany pathological processes of different etiology. Some typical alterations observed in OCT patterns are characteristic of concrete pathologies. This information can be used to indicate the fact of alterations occurring in the organs, to evaluate these alterations qualitatively, and, an important point, to accurately localize the pathological area.

24.4 OCT IN MINIMALLY INVASIVE SURGERY AND EVALUATION OF TREATMENT RESULTS

Optical coherence tomography can be used to monitor evolving changes in the human body caused by different types of treatment. In recent years, various organ-preserving methods, such as cryoapplication, laser vaporization, and electro-excision have found more widespread use in gynecological practice. Therefore, the need to evaluate the effectiveness of pathological tissue removal and monitor long-term results for early detection of the disease recurrence is of great importance. To analyze the OCT capabilities for monitoring treatment adequacy, a dynamic OCT study of the uterine cervix was undertaken after various types of treatment.

Typical response of biotissue to damage agents are well known. An immediate response of living tissue to intervention is intensive vasodilation, leading to edema with subsequent development of a limited zone of dystrophy and necrosis. Restorative processes further lead to regeneration of tissue, an important criterion of recovery. We performed a series of OCT studies to observe the results of cryodestruction of the uterine cervix. In case of cervical ectopy treatment, the pathologically altered tissue was frozen to −160–180°C by application of a tip with circulating nitrogen vapor. OCT information on the development of the response of the uterine cervix to cryoapplication (Fig. 23) correlates well with the known morphological data: Immediately after cryoapplication, swelling occurs; within 24 h the development of cryonecrosis begins; and during the next six weeks healing takes place [13].

One of the minimally invasive treatments of the uterine cervix is laser vaporization. In the gynecological clinic of the Nizhny Novgorod Medical Academy, such operations are performed using a pulsed YAG:Nd laser with radiation at a wavelength of 1.44 μm. OCT examination (Fig. 24) of laser-treated regions showed tissue alterations resembling those in cryodestruction. However, in cryodestruction the epithelial integrity is not broken, whereas in laser vaporization a tissue defect occurs. OCT can measure its depth, clearly determine the demarcation line, and evaluate the reaction of surrounding tissues. It is known that the size of a zone of collateral damage is highly variable depending on the type of tissue, the type of pathological process, the method of treatment, the instrument modification, and

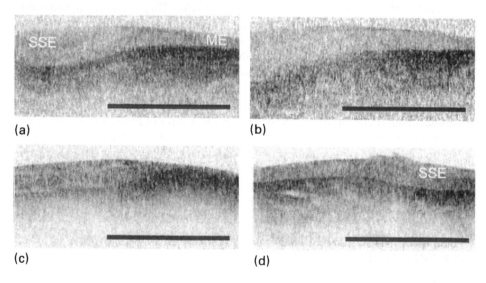

Figure 23   Optical coherence tomographic images of cervix. (a) Before cryoapplication, demonstrating transition of stratified squamous epithelium (SSE) to metaplastic epithelium ME; (b) immediately after cryoapplication with development of tissue swelling; (c) two days later, with development of necrosis (to the right) and collateral inflammation (to the left); (d) six weeks later, demonstrating recovery of SSE. Images (c) and (d) are averaged over three frames.

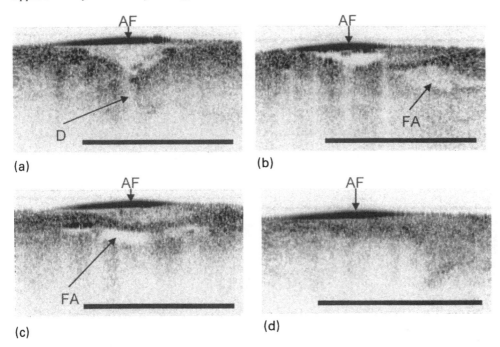

Figure 24 Optical coherence tomographic images of the cervix (a) immediately after laser vaporization with a tissue defect (D); (b) 5 min later with a decrease of the defect due to swelling of surrounding tissue and fluid accumulation (FA); (c) 10 min later, with further development of edema; (d) one day later, with formation of necrosis (unstructured highly scattering zone). A black narrow stripe repeated similarly in all tomograms is an artifact (AF) due to mirror reflection form the OCT tip window.

the choice of treatment parameters [13]. Based on OCT examination, one can evaluate the influence of various manipulation on living tissue, perform a comparative analysis of these manipulations, and hence choose the most effective mode of treatment.

Organ-preserving operations set up a number of requirements, such as minimal traumatization of healthy tissue and, more important in oncology, adequate excision of the pathological area. In precancer and preinvasive cancer of the uterine cervix in women of reproductive age, a pathological area can be excised by the use of various instruments such as a cold knife, laser scalpel, or electroloop. Treatment is deemed effective if histological study of the removed area does not reveal cancer cells at the borders of the tissue section. Currently, electroexcision of the uterine cervix is most widely used in gynecological practice. Unfortunately, electrotrauma causes such pronounced changes in the tissue that often it is difficult to evaluate the excised material morphologically. To our mind, OCT can ensure more accurate evaluation of the effectiveness of tissue removal by examining the edges of the postoperative wound. When an optical pattern of healthy epithelium is detected at the borders of the tissue section, one can speak of adequate removal of the pathological area. Because OCT is able to acquire useful information in real time, it can be used for evaluation intraoperatively. The following clinical case illustrates this OCT application.

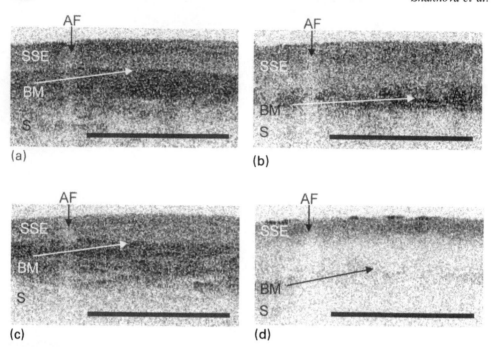

Figure 25 Tomograms of cervical mucosa, demonstrating intraoperative application of OCT (patient M.S.). (a) Healthy area before treatment; (b) zone of punctation with hyperplasia of SSE and deformation of BM, before treatment; (c) margin of wound with normal mucosa and signs of collateral inflammation in stroma, immediately after excision; (d) margin of wound with abnormal mucosa characterized by epithelial hyperplasia and deformation of basement membrane with signs of collateral swelling, immediately after excision. Image (d) served as an additional argument for repeated excision. The light vertical stripe repeated similarly in all tomograms is an artifact due to contamination of the OCT probe surface.

In patient M.S., 28 years old, cytological screening revealed CIN III. Colposcopic study showed abnormal findings with punctation, zones of open glands, and excessive vascularization. Tomograms taken from the zone of punctation demonstrated structural alterations, hyperplasia of the epithelium, and reaction of underlying stroma (Figs. 25a and 25b). Electroexcision of the uterine cervix was undertaken, followed by OCT examination of the borders of the wound. In the majority of tomograms epithelium was normal in the area adjacent to the section line (Fig. 25c) except for one region topically corresponding to the boundary with punctation. The OCT image of this region is shown in Fig. 25d. This intraoperative OCT information served as an additional argument for repeated excision.

Along with the intraoperative application, OCT can also be useful for postoperative monitoring of the recovery processes and evaluation of their completeness and timeliness. For instance, a distinctive feature of laser therapy is early healing, as confirmed by OCT. Three weeks after laser vaporization, OCT tomograms demonstrate recovery of the epithelial structure with some signs of inflammation (Fig. 26a), whereas after cryoapplication the reparation process is completed only in six weeks (Fig. 23d), similar to the case of electroexcision (Fig. 26b). Dynamic postoperative

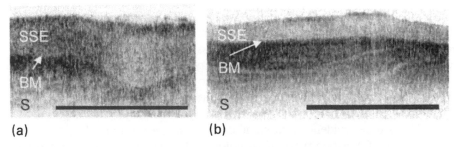

Figure 26 Tomograms demonstrating postoperative OCT control. Images of treated cervix (a) 3 weeks after laser vaporization and (b) 6 weeks after electroexcision show regeneration of normal epithelium with signs of reactive inflation. In (a), a light rounded formation is sclerosis in the focus of laser application. In (b), fluid accumulation in stromal tissue is shown by light stripes. Image (b) is averaged over three frames

OCT imaging can not only control the reparative processes but also helps to assess long-term results of surgical treatment. We demonstrate this OCT application with the following clinical case.

> A 25-year-old female patient G.A. complained of bleeding on coitus. A diagnosis of precancer of the uterine cervix was made based on cytological data. Colposcopy revealed an atypical zone of transformation. Biopsy confirmed the diagnosis of uterine cervical precancer, verified morphologically as CIN III. OCT revealed regions of local destruction of the basement membrane, which made us suspect a microcarinoma of the uterine cervix. Electroconization of the uterine cervix was performed. Histological study confirmed the diagnosis of microcarcinoma. The patient was repeatedly examined with colposcopy and OCT imaging. In seven months of follow-up, colposcopic study revealed tiny changes of a small region of exocervix. These changes were thought to be signs of cervicitis. In OCT images of this region, the epithelial structure was seen to have changed. A repeated excision was performed. Histological study of the excised region revealed CIN III. Further follow-up examinations with both colposcopy and OCT showed complete recovery of the epithelium of the uterine cervix. At present, the patient is healthy, she has become pregnant, and the course of pregnancy shows no complications. We plan to follow this case with OCT.

Thus, the capability of OCT to obtain in vivo, in real time and noninvasively, information on the response of biological tissue to damaging agents is of considerable practical importance. OCT has proven to be useful for the intra- and postoperative control of the adequacy of treatment and monitoring of healing processes during long-term follow-up for detection of disease recurrence.

24.5 CONCLUSION

The trends of contemporary medicine to use minimally invasive organ-preserving methods of treatment are driving a demand for new diagnostic techniques. Optical coherence tomography emerged as a new bioimaging modality to meet all the main requirements that a modern diagnostic technique should satisfy, such as a large amount of novel diagnostic information, high speed of data acquisition, and portable and easy-to-use devices. Due to all these advantages, OCT is promising to find a place in some areas of medical practice.

In this chapter, we presented OCT capabilities in gynecology. We demonstrated that OCT data on the tissue structure of female genital organs and the precise dimensions of the tissue components can be successfully used to evaluate the functional states of the female body. In particular, it may be utilized to monitor changes in hormonal activity and to follow the course of hormonal therapy.

In vivo detection of structural alterations caused by pathological processes is, in our opinion, of essential interest to practicing physicians from several points of view. First, OCT studies evidence that some definite changes in optical patterns of tissue are indicative of concrete types of pathologies. Hence, OCT has the potential to contribute to making a differential diagnosis. Second, OCT can indicate exactly margins of a pathological zone, which is particularly useful for guiding target biopsy. Finally, the capability of OCT to evaluate the state of the assessment membrane of epithelium and determine, with high precision, the linear dimensions of a lesion can help in further clinical applications to assess the extent of pathology and the stage of the disease.

Another interesting application of OCT in the future may be in intraoperative and postoperative control. When used intraoperatively, OCT may serve as a useful tool to control the effectiveness of tissue removal and to correct, if necessary, the extent of tissue excision immediately in the course of an operation, not waiting for the results of histological study. In an early postoperative period, OCT can be applied to estimate whether the reparative processes are effective and timely, and during a longer follow-up OCT can ensure early detection of recurrence of a disease.

In conclusion, it is important to note that OCT imaging, though treated by the scientific community very enthusiastically, should not be thought of as a replacement for currently available diagnostic techniques. Before OCT finds widespread application in clinical practice, a thorough scientific investigation remains to be done to work out unambiguous and commonly adopted ways to interpret recorded images, to determine definitive OCT criteria of various pathologies, etc. New technical improvements are also desirable. In spite of all this, we believe that OCT imaging will soon find a place as an interesting complementary method among medical diagnostic modalities.

REFERENCES

1. van Niekerk WA, Robiniwich M, Nozawa S, et al. Colposcopy, cervicography, speculoscopy and endoscopy. Cytology Towards the 21 Century: An International Expert Conference and Tutorial. Acta Cytol 42:33–49, 1998.
2. Huang D, Wang J, Lin CP, Shuman JS, Stinson WG, Chang W, Hee MR, Flotte T, Gregory K, Puliafito CA, Fujimoto JG. Optical coherence tomography. Science 254:1178, 1991.
3. Sergeev AM, Gelikonov VM, Gelikonov GV, Feldchtein FI, Kuranov RV, Gladkova ND, Shakhova NM, Snopova LB, Shakhov AV, Kuznetzova IA, Denisenko AN, Pochinko VV, Chumakov YuP, Streltzova OS. In vivo endoscopic OCT imaging of precancer and cancer states of human mucosa. Opt Express 1(13):432–440, 1997; *http://epubs.osa.org/oearchive/pdf/2788.pdf*
4. Feldchtein FI, Gelikonov VM, Gelikonov GV, Kuranov RV, Sergeev AM, Gladkova ND, Shakhov AV, Shakhova NM, Snopova LB, Terent'eva AB, Zagainova EV, Chumakov YuP, Kuznetzova IA. Endoscopic applications of optical coherence tomography. Opt Express 3(6):257–270, 1998; *http://epubs.osa.org.oearchive/pdf/5788.pdf*

5. Pitris C, Goodman A, Boppart SA, Libus JJ, Fujimoto JG, Brezinski ME. High-resolution imaging of gynecologic neoplasms using optical coherence tomography. Obstet Gynecol 93(1):135–139, 1999.
6. Ross MH, Romrell LJ, Kaye GI. Histology. A Text and Atlas. 3rd ed. Baltimore: Williams and Wilkins, 1995.
7. Coppleson M, Monaghan JM, Morrow CP, Tattersall MH. In: M Coppleson, ed., Gynecologic Oncology. 2nd ed. New York: Churchill Livingstone, 1992.
8. Gelikonov VM, Gelikonov GV, Gladkova ND, Leonov VI, Feldchtein FI, Sergeev AM, Khanin YaI. Optical fiber interferometer and piezoelectric modulator. US Patent 5835642 (1998).
9. Rusakevich PS. Background and Precancer Diseases of Uterine Cervix. Minsk: Vysshaya shkola, 1998.
10. Leppert PC. Proliferation and apoptosis of fibroblasts and smooth muscle cells in rat uterine cervix throughout gestation and the effect of the antiprogesterone on a pristone. Am J Obstet Gynecol 178(4):713–723, 1998.
11. Cartier R. Practical Colposcopy. New York: Gustav Fisher Verlag, 1984.
12. Creasman WT, Zaino RJ, Major FJ et al. Early invasive carcinoma of the cervix (3 to 5 mm invasion): Risk factors and prognosis. A gynecologic oncology group study. Am J Obstet Gynecol 178(1):62–65, 1998.
13. Wright VC, Lickrish GM, Shier RM. Basic and Advanced Colposcopy. Houston: Biomedical Communications, 1995, Parts I, II.

25

Gastrointestinal Applications of Optical Coherence Tomography

NORMAN S. NISHIOKA, STEPHAN BRAND, BRETT E. BOUMA, GUILLERMO J. TEARNEY, and CAROLYN C. COMPTON

Harvard Medical School and Wellman Laboratories of Photomedicine, Massachusetts General Hospital, Boston, Massachusetts

25.1 INTRODUCTION

There are many compelling reasons for developing OCT imaging systems for use in the gastrointestinal tract. Modern gastrointestinal endoscopic instruments provide ready access to the mucosal surface of the esophagus, stomach, duodenum, colon, rectum, and terminal ileum and with specialized instrumentation such as choledo-choscopes and enteroscopes it is possible to directly visualize portions of the pancreatic duct, bile ducts, and jejunum. Furthermore, the majority of gastrointestinal disease processes are mucosal in origin, so access to the mucosal aspect of the gastrointestinal tract is especially important from a clinical perspective. However, despite the great facility with which the gastrointestinal mucosa can be visualized, current endoscopes have certain limitations. For example, typical magnifications provided by endoscopes are approximately 10–25× and spatial resolution is typically limited to approximately 100 μm. Even specialized zoom endoscopes with magnifications of up to 100× have spatial resolutions no better than 50 μm. All images produced by standard endoscopes are by necessity limited to examination from the mucosal surface. Thus, essentially no information about the depth of an object or its three-dimensional character is available during routine endoscopy.

Endoscopic ultrasound (EUS) has greatly enhanced the ability to discern the depth of lesions and has provided means of imaging structures outside the gastrointestinal tract such as the pancreas, lymph nodes, and liver with great accuracy. Standard EUS instruments operate at a frequency of 7.5 MHz with a corresponding resolution of approximately 340 μm (in water). This relatively low operating frequency permits good depth of penetration into tissue, and structures many centimeters beneath the probe can be clearly visualized. High frequency ultrasound probes are available although not widely used. These instruments have operating frequencies as high as 25 MHz and can provide resolution as low as $110\,\mu$m in the axial direction and $240\,\mu$m in the lateral direction [1]. It is important to note that resolution specified for OCT systems is measured in air. To determine the effective resolution of OCT systems in water or tissue, the resolution measured in air must be divided by the index of refraction. An OCT system with a resolution of $10\,\mu$m measured in air would, for example, have a $7\,\mu$m resolution in water. OCT provides higher spatial resolution than EUS but lower depth of penetration (see Table 1). Thus, using current technology, OCT and EUS are quite complementary in their imaging capabilities, and OCT is unlikely to replace EUS as a routine imaging procedure.

From an operational standpoint, OCT has two characteristics that may make it easier to use and interpret than EUS. First, EUS requires that an acoustic match between the transducer and tissue be present. In general, this means that water must be interposed between the instrument and the tissue surface. Techniques for doing this include operating in a pool of water or in a situation where water is flowing or by wrapping a water-filled balloon around the transducer. In contrast, OCT can operate with either a water or air interface, making it simpler to use from a technical standpoint. Another difference between OCT and EUS is in the interpretation of images. Ultrasound images are difficult to untrained gastroenterologists to interpret, as these practitioners are not accustomed to viewing images based on differences in acoustic impedance. Thus, a significant learning curve exists for EUS, and most practitioners have taken specialty training in its use; training periods of a year or more are typical. Thus, even large gastrointestinal endoscopy groups have no more than one or two individuals trained in performing and interpreting EUS. On the other hand, OCT imagery has the potential to be more widely accepted. The images provided by OCT closely mimic histopathology, and as spatial resolution improves in future instruments this match with histopathology will increase. Because most gastroenterologists have at least passing familiarity with the histopathological appearance of gastrointestinal tract structures, it is possible that the transition to interpreting OCT images will be easier than that of interpreting EUS images.

Table 1 Comparison of OCT and Conventional EUS

	OCT	EUS
Typical configuration	Catheter	Specialized endoscope
Penetration depth	2 mm	5 cm
Spatial resolution (in water)	$7\,\mu$m	$110\,\mu$m (25 MHz)
Image analog	Histopathology	Ultrasound
Coupling medium	Air or water	Water
Doppler	Possible	Available

25.2 IN VITRO STUDIES

There have been several reports of OCT imaging performed on in vitro specimens. Although the results of these studies are of limited clinical value because of the use of nonliving tissue, they are important because they form the basis of our present understanding of the potential ability of OCT to image GI tract structures. For example, Izatt and coworkers [2,3] described the use of a mechanically scanned fiber-based OCT device to obtain images of porcine esophagus in vitro. This system was not designed for clinical use and required 100 s to acquire a single image. In the esophagus, three distinct layers were identified based on correlation of the measured thicknesses of the layers with fixed histological sections [2]. These layers were felt to represent squamous epithelium, lamina propria, and muscularis mucosa. The squamous epithelium was seen as a highly scattering layer, while the lamina propria demonstrated much less backscatter. In vivo OCT studies by our group [4,5] and studies by Sergeev et al. [6] showed a different backscatter pattern with a highly scattering lamina propria and a much less scattering squamous epithelium. In the in vitro study, the submucosa and muscularis propria were poorly visualized due to attenuation of the incident light beam below detectable levels [2]. In this report, OCT imaging was also performed in vitro on a segment of stomach from a patient with gastric cancer. The normal stomach appeared similar to the esophageal images in that the mucosa and lamina propria were readily recognized. Areas of the stomach affected by adenocarcinoma were seen as an area of increased backscatter. In a sample of normal human colon, the mucosa, muscularis mucosa, and submucosa could be identified. Interestingly, colonic crypts that were readily seen in histological sections were not resolved by OCT. Although the imaging system was not suitable for clinical use, this study demonstrated the potential of OCT to image the superficial layers of the gastrointestinal tract.

In a similar study, Tearney et al. [7] reported on an in vitro experience using autopsy specimens. The fiber-optic sample arm of an OCT device was mechanically scanned across the tissue in an acquisition period of 45 s. This system was also unsuitable for clinical use. Postmortem images of the esophagus were similar to those reported by Izatt et al. [2]. The upper portion of the mucosa appeared homogeneous in the OCT images. The muscularis mucosa was more reflective than the mucosa in these experiments. Colonic inflammation was characterized by an area of high backscatter, and disruption of the crypt architecture was also evident. In another study, the same group of investigators examined OCT images of the pancreatic and biliary ducts obtained from autopsies [8]. OCT images of the common bile duct (CBD) demonstrated the ability of OCT to resolve the various layers of the CBD. In addition, the glands of the ducts and their associated ductules could be identified. Images of the pancreatic duct revealed that the ductal epithelium as well as the periductal pancreatic tissue and islet cells could be visualized [8].

25.3 IN VIVO IMAGING IN ANIMALS

Tearney et al. [9] described in vivo OCT imaging in rabbits. This report was important because it demonstrated that it was possible to develop an OCT system with the potential for clinical use. The light source used to obtain these images was a mode-locked chromium : forsterite laser operating at a wavelength of 1280 nm.

Unfortunately, this source is not sufficiently portable for routine clinical use. Images of the rabbit esophagus revealed visualization of the mucosa, submucosa, inner muscular layer, outer muscular layer, serosa, and adventitial structures. However, the rabbit esophagus is considerably thinner than the human esophagus, and therefore these observations may not directly correlate with human clinical studies. In addition, the animal model is limited by the lack of a variety of disease states such as dysplasia and neoplasia, and thus it is not possible to determine the true clinical efficacy of OCT from animal studies.

25.4 CLINICAL STUDIES

25.4.1 Technology

To date, three different strategies for deploying endoscopic OCT scanning in vivo have been described. Although all three approaches have used catheters designed to be delivered via the instrument channel of a gastrointestinal endoscope, the scanning methods have been different. Sergeev and coworkers have demonstrated the use of a forward-viewing catheter in which the lateral scanning is performed at the distal end of the catheter. Scanning is accomplished by a tiny mirror driven by a galvanometer. The scanning rate is 30 cm/s and produces a 200 × 200 pixel image in 1 s. Image size was approximately 1.7 mm wide and 1.2 mm deep. The catheter terminates in a window. Operating wavelength was 830 nm. A group at Case Western Reserve working in conjunction with the Olympus Corporation [2] developed a radial scanning OCT catheter. The catheter is 2.4 mm in diameter and provides a 360° sector scan perpendicular to the catheter. The frame rate is 6.7 fps. Our group at Massachusetts General Hospital has reported the use of a linear scanning OCT system [10]. This catheter probes tissue perpendicular to the catheter while the optics are scanned in a linear fashion along the longitudinal axis of the catheter.

A brief comparison of the three systems is presented in Table 2.

25.4.2 Pilot Studies of OCT in Humans

The first reported in vivo demonstration of OCT in the human gastrointestinal (GI) tract occurred in 1997. Sergeev et al. [6] described a preliminary experience in four patients undergoing upper GI endoscopy. They were able to identify five layers within the normal esophagus. They tentatively identified these layers as mucosa (squamous epithelium), lamina propria, muscularis mucosa, submucosa, and muscularis propria. Correlation was based on approximate correlation with

Table 2 Comparison of OCT Systems

	MGH	Case Western	Institute of Applied Physics of RAS
Scanning	Longitudinal	Radial	Transverse
Operating wavelength	1300 nm	1300 nm	830 nm
Frame rate	4 Hz	6.7 Hz	1 Hz
Scan size ($w \times d$)	5.5 mm × 2.5 mm		1.7 mm × 1.2 mm

biopsy material based on known thicknesses of these layers, but no histological sections of the corresponding OCT images were provided in this study. Furthermore, the biopsy specimens would not have included all layers visualized by OCT and therefore would be of limited value in definitively identifying the tissue layers seen with OCT. In the gastric antrum, a similar analysis suggested that OCT could resolve the mucosa (Columnar epithelium), lamina propria, and muscularis mucosa. Other features that may have been resolved included glands, gastric pits, and blood vessels. OCT imaging of an esophageal cancer and a gastric cancer revealed a greater number of blood vessels within the tumor mass, suggesting the presence of increased vascularity. In addition, increased backscatter was observed from the epithelial layer of the tumors, which may have resulted from a greater nuclear density.

Two other groups have since reported larger clinical experiences with OCT in the GI tract. Sivak et al. [11] reported their initial experience in 38 patients. Images of normal tissue were obtained from the esophagus, stomach, duodenum, terminal ileum, and colon. The normal esophagus was visualized as a five-layer pattern. Structures thought to represent glands and blood vessels were seen in the fourth layer, so this layer was felt to represent the submucosa. This assignment of layers was in agreement with the experience of Sergeev et al. [6]. In the stomach and small intestine, gastric pits and duodenal villi could be identified. This group also determined that a probe with a 1 mm focal point appeared to provide optimal image quality.

Our group at the Massachusetts General Hospital also reported its initial experience in the first 30 patients [4]. Our experience has since increased to more than 100 patients. A brief description of the OCT appearance of normal gastrointestinal tissue is given in the following sections.

Esophagus—Normal Esophageal Squamous Mucosa

It was possible to differentiate normal esophageal squamous epithelium from gastric mucosa in all patients that have been investigated by OCT in our institution. OCT images of normal esophageal mucosa are characterized by a layered anatomy. Five anatomical layers can be clearly delineated in the OCT images (Figs. 1 and 2). These layers represent epithelium, lamina propria, muscularis mucosae, submucosa, and muscularis propria. The different layers were distinguished by the relative difference in the intensity of their backreflection. An intense backreflection is denoted by a darker gray scale in the OCT images. Depth measurements performed on in vitro OCT images of cadaveric specimens and their corresponding histology were used to identify the layered structures visible in the OCT images (Fig. 1). The OCT image penetration depth in the esophagus is approximately 1.5–2.0 mm.

Stomach—Normal Gastric Tissue

In vivo OCT images of normal gastric tissue show marked differences between esophageal squamous epithelium and gastric epithelium, which reflects the different histological anatomy (see Table 3). The layered architecture of squamous epithelium cannot be seen in OCT images of gastric tissue. Instead, the gross architecture of gastric pits and crypts is visible in the OCT images (Fig. 3). Thus, in contrast to the horizontally oriented layered architecture of squamous epithelium, the tissue orientation of gastric tissue is vertical in the OCT images. Also, the penetration depth of

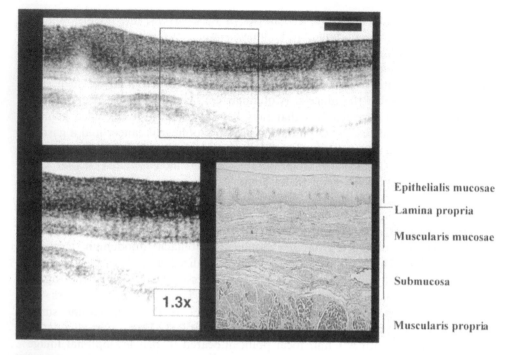

Epithelialis mucosae
Lamina propria
Muscularis mucosae

Submucosa

Muscularis propria

Figure 1 Esophageal squamous epithelium (ex vivo).

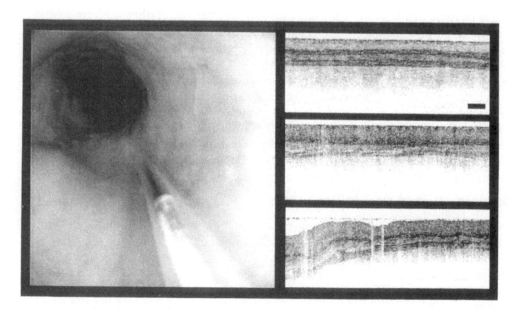

Figure 2 Esophageal squamous epithelium (in vivo).

Table 3 OCT Features of Squamous Epithelium and Gastric Mucosa

OCT features	Squamous epithelium	Gastric mucosa
Main feature	Different tissue layers	Crypts and pits
Layer architecture?	Yes (five layers)	No
Tissue orientation	Horizontal	Vertical
OCT penetration depth	High	Low
Image contrast	Varies from layer to layer	High on mucosal surface, low in deeper structures

OCT images of the stomach (750 μm) is less than that of the esophagus, which usually limits visualization to the gastric mucosa.

Gastroesophageal Junction

The abrupt histological change from esophageal squamous mucosa to gastric mucosa at the gastroesophageal junction can be observed by OCT (Fig. 4). The horizontal, layered tissue architecture of the squamous epithelium can be easily differentiated from the vertical "crypt-and-pit architecture" of the stomach. Although the layered architecture of the squamous epithelium is visible at the gastroesophageal junction, the differences in the backscattering of the different layers are usually not so pronounced as in the proximal csophagus.

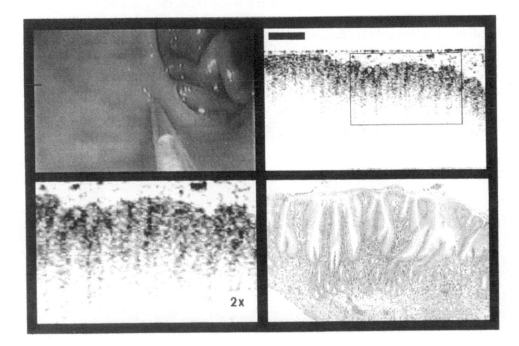

Figure 3 Gastric mucosa.

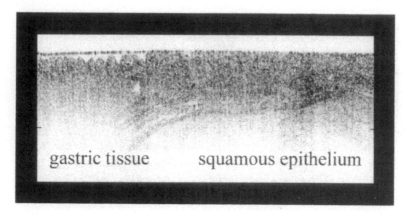

Figure 4   Gastroesophageal junction.

Duodenum

Characteristics of the duodenal mucosa evidenced in OCT images are different from those of other tissue types. OCT can visualize the gross anatomical structures of duodenal mucosa including duodenal villi and crypts of Lieberkühn (Fig. 5). The OCT image shown in Fig. 5 was obtained with close contact between the OCT probe and the duodenal mucosa. Thus, the duodenal villi appear compressed, and crypts are only indirectly visualized as dark vertical stripes.

Colon

Optical coherence tomographic images of the colon show the gross morphology of the colon, including the mucosa, muscularis mucosa, and submucosa (Fig. 6). Visualization of fine cellular details and single colonic crypts is beyond the resolution of OCT, although in some cases dark vertical lines in the superficial mucosa indicate the location of crypts.

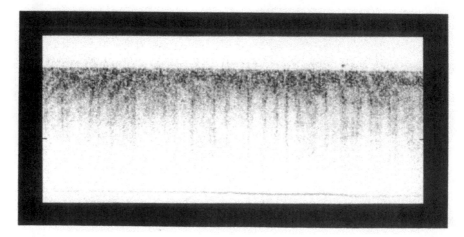

Figure 5   Duodenal mucosa.

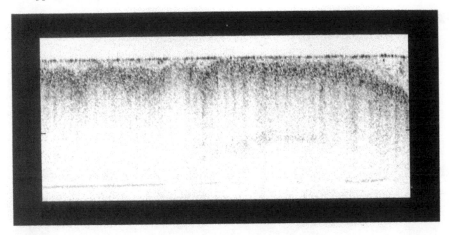

Figure 6 Normal colonic mucosa.

25.5 POTENTIAL CLINICAL APPLICATIONS OF OCT

The studies performed with OCT to date have all been preliminary survey studies, and the number of patients with abnormal tissue that have been imaged remains very small. Thus, no clear clinical use of OCT in the GI tract has yet evolved. Nonetheless, the experience has been sufficient to suggest possible uses of OCT in the GI tract. It is beyond the scope of this chapter to speculate on all the potential applications of OCT in the GI tract, but several of the more promising applications will be mentioned briefly.

25.5.1 Identification of Abnormal Mucosa

Although images of fine cellular detail within gastrointestinal tissue is beyond the resolution of current OCT technology, information about tissue architecture is readily apparent in the images. The best studied example of this is in Barrett's epithelium.

Barrett's Esophagus

Barrett's esophagus occurs in the esophagus when the normal squamous epithelial lining of the esophagus is replaced by columnar epithelium. Although historically three types of Barrett's epithelium have been described, only one type is important clinically. This so-called specialized columnar epithelium or intestinal metaplasia is the only type of Barrett's epithelium that is known to have malignant potential. Thus, intestinal metaplasia in the esophagus has become synonymous with Barrett's epithelium. In our experience, the identification of Barrett's epithelium is readily apparent by OCT. In this setting, the laminar appearance of normal squamous mucosa contrasts quite clearly with the columnar architecture of Barrett's epithelium. In addition, Barrett's epithelium shows distinct features that make differentiation of Barrett's epithelium from gastric mucosa by OCT possible (Fig. 7). OCT images of gastric mucosa show a small penetration depth, a regular "crypt-and-pit architecture" and a vertical tissue orientation. In Barrett's esophagus the regular crypt-and-pit architecture is lost, and the penetration depth of OCT is deeper than in gastric tissue. In addition, the mucosal surface of Barrett's

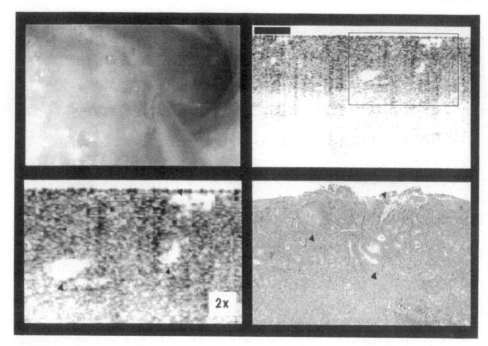

Figure 7   Barrett's esophagus.

epithelium is usually very irregular. However, this feature can be observed only in cases where there is no direct contact between the OCT probe and the mucosal surface (Fig. 8). Direct contact between the OCT probe and the mucosal surface usually leads to a flattening of the mucosal surface (Fig. 7). Thus, off-surface imaging provides more detailed information of the mucosal surface and is helpful in differentiating Barrett's epithelium from gastric mucosa. In most Barrett's patients, mucosal glands have been visualized by OCT (Fig. 7). The glands

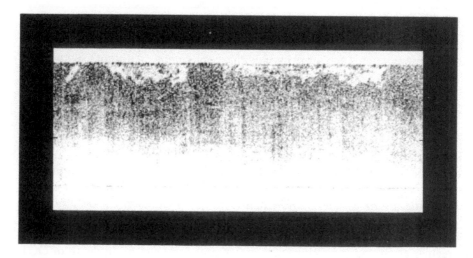

Figure 8   Irregular mucosal surface in Barrett's esophagus.

could be recognized as either pockets of low reflectance below the epithelial surface or invaginations through the epithelium. Observation of deeper structures such as the muscularis mucosae was typically not possible due to the loss of signal or shadowing arising from strong scattering within the metaplastic epithelium. In addition, distinct tissue layers such as that seen in squamous epithelium are usually absent in Barrett's epithelium.

Identification of Barrett's epithelium is not usually a clinically challenging problem for the endoscopist as the pearly white squamous mucosa also contrasts nicely with the pinker, salmon color of Barrett's epithelium. However, this distinction is made endoscopically by visualizing the squamocolumnar junction and using the contrast at this level as a guide. Thus, the endoscopic appearance of Barrett's esophagus is based on a relative difference in mucosal color and texture. We have had occasions where the squamocolumnar junction was not obvious endoscopically due to the extensive length of Barrett's epithelium. In this situation, OCT imaging was useful because it demonstrated that the esophageal mucosa had been replaced by Barrett's epithelium. In addition, it is endoscopically difficult to visualize the distal border between normal gastric tissue and Barrett's epithelium. This differentiation is usually made by visualization of the gastric folds, which is only a rough estimation. We have been able to image the transition zone from normal gastric tissue to Barrett's epithelium (Fig. 9) in several patients. Based on these preliminary findings, we believe that the criteria listed in Table 4 can be used to identify the transition zone from Barrett's epithelium to gastric tissue. These characteristics might also be useful for identifying patients with small amounts of intestinal metaplasia in the distal esophagus ("ultrashort" Barrett's).

Barrett's esophagus with and without dysplasia has been studied with OCT. Dysplasia is defined by cytological and architectural changes. Cytological features (e.g., nuclear size and shape, nuclear-to-cytoplasmic ratio, nuclear stratification) are beyond the resolution of OCT. However, subcellular changes, such as an increased nuclear-to-cytoplasmic ratio, may alter the light reflection characteristics of Barrett's epithelium and thereby lead to enhanced contrast in OCT images of dysplastic Barrett's epithelium. This contrast could potentially be used for the detection of dysplasia and is the focus of ongoing studies. In addition, we observed changes in the glandular architecture (irregular shaped, cribriform glands) in high-grade dysplasia, which may be specific for dysplastic Barrett's epithelium (see 25.5.2). Larger trials will be necessary to confirm the sensitivity and specificity of these features for diagnosing high-grade dysplasia.

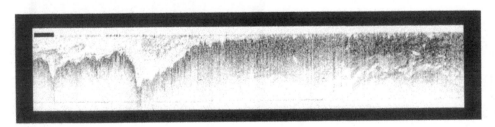

Figure 9   Junction of gastric mucosa (left) and Barrett's metaplasia (right).

Table 4 OCT Features of Barrett's Epithelium and Gastric Mucosa

OCT features	Barrett's epithelium	Gastric mucosa
Main feature	Loss of regular crypt-and-pit architecture	Crypt-and-pit architecture
Mucosal surface	Irregular	Regular crypts and pits
Image contrast	Inhomogeneous	High contrast on mucosal surface, low contrast in deeper layers
Image depth	Medium to high	Low
Tissue orientation	Irregular, deeper layers at the transition zone often horizontally oriented	Vertical
Glands	Frequent	Occasional

Gastritis

Gastritis is a generic term that refers to the presence of inflammation within the gastric wall. It is a very common condition and can be produced by a wide variety of factors, including medications, infection, trauma, gastric acidity, and autoimmune diseases. Gastritis is detected endoscopically by the appearance of erythema, which is typically patchy in distribution. Areas of negative gastritis can be differentiated from normal gastric mucosa by OCT by increased backscattering from the mucosal layer with a more pronounced crypt-and-pit architecture than in normal gastric tissue (Fig. 10). Although OCT appears to be fully capable of identifying the presence of gastritis, the clinical value of this capability is unclear.

Celiac Disease

The villous architecture of the duodenum is readily apparent in OCT images (Fig. 5). This observation suggests that OCT maybe useful in screening patients for disease conditions characterized by atrophy of the villous architecture. Thus, diseases such as celiac disease might be readily ruled out by OCT imaging of the duodenal mucosa,

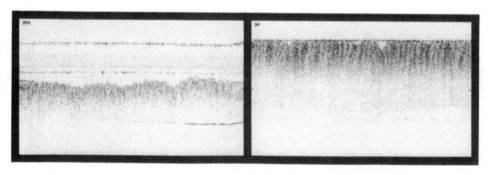

Figure 10 Normal gastric mucosa (left) and mucosa with gastritis (right).

which might make it unnecessary to obtain biopsies to rule out villous atrophy. On the other hand, the finding of villous atrophy is not specific for any disease, and it is therefore unlikely that OCT will obviate the need to obtain biopsies in the presence of villous atrophy.

Inflammatory Bowel Disease

Inflammatory bowel disease typically involves the mucosal surface of the GI tract. The involvement can occur anywhere along the GI tract from the mouth to the anus. In general, the presence of mucosal inflammation can be readily identified during routine endoscopic procedures. However, assessing the degree of inflammation can be assessed only qualitatively. Because the thickness of the mucosa can be accurately measured by OCT, this may provide a useful measure of disease activity, particularly in ulcerative colitis. The issue of screening for dysplasia in patients with chronic ulcerative colitis is discussed briefly in the following section.

25.5.2 Identification of Dysplasia

Most proponents of OCT have suggested that it may have the potential to identify dysplasia during endoscopy. Potential uses would be to screen patients with Barrett's esophagus and chronic ulcerative colitis. From a clinical perspective, this is a particularly important potential use of OCT because areas of dysplasia are typically indistinguishable from surrounding tissue without dysplasia during endoscopy. Thus, the current practice is to obtain random biopsies looking for foci of dysplasia. Obviously, this approach carries with it a significant chance that a sampling error will be made and therefore a real-time method of identifying areas of dysplasia or targeting those areas most suspicious for harboring dysplasia would be of great benefit. In principal, OCT could improve the diagnostic yield of such screening procedures. However, no one has yet shown either in vivo or in vitro that current OCT imaging techniques have sufficient resolution to differentiate dysplastic from nondysplastic epithelium. In the MGH experience with patients with Barrett's epithelium, it has not been possible to reliably differentiate Barrett's epithelium with high-grade dysplasia from Barrett's epithelium without dysplasia using simple visualization of OCT images. Because the resolution of current OCT devices is insufficient to resolve structures at the cellular level, it is likely that the identification of dysplasia will need to derive out of gross structural features. Thus, architectural features rather than cytological features will need to be identified as markers of dysplasia. In certain cases of Barrett's with high-grade dysplasia we have observed glandular architecture of disordered and chaotic appearance. Other features that may be indicators for high-grade dysplasia are an irregular shape of the glands and a cribriform pattern of the glandular architecture (Fig. 11). This finding is also seen in histological sections and may be a relatively specific marker of high-grade dysplasia. However, the sensitivity of this feature for identifying areas of high-grade dysplasia is unknown.

It should be noted that alternative approaches for identifying dysplasia are being actively pursued. These methods include dye spraying of the mucosa with agents such as methylene blue at the time of endoscopy to selectively stain various tissue types, fluorescence measurements, and the use of fluorescent markers such as protoporphyrin IX derived from orally administered 5-aminolevulinic acid. Whether

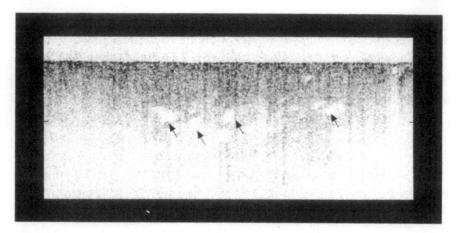

Figure 11 Barrett's esophagus with high-grade dysplasia (arrows indicate dysplastic glands).

OCT or any of these alternative approaches will ultimately prove to be clinically useful for detecting dysplasia in Barrett's esophagus is not yet known.

Colonic Polyps

Optical coherence tomography may have the potential for differentiating colonic polyps. The most common types of colonic polyps are hyperplastic (nonadenomatous) and adenomatous polyps. Hyperplastic polyps are non-neoplastic hyperproliferative lesions characterized by the failure of mature epithelial cells to detach normally. Adenomatous polyps are benign neoplasms consisting of poorly differentiated epithelial cells with different degrees of dysplasia and are known to be premalignant. The vast majority of colorectal carcinomas are thought to arise from adenomatous polyps. The incidence of colorectal carcinomas in the United States is second only to that of lung cancer. The ability to identify polyp types during endoscopy is of potential clinical importance because early detection of premalignant lesions is important in the treatment of patients. The ability to distinguish adenomatous from hyperplastic polyps in vivo could significantly reduce complications and costs associated with polypectomy. In our limited experience, OCT appears to have the potential to identify the differences in the mucosal surface of normal colonic mucosa and colonic polyps (Fig. 12). However, the OCT data are too preliminary to determine if OCT will have the potential to distinguish adenomatous from hyperplastic polyps.

Cancer Staging

The majority of gastrointestinal cancers originate in the mucosal layer of the intestine, and this makes detection and staging of mucosal cancers by OCT particularly attractive. In most but not all instances, the tumor is readily evident at the time of endoscopy. However, the depth of invasion is not discernible by conventional endoscopic methods and the depth of invasion is particularly important as it has significant consequences for management. Currently, cancer staging is most frequently done by EUS. Although EUS can accurately stage most tumors, superficial tumors

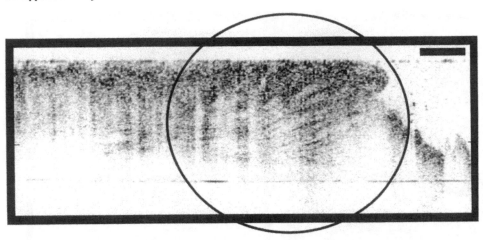

Figure 12 Colonic hyperplastic polyp.

may be difficult to stage accurately using current EUS technology. This is particularly true of squamous cell carcinomas of the esophagus, where the echogenicity of superficial squamous cell cancers is not significantly different from that of surrounding normal squamous mucosa. It is in this subset of superficial tumors that staging is crucial.

The advent of endoscopic mucosectomy techniques and other local therapies such as photodynamic therapy has made it important to accurately stage superficial tumors because endoscopic methods may be adequate therapy for tumors confined to the mucosal layer. OCT may ultimately prove valuable as a tool for selecting those patients suitable for local endoscopic therapy. In addition, OCT may be able to evaluate the tumor site following resection to ensure that the resection margins are free of gross tumor. Figure 13 shows an OCT image of an esophageal adenocarcinoma arising from Barrett's epithelium. Figure 14 is an OCT image of a gastric adenocarcinoma. In both cases the distortion of the normal tissue morphology is readily apparent in the OCT images. In the gastric adenocarcinoma only the mucosal layer has been imaged by OCT because of an increased backscattering of the mucosal tumor cells, which limits the penetration depth of OCT and may limit its value for tumor staging. Because only a few carcinomas have been studied by OCT to date, these observations need further investigation.

25.5.3 Submucosal Lesions

Although the majority of clinically significant abnormalities of the GI tract originate in the mucosa, several important regions reside beneath the mucosal layer. For example, varices are dilated veins of the GI tract that reside primarily below the mucosa and occur in response to increased pressure within the portal system. They are frequently seen in patients with chronic cirrhosis of the liver. Varices can occur anywhere within the GI tract, but the majority of clinically important ones are located in the esophagus and stomach. OCT clearly has the potential to locate and identify varices as well as provide quantitative information about them. For example, the size and depth of the varices could be known with high accuracy.

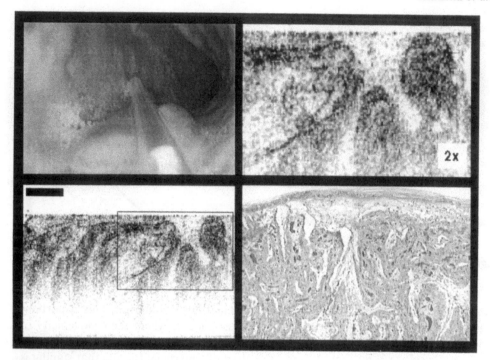

Figure 13   Esophageal adenocarcinoma.

Furthermore, if Doppler methods were incorporated into the OCT system, information about flow through the varix would be available. Quantitative measures of varices may be useful for directing and selecting endoscopic management as well as forecasting the risk of future complications

Benign tumors of the GI tract often occur in the submucosal and muscular layers of the GI tract. For example, lipomas are fatty tumors of the GI tract that are frequently seen in the colon. They carry no inherent risk but can be difficult to remove endoscopically. Thus, lipomas are generally not resected. OCT may be a convenient way to quickly identify a polyp as a submucosal lipoma so that the endoscopist can be confident that leaving the lesion behind would be of no clinical consequence. Leiomyomas are benign tumors arising from the muscular layers of the GI tract that are noted endoscopically as a smooth mass lesion arising from the wall of the GI tract. Even using EUS methods, it is not possible to reliably differentiate a

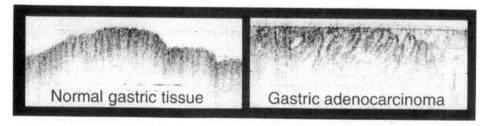

Figure 14   Gastric adenocarcinoma.

benign leiomyoma from its malignant counterpart, the leiomyosarcoma. This is obviously an important distinction. Whether OCT could provide useful information in this clinical setting is unknown, but as the depth of penetration of OCT devices improves, there is the possibility of using OCT to assist in making this important distinction.

25.5.4 Pancreatic Ducts and Bile Ducts

Although images of the pancreaticobiliary tree have been obtained in vitro [8], no images of pathological conditions of these ducts have been acquired and no OCT images of these structures have yet been obtained in humans. Minor modifications of current OCT technology would be adequate to acquire images of the pancreatic and common bile ducts clinically. Whether such images would be clinically useful and whether the images would provide information not available from conventional methods such as EUS, endoscopic retrograde cholangiopancreatography (ERCP), and cholangiopancreatoscopy is unknown.

25.6 SAFETY CONSIDERATIONS

The tolerance of the gastrointestinal tract to light is unknown, and no safe limits for light exposure to the mucosal surface have been identified. Most investigators have used the ANSI standards for skin with the knowledge that gastrointestinal mucosa may very well have a significantly different tolerance to light than skin. Another approach has been to use laser ablation thresholds as a very crude guide. However, it is known that significant tissue injury can occur at light doses well under ablation threshold. Finally, investigators have sought to define a lower limit to the safelight doses in the gastrointestinal tract by estimating the light output produced by gastrointestinal endoscopes. Because light exposure to the gastrointestinal mucosa during routine endoscopy is not known to produce any deleterious effects, it is reasonable to assume that the light dose applied during these procedures is a conservative estimate of the lower limit of light tolerance by the gastrointestinal tract. These estimates have indicated a surprisingly high tolerance of the gastrointestinal tract to light, because the light delivered during endoscopic procedures can easily exceed the ANSI standards for skin [13,14]. Unfortunately, no safety information is available at the infrared wavelengths currently used in OCT instruments, because standard endoscopic light sources deliver only visible light. Nonetheless, despite the lack of firm data supporting the safety of the light doses delivered during OCT measurements, the dose of light is relatively small and unlikely to produce any significant injury.

Optical coherence tomographic devices currently used in gastrointestinal endoscopy use a through-the-scope approach in which the OCT catheter is passed through the instrument channel of a standard endoscope. Passage of devices through the endoscope's instrument channel is a standard part of gastrointestinal procedures and can be done with essentially no additional risk. Thus, it has been generally accepted that OCT imaging adds no additional risk to endoscopic procedures. No complications resulting from OCT imaging of the gastrointestinal tract have been reported.

25.7 FUTURE DIRECTIONS

Current OCT systems are far from optimized for use in the GI tract. The present systems have been designed using a highly empirical approach. Educated guesses based on tissue optical properties have been used to select operating parameters. For example, the optimal wavelength for imaging the GI tract is unknown. In general, near-infrared wavelengths have been used because the tissue penetration of light at these wavelengths is superior to shorter wavelengths and suitable low coherence light sources are available. Furthermore, previous in vitro studies have suggested that varying wavelength produces only modest changes in image quality [12]. Nonetheless, for specific clinical applications, it is conceivable that varying the wavelength used could significantly enhance the clinical performance of OCT. Furthermore, as newer light sources become available, image quality will likely improve to the point that it is possible to resolve certain details of cellular architecture. In a similar fashion, the OCT systems in use all have taken slightly different approaches to catheter design. Which approach for scanning and which design of the optical elements (e.g., confocal parameter) will be optimal for any given clinical application is unknown at this point. It is likely that no single approach will be optimal for all endoscopic applications.

For many years, endoscopists have routinely used a variety of dyes to enhance the visualization of mucosal lesions at the time of endoscopy. It is reasonable to assume that dyes could similarly enhance the visualization of GI tract tissue by OCT. Essentially nothing is known about what role contrast agents might play in OCT imaging, but it may be possible to use any of a large number of dyes or other optical contrast agents to improve the selectivity and sensitivity of OCT. This is an area of investigation that holds significant future promise.

The addition of Doppler techniques to OCT systems has been demonstrated, although OCT Doppler images of the GI tract in humans have yet to be demonstrated. Nonetheless, the use of Doppler methods should provide clinically useful information about blood flow and perfusion to the GI tract.

From a clinical perspective, the clinical use of endoscopic OCT in the GI tract is very much in its infancy. Like any new technology it is not yet clear in which clinical settings the technology will prove to be cost-effective. Careful prospective clinical studies will need to be performed to establish the clinical utility of OCT. In the current healthcare environment of strict cost containment, these studies will be crucial to the acceptance of OCT as a routine clinical tool.

25.8 CONCLUSIONS

The feasibility of OCT imaging in the GI tract of humans during routine gastrointestinal endoscopy has been demonstrated conclusively. High resolution images of the GI tract have been obtained with these systems and have provided the highest resolution endoscopic images of the GI tract ever achieved. The overall clinical experience with OCT is still very limited, with well under 200 patients having been examined worldwide. Nonetheless, the preliminary experience has been very positive, and as the clinical experience grows it is very likely that OCT will find an important clinical niche in the endoscopic armamentarium.

REFERENCES

1. Wiersema MJ, Wiersema LM. High-resolution 25-megahertz ultrasonography of the gastrointestinal wall: Histological correlates. Gastrointest Endosc 39:499–504, 1993.
2. Izatt JA, Kulkarni MD, Wang H-W, Kobayashi K, Sivak MV Jr. Optical coherence tomography in gastrointestinal tissues. IEEE J Selected Topics Quant Electron 2:1017–1028, 1996.
3. Kobayashi R, Izatt JA, Rulkarni MD, Willis J, Sivak MV Jr. High-resolution cross-sectional imaging of the gastrointestinal tract using optical coherence tomography: Preliminary results. Gastrointest Endosc 47:515–523, 1998.
4. Bouma BE, Tearney GJ, Compton CC, Nishioka NS. Endoscopic optical coherence tomography of the gastrointestinal tract. Gastrointest Endosc 49:AB152, 1999.
5. Bouma BE, Tearney GJ, Compton CC, Nishioka NS. High-resolution imaging of the human esophagus and stomach in vivo using optical coherence tomography. Gastrointest Endosc 51:467–474, 2000.
6. Sergeev AM, Gelikonov VM, Gelikonov GV, et al. In vivo endoscopic OCT imaging of precancer and cancer states of human mucosa. Opt Express 1:432–440, 1997.
7. Tearney GJ, Brezinski ME, Southern JF, Bouma BE, Boppart SA, Fujimoto JG. Optical biopsy in human gastrointestinal tissue using optical coherence tomography. Am J Gastroenterol 92:1800–1804, 1997.
8. Tearney GJ, Brezinski ME, Southern JF, Bouma BE, Boppart SA, Fujimoto JG. Optical biopsy in human pancreatobiliary tissue using optical coherence tomography. Dig Dis Sci 43:1193–1199, 1998.
9. Tearney GJ, Brezinski ME, Bouma BE, Boppart SA, Pitris C, Southern JF, Fujimoto JG. In vivo endoscopic optical biopsy with optical coherence tomography. Science 276:2037–2039, 1997.
10. Bouma BE, Tearney GJ. Power-efficient nonreciprocal interferometer and linear scanning fiberoptic catheter for optical coherence tomography. Opt Lett 24:531–533, 1999.
11. Sivak MV Jr, Kobayashi K, Izatt JA, Rollins AM, Ungarunyawee R, Chak, A, Wong RCK, Isenberg GA. In-vivo high-resolution cross-sectional imaging of the human gastrointestinal tract using optical coherence tomography. Gastrointest Endosc 49:AB159, 1999.
12. Bouma BE, Nelson LE, Tearney GJ, Jones DJ, Brezinski ME, Fujimoto JG. Optical coherence tomographic imaging of human tissue at $1.55\,\mu m$ and $1.81\,\mu m$ using ER- and TM-doped fiber sources. J Biomed Opt 3:76–79, 1998.
13. Nishioka NS, Schomacker KT. Mucosal exposure to light during routine endoscopy. Gastrointest Endosc 49:456–461, 1999.
14. American National Standards Committee, American National Standards Institute for the Safe Use of Lasers. ANSI Z136.1-1993. Orlando, FL: Laser Institute of America, 1993:71.

26

Optical Coherence Tomography in Cardiology

**GUILLERMO J. TEARNEY, BRETT E. BOUMA, M. S. SHISHKOV,
K. SCHLENDORF, S. HOUSER, D.-H. KANG, H. T. ARETZ,
T. J. BRADY, and I.-K. JANG**

*Harvard Medical School and Wellman Laboratories of Photomedicine,
Massachusetts General Hospital, Boston, Massachusetts*

26.1 INTRODUCTION

Every year, approximately 1.5 million patients in the United States suffer an acute myocardial infarction (AMI) [1]. Despite an intense effort to improve early recognition and management of the patients, mortality from AMI remains high, approaching 30% of all cases, 60% of which occur prior to hospitalization [1]. When a patient has survived the initial stage and reaches a hospital, the treatment is either thrombolytic therapy or primary angioplasty. Although antegrade flow of the culprit vessel is often restored, a significant number of the patients retain left ventricular dysfunction and develop heart failure with an increased mortality. Therefore, it is crucial to detect vulnerable coronary atheromatous plaques prior to their rupture or erosion to prevent irreversible myocardial damage.

Rupture or erosion of a coronary atherosclerotic plaque usually causes AMI. Subsequently, a thrombus forms and blocks blood flow to the myocardium, causing myocardial cell death. Atherosclerotic plaques differ in composition and vulnerability. As the name atherosclerosis implies, *atheromatous gruel* (lipid-rich and soft) and *sclerotic tissue* (collagen-rich and hard) are the two main components of coronary plaques. Atheromatous gruel is dangerous because it is soft and vulnerable to rupture. The gruel is separated from the vascular lumen by a fibrous cap. This fibrous cap varies greatly in thickness, strength, stiffness, and cellularity, but it is often its "shoulder regions," the junctions between the cap and the adjacent more normal intima, that are thinnest and most heavily infiltrated by macrophage foam cells [2,3].

693

These shoulder regions are also points of maximal stress and therefore are at high risk for rupture. The three most important factors for vulnerability of plaques are thin fibrous caps, amount and composition of lipid gruel, and the amount and activity of macrophages [2,3].

Another mechanism that contributes to plaque rupture is an external trigger. Triggers for plaque rupture may be hemodynamic and mechanical stresses due to "surges in sympathetic activity," resulting in increases in blood pressure, heart rate, myocardial contractility, coronary flow, and coronary tone [4]. These extrinsic factors have been elucidated through studies correlating the onset of AMI with specific times within the circadian rhythm. However, plaque vulnerability seems to play a much more important role in rupture than triggers, because only vulnerable plaques are prone to rupture, and most myocardial infarctions occur during normal daily activities without an obvious precipitating cause [5].

It is generally accepted that plaques with a fibrous cap thickness of less than 30–65 μm are prone to rupture [2,3]. When the amount of lipid makes up more than 60% of plaque volume, the plaque is considered vulnerable [6]. Since two of the three determinants of plaque vulnerability are structural abnormalities, a high resolution imaging technique should be able to detect plaques vulnerable to rupture. Currently available modalities for imaging or for detecting plaques are intravascular ultrasound (IVUS) and magnetic resonance imaging (MRI). Although IVUS is widely used in interventional cardiology to obtain local structure including reference vessel diameter and localization of calcium and to confirm stent deployment, its low resolution ($\sim$ 100 μm using a 30 MHz probe) does not allow visualization of the fine structures of plaques [7–13]. MRI has a resolution similar to that of IVUS ($\sim$ 100 μm) and therefore does not allow discrimination of different components of plaques [14–16].

The high resolution capabilities of optical coherence tomography (OCT) make it a promising imaging technology for diagnosing vulnerable plaques in the coronary vasculature. Moreover, the limited penetration of OCT ($\sim$ 2 mm) is of little consequence in the coronary arteries, because the average normal vessel wall thickness is on the order of several millimeters. Important pioneering work has been performed by the group at the Massachusetts Institute of Technology demonstrating the feasibility of performing OCT to diagnose arterial pathology. Experiments performed in vitro have shown that OCT is capable of resolving clinically relevant architectural morphology, including fibrous caps, lipid-laden pools, and calcifications [17–19]. In addition, direct comparisons between in vitro OCT images and IVUS have demonstrated superior resolution and contrast in OCT images [19,20]. A recent study, using a 1 mm diameter (3.2 F) OCT catheter, has shown the adverse effects of blood on OCT imaging and the capability to image the wall of a rabbit aorta in vivo [21]. These experiments have defined a high-impact clinical application for OCT and serve as a solid foundation for investigators performing larger studies to evaluate the use of OCT for detecting vulnerable plaques.

In our laboratory, we have constructed a catheter-based OCT system suitable for clinical use. The remainder of this chapter describes results we have obtained using this system for imaging cadaveric human coronary arteries and porcine coronary arteries in vivo. We hope that our results, along with the efforts of other investigators, will help take this imaging technology one step further toward application of OCT in patients.

26.2 OCT SYSTEM OVERVIEW

The OCT system developed for this study used a power-efficient nonreciprocal Mach–Zehnder interferometer similar to that described in Chapter 6 [22]. The optical source power was 5 mW, centered at 1300 nm, with a bandwidth of 70 nm, giving an axial resolution of $10\,\mu m$. A high speed phase control delay line was used for coherence gating and was capable of performing 2000 axial scans per second [23]. Images were acquired at either 8 frames per second (fps) (250 angular pixels × 250 radial pixels) or 4 fps (500 angular pixels × 250 radial pixels). OCT images were displayed in real time using an inverse gray-scale lookup table and digitally stored.

Both a 2.0 mm(7 F) and a 1.0 mm (3.2 F) diameter catheter were constructed. Each catheter consisted of a single-mode optical fiber within a wound stainless steel cable [24]. At the distal tip of the fiber, a gradient index lens and a microprism were used to produce a focused output beam that propagated transversely to the catheter axis [24]. The transverse resolution provided by the distal optics was $25\,\mu m$. Surrounding the mechanical and optical components was a transparent, sealed plastic sheath. For the 3.2 F catheter, the sheath was designed to incorporate a guidewire in a monorail configuration (Fig. 1). All the mechanical properties of this catheter are comparable with the IVUS 3.2 F catheter. The proximal end design was similar to those described in previous publications [24,25]. The stainless steel cable that carried the fiber and the focusing optics was cemented to an FC fiber-optic connector that could be attached to and detached from the rotating end of the rotational coupler (Fig. 1). The coupler consisted of two gradient index (GRIN) lens collimators separated by an air gap precisely aligned to ensure maximal throughput. A stabilized electric motor was used to spin the rotating end of the coupler (4–8 Hz) with the catheter through a belt drive. The rotating coupler, the motor, and the drive were enclosed in a compact (12 cm × 5 cm) handheld unit compatible with the requirements of the cardiology suite (Fig. 1).

26.3 EX VIVO OCT IMAGING OF HUMAN CORONARY ARTERIES

Cadaveric coronary artery segments ($n = 42$) were obtained from 11 patients and stored in phosphate-buffered saline. The segments were marked with a suture through the lumen of the artery and imaged using a 3 F or 7 F OCT catheter with a pullback length of 5 mm. After imaging, the location of the suture was marked by India ink applied to the outer surface of the adventitia. Histological

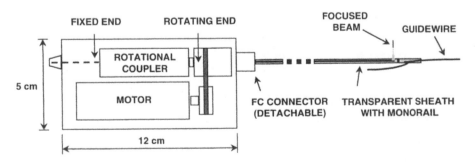

Figure 1 Schematic of the OCT catheter.

sections were obtained every $50\,\mu m$ and stained with either hematoxylin and eosin (H&E) or Movat's Pentachrome. OCT images were compared to histology for identification of discrete morphological parameters. Fibrous cap thicknesses were measured by OCT and histology, and the correlation was determined by Pearson's correlation coefficient r.

In all nonatheromatous artery segments ($n = 17$), differentiation of the intima, media, and adventitia was possible due to differences in backscattering from these layers (Fig. 2). In all nonatheromatous segments, the medium was less backscattering than either the intima or the adventitia (Fig. 2). Because the study population from cadavers was heavily weighted toward advanced age, intimal hyperplasia was identified in all OCT images of the nonatheromatous segments (Fig. 2). The internal and external elastic lamina were infrequently identified as discrete morphological entities. More often, the location of the internal and external elastic lamina could be inferred as the boundary between the antomatical layers of the artery. Absence of a layered structure was seen in all of the coronary arteries with atheroma ($n = 25$) (Figs. 3–5). Calcifications within the plaques ($n = 11$) were identified by the presence of high backscattering at the interfaces between calcification and the surrounding tissue, a low backscattering heterogeneous interior, and increased imaging penetration depth (Fig. 4). However, based on these static images, the appearance of many coronary arteries with calcifications is very similar to that of atheromatous plaques with thin caps. Lipid pools ($n = 15$) were identified by the presence of heterogeneous low-backscattering areas (Fig. 5). Some images also contained evidence of neovascularization, seen as well-defined areas of low backscattering (vessels) within the lipid core of the plaque (Fig. 5). A reliable match between the OCT images and histology was found in 10/25 of the atheromatous specimens. Fibrous caps were measured by OCT ($30–450\,\mu m$), and cap thicknesses correlated well with histology ($r = 0.98$) in the 10 specimens with a reliable OCT–histology correspondence.

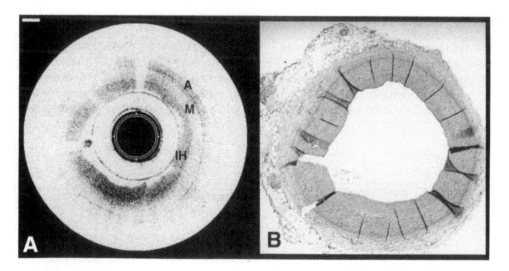

Figure 2   (A) Optical coherence tomograhic image of a coronary artery with intimal hyperplasia (IH). The media (M) and adventitia (A) are also clearly seen. (B) Corresponding histology (H&E). Scale bar, $500\,\mu m$.

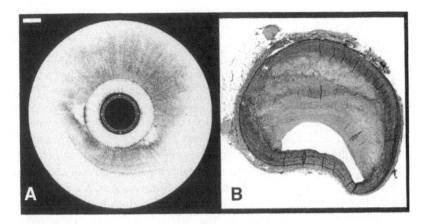

Figure 3   (A) Optical coherence tomographic image of a coronary artery with a large, eccentric fibrous plaque (P). (B) Corresponding histology (Movat's pentachrome). Scale bar, 500 μm.

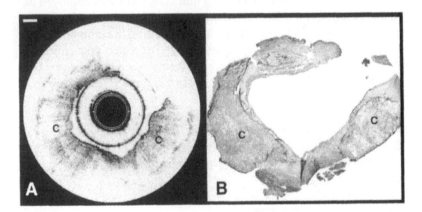

Figure 4   (A) Optical coherence tomographic image showing intimal and medial calcifications (C). (B) Corresponding histology (Movat's pentachrome). Scale bar, 500 μm.

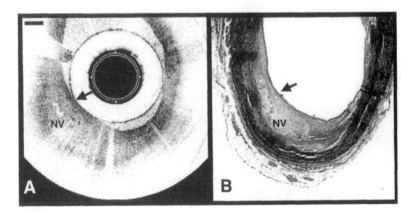

Figure 5   (A) Optical coherence tomographic image of an atheromatous plaque with a thin fibrous cap (arrow). Note the presence of neovascularization (NV) within the lipid core. (B) Corresponding histology (Movat's pentachrome). Scale bar, 500 μm.

26.4   IN VIVO OCT IMAGING OF PORCINE CORONARY ARTERIES

Three ($n = 3$) pigs with an average weight of 50 kg were used in the study. The swine were anesthetized (Telazol IM 40 mg/kg, Xylazine 1 mg/kg, and Thiopental 20–25 mg/kg), intubated, and artificially ventilated (isoflurane 1–2%). Lidocaine (100 mg) and heparin (250 U/kg) were also administered. An 8 F introducer was placed in the femoral artery, and a guide catheter was advanced to the coronary ostia. Under fluoroscopic guidance, each coronary artery was identified by contrast injection. Using standard angioplasty techniques, a guidewire was advanced into each coronary artery and 3.2 F IVUS (30 MHz CVIS, Sunnyvale, CA) imaging was performed. Next, the OCT catheter was advanced over the guidewire, and OCT imaging was conducted. Visualization of the arterial wall was attempted using 8–10 cm^3 normal saline flush through the guide catheter. After all three coronary arteries were imaged, an intimal dissection was crated using an oversized balloon catheter with a pressure of 12 atm for a duration of 30 s and imaged by IVUS and OCT. Following the dissection, a 4.0 × 16 mm NIR stent was deployed at 16 atm and imaged by IVUS and OCT. All fluoroscopic, IVUS and OCT images were recorded on Super-VHS videotape. After the procedure, the animals were euthanized (pentobarbital 100 mg/kg). The hearts were prosected and injected with formaldehyde for further histological processing. Guidelines of the Massachusetts General Hospital Subcommittee on Research Animal Care were followed for handling of the pigs.

As mentioned in previous publications [21], blood caused significant optical attenuation between the outer catheter sheath and the coronary artery wall. As a result, without saline purging, OCT images enabled clear visualization of the artery wall only when the catheter sheath was in close proximity to the tissue (Fig. 6).

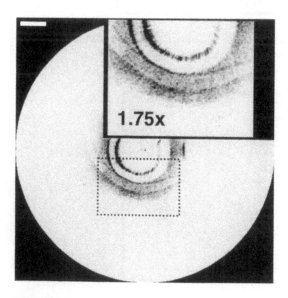

Figure 6   Optical coherence tomographic image of the porcine coronary artery (in vivo) without a saline purge. Identification of the intima (I), media (M), and adventitia (A) is possible when the catheter is in close proximity to the vessel wall. Scale bar, 500 μm.

Clearer visualization of the entire vessel was achieved with a saline flush through the guide catheter (Fig. 7). Arterial selectivity of the flush was a major contributing factor in the ability to image the entire vessel during a purge. In approximately 50% of the saline flushes, the flush was not selective and did not allow identification of the entire vessel wall. When successful, purging allowed the duration of unobstructed image to range from 2 to 5 s. When the vessel was clearly visualized, the intima, media, and adventitia of the coronary artery wall could be easily differentiated (Figs. 7 and 8), in contrast to the IVUS image (Fig. 8b). Motion artifacts caused by the beating heart were significant at 4 fps and resulted in a misregistration of the image for one full revolution of the catheter (Fig. 7). Imaging at 8 fps showed a reduction of motion artifacts and proper registration of the image (Fig. 8a).

Optical coherence tomographic images of dissections allowed subtler changes to be identified than those seen by IVUS. Small abnormalities including pockets of disrupted intima and media could be clearly resolved in OCT images (Figs. 9a and 9b) and were not seen by IVUS (Fig. 9c). OCT images also enabled the precise microanatomical location of the arterial wall damage to be identified (Figs. 9a and 9b). In addition, OCT allowed fragments of detached intima and media to be seen within the lumen of the vessel (Fig. 9b).

The high resolution capabilities of OCT also enabled superior imaging of stent deployment compared to IVUS. Determination of the exact relationship between the anatomical layers of the coronary artery wall and the struts of the stent was possible using OCT (Fig. 10a). The struts of the stents were visible in the IVUS images but with significantly less resolution (Fig. 10b).

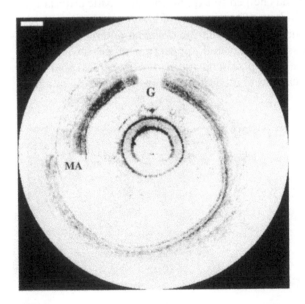

Figure 7 Optical coherence tomographic image of the porcine coronary artery (in vivo, 4 fps) with a saline purge. Note the position of the guidewire (G). Note the motion artifact (MA), present at 9 o'clock, representing misregistration of the catheter following one complete rotation. Scale bar, 500 μm.

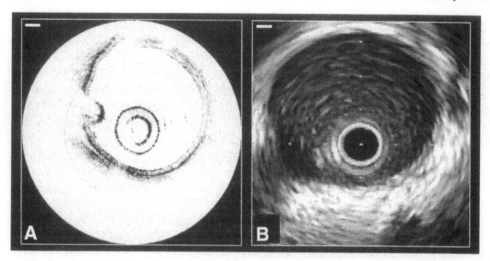

Figure 8   (A) Optical coherence tomographic image of a coronary artery (in vivo) acquired with a saline flush at 8 fps, showing the relative absence of motion artifacts. (B) Corresponding IVUS image. OCT scale bar, 500 µm; IVUS tick marks, 1 mm.

26.5   DISCUSSION

Optical coherence tomographic imaging and histopathological correlation of a large number of coronary arteries in vitro is an important step that must be performed in order to understand in vivo OCT images of human atheromatous pathology. Our study of 42 coronary artery segments has helped to expand the diagnostic criteria for clinically relevant atheromatous pathology. The presence of a layered structure with a thickened intima and a discrete media and adventitia was characteristic of non-atheromatous coronary arteries. Loss of the layered appearance of the OCT image always correlated with either the presence of calcifications of atheroma. Lipid-rich atherosclerotic plaques with fibrous caps were identified in many of the OCT images,

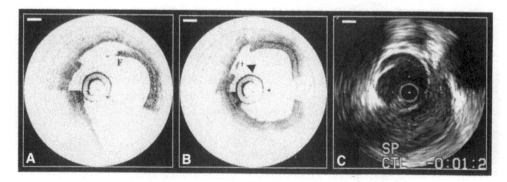

Figure 9   (A) Optical coherence tomographic image of the porcine coronary artery dissection (in vivo) with a saline purge shows the presence of a flap (F). (B) OCT image of the dissection showing tissue within the lumen. (C) Corresponding IVUS image. OCT scale bars, 500 µm; IVUS tick marks, 1 mm.

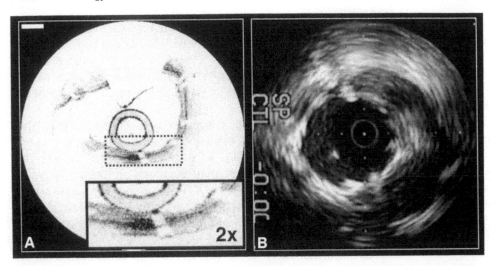

Figure 10 (A) Optical coherence tomographic image of the porcine coronary artery stent (in vivo) with a saline purge. (B) Corresponding IVUS image. OCT scale bar, 500 μm; IVUS tick marks, 1 mm.

and the measurements of cap thickness correlated well with histology. The similarities between many images of calcified coronary arteries and thin capped plaques may present a diagnostic dilemma. However, it is likely that with real-time imaging the different temporal mechanical dynamics of these two entities will enable their differentiation.

The feasibility of performing OCT in living coronary arteries has been demonstrated in the porcine experiments. Layers of the normal swine coronary artery could be clearly identified, and the imaging penetration depth was through the intima. These results, in combination with previous published work [17–21], support the use of OCT for the early detection of vulnerable plaques. In addition, OCT enabled visualization of small disruptions within the intimal and medial dissections that could not be identified by IVUS. The ability of OCT to image small areas of arterial wall damage opens up the possibility of using OCT as a tool for determining the appropriate management of dissections. Finally, the OCT images of the coronary arterial stent indicate that this technology maybe used to more accurately aid the cardiologist in measuring stent apposition following deployment.

Two major technical difficulties, motion artifacts and removal of blood from the field of view, must be addressed before useful application of this technology in patients. Motion artifacts at 4 fps frequently caused misregistration in the OCT image. The motion artifacts at 8 fps were less noticeable but still present, warranting further development to increase the speed of OCT systems. OCT imaging without saline purging allowed visualization of only a small sector of the arterial wall due to attenuation of the light by blood. Saline flushing allowed visualization of the entire wall in approximately 50% of all attempts, depending on the vessel size and the position of the guiding catheter. In the other cases, imaging was suboptimal due to the poor selectivity of the flush. This situation may be remedied by purging through a smaller diameter guide catheter. However, even when flushing was successful, the maximum time for optimal imaging was only 5 s. Alternatives to flushing include proximal occlusion, such as that used in angioscopy [26]. The use of eccentric catheters without purging would force the OCT catheter to be in contact with the arterial wall. Although this would allow visualization of only a portion of the vessel wall at a time, the remainder of the vessel could be visualized by rotating the catheter sheath.

Optical coherence tomography shows great promise in cardiology. The resolution of OCT images is superior to that of other available intravascular imaging modalities, and the depth of penetration of OCT imaging is sufficient to view the clinically relevant features in atheromatous plaques. Research performed by other investigators and this laboratory have advanced OCT technology and categorized OCT images of vascular pathology to the point where studies to assess clinical viability can be performed. However, in vivo OCT imaging of coronary arteries is still at a very early stage. Technical difficulties such as scan speed and obstruction of view by blood must be overcome. Moreover, localizing the OCT catheter to a region of potential plaque vulnerability has not been addressed. Because of the potential impact of this technology in cardiology, it is likely that an influx of resources and new investigators will solve these issues and OCT will emerge as an important diagnostic modality for preventing acute myocardial infarction.

ACKNOWLEDGMENTS

This study was supported by a grant from the Center for Innovative Minimally Invasive Therapy, Boston, MA. We also thank the laboratory of Dr. David Torchiana for the use of his animal facilities and James Titus and Dr. Jennifer White for their invaluable assistance and expertise. Finally, we thank Sven Holden for his excellent work processing the histology specimens.

REFERENCES

1. American Heart Association. Heart and Stroke Facts: 1996, Statistical Supplement. Dallas, TX: Am Heart Assoc, 1996.
2. Falk E. Why do plaques rupture? Circulation 96:III30–III42, 1992.
3. Lee RT, Libby P. The unstable atheroma. Arterioscler, Thromb, Vasc Biol 17:1859–1867, 1997.
4. Muller JE, Tofler GH, Stone PH. Circardian variation and triggers of onset of acute cardiovascular disease. Circulation 79:733–743, 1989.
5. Fuster V, Badimon L, Badimon JJ, Chesebro JH. The pathogenesis of coronary artery disease and the acute coronary syndromes. N Engl J Med 326:242–250, 310–318, 1992.
6. Loree HM, Tobias BJ, Gibson LJ, Kamm RD, Small DM, Lee RT. Mechanical properties of model atherosclerotic lesion lipid pools. Arterioscler Thromb 14:230–234, 1994.
7. Yock PG, Fitzgerald PJ, Linker DT, Angelsen BA. Intravascular ultrasound guidance for catheter-based coronary interventions. J Am College Cardiol 17:39B–45B, 1991.
8. Yock PG, Fitzgerald PJ. Intravascular ultrasound: State of the art and future directions. Am J Cardiol 81:27E–32E, 1998.
9. Colombo A, Hall P, Nakamura S, Almagor Y, Maiello L, Martini G, Gaglione A, Goldberg SL, Tobis JM. Intracoronary stenting without anticoagulation accomplished with intravascular ultrasound guidance [see Comments]. Circulation 91:1676–1688, 1995.

10. Stone GW, Hodgson JM, St Goar FG, Frey A, Mudra H, Sheehan H, Linnemeier TJ. Improved procedural results of coronary angioplasty with intravascular ultrasound-guided balloon sizing: The CLOUT Pilot Trial. Clinical Outcomes With Ultrasound Trial (CLOUT) Investigators. Circulation 95:2044–2052, 1997.

11. Peters RJ, Kok WE, Havenith MG, Rijsterborgh H, van der Wal AC, Visser CA. Histopathologic validation of intracoronary ultrasound imaging. J Am Soc Echocardiol 7:230–241, 1994.

12. Frimerman A, Miller HL, Hallman M, Laniado S, Keren G. Intravascular ultrasound characterization of thrombi of different composition. Am J Cardiol 73:1053–1057, 1994.

13. Peters RJ, Ge J, Linker DT, Visser CA, Yock PG. Observer agreement on qualitative analysis of intracoronary ultrasound images. Circulation 90:551, 1994.

14. Baer FM, Theissen P, Crnac J, Schmidt M, Jochims M, Schicha H. MRI assessment of coronary artery disease. Rays 24:46–59, 1999.

15. van der Wall EE, Vliegen HW, de Roos A, Bruschke AV. Magnetic resonance imaging in coronary artery disease [see Comments]. Circulation 92:2723–2739, 1995.

16. Zimmermann-Paul GG, Quick HH, Vogt P, von Schulthess GK, Kling D, Debatin JF. High-resolution intravascular magnetic resonance imaging: Monitoring of plaque formation in heritable hyperlipidemic rabbits. Circulation 99:1054–1061, 1999.

17. Brezinski ME, Tearney GJ, Bouma BE, Izatt JA, Hee MR, Swanson EA, Southern JF, Fujimoto JG. Optical coherence tomography for optical biopsy: Properties and demonstration of vascular pathology. Circulation 93:1206–1213, 1996.

18. Brezinski ME, Tearney GJ, Bouma BE, Boppart SA, Hee MR, Swanson EA, Southern JF, Fujimoto JG. Imaging of coronary artery microstructure (in vitro) with optical coherence tomography. Am J Cardiol 77:92–93, 1996.

19. Brezinski ME, Tearney GJ, Weissman NJ, Boppart SA, Bouma BE, Hee MR, Weyman AE, Swanson EA, Southern JF, Fujimoto JG. Assessing atherosclerotic plaque morphology: Comparison of optical coherence tomography and high frequency intravascular ultrasound. Heart 77:397–403, 1997.

20. Tearney GJ, Brezinski ME, Boppart SA, Bouma BE, Weissman NJ, Southern JF, Swanson EA, Fujimoto JG. Images in cardiovascular medicine. Catheter-based optical imaging of a human coronary artery. Circulation 94:3013, 1996.

21. Fujimoto JG, Boppart SA, Tearney GJ, Bouma BE, Pitris C, Brezinski ME. High resolution in vivo intra-arterial imaging with optical coherence tomography. Heart 82:128–133, 1999.

22. Bouma BE, Tearney GJ. Power-efficient nonreciprocal interferometer and linear-scanning fiber optic catheter for optical coherence tomography. Opt Lett 24:531–533, 1999.

23. Tearney GJ, Bouma BE, Fujimoto JG. Phase and group delay relationships for the phase control rapid-scanning optical delay line. Opt Lett 1997.

24. Tearney GJ, Boppart SA, Bouma BE, Brezinski ME, Weissman NJ, Southern JF, Fujimoto JG. Scanning single-mode fiber optic catheter-endoscope for optical coherence tomography. Opt Lett 21:1–3, 1996.

25. Tearney GJ, Brezinski ME, Bouma BE, Boppart SA, Pitris C, Southern JF, Fujimoto JG. In vivo endoscopic optical biopsy with optical coherence tomography. Science 276:2037–2039, 1997.

26. Uchida Y, Fumitaka N, Tomaru T, Morita T, Oshima T, Sasaki T, Morizuki S, Hirose J. Prediction of acute coronary syndromes by percutaneous coronary angioscopy in patients with stable angina. Am Heart J 130:195–203, 1995.

27

Capabilities of Optical Coherence Tomography in Laryngology

N. D. GLADKOVA and A. V. SHAKHOV

Nizhny Novgorod Medical Academy, Nizhny Novgorod, Russia

FELIX I. FELDCHTEIN

Institute of Applied Physics, Nizhny Novgorod, Russia

27.1 INTRODUCTION

Optical coherence tomography (OCT) was proposed a decade ago as a novel method for biotissue examination [1] that potentially provides noninvasive imaging of subsurface tissue structures in the near-infrared range with spatial resolution of several micrometers. From the very beginning, mucous membranes of internal organs attracted considerable attention as a promising application area for OCT. However, it was not until the implementation in 1997 of an endoscopic OCT (EOCT) instrument compatible with the standard clinical endoscopic equipment [2] that clinical trials were put on a real basis, since then resulting in the examination of hundreds of patients with abnormalities in the gastrointestinal, respiratory, urinary, and genital tracts [3].

In earlier studies [2] it was demonstrated that OCT is informative in the case of tissue covered with nonkeratinized epithelium separated from underlying stroma by a smooth basement membrane. OCT provides objective information on mucosal structure because of the optical backscattering coefficient of different tissue layers. In particular, different scattering properties of the epithelium and stroma provide visualization of the position and integrity of the basement membrane. The spatial resolution of OCT is sufficient to reveal such microstructural elements of mucosa as blood vessels and glands. Differences in thickness and transparency of the epithelium, the content of connective tissue, and the architecture of the basement membrane may lead to differences in the appearance of OCT images in specific regions of the larynx. Information on tissue structure provided by OCT can be used in the detection of tumors and tumorlike lesions that violate or change these structures. Our OCT device, which has a spatial resolution of 10–20 μm, cannot directly detect the cellular level of changes in high-grade dysplasia or carcinoma. However, OCT can still reveal some peculiarities of epithelial malignancy at the level of tissue architecture, such as abnormal cell concentrations that lead to the loss of orientation of epithelium and stroma. OCT also can detect changes in optical properties of malignant epithelium and increased vascularization of the lamina propria and submucosa. Thus, there are good reasons to believe that OCT will be successfully used in the diagnosis of laryngeal diseases. Of importance is that the majority of laryngeal diseases originate from the epithelium, the basement membrane, and the subepithelial connective tissue.

In this chapter we will concentrate on the results of clinical studies performed at the Department of Otorhinolaryngology of the Nizhny Novgorod Regional Hospital using an OCT device (Fig. 1) developed at the Institute of Applied Physics. A description of this device with advanced capabilities for in vivo endoscopic applications can be found elsewhere [2–4].

The probing low coherent light was generated by a superluminescent semiconductor diode operating at a center wavelength of 830 nm, with a full width at half-maximum (FWHM) spectral bandwidth of 25 nm and output power of 1.5 mW. The in-depth resolution was $\sim 15\,\mu$m in free space units; the lateral one, 20 μm. In-depth

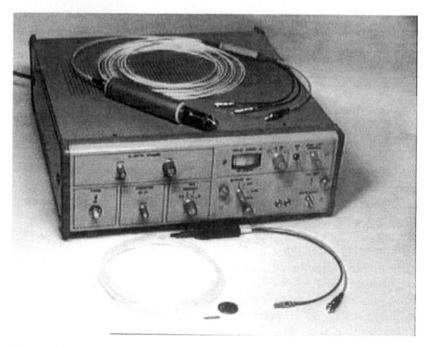

Figure 1 Compact fiber-based OCT device. The scale is given by a U.S. quarter in the foreground.

scanning was performed with a piezofiber modulator [5] with a scanning range of 1–2 mm (free space units) and a scan rate of 70–150 Hz, resulting in a typical acquisition time for a 200 × 200 pixel image of 1.5–3 s. All acquired OCT images are represented in the inverse gray-scale palette, where a darker gradation corresponds to a higher intensity of backscattered light (analogous to echo-positive regions in ultrasonography). The scale is given by a 1 mm bar, and the vertical scale is normalized with the assumption that the average group refractive index of mucosa is 1.4 [6]. The galvanometer-type probe with an outer diameter of 2.7 mm (Fig. 2) delivered ∼ 0.5 mW of the optical power to the tissue and provided lateral scanning over 1.6 mm. The majority of OCT images presented here (all except Figs. 14, 16–19, 22a, 22d, and 22e) were averaged over three frames.

Endoscopic OCT imaging was combined with direct operative laryngoscopy, i.e., the probe was introduced into the lumen of a laryngoscope to approach examined areas of laryngeal mucosa. Figure 3 shows a general view of the procedure when a surgeon is carrying out microlaryingoscopy in combination with OCT. In particular, in vivo imaging of regions that were subjected further to excisional biopsy and histological examination was performed to set up correspondence between OCT and morphological features.

27.2 OCT IMAGING OF HEALTHY LARYNGEAL TISSUE

The larynx is a portion of the respiratory tube connecting the pharynx with the trachea. Its walls do not collapse during breathing because of the presence of several cartilage structures connected to each other with joints and ligaments and multiple muscles. Due to this, the larynx is easily amenable to examination with rigid endoscopic equipment as well as with instruments for endoscopic optical coherence tomography (EOCT).

In this chapter we will concentrate on the most important structures of the larynx [7] shown in Fig. 4 [8]: the epiglottis (*1*), the false (vestibular) folds (*2*), the true vocal folds (*3*), the laryngeal ventricle (*4*), the anterior (*5*) and posterior (*7*), commissures and the subglottal space (*6*). The larynx performs numerous functions, the most important among them being respiratory, voice-producing and protective. These functions bring some specificity to the structure of each portion [9]. In parts subjected to intense mechanical irritation, laryngeal mucosa is lined with nonkeratinized stratified squamous epithelium (SSE), whereas in other parts it is lined with stratified columnar epithelium (SCE) or pseudostratified ciliated epithelium (PSE).

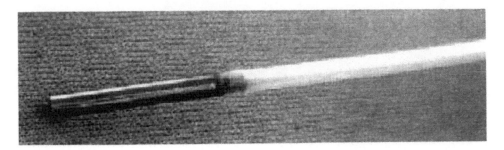

Figure 2   Endoscopic OCT probe with internal lateral scanning.

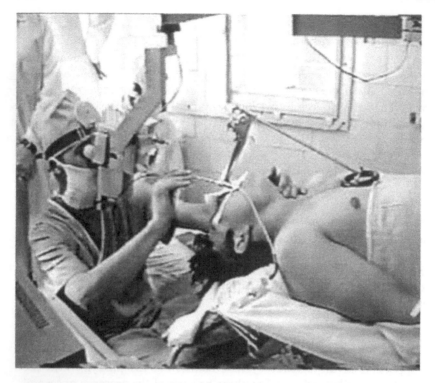

Figure 3 General view of the OCT imaging procedure combined with microlaryngoscopy.

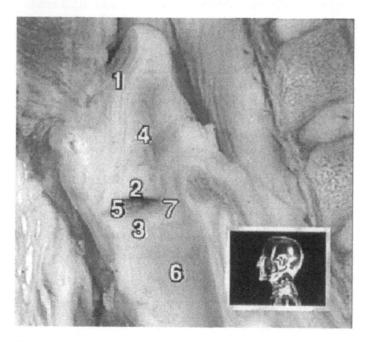

Figure 4 Schematic of the larynx. *1*, Epiglottis, *2*, false (vestibular) fold; *3*, true vocal fold; *4*, laryngeal ventricle; *5*, anterior commissure; *6*, subglottal space; *7*, posterior commissure. (From Ref. 8.)

The lamina propria (LP) of mucosa consists of well-vascularized loose connective tissue with different features in the different portions of the larynx. On the anterior surface of the epiglottis, in the arytenoid cartilages, aryepiglottal folds, and ventricles, and in the area of the false vocal folds the LP is very loose. In deep layers of LP there are numerous mixed protein-mucous glands (GL) and, sometimes, lymph nodes called laryngeal tonsils. In other parts of the larynx LP is more dense and there are few GL and no lymphoid tissue at all. The submucosal layer is absent in the larynx [10].

Owing to easy access and a distinct stratified structure, the larynx is a favorable subject for EOCT imaging. Optical images of the larynx have good contrast and are concise. In order to get some point of reference, in vivo OCT images of normal mucosa were obtained from different portions of the larynx. For this reason, regions of mucosa were imaged that, according to clinical and morphological examination, were not affected by any pathological process. Based on the images of mucosa of the epiglottis ($n = 5$), vestibular folds ($n = 7$), true vocal folds ($n = 7$), laryngeal ventricles ($n = 6$), anterior and posterior commissures ($n = 5$), and the subglottis ($n = 4$) that were made in 28 patients during laryngoscopic study, a collection of OCT images of normal human mucosa in different laryngeal portions was compiled. In doubtful cases excisional biopsy was taken; however, obtained histological material was sufficient to evaluate the state of the organ but too small and fragmented to be demonstrated as parallel histology. To see the correlation between OCT and typical morphological features of the mucosa in different portions of the larynx we used laryngeal tissue taken postmortem from seven people who had died of diseases not associated with pathologies in the larynx. Postmortem samples were not imaged by OCT because of poor contrast in dead tissues. The structures in OCT in vivo images of normal tissues, presented in Figs. 5–12, such as epithelium, lamina propria, basement membrane, blood vessels, and glands with ducts were identified on the basis of typical histology and typical morphometrical parameters of these structures (depth, size, elongation, frequency per unit area).

Figure 5a is a tomogram of the lower lingual epiglottis; Fig. 6a is a tomogram of the middle laryngeal epiglottis. Figures 5b and 6b show typical histology of the linguals and laryngeal epiglottis, respectively. In the lingual part (Fig. 5) the epithelium is SSE. Its thickness may vary from 100 to 300 μm; in this tomogram the SSE appears as a poorly backscattering strip 150 μm thick. Morphologically, the basement membrane (BM) is almost entirely even, with rare small appendages. The epithelium in the middle laryngeal epiglottis (Fig. 6), being part of the lining of the respiratory tract, is SCE. In contrast to the PSE of the subglottis and trachea where the number of nuclear rows is typically three, in the respiratory epithelium of the epiglottis there are six or seven nuclear rows. Due to this, the thickness of the SCE is 70–100 μm (with 100 μm in the OCT image), which is close to that of the SSE. The basement membrane is even along practically the entire length and has no appendages. The cartilaginous plate of the epiglottis (Figs. 5b and 6b) is deep (600–1600 μm) and cannot be visualized by OCT. The cartilage is known to be covered with perichondrium that consists of dense fibrous connective tissue. This tissue merges into lamina propria that contains loose fibrous connective tissue. Because of the similar optical properties of these two connective tissues, they are poorly differentiated with OCT. In the tomograms they are seen as a single highly

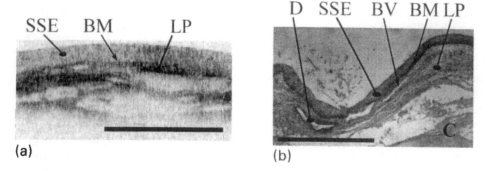

(a)

(b)

Figure 5 Normal lower lingual epiglottis. (a) Tomogram; (b) typical histology. Here and in later figures the following abbreviations are used: SSE, stratified squamous epithelium; LP, lamina propria of mucosa; BV, blood vessel; D, duct of a protein-mucous gland; BM, basement membrane; C, cartilage. Light areas in the OCT image can be either blood vessels or gland ducts. Bar size is 1 mm.

backscattering band whose width and brightness vary in different parts of the larynx. For instance, LP in the lingual epiglottis (Fig. 5b) is more loose than in the laryngeal epiglottis (Fig. 6b) and contains a large number of blood vessels (BV) with a diameter of 50–200 μm. These BV are seen in the OCT images as light areas of different shapes (Figs 5a and 6a). In LP of the lingual epiglottis (Fig. 5b), along with blood vessels there are mucous-protein glands (GL) with ducts. Typically, no distinct OCT features can reliably distinguish BV from GL or ducts, because both look like poorly backscattering cavities. Figure 7 shows the mucosa of the upper larynx around the arytenoid cartilages: tomogram (Fig. 7a) and histology (Fig. 7b). Clearly differentiable by OCT are poorly backscattering SSE of 100 μm thickness and the highly backscattering and well-vascularized LP that merges into the perichondrium.

The false (vestibular) (Fig. 8) and true (Fig. 9) vocal folds, being most often subjected to tension, are covered by SSE ranging from 80 to 250 μm in thickness. In the OCT images it is also seen as a poorly backscattering stripe. The basement

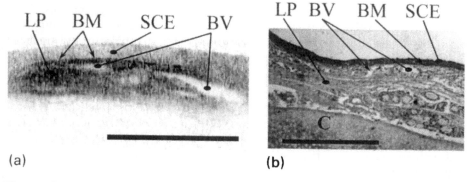

(a)

(b)

Figure 6 Normal middle laryngeal epiglottis. (a) Tomogram; (b) typical histology. SCE = stratified columnar epithelium.

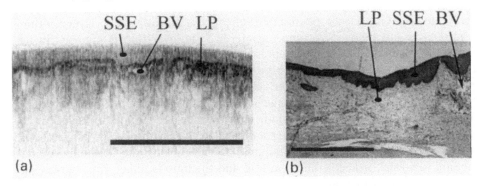

Figure 7 Normal mucosa on top of arytenoid cartilages. (a) Tomogram; (b) typical histology.

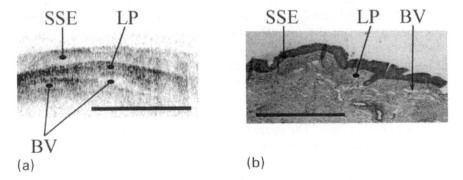

Figure 8 Normal false (vestibular) folds. (a) Tomograms; (b) typical histology.

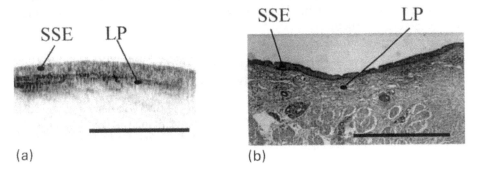

Figure 9 Normal true vocal folds. (a) Tomograms; (b) typical histology.

membrane is typically smooth; the papillae are poorly developed. The base of the false vocal folds is a highly vascularized (vessels are up to 150 μm in diameter) loose connective tissue. Lamina propria of the vestibular folds and of the vestibular portion of the larynx extends to the supraglottal fatty tissue. This facilitates the quick growth of tumors deeper in to the larynx and the epiglottis. The imaging depth of the normal vestibular folds with our device is no less than 0.8 mm, which allowed us to observe the connective tissue with large blood vessels. The true vocal folds (Fig. 9) normally have no GL. Elastic fibers of LP of mucosa consist of two layers: a thin superficial layer just below SSE, and an intermediate layer that is attached in its depth to a striated vocal muscle. The presence in the lamina propria of dense well-organized clusters of elastic fibers can produce high backscattering. The muscle is usually 300–400 μm deep from the surface and is not seen because of poor back-scattering in OCT images. The "Reinke's space" is usually defined as a potential space between the two layers of elastic fibers of the true vocal fold, i.e., between the superficial layer and intermediate layer attached to vocal muscle. This space is of great importance from the functional point of view. Being the first barrier and responding to edema, it keeps the vocal fold and the muscle intact, thus preserving the voice production function.

The laryngeal ventricle (Fig. 10) is an area of widening of the lumen of the larynx between two rows of folds. It is lined with relatively thin (30–80 μm) PSE with underlying thin (150–200 μm) LP. As a rule, the LP adjoins the vocal muscle or directly adjoins the thyroid cartilage. So the depth of imaging in this laryngeal portion is no more than 270–300 μm. The anterior commissure (Fig. 11) is lined mainly with PSE 40–60 μm in thickness, though in some regions it may be covered by SSE. Tomographically, these two types of epithelium have no specific OCT signs except thickness. The posterior commissure (Fig. 12) is lined with SSE up to 250 μm in thickness. Their lamina propria, as in the case of the false folds, consists of loose well-vacularized fibrous connective tissue, making these portions of the larynx vulnerable to the growth of tumors. The subglottis (Fig. 13) performs only the respiratory function, so it is lined with PSE no more than 30–70 μm thick. Because thin LP usually merges into the perichondrium of the cricoid cartilage, the imaging depth of this portion of the larynx, as well as of the laryngeal ventricle mucosa, is only ∼ 300 μm.

Thus, OCT imaging can easily detect specific morphological features of normal mucosa in different portions of the larynx by detecting the difference in scattering properties of mucosal structures.

27.3 OCT IMAGING OF PATHOLOGICAL PROCESSES OF DIFFERENT ORIGINS IN THE LARYNX

Optical coherence tomography can be successfully used in the diagnosis of pathological processes of different origins in the larynx. Such factors as the close location of

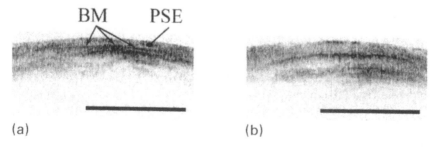

(a)   (b)

Figure 10 Tomograms of normal mucosa of laryngeal ventricles. PSE = pseudostratified columnar epithelium.

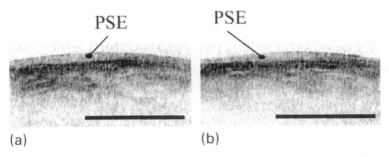

Figure 11   Normal mucosa of anterior commissure.

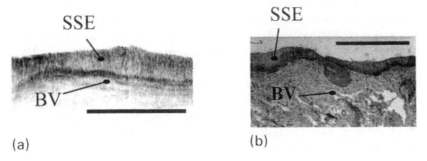

Figure 12   Normal mucosa of posterior commissure. (a) Tomogram; (b) typical histology.

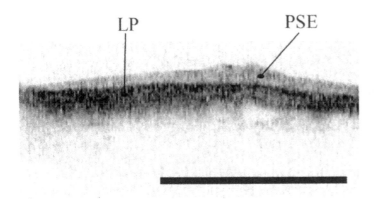

Figure 13   Normal mucosa of the subglottal space.

the larynx to the outer environment, hence a high probability of contact with infectious and noninfectious agents, as well as high functional activity frequently accompanied by overtension and traumatization of the ligamentous apparatus precondition a high rate of development of various laryngeal diseases. It is known that the frequency of cancerous processes in the larynx is high, being 5% of that of all carcinomas in other organs. Note that the most frequent (98%) are tumors of epithelial origin, i.e., squamous cell carcinoma [11,12]. Clearly, early cancer diagnosis, i.e., diagnosis of cancers in intraepithelial stages or cancer in situ, is of particular importance. Timely diagnosis of limited cancer provides an opportunity for organ-preserving surgical treatment, which allows the patient to retain the respiratory, voice production, and protective functions of the larynx. Fortunately, early cancerous and many precancerous conditions are characterized by hoarseness, a clinical symptom evident enough to lead to consultation with an otorhinolaryngologist.

An endoscopic OCT study was undertaken in 35 patients with abnormalities of different origins in the larynx. Various forms of laryngitis were diagnosed in nine patients, carcinoma was diagnosed in 19 patients, vocal nodules were diagnosed in another six patients, and a glandular mucosal cyst in the region of the vocal fold was diagnosed in one patient. Of the 19 cases with carcinoma, seven patients were followed after a course of radiation therapy and were monitored by EOCT to determine in vivo the effect of ionizing radiation on laryngeal mucosa. Diagnoses were made on the basis of clinical information, including fibrolaryngoscopic and direct microlaryngoscopic data, and were further confirmed morphologically. OCT was a supplementary technique and was combined with direct microlaryngoscopy. The EOCT study of the laryngeal mucosa was accomplished by inserting the EOCT probe through the lumen of a laryngoscope. In vivo images of laryngeal tissue were obtained. These tissue regions underwent further excisional biopsy and histological examination to make a diagnosis and to set up correspondence between OCT images and morphological features. As in the case of normal mucosa of the larynx, excisional biopsy was sparing. The tissue sections for biopsy were quite informative for evaluating the state of the organ but too small to demonstrate them as parallel histology. This explains the small number of parallel histological data presented in this section.

27.3.1 OCT Capabilities for Evaluation of the Epithelium in the Larynx

As indicated earlier, different portions of the larynx are lined with different types of epithelium, that is SSE, SCE, or PSE (respiratory). The major histological difference between them is the presence of respiratory cells that cannot be visualized with current OCT technology. OCT is able to detect differences in the thickness of the epithelium, which in normal laryngeal mucosa may vary within 30–300 μm. Note that the OCT resolution is enough to detect epithelium up to 10–15 μm thick. A decrease in the thickness of the epithelium is known to be evidence of atrophy. We will demonstrate some tomograms taken from different portions of the larynx that reveal signs of atrophic epithelium. Figure 14a exhibits an OCT image of epithelial atrophy of vocal folds in a patient with chronic atrophic laryngitis. OCT signs of the atrophy are a decrease in the thickness of SSE down to 35 μm in comparison with 80–250 μm in normal epithelium and an excessive number of large blood vessels up to 150 μm in diameter in the superficial layer of LP. Figures 14b and 14c are tomograms showing severe epithelial atrophy of the laryngeal epiglottis and vestibular folds. Atrophy of the epithelium here is a consequence of radiation therapy that affects the mucosa of intact portions in patients with laryngeal carcinoma. According to the morphological information, the epithelium is less than 10 μm thick and hence cannot be seen by OCT. Note also that in Fig. 14c a strongly widened mucous gland with ducts is clearly seen.

Keratosis of epithelium (KE) of the vocal fold in a patient with mycotic laryngitis is illustrated in Fig. 15a. An OCT sign of KE is more intense backscattering

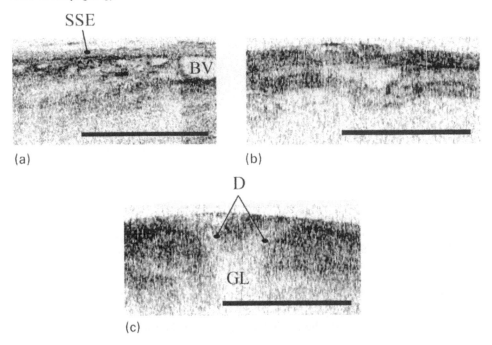

Figure 14 Atrophic SSE in different portions of the larynx is seen in these tomograms by a severe decrease in thickness (a) up to complete disappearance (b,c). Tomogram (c) shows a pathologically dilated mucous gland (GL) with open ducts (D) in a patient after a course of radiation therapy.

from epithelial tissue. Figure 15b is a tomogram of a region of vestibular fold mucosa with signs of KE (high backscattering from the tissue surface), of papillomatous hyperplasia of epithelium (an increase in the thickness up to $450\,\mu$m), and of parakeratosis of epithelium (PKE) (areas of poor backscattering). All these features are caused by the effect of radiation therapy on intact mucosa. Apart from KE, there is also another pathology in laryngeal mucosa that increases backscattering from the epithelium. We examined a case of fibrin laryngitis (Fig. 16). The highly backscattering turbid fibrin deposits on the vocal folds alter the configuration of the epithelial surface and obstruct imaging of underlying structures.

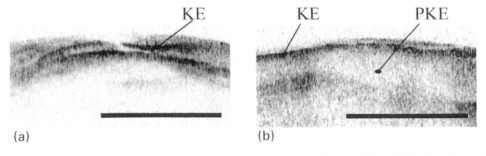

Figure 15 Tomograms of mucosa of (a) vocal fold and (b) vestibular fold with signs of keratosis of the epithelium (KE) in a patient with myotic laryngitis and KE and parakeratosis of the epithelium (PKE) in a patient after a course of radiation therapy.

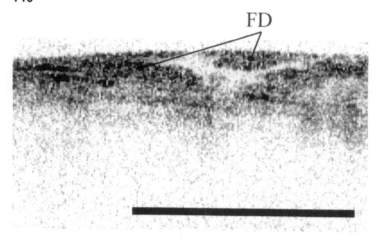

Figure 16   Fibrous laryngitis of the vocal folds. FD = fibrin deposits.

Thus, OCT of laryngeal mucosa allows imaging of different abnormalities in the epithelium such as atrophy, KE, and PKE, which are evidenced in OCT images by changes in the thickness of the epithelium and/or in the intensity of backscattering.

27.3.2   OCT Imaging of Inflammatory Processes in the Larynx

A nonspecific reaction of the human body, inflammation is known to have common morphological signs irrespective of its causes (infectious agents, exposure to radiation, etc.). These signs include edema and cellular infiltration of connective tissue in the active stage, and sclerosis (fibrosis) as the outcome of the process [13]. OCT imaging can detect structural alterations in connective tissue of the laryngeal mucosa that are characteristic of inflammation.

Morphologically confirmed regions of fluid accumulation in the vocal fold in a patient with acute edematous laryngitis (Fig. 17) are seen in the OCT images as light (poorly backscattering) areas with indistinct and uneven borders. It should be noted that edema affects the Reinke's space, which is filled with loose fibrous connective

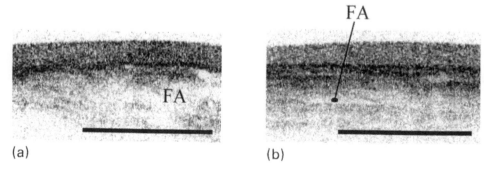

(a)   (b)

Figure 17   Edema of vocal fold in a patient with acute edematous laryngitis. FA = fluid accumulations in the Reinke's space.

tissue. This leads to thickening of the LP of mucosa in comparison with normal mucosa of the vocal fold (Fig. 14). We also studied after-effects of radiation therapy on intact vocal fold mucosa in patients with laryngeal carcinoma. It is known that an immediate effect of radiation therapy on the mucous membrane is the development of edema and cellular infiltration of connective tissue. OCT signs of these reactions are indicated in Fig. 18. Edematous fluid accumulation appears as poorly backscattering regions, and cellular infiltrate is seen as highly backscattering regions. These OCT signs are universal for different tissues. For example, we observed such regions previously in inflamed dermis, where they were demonstrated with parallel histology [14].

Long-term effects of ionizing radiation are deep fibrosis of lamina propria with cellular reaction and pronounced hypertrophy of glands [15]. Such alterations are seen in OCT images as increased backscattering from the subepithelial layer as an OCT sign of fibrosis and as reduced scattering from expanded laryngeal glands filled with mucous secretion (Fig. 19). In some cases a pronounced atrophy of mucosal epithelium in the larynx, along with the above aftereffects, was noted in patients 4–5 years following a course of effective radiation therapy (Figs. 14b and 14c). For comparison, normal mucosa of the vestibular folds is shown in Fig. 8a.

27.3.3 OCT Monitoring of Tumors and Tumor-Like Lesions

The capability of OCT to differentiate between epithelium and underlying connective tissue to evaluate their state as well as the state of the basement membrane allows application of this imaging technique for the diagnosis of tumors and tumor-like lesions. Our OCT device, which has a spatial resolution of 10–20 μm, cannot detect directly the cellular layer of changes in high-grade dyspasia or carcinoma. However, OCT can reveal some peculiarities of epithelial malignancy at the level of tissue architecture, such as an abnormal concentration of cells that leads to the loss of epithelium and stroma orientation. OCT also can detect changes in optical properties of malignant squamous epithelium (MSE) and increased vascularization of the lamina propria.

In our OCT study, in 19 cases of morphologically confirmed invasive cancer of the vocal folds all OCT images indicate a lack of regular structure of mucosa and an appearance of areas of high backscattering from the tumor. Figure 20

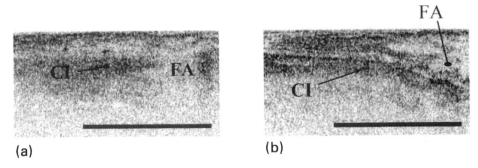

(a) (b)

Figure 18 Edema of vocal fold and cellular infiltration (CI) in a patient after a course of radiation therapy.

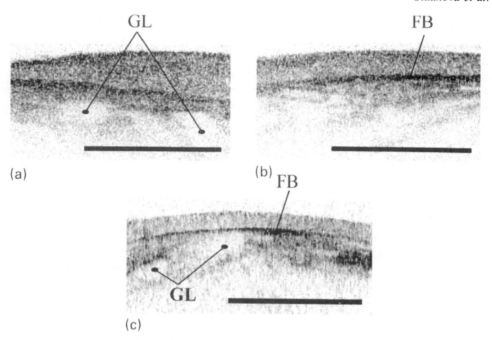

(a)   (b)

(c)

Figure 19 Fibrosis (FB) of the lamina propria of mucosa and hypertrophy of laryngeal glands (GL) in the vocal fold in a patient after a course of radiation therapy.

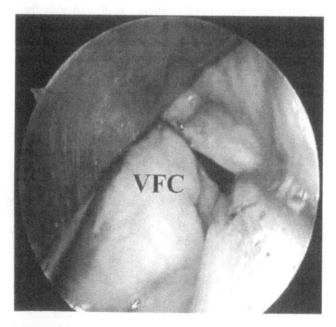

Figure 20 Laryngoscopic view of an invasive cancer of vocal fold. VFC = vocal fold carcinoma.

shows a laryngoscopic view of the larynx with an invasive cancer of the vocal fold. Figure 21 exhibits tomograms and parallel histology of the vocal fold in a patient with squamous cell carcinoma with invasion of more than 1 mm. Clusters of cells of the MSE alter the typical mucosal architecture and, in addition, have optical properties that differ from those of the normal mucosa, as can be easily seen in the OCT image. Although OCT images cannot provide information on specific morphological features of a tumor, a complete lack of structural form on OCT can, in some cases, be used in cancer diagnosis together with data obtained with conventional techniques (endoscopic and cytological studies). Additionally, OCT imaging of invasive cancerous tumors may indicate specific features such as an excessive number of large blood vessels (diameter more than 50–70 μm) at small depths (Fig. 21b).

It is known that the most objective information for specific cancer diagnostics is provided by histological examination of biopsy material. An inaccurate choice of biopsy sites is one of the causes of misdiagnosis in oncology. Traditional endoscopic techniques used in combination with microlaryngoscopy that provides a two- to eight-fold magnification can detect the boundaries of the pathological processes on the basis of only subjective criteria such as color and surface pattern. In the OCT images taken in six patients with carcinoma of the vocal folds (Fig. 22), the transition from abnormal to healthy epithelium is clearly visualized. In contrast with visual border detection, OCT can show structural changes at the boundary between normal tissue and the tumor, increasing reliability, objectivity, and accuracy. The exact localization by OCT of pronounced structural alterations and a focus of pathological changes allows guidance of excisional biopsy and minimization of diagnostic errors. Hence, OCT data can be used in detecting boundaries of pathological

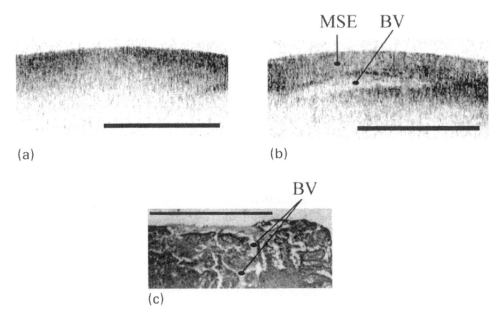

Figure 21 Invasive cancer of vocal fold. (a) Structureless OCT image; (b) OCT image with a large vessel; (c) parallel histology. MSE = malignant squamous epithelium.

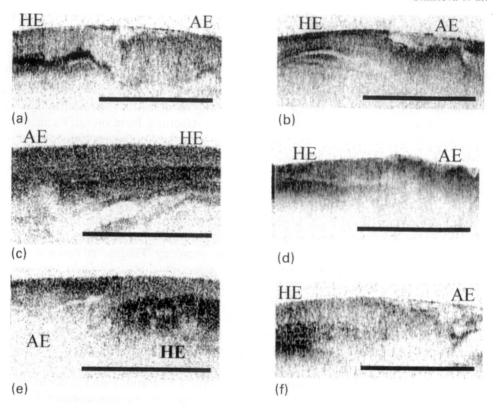

Figure 22 Boundary between healthy epithelium (HE) and abnormal epithelium (AE) in six different patients with invasive cancer of the vocal fold.

zones. The clinical importance of this OCT capability is evident in at least three cases:

1. In endophytic cancer, where, in contrast to exophytic cancer, it is difficult to determine the real size of a tumor, a parameter that is essential for determining the stage of the pathological process and, hence, for an adequate choice of treatment.
2. When a tumor is small, i.e., when it is possible to perform surgical procedures that can preserve not only an organ but its functions as well. In this case the accurate identification of tumor boundaries enables its effective removal under intraoperative control by OCT.
3. For guidance in various types of microsurgical operations with laser, cryo-, electro-, and other applications.

Thus, OCT has the capability to indicate exactly the margin of an area with structural alterations and therefore can provide an accurate map for excisional biopsy. This technique may also enable more effective surgical operations with higher precision of tissue removal.

Noninvasive differential diagnosis of neoplastic and benign lesions is very important and difficult. Our experience with OCT imaging for these purposes demonstrated some positive results. In the following we will present a specific example of OCT capabilities for this clinical application.

Two patients had a small abnormal process slightly altering the profile of vocal fold mucosa. A diagnosis was made to differentiate between a polyp, a glandular mucosal cyst, and a neoplasia of the vocal folds on the basis of microlaryngoscopic data. The clinical diagnosis was confirmed by histology of biopsy sections obtained from the pathological regions. In one patient, the morphological study of the biopsy material (Fig. 23b) confirmed the diagnosis of a polyp of the vocal fold, the so-called vocal nodule, which is characterized by slightly atrophic squamous epithelium, fibrinoid alterations, micromathosis, and stromal edema. OCT provided two optical patterns, which differed from the norm and had (in contrast to carcinoma) clear individual features. Figure 23a is a tomogram clearly indicating the epithelial layer of 50–100 μm thickness and an underlying poorly backscattering area without any distinct borders that correspond to alterations in stroma described earlier. In the other patient, a cyst of the mucous gland of the larynx was morphologically diagnosed. In the tomogram (Fig. 24), under a normal epithelium there is a rounded, poorly backscattering cavity with a sharp border, which is typical for fluid retention formations such as laryngeal cyst. Thus, different optical properties of the revealed formations and the presence of their structural forms in the OCT patterns (in contrast to malignant tumors) provided additional important information for laryngoscopic study, allowing us in the future to make a differential diagnosis immediately during the course of the study.

27.4 CONCLUSIONS

The already existing clinical devices acquire images of mucosa with a resolution as good as 10–15 μm, thus allowing identification of epithelium, underlying connective tissue with vessels and glands, and cartilage and proper muscles of the larynx. A depth of imaging of up to 1.5 mm is sufficient for evaluation of these structures. OCT is a noninvasive technique that avoids trauma and has no side effects because it utilizes radiation in the near-infrared with a power of approximately 1 mW. A high rate of image acquisition allows minimization of errors caused by involuntary movements of the object and the operator. OCT is capable of measuring exact dimensions of structures, which is important for diagnosing some pathological conditions and for specifying quantitative criteria of image interpretation.

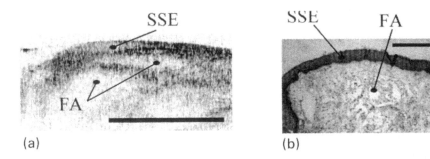

(a) (b)

Figure 23 Edematous polyp (vocal nodule) of the vocal fold. (a) Tomogram; (b) parallel histology.

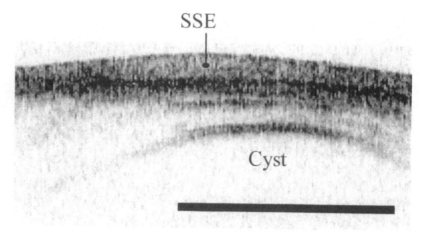

Figure 24 Cyst of the vocal fold.

Optical coherence tomographic imaging of normal mucosa in different portions of the larynx reflects some specific inherent features of its morphological structure. The visualization is possible due to the difference in optical properties of
mucosal structures. The distinct layer-to-layer structure makes the larynx an excellent subject for OCT study and allows reliable differentiation between optical images
of normal and pathologically altered tissue.

Easily amenable to OCT is the epithelium–connective tissue system, so it is
possible to assess the state of epithelium and connective tissue and their interrela-
tionship. Among pathologies of epithelium detectable by OCT are atrophy, keratosis, and parakeratosis, which are seen in OCT images by changes in thickness and/or
intensity of backscattering. In the stroma, OCT can detect such alterations as edema
and cellular infiltration of the connective tissue at the active stage of inflammation,
and fibrosis as the outcome of the process.

The structural information obtainable with OCT can be used to detect tumors
and tumor-like lesions that change or alter tissue structure. OCT can be successfully
applied to the diagnosis of neoplastic processes because of its high spatial resolution
and its ability to differentiate between epithelium and underlying connective tissue as
well as to define their state and the state of the basement membrane. In cases of
morphologically confirmed invasive cancer of the vocal folds, the OCT images reveal
a loss of structure and an appearance of areas of intense backscattering from tumorous tissue. OCT images do not provide information on specific morphological features of the tumor, but such OCT signs as complete lack of mucosal structure can be
used in cancer diagnostics together with data obtained with the traditional techniques of endoscopy and cytology.

Histological examination of biopsy material is widely recognized as the most
objective method for cancer detection. An inaccurate choice of biopsy site often
leads to errors in cancer diagnostics. The loss of normal structural form occurs at a
border between healthy tissue and a tumor. Precise localization by OCT of most
pronounced structural alterations, a focus of pathological alterations, helps to
guide biopsy and hence minimize diagnostic errors. In some cases, OCT can distinguish between pathological processes of differing origin, for example, inflamma-

tion and neoplastic processes, and between some tumors and tumor-like lesions if the latter exhibit distinct structural form in the OCT images, which clearly differentiates them from malignant tumors. The capability of OCT to indicate linear dimensions of tumorous tissue may be of great help in guidance of organ-preserving operations when highly precise removal of tissue is required. OCT can be useful for monitoring evolving changes in the pathological process during treatment. OCT monitoring of the state of laryngeal tissue can reliably evaluate the effectiveness of treatment and, if necessary, make timely corrections during the course of treatment, a capability especially important when radiation therapy is undertaken.

In summary, OCT has been demonstrated to be a highly promising technology for diagnosing pathological processes in the larynx to improve diagnostic capabilities to a qualitatively higher level.

REFERENCES

1. Huang D, Wang J, Lin CP, Shuman JS, Stinson WG, Chang W, Hee MR, Flotte T, Gregory K, Puliafito CA, Fujimoto JG. Optical coherence tomography. Science 254:1178, 1991.
2. Sergeev AM, Gelikonov VM, Gelikonov GV, Feldchtein FI, Kuranov RV, Gladkova ND, Shakhova NM, Snopova LB, Shakhov AV, Kuznetzova IA, Denisenko AN, Pochinko VV, Chumakov YuP, Streltzova OS. In vivo endoscopic OCT imaging of precancer and cancer stages of human mucosa. Opt Express 1(13):432–440, 1997. *http://epubs.osa.org/oerachive/pdf/2788.pdf*
3. Feldchtein FI, Gelikonov VM, Gelikonov GV, Kuranov RV, Sergeev AM, Gladkova ND, Shakhov AV, Shakhova NM, Snopova LB. Terent'eva AB, Zagainova EV, Chumakov YuP, Kuznetzova IA. Endoscopic applications of optical coherence tomography. Opt Express 3(6):257–270, 1998. *http://epubs.osa.org.oearchive/pdf/5788.pdf.*
4. Sergeev AM, Gelikonov VM, Gelikonov GV, Feldchtein FI, Gladkova ND, Kamensky VA. Biomedical diagnostics using optical coherence tomography. OSA TOPS Adv Opt Imaging Photon Migrat 2:196–199, 1996.
5. Gelikonov VM, Gelikonov GV, Gladkova ND, Leonov VL, Feldchtein FI, Sergeev AM, Khanin YaI. Optical fiber interferometer and piezoelectric modulator. US Patent 5835642 (1998).
6. Tearney GJ, Brezinski ME, Bouma BE, Hee MR, Fujimoto JG. Determination of the refractive index of highly scattering human tissue by optical coherence tomography. Opt Lett 20(21):2258–2260, 1995.
7. Hast MH. Anatomy of the larynx. In: GM English ed. Otolaryngology, Vol 3. Philadelphia: Lippincott, 1993.
8. University of Arkansas for Medical Sciences. The Anatomy Project. *http://anatomy.uams.edu./htmlpages/anatomyhtml/atlas_html/rsa3p*14.*html.* Parthenon Publishing Group, 1997.
9. Sasaki CT, Driscoll BP, Gracco C. Anatomy and physiology of the larynx. In: JJ Ballener, JB Snows, eds. Otorhinolaryngology. Head and Neck Surgery. Baltimore: Williams and Wilkins, 1996:422–437.
10. Ham AW, Cormack DH. Histology. Philadelphia: Lippincott, 1979.
11. Paches AI. Tumors of Head and Neck. Moscow: De-Jure, 1996:346–378.
12. Castellanos PF, Spector JG, Kaiser TN. Tumors of the larynx and laryngopharynx. In: JJ Ballenger, JB Snow, eds. Otorhinolaryngology. Head and Neck Surgery. Baltimore: Williams and Wilkins, 1996:585–604.

13. Koufman JA. Infections and inflammatory diseases of the larynx. In: JJ Ballenger, JB Snow, eds. Otorhinolaryngology. Head and Neck Surgery. Baltimore: Williams and Wilkins, 1996:532–555.

14. Gladkova ND, Petrova GA, Nikulin NK, Radenska-Lopovok SG, Snopova LB, Chumakov YuP, Nasonova VA, Gelikonov VM, Gelikonov GV, Juranov RV, Sergeev AM, Feldchtein FI. In vivo optical coherence tomography imaging of human skin: Norm and pathology. Skin Res Technol 6:6–16, 2000.

15. Chandler JR. Radiation fibrosis and necrosis of the larynx. Ann Otorhinolarynx 88:509, 1979.

28

Optical Coherence Tomography in Urology

F. KOENIG

Charité Medical School, Humboldt University Berlin, Berlin, Germany

GUILLERMO J. TEARNEY and BRETT E. BOUMA

Harvard Medical School and Wellman Laboratories of Photomedicine, Massachusetts General Hospital, Boston, Massachusetts

28.1 INTRODUCTION

28.1.1 Background

The introduction of charge-coupled device (CCD)-based intraluminal endoscopic imaging of the urinary tract surface has led to substantial reductions in the morbidity and mortality associated with disorders in this organ system. However, the relatively low resolution and the inability to image the structure of tissue below the luminal surface frequently limit endoscopic imaging. A technology able to obtain high resolution, cross-sectional images of tissue could substantially improve the diagnosis and treatment of urinary tract disorders.

Transitional cell carcinoma (TCC) is the second most common malignancy of the genitourinary tract. In 1997 the incidence was 16.8 cases per 100,000 people in the United States, an increase from 14.6 per 100,000 in 1973 [1]. Fortunately, the mortality rate decreased from 4.1/100,000 in 1973 to 3.2/1000,000 in 1997. The majority (up to 65%) of urothelial tumors are low grade and superficial when the patient first presents to the urologist, but despite adequate transurethral resection of the primary bladder lesion (TURB) the recurrence rate is particularly high, 37–77%, depending on the tumor stage and grade. Incomplete resection of the primary lesion has been proven to be one of the reasons. In addition, concomitant overlooked micropapillary lesions, dysplasia, or carcinoma in situ (CIS) as well as disseminated tumor cells could lead to the tumor relapse. Up to one-third of the recurrent tumors will progress to a higher stage and/or grade that requires more invasive treatment. It is well known that patients with stage T1 tumors (invading the lamina propria) have a poorer prognosis than those with Ta tumors (confined to the urothelium) and that patients with G3 lesions (dedifferentiated) have a higher chance of tumor recurrence and/or progression than those with (well-differentiated) G1 lesions [2,3]. It is also known that about 50% of patients with low stage, low grade TCC have concomitant urothelial dysplasia, either CIS or higher differentiated forms of dysplasia [4,5]. Up to 80% of the patients who are found to have CIS in addition to a low stage, low grade lesion have an associated invasive carcinoma within 4 years. If any other dysplastic lesion is found adjacent to multiple tumors that involve the lamina propria, invasion will occur in 30% of these patients within 4 years [5]. Unfortunately, early malignant and dysplastic lesions are often barely visible or are invisible because their appearance is similar to that of inflamed or normal tissue.

Histologically determined stage and grade of resected tumor tissue are still the gold standard in the diagnosis of urothelial carcinoma and the main prognostic factors dictating subsequent treatment. Although these treatment decisions are sometimes vital for the patient, it has been shown that staging and grading performed by the pathologist are highly subjective and the results vary between different investigators and institutions. In addition, in order to determine the stage of a carcinoma it is necessary to identify or exclude muscle invasion, which sometimes is not possible due to thermal damage of the resected tissue or due to nonrepresentative biopsies missing the area of the deepest tumor infiltration. This leads to understaging in up to 30% of high risk (G3) lesions. It is also well known that within histologically determined subgroups of TCC the biological behavior of tumors is heterogeneous, with different malignancy potential, including growth pattern, risk of progression and metastasis. Furthermore, the response to local or systemic treatment modalities (BCG, chemotherapy, radiotherapy) is not predictable. Some patients with highly aggressive tumors may need adjuvant treatment following radical cystectomy. As a result of these diagnostic dilemmas in urology, there is an enormous interest in developing independent tumor markers, determining prognostic factors, and, especially, devising new diagnostic imaging techniques.

Another area of interest is the reduction of morbidity during and following the removal of hypertrophic prostatic tissue, referred to as transurethral resection of the prostate (TURP), one of the most common of all surgical procedures. As men age, the prostate grows (hypertrophies) and often obstructs urination. When a TURP is performed, this tissue is removed with an endoscope-based surgical device. In a low but significant percentage of these procedures, impotence (sexual dysfunction or incontinence (inability to control urination) result from damage to the external sphincter and small adjacent nerves. These complications would be avoided if any imaging technique that was able to image the structure of tissue below the luminal surface existed.

28.1.2 Current Imaging Modalities

Since the introduction of Hopkins rod lenses, not much has changed with regard to the optics of today's cystoscopes. Modern color CCD cameras attached to the endoscope give excellent magnified images of the bladder surface and allow the detection of very small tumors. However, as shown by several studies, flat and micropapillary lesions are still missed during standard while light cystoscopy and at least partially lead to the high recurrence rate.

To improve the diagnosis of dysplastic and early malignant lesions including CIS, several groups in the United States and Europe are currently using 5-aminolevulinic acid (ALA) to enhance the diagnosis of bladder carcinoma [6–8]. The results of these clinical studies indicate a sensitivity of up to 97% and a specificity around 60% for ALA-based photodetection (PD) of malignant bladder lesions [6]. Photodetection of malignancies is based on the fluorescence of dyes (fluorophores) that localize preferentially in neoplastic tissue. Porphyrins and other tetrapyrroles are the most exploited group of dyes for PD and photodynamic therapy (PDT). The use of hematopophyrin (Hp) as a fluorophore and photosensitizer was described as early as 1913 [9]. Porfimer sodium (Photofrin), a purified form of hematopophyrin derivative (HpD), is approved for PDT in several countries and is currently the only approved PDT drug in the United States. In principle, Photofrin could be used for PD. However, it has the disadvantage of causing skin photosensitization that can last for several weeks. In contrast, intravesical instillation of ALA, first described in 1993 by Baumgartner et al. [10], shows no systemic side effects and leads to an increase of protoporphyrin IX (PPIX) in neoplastic bladder lesions. ALA is a precursor of PPIX, which is in turn the immediate precursor of heme in the biosynthetic pathway for heme. Because heme-containing enzymes are required for aerobic energy metabolism, all mammalian nucleated cells have the capacity to synthesize heme. PPIX is an endogenous photosensitizer that fluoresces red under excitation with blue light. For PD of bladder carcinoma, 50 mL of a 3% ALA solution is instilled intravesically 2–3 h prior to cystoscopy. The detection system used to capture and to display PPIX fluorescence images consists of a standard cystoscopic xenon light source with the addition of an internal filter assembly, which passes primarily blue light (200–400 mW at 425 nm with a full width at half-maximum of ~ 50 nm). A foot pedal allows the surgeon to conveniently switch between standard white light and blue light, which are used for illumination or fluorescence excitation of the bladder surface, respectively. In order to visualize the red fluorescence light, a yellow filter is incorporated in the cystoscope to block most of the blue excitation light. The bladder is studied primarily with the naked eye or by using a color CCD camera with integrating capability. Images from the CCD camera are displayed on a standard color monitor. According to a recently published study investigating 1460 bladder biopsies, 57% of CIS and 32% of all neoplastic lesions have been overlooked by standard white light cystoscopy and could be identified solely by their PPIX fluorescence [11].

Intravesical ultrasound was first described in 1974 and is used primarily for staging of bladder carcinoma, that is, its depth of invasion [12]. To date, flexible 20 MHz scanners with an outer diameter of only 2 mm (UM-4R, UM-4R-proto, Olympus) can be passed through the working channel of an endoscope. It has been shown that the use of these miniature probes allows in vivo staging of urothelial carcinoma. In a recent pilot study including 51 patients, muscle invasion of tumors (T2) was clearly identified [13]. According to histopathological diagnosis, 92% of the 52 investigated bladder lesions (33 Ta/1, 14 T2, and five T3 tumors invading the adipose tissue surrounding the bladder) could be staged correctly by applying intravesical ultrasound. Only two carcinomas were staged as superficial while pathology revealed muscle invasion. One T3 and one Ta/1 tumor staged by ultrasound were classified as T2 by the pathologist. Due to the limited resolution, Ta and T1 tumors could not be distinguished. No cases of CIS were included in this initial study.

To date, the resolution of other imaging techniques such as X-ray radiography, standard magnetic resonance imaging (MRI), and computed tomography (CT) is too low for a reliable determination of tumor invasion. The detection of CIS as well as other flat or micropapillary lesions is not possible. A thin-section helical CT scan is able to detect bladder tumors down to 0.3 cm in size but cannot replace cystoscopy for detection and follow-up of urothelial carcinoma [14,15]. In a study comparing the diagnostic potential of CT scans and transrectal ultrasound (TRUS), the latter technique was superior in detecting superficial and infiltrating tumors [16]. Results of experimental studies investigating the staging of bladder carcinoma by MR imaging following administration of diethylenetetraminepenta acetic acid chelate of gadolinium (DTPA Gd) are promising. The normal bladder wall was visualized and shows three layers: an inner thin layer of low intensity, a middle layer of marked enhancement, and a thick outer layer of intermediate intensity. In a preliminary clinical study, MRI invariably allowed accurate staging of bladder tumors in 13 patients [17].

In conclusion, none of the discussed imaging techniques can replace cystoscopy and histology for the staging of urothelial cancer. The ALA method improves standard white light cystoscopy by increasing the detection rate of flat malignant lesions and small satellite tumors. Intravesical ultrasound and MR imaging may allow noninvasive staging of bladder carcinoma in the future. However, large-scale clinical studies are necessary to validate the true diagnostic potential of these new methods.

28.1.3 Clinical Relevance

In the past, in addition to the resection of the primary tumor, random biopsies were recommended to detect invisible hard-to-find lesions like CIS. More recent studies have shown that these invasive biopsies are of limited value for the patient [18]. The ALA fluorescence cystoscopy is a very sensitive orientational method that allows localization of nearly all malignant and dysplastic lesions. However, the specificity of 60% for this method is low. False positive results are mainly caused by inflammation of the urothelium leading to a high number of useless biopsies taken from nonmalignant areas.

In order to reduce and optimize bladder biopsies, new methods should be able to identify the morphological differences between malignant and nonmalignant lesions. In contrast to inflammatory changes, malignant lesions are characterized by hyperproliferation that leads to an increase in the thickness of the urothelium. Less than 10% of hyperproliferative areas are benign. However, high grade (dedifferentiated) flat tumors like CIS tend to exfoliate cells into urine, which leads to a reduction of urothelial layers. Occasionally the urothelium is completely denuded.

Besides the difficulties regarding the detection of flat malignant lesions, it is most relevant to determine the depth of invasion. Once a bladder tumor has invaded the muscular layer of the bladder wall, radical cystectomy is indicated in order to prevent metastatic spread of the disease. An optical method that could noninvasively predict muscle infiltration would spare the patient the TURB prior to a radical operation and subsequently might lower the risk of metastasis by preventing tumor cell seeding.

Transitional cell carcinoma occurs not only in the urinary bladder but also in the ureter and the urine-collecting system of the kidney. Detection of malignant lesions in the narrow ureter and the kidney poses several problems. The diameter of an ureteroscope is small, and therefore the vision of the surgeon is limited. In addition, the miniature probes used for biopsies and resections are difficult to handle.

In summary, the disturbed architecture of the neoplastic urothelium is a "diagnostic marker" and could be targeted by new optical systems. OCT has the potential of detecting the described morphological differences and hopefully can help to differentiate flat neoplastic and inflammatory lesions by providing cross-sectional images. In addition, because the penetration depth of OCT is between 2 and 4 mm, it is hoped that muscle invasion of TCC can also be determined. Furthermore, as a fiber-based method, OCT can be integrated into ureteroscopes for imaging the upper urinary tract.

Finally, an imaging technology like OCT, which can yield resolutions in the micrometer range, can potentially provide information on tissue microstructure that would enable localization of the prostatic capsule and aid in preventing damage to the neurovascular bundles and the external sphincter during TURP.

28.2 METHODS

This chapter presents a summary of three studies performed on human urological tissues: (1) ex vivo autopsy tissue specimens, (2) cystectomy specimens, and (3) in vivo human bladders. The OCT system used for the autopsy specimens was constructed at the Massachusetts Institute of Technology for ex vivo studies (see Chapters 19, 21, and 23). The OCT system used for the surgical cystectomy specimens was developed by the group in Lübeck (Ralf Engelhardt et al., Medical Laser Center Lübeck, Germany) and is described in detail in Chapter 20. For the in vivo work in the bladder, the system was identical to that used for the studies in the gastrointestinal tract by researchers at the Massachusetts General Hospital (Chapter 25).

28.2.1 Autopsy Specimens

Normal urological tissue including the prostatic urethra, prostate, bladder, and ureters was obtained within 5 h of the initiation of autopsy. More than 20 samples from five patients were examined. The tissues were dissected to dimensions of approximately 10 mm × 5 mm and imaged with the luminal surfaces exposed. During imaging, the tissues were partially immersed in isotonic saline to prevent dehydration. Imaging was performed through air at room temperature. The position of the beam on the sample was monitored using a visible light-guiding beam (633 nm helium-neon laser) that was coincident with the 1300 nm infrared OCT beam on the sample. The imaging planes were marked using small injections of dye. The samples then underwent routine histological processing. Samples were immersed in 10% buffered formalin for 48 h. The tissues were then processed for standard paraffin embedding. Thin (5 μm) sections were cut at the marked imaging sites and stained with hematoxylin and eosin (H&E).

28.2.2 Cystectomy Specimen

In order to study invasive bladder carcinoma a complete cystectomy specimen was first fixed in formalin, later cut open, and then imaged with the luminal surface exposed. Except for the incision to open the bladder, the specimen was left intact to mimic the in vivo situation. The imaging planes were marked using thin 3-0 PDS (surgical suture material). After the OCT images were acquired, the sample underwent routine histological processing including standard paraffin embedding. Thin (5 μm) sections were cut at the marked imaging sites and stained with hematoxylin and eosin (H&E).

28.2.3 In Vivo Bladder

A total of five patients undergoing routine cystoscopy were imaged with the OCT system. The OCT catheter was gas-sterilized. Following endoscopic inspection, the OCT catheter was inserted through the access port of the cystoscope. The cystoscope camera output aided in guiding the OCT catheter to specific regions of interest. The OCT image acquisition rate of 4 frames per second (fps) was sufficient to avoid motion artifacts. Following the acquisition of several images at one location, the OCT catheter was removed, a biopsy probe was inserted through the access port, and a mucosal biopsy at the imaging site was performed. Biopsy specimens were immersed in 10% buffered formalin and submitted for routine histological processing, hematoxylin and eosin (H&E) staining, and histopathological evaluation.

28.3 RESULTS

28.3.1 Autopsy Specimens

Prostatic Urethra

Optical coherence tomography enables visualization of the architectural microstructure of the prostatic urethra and the periurethral prostate (Figs. 1 and 2).

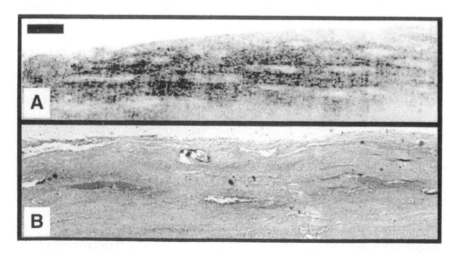

Figure 1 Autopsy specimen. (A) OCT image of the prostatic urethra. (B) Corresponding histology visualized with hematoxylin and eosin (H&E). Scale bar, 500 μm. (From Ref. 19.)

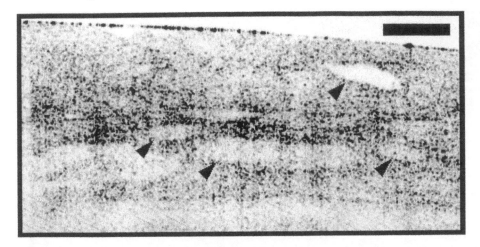

Figure 2 Autopsy specimen. OCT image of the periurethral prostate, showing the presence of prostatic glands (arrowheads). Scale bar, 500 μm. (From Ref. 19.)

Differentiation between the prostatic urethra and the prostate is possible due to the different backreflection characteristics of the two tissue types. Paraurethral gland ducts can be visualized within the urethra (Fig. 2). Prostatic glands can be identified in both images (Figs. 1 and 2) and demonstrate the capability to image completely through the urethra to the prostate. Areas of relatively low backscatter within the prostatic glands represent the presence of prostatic secretions. Because the resolution of the OCT system used in this study was 16 μm, the epithelium of the urethra is not resolved.

Neurovascular Bundle

The high resolution of OCT allows imaging of neurovascular bundles near the capsule at the prostate/adipose tissue border. In Fig. 3, a portion of the prostate has been excised and imaged. The prostate tissue appears relatively homogeneous at this resolution. The outlines of entire adipose cells can be visualized in this OCT image. A neurovasular bundle can be seen within the adipose tissue adjacent to the prostate (Fig. 3). Neurovascular bundles appear to have a high backreflection intensity relative to that of the surrounding adipose tissue. Thus, OCT provides high contrast between neurovascular bundles and adipose tissue at the prostate/adipose border.

Prostatic Capsule

Optical coherence tomographic images of the exterior surface of the prostate demonstrate the capability of OCT to resolve and locate the prostatic capsule (Fig. 4). Differentiation of the collagenous layers of the capsule is made possible by the differences in backreflection between the capsule and the prostate. The axial thickness of the capsule in the image can be measured from the OCT image and is approximately 50 μm. Figure 4 also shows an artery below the fibrous capsule. Microstructures visible within the artery include the enigma and media of the vessel.

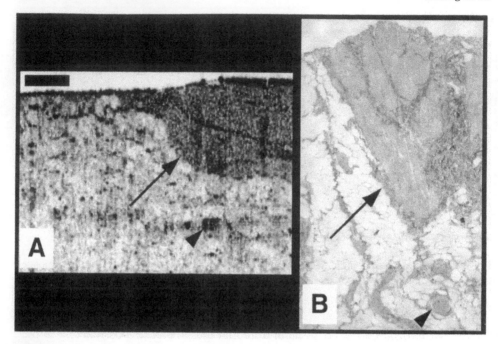

Figure 3 Autopsy specimen. (A) OCT image of periprostatic adipose tissue, showing the border between the prostate and periprostatic adipose tissue (arrow). neurovascular bundles (arrowhead) are seen within the periprostatic adipose tissue. (B) Corresponding histology (H&E). Scale bar, 500 μm. (From Ref. 19.)

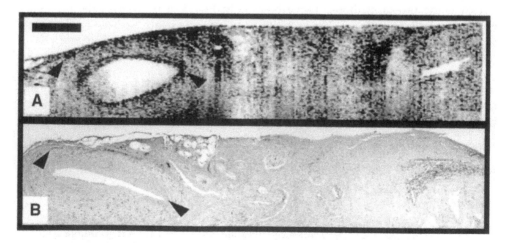

Figure 4 Autopsy specimen. (A) OCT image of the prostatic capsule (arrowhead), demonstrating a pericapsular artery (arrowhead). (B) Corresponding histology (H&E). Scale bar, 50 μm. (From Ref. 19.)

Bladder and Ureter

Different anatomical layers in the bladder can be identified in the OCT image, including the urothelium, submucosa, and muscularis propria (Fig. 5). OCT images of the ureter demonstrate the capability of OCT to resolve the urothelium, muscular layers, and adventitia (Fig. 6). Differentiation of these layers is made possible by visualization of the different backreflection characteristics within each layer.

28.3.2 Invasive Bladder Carcinoma (Cystectomy Specimen)

The images were obtained from obviously malignant sites (Fig. 7) and adjacent normal areas, which was later confirmed by histology (Fig. 8). Normal areas of the mucosa are seen to have a layered structure corresponding to the urothelium, submucosa, and muscular layers (Fig. 8). In contrast to the normal bladder, the OCT image of invasive carcinoma demonstrates a loss of the layered structure of normal bladder mucosa and marked architectural disorganization of the mucosa (Fig. 7). Invasive tumors appear to have a different backreflection intensity relative to that of the adjacent normal tissue. The depth of invasion into the muscularis by the tumor can also be appreciated (Fig. 7).

28.3.3 In Vivo Bladder

Optical coherence tomographic images of the prostatic urethra acquired in vivo show morphological features similar to those of ex vivo images, including periurethral prostatic glands and ducts containing secretions with relatively low backscatter

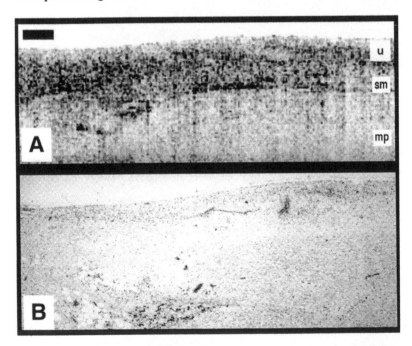

Figure 5 Autopsy specimen. (A) OCT image of the bladder mucosa, allowing visualization of urothelium (u), submucosa (sm), and muscularis propria (mp). (B) Corresponding histology (H&E). Scale bar, 500 μm. (From Ref. 19.)

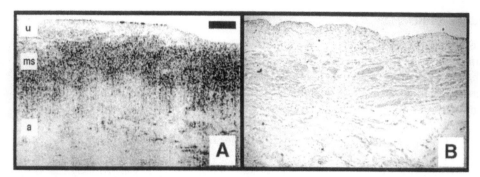

Figure 6 Autopsy specimen. (A) OCT image of the ureter, showing the urothelium (u), muscularis (ms), and adventitia (a). (B) Corresponding histology (H&E). Scale bar, 500 μm. (From Ref. 19.)

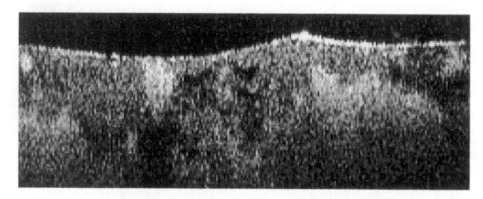

Figure 7 Cystectomy specimen. OCT image of invasive transitional cell carcinoma.

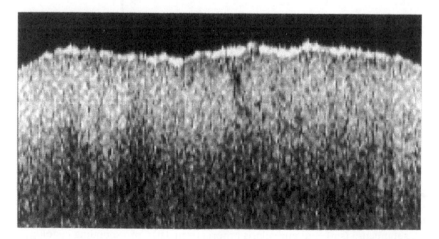

Figure 8 Cystectomy specimen. OCT image of normal bladder mucosa.

(Fig. 9). The bladder mucosa images obtained in vivo, however, demonstrate a striking degree of contrast between the urothelium and the underlying connective tissue (Fig. 10), as opposed to the ex vivo data (Figs. 5 and 7). In Fig. 10, the urothelium has much less backscattering than the underlying lamina propria, allowing for precise determination of the urothelial thickness. Finally, OCT images of a papillary TCC show marked surface irregularity and architectural disorganization (Fig. 11). The layered structure of the normal urothelium is absent, and fronds of papillary epithelium are visualized emanating from the surface (Fig. 11). Note, however, that the OCT imaging penetration depth through these papillary fronds is diminished, making it difficult to discern the muscular layers of the bladder mucosa (Fig. 11).

28.4 CONCLUSIONS

The results of ex vivo and initial in vivo studies demonstrate the high resolution imaging capabilities of OCT at shallow tissue depths. Due to differences in light backscattering, the cross-sectional images show a striking degree of contrast between

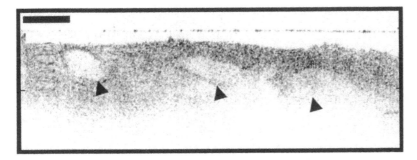

Figure 9 Periurethral prostate (in vivo). OCT image shows presence of prostatic glands containing secretions (arrowheads).

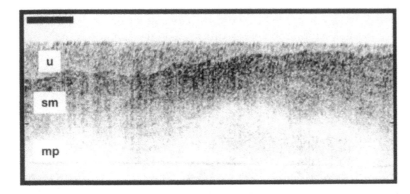

Figure 10 Bladder (in vivo). OCT image shows the high degree of contrast between the urothelium (u), the underlying submucosa (sm), and the muscularis propria (mp). Scale bar, 500 μm.

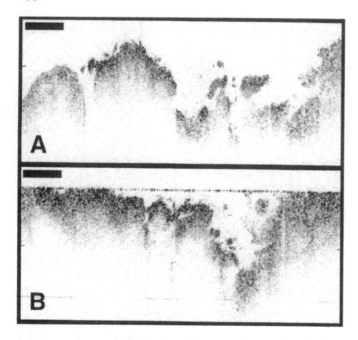

Figure 11   Bladder (in vivo). (A, B) OCT images of papillary transitional cell carcinoma. Scale bars, 500 μm.

the urothelium and the underlying connective tissue. Although additional studies still need to be performed to assess clinical utility in the field of urology, images of the urinary tract suggest a potential role for OCT in the staging and detection of flat neoplastic lesions (e.g., CIS) of the urothelium as well as residual carcinoma following transurethral resection of the primary lesion. In addition, if OCT were capable of differentiating flat neoplastic from inflamed urothelium, it could improve the low specificity of fluorescence cystoscopy (ALA).

Because of the limited penetration depth of this imaging modality, the use of OCT for tumor staging does not appear possible for papillary lesions or tumors beyond a depth of 3 mm. However, in the clinical field of urology, the true diagnostic potential as well as other applications of OCT need to be demonstrated in large-scale clinical studies. Possibly, in combination with other imaging techniques such as intraluminal ultrasound, MRI, or CT, OCT will allow precise in vivo staging of all forms of urothelial carcinoma in the urethra, bladder, or upper urinary tract.

REFERENCES

1. Ries LAG, Kosary CL, Hankey BF, Miller BA, Clegg L, Edwards BK. SEER Cancer Statistic Review, 1973–1996. Bethesda, MD: Natl Cancer Inst, 1999.
2. Kiemeney LA, Witjes JA, Heijbroek RP, Verbeek AL, Debruyne FM. Predictability of recurrent and progressive disease in individual patients with primary superficial bladder cancer. J Urol 150:60, 1993.
3. Heney NM, Ahmed S, Flanagan MJ, Frable W, Corder MP, Hafermann MD, Hawkins IR. Superficial bladder cancer: Progression and recurrence. J Urol 130:1083, 1983.

4. Althausen AF, Prout GR Jr, Dal JJ. Non-invasive papillary carcinoma of the bladder associated with carcinoma in situ. J Urol 116:575, 1976.

5. Wolf H, Olsen PR, Fischer A, Hojgaard K. Urothelial atypia concomitant with primary bladder tumor. Incidence in a consecutive series of 500 unselected patients. Scand J Urol Nephrol 21:33, 1987.

6. Kriegmair M, Baumgartner R, Knüchel R, Stepp H, Hofstädter F, Hofstetter A. Detection of early bladder cancer by 5-aminolevulinic acid induced prophyrin fluorescence. J Urol 155:105, 1996.

7. Jichlinski P, Forrer M, Mizeret J, Glanzmann T, Braichotte, D, Wagnieres G, Zimmer G, Guillou L, Schmidlin F, Graber P, van den Bergh H, Leisinger HG. Clinical evaluation of a method for detecting superficial transitional cell carcinoma of the bladder by light-induced fluorescence of protoporphyrin IX following topical application of 5-aminolevulinic acid: Preliminary results. Laser Surg Med 20:402, 1997.

8. Koenig F, McGovern FJ, Larne R, Enquist H, Schomacker KT, Deutsch TF. Diagnosis of bladder carcinoma using protoporphyrin IX fluorescence induced by 5-amionolaevulinic acid. Br J Urol 83:129, 199.

9. Meyer-Betz F. Untersuchungen über die biologische (photodynamische) Wirkung des Hämatopophyrins under anderer Derivate des Blut- und Gallenfarbstoffs. Deut Arch Klin Med 112:476, 1913.

10. Baumgartner R, Kriegmair M, Stepp HG, Lumper W, Heil P, Riesenberg R, Stocker S, Hofstetter AG. Photodynamic diagnosis following intravesical instillation of aminolevulinic acid (ALA): First clinical experiences in urology. In: TJ Dougherty, ed. Optical Methods for Tumor Treatment and Detection, Mechanisms and Techniques in Photodynamic Therapy. II. Proc SPIE 1881:20–25, 1993.

11. Zaak D, Stepp H, Baumgartner R, Kriegmair M, Hofstetter A. Endoscopic detection of urinary bladder cancer with 5-aminolevulinic acid based fluorescence endoscopy. J Urol 161(suppl)170, 1999.

12. Holm HH, Northeved AA. Transurethral ultrasonic scanner. J Urol 111:238, 1974.

13. Uchida K, Akaza H. Intraluminal ultrasonography in urology. Endoscopy 30:A14, 1998.

14. Hussain S, Loeffler JA, Babayan RK, Fenlon HM. Thin-section helical computed tomography of the bladder: Initial clinical experience with virtual reality imaging. Urology 50:685, 1997.

15. Merkle EM, Wunderlich A, Aschoff AJ, Rilinger N, Gorich J, Bachor R, Gottfried HW, Sokiranski R, Fleiter TR, Brambs HJ. Virtual cystoscopy based on helical CT scan data sets: Perspectives and limitations. Br J Radiol 71:262, 1998.

16. Caskurlu T, Tasci AL, Sevin G, Cek M, Carbone A, Gezeroglu H. The role of transrectal echography (TRE) in the evaluation and staging of bladder tumors: Comparison with suprapubic echography and computerized axial tomography (CAT). Arch Ital Urol Androl 70:1, 1998.

17. Takeda K, Kawaguchi T, Shiraishi T, Kobayashi S, Hayashi N, Yanagawa M, Tochigi H, Sakuma H, Kawamura J, Nakagawa T. Normal bladder wall morphology in Gd-DTPA-enhanced clinical MR imaging using an endorectal surface coil and histological assessment of submucosal linear enhancement using [^{14}C]Gd-DOTA autoradiography in an animal model. Eur J Radiol 26:290, 1998.

18. Kiemeney LA, Witjes JA, Heijbroek RP, Koper NP, Verbeek AL, Debruyne FM. and the members of the Dutch South-East Co-operative Urological Group. Should random urothelial biopsies be taken from patients with primary superficial bladder cancer? A decision analysis. Br J Cancer 73:164, 1994.

19. Tearney GJ, Brezinski ME, Southern JF, Bouma BE, Boppart SA, Fujimoto JG. Optical biopsy in human urologic tissue using optical coherence tomography. J. Urol. 57:1915, 1997.

Index